The
Chemistry
of
Success

Six Secrets of
Peak Performance

Susan M. Lark, M.D.

James A. Richards, M.B.A.

BAY
BOOKS

Bay Books is an imprint of Bay Books & Tapes, Inc., 555 De Haro St., No. 220, San Francisco, CA 94107

Cover design: Nita Ybarra
Interior design: Tasha Hall
Typesetting: Jeff Brandenburg
Copy editors: Brian Jones and Carolyn Miller
Proofreader/indexer: Ken Della Penta

Library of Congress Cataloging-in-Publication Data

Lark, Susan M., 1945–
    The chemistry of success : six secrets of peak performance / Susan M. Lark, James A. Richards.
        p.   cm.
    Includes bibliographical references and index.
    ISBN 1-57959-501-4 (hc : alk. paper)
    1. Health. 2. Metabolism. 3. Biochemistry. I. Richards, James A., M.B.A. II. Title
RA776.5.L3226   1999
613—dc21   99–35728
                                                                          CIP

Printed in the United States
10 9 8 7 6 5 4 3 2 1
Distributed by Publishers Group West

We dedicate this book to our daughter, Rebecca, and to our mothers, Ruth and Doris, with much love. In fond memory of our fathers, Joseph and Harold.

It is also dedicated to all of those people who are committed to performing to their very best throughout their lives.

CONTENTS

ACKNOWLEDGMENTS

We both wish to thank the following individuals for their exceptionally dedicated and persistent work on the book:

Our wonderful and supportive publishers, Robert Manley and James Connolly, who made this book the very best it could possibly be.

Clancy Drake for her terrific editorial direction.

Erika Sloan, our dynamic and gifted marketing manager.

Amy Armstrong for providing the beautiful design work for the book.

Laura leGrand for her fine editorial support.

Brian Jones and Carolyn Miller for their excellent editing of the book and their attention to detail, which greatly improved the quality and readability of the book.

Molly Siple, our research assistant, who worked long and hard hours. We feel great appreciation for her excellent work and willingness to go the extra mile.

Torrie Randall, who provided very helpful editing in the early stage of the book's development.

Dolores Shaw, our personal assistant, whose tireless energy and great organizational skills helped to keep our operation going while writing this book.

Finally, to all of those researchers and scientists whose work and research studies related to this project and without whom this book would not have been possible.

INTRODUCTION

THIS BOOK GREW out of a series of questions that first began to puzzle us more than two decades ago: Why do many highly successful people have abundant energy and the determination and focus to succeed while sometimes ignoring many of the rules of good health? Might these individuals have a chemical makeup that differs substantially from that of the rest of the population? Is there in fact a "chemistry of success," and if so, can it be restored in individuals who have lost it or created in those who never possessed it?

Both Susan, as a physician specializing in preventive medicine, and Jim, as a businessman often working in the health care field, suspected that there is such a chemistry of success. Both of us have observed it in politicians who maintain grueling schedules, traveling constantly, and often eating rich, unhealthy food on the banquet circuit, yet still have boundless energy. We have also seen it in athletes who play an intense game at their maximum level of physical exertion, perhaps even sustaining bruises and other minor injuries, yet manage to recover quickly enough to play equally well the next night. For many years, we have admired the energy and stamina of successful businessmen and -women whose work requires them to travel extensively, participate in endless meetings, socialize with customers late into the evening—yet still be fresh for an early-morning breakfast with an important client. We have also marveled at the productivity and creativity of many top-notch scientists, artists, and writers.

Even more amazing to us has been our observation that that, unlike most people, these peak performers rarely seem to get sick during the prime of their careers, despite having much more demanding schedules than most of us. They are frequently in the news, maintain busy and complicated work and personal lives, and are often seen prominently at social events, charity functions, and the opening nights of the theater and opera.

Many of these individuals display lifestyle habits that should undermine or destroy the strong constitutions they obviously were born with.

Both of us have also personally known a number of people who have achieved most of their goals and expectations and have lived their lives to the fullest while displaying the same lifestyle contradictions as their more publicly prominent counterparts. All of these individuals possess one or more special traits: They have more vigor, energy, or athletic ability, better social skills, more natural exuberance, or greater intellectual gifts than anyone else around them. They are always able to perform at levels that far outshine their peers. They never seem to get tired, function well on very little sleep, and rarely get sick. These natural peak performers are grateful for their energy and resilience, yet they have no idea how or why they are able to accomplish so much.

IT'S NOT ALL IN YOUR HEAD

In the course of our research, we have read dozens of books on success and peak performance. These books do not begin to explain all of the contradictions that we have observed among both prominent public figures and our most successful friends and clients. Virtually none of the books even mention health as a factor necessary for success. The few books that do make no mention of which functions of the body are involved in peak performance.

All the books state that a positive mental attitude is the most important determinant of success. Psychologists, social scientists, and many others who have studied predictors of success believe that it all comes down to mental programming: Highly successful people are thought to have better mental programming than less successful people. Hundreds of books have discussed "the winner's mind" and have concluded that such a thing exists. Many of the self-help books, tapes, and seminars that have been developed to assist people in reaching their life goals assert that if you simply model the thought processes of very successful people, you can attain the same high level of success.

We both recognize the critical importance of positive mental programming and have personally found a number of these books relevant and useful. However, we eventually began to question the argument that good mental programming alone determines success. Susan's twenty-four years of clinical practice and Jim's thirty years of observation of the business world suggest that more than positive mental programming is needed to explain the capabilities for maximum achievement that some exceptional people possess.

WHAT JIM LEARNED ABOUT PEAK PERFORMERS IN THE BUSINESS WORLD

When I graduated from Stanford's Graduate School of Business, I joined Lehman Brothers, one of the leading investment banking and brokerage firms in the United States. I worked there throughout the 1970s, which was a very difficult period in the securities business, characterized by a decade-long bear market and the worst stock market decline since the Great Depression. In addition, there were severe financial and political shocks created by the Arab oil embargo, very high inflation and interest rates coupled with low economic growth ("stagflation"), and the infamous Watergate scandal, which culminated in President Nixon's resignation. So I was in a good position to observe people trying to succeed in an extraordinarily challenging environment.

I have always been interested in the characteristics of successful people and have read a number of the classic books on success such as Napoleon Hill's *Think and Grow Rich* and James Allen's *As a Man Thinketh*. I incorporated the ideas espoused in these books into my personal philosophy after observing that many successful people seem to follow and even exemplify these ideas. However, no matter the mental and social abilities of these individuals, not all of them rose to the very top of the heap. There were always a select few who excelled above the equally bright and hard-working people around them, and I found myself wondering what special traits these peak performers had that others did not.

Over time, I realized that what these people have is boundless energy and stamina. They also seem to be immune to—and recover quickly from—the minor illnesses, allergies, and chronic ailments that plague much of the population and cause significant discomfort and loss of productivity. In addition, many of these individuals have the ability to get by for sustained periods on little sleep. They can eat almost anything and still maintain a high level of energy, and they recover quickly from late nights of drinking and socializing. They survive and even thrive on a schedule that includes nearly constant travel.

Often, they are able to outlast their coworkers or competitors simply because they are the last man standing. They just keep showing up and doing those repetitive tasks that eventually lead to success. They persist until people say yes. When they make mistakes or even fail, they pick themselves up and simply start over—again and again, until they learn the lessons they need to attain their goals. These people are relentless, indefatigable; they just outlast their competition. I have wondered for years what physical or chemical functions they have that allow them to perform in this manner.

WHAT SUSAN LEARNED ABOUT PEAK PERFORMANCE AS A PHYSICIAN

Like Jim, I have been fascinated by peak performers for years; as a doctor, I have thought about this topic from a medical viewpoint. While Jim was working with and observing peak performers, people at the top of their game professionally and personally, I spent many years as a physician working with people who, because of their health issues, were often just getting by in terms of their level of performance. After twenty-four years of working with patients, I am convinced that peak performance involves more than simply a positive mental attitude. Because my field is preventive medicine and involves a significant amount of time spent both counseling and educating my patients as to how they can best modify their health habits, I have always scheduled very long initial and follow-up visits. I normally spend one to one-and-one-half hours at the first visit finding out not only about my patient's physical and emotional symptoms but also about how they are handling their career and personal lives. After working with thousands of patients, I began to understand that many of them were unable to perform effectively in many areas of their lives.

Many of the patients I've seen in my practice are bright, well-educated people with a variety of interesting and demanding careers, and with many emotional and spiritual resources. They have been engineers, computer programmers, artists, writers, teachers, psychologists, homemakers, lawyers, and other Silicon Valley professionals of all stripes. They have also tended to be people who will seek counseling or spiritual guidance if they feel they need it, and who will incorporate meditation and other stress-relieving practices into their lives. In short, they are, on the whole, people who seemed to be mentally well programmed for success, yet they have frequently felt that they were not performing to their own expectations in either their professional, their personal, or their social lives.

What I observed was that chemical imbalances were often as much (if not more) of a determinant than emotional problems in people's inability to live and perform as fully as they had hoped. They complained of symptoms like brain fog that wouldn't go away; an ongoing lack of physical energy; colds, flus, and respiratory infections that lingered for weeks and allergy symptoms that persisted for months; poor digestive function; headaches; muscle and joint aches and pains; and many other chronic physical problems. Some of my other patients reported feelings of anxiousness or agitation, as well as an inability to make decisions calmly. These symptoms, as well as many others, are typical of the type of complaints that I have heard over the years from patients—problems that affected their ability to perform to their own expectations in their careers and in their personal and social lives.

Many of my patients seemed, as a result of these symptoms, to be suffering from what I call the Law of Diminishing Expectations. As their chemical imbalances and physical symptoms worsened, they were less able to meet the demands of their careers, participate in the sports they enjoyed, or even handle their social relationships. They contracted their activities to meet their diminished capability in the various areas of their lives. Unfortunately, they often found that they had to discontinue many of the activities that they enjoyed the most in order to be able to carry out the tasks necessary for their own survival. They would make every effort to continue showing up at work so that they could earn a paycheck and take care of their family, but sometimes not do much else. They also stated that when they had been physically healthier, their ability to pursue and attain their goals had been much greater.

It became obvious to me that the law of diminishing expectations affects millions of other people besides my patients. All of us either have to perform or choose to perform in various areas of our lives. Most of us have job or family responsibilities that must be met if we are to continue to function as productive members of society. There are also many activities we choose to do, such as reading, playing with our children, enjoying a healthy sexual relationship and love life, listening to music, gardening, producing artistic creations, or participating in sports and games. Yet many people lack the firepower necessary to go about their daily tasks and activities with the same level of zest and vitality that natural peak performers are gifted with. I wanted to know what that special something is that peak performers have in abundance but that so many of us lack, to greater or lesser degrees. I also wanted to understand how it related to the chemical and physical makeup of the body and to find out if it was something that could be restored.

To understand the mechanisms of this problem better, I reviewed the research on the relationship of peak performance traits (such as physical vitality and stamina, mental clarity and acuity, and the ability to get along with people) to various aspects of health in fields as diverse as internal medicine, geriatrics, and psychiatry. I also looked at other cultural models and even studied the research on Paleolithic human beings to better understand which physical and chemical determinants were most important for peak performance and health.

I was intrigued to find that the observation that some people are born with greater reserves of energy and vitality than the rest of the population has been recognized for thousands of years in traditional healing models. In Asian medicine, the energy that you are born with is called *jing*. Jing is the vital force that we inherit from our parents and ancestors; it determines our individual constitution and level of health. Our innate resistance to disease, our reproductive health, our level of energy, and even our longevity are determined by how much jing we are born with. It is like money in a bank, and we are constantly drawing down on our reserves. Once it is used up, we have exhausted our life force. The ancient Indian or Ayurvedic health model recognizes a similar concept, called *prana*, the spark of life.

I also found that a more recent version of this theory was developed nearly seventy years ago by Hans Selye, the famous Canadian physiologist, whose groundbreaking research led to the modern theories of how the body adapts to stress. He developed the concept of *adaptation energy*. This term describes the differences in people's innate ability to handle the various stresses they encounter throughout their lives. These stresses can include heavy physical exertion, emotional wear and tear, and climatic changes. When people are endowed with a high level of adaptation energy, they are able to handle stress more effectively and are more resistant to physical breakdown and even disease. As described in Selye's own words from his book *The Stress of Life*, "It is as though, at birth, each individual inherited a certain amount of adaptation energy, the magnitude of which is determined by his genetic background, his parents ... in any case, there is just so much of it, and he must budget accordingly."

After reading thousands of research articles on the link between various aspects of peak performance and health and after working with thousands of patients in my clinical practice, I began to see some clear patterns. I realized that a number of essential chemical functions directly affect our ability to perform at peak levels in every area of life. I also found that these same chemical functions are necessary for optimal health and resistance to disease.

As a physician specializing in clinical nutrition and preventive medicine, I have also always been very interested in how people can support and restore these functions themselves by means of nutrition- and lifestyle-based therapies. There is a tremendous amount of research in the medical literature supporting such therapies. Over the years I have used much of this growing body of information to help put together the nutritional and lifestyle-based programs for my patients. Many of my patients have found these programs to be very helpful. Our friends, family members, and business associates have also benefited from this information.

THE SIX CHEMICAL FUNCTIONS NEEDED FOR PEAK PERFORMANCE AND HEALTH

To function as a peak performer and to enjoy optimal health, an individual must be able to efficiently do the following six things:

1. Regulate the body's acid/alkaline balance.

2. Produce digestive enzymes.

3. Detoxify pollutants and other toxic chemicals as well as one's own waste products.

4. Oxygenate tissues and cells.

5. Neutralize the chemical imbalances caused by stress.

6. Produce sex hormones.

The more of these functions an individual has intact and operating efficiently, the more capable of peak performance he or she will be.

You will be learning about these functions and how to keep them in excellent working condition as you read this book. The techniques that we describe on how to restore and maintain each of these functions are very effective and easy to implement. They will give you the tools you need to perform to your own goals and expectations. The book also provides essential information on how to relieve and prevent many common health problems by restoring the six chemical functions needed for success.

THE EIGHT TRAITS OF PEAK PERFORMERS

The six chemical functions are crucial in supporting eight traits that are essential components of peak performance and success:

1. Physical vitality and stamina.

2. Mental clarity and acuity.

3. Determination and perseverance in pursuing goals.

4. The ability to get along with other people.

5. The ability to remain calm under pressure.

6. Optimism and vision.

7. Speedy recovery from illness, injury, and exertion.

8. Resistance to illness.

The last two traits are usually not mentioned in books on success, but colds, flus, allergies, digestive problems, muscle and joint aches and pains, accidents and injuries, and many other common health problems take an extraordinary toll on people's ability to perform successfully in any task or endeavor. These eight traits form the foundation of this book; let us now briefly describe each of them.

1 Physical vitality and stamina

Highly successful people have deep reservoirs of energy that allow them to persevere and meet their goals, no matter how difficult. They have the ability, when necessary, to tolerate grueling work or training conditions.

Peak performers can work long hours, travel extensively, meet tight deadlines, and engage in rigorous athletic or other training. Their high level of physical energy also allows them to enjoy a rich and varied life. They are able to engage in an active social life, learn a new language, take up a new sport, or start a new business venture. Individuals with less physical energy and stamina are much more limited in the types and variety of activities that they can engage in.

◀2 Mental clarity and acuity

Peak performers have the ability to think clearly and analytically and to solve problems effectively. They also possess a sharp memory and can recall names, facts, and other details easily. This mental edge is mandatory for success in virtually any career—whether you are a quarterback reading a defense, a scientist interpreting data, or a CEO doing strategic planning. One hundred years ago, there were still many jobs that depended on brawn rather than brains. This is no longer true in today's modern world, where most of these "muscle" jobs are now done by robotic and other heavy equipment. Most careers are now based on the accumulation of knowledge.

◀3 Determination and perseverance in pursuing goals

Highly successful people tend to stay focused on their goals and aspirations until they accomplish them, at which time they set new ones. These individuals have the energy, stamina, and excellent health necessary to persevere and keep changing their strategies and tactics until they finally get it right. Even if these individuals begin with poor mental programming, they will keep learning from their mistakes until they reach their goals.

◀4 The ability to get along with other people

Peak performers are able to get along with their superiors as well as their co-workers, their instructors as well as their fellow students. They know how to listen, take feedback, and deliver their messages in a socially acceptable manner. They also tend to have positive relationships with their family and friends. They do not usually react with inappropriate anger, upsets, fear, or anxiety in their dealings with others. In addition, highly successful people are able to handle all types of social demands. Participation in social and business functions often involves eating many rich meals and doing a fair amount of social drinking (if they enjoy alcoholic beverages). Highly successful people are able to attend and participate in these events, digest the rich food, metabolize the alcohol—and still be in the office early the next day, as if after a routine night at home. Their ability to socialize and maintain good long-term relationships is a great asset they use for both their personal enjoyment and business advancement.

5 The ability to remain calm under pressure

Many people are able to perform reasonably well when the level of stress is minimal. However, peak performers are able to stay calm, centered, and focused when the stress level is increased because of major deadlines, crucial negotiations, the determining moments in a sporting event, or unexpected events such as mechanical breakdowns or natural disasters. Those people who can remain calm during periods of high stress are more likely to demonstrate good judgment and solve problems in a logical and impartial manner.

6 Optimism and vision

Many of life's great leaders, coaches, CEOs, teachers, and athletes have been optimists. For them, there is always a way to solve a problem, create an opportunity, recover from a setback, or come back to win an important game in the final minutes; nothing is impossible. They know they are going to achieve their goals. They simply do not take no for an answer. They can visualize how the future will develop and what steps they need to take to get there. Optimists inspire themselves and the people around them to exceed their limitations.

7 Speedy recovery from illness, injury, and exertion

Peak performers have the ability to recover rapidly from strenuous physical exertion, mental or emotional stress, illness, allergy symptoms, injury, or major or minor surgery. When these individuals are injured on the job, begin to come down with a minor illness, or sustain an injury in an athletic event, they are able to heal rapidly and are back in the game much more quickly than the average person. Professional athletes provide an excellent example of this trait. Their ability to recover from illness, injury, and hard physical exertion, as much as their athletic prowess, is a prerequisite for sustaining a long career. Businesspeople who are able to recover quickly from minor ailments like colds and flus or from injuries incurred on the job or while engaging in sports are natural peak performers who can easily maintain or resume their normal schedules. They are able to meet deadlines, attend meetings, and keep to demanding travel schedules much better than most people.

◀8 Resistance to illness

Maximum achievers are able to withstand grueling work demands and deadlines, excessive social commitments, frequent travel, and emotional stress and still remain in excellent health. They also do not experience the loss of productivity and time away from work that dealing with chronic illnesses causes. Unfortunately, millions of individuals are unable to withstand the physical and emotional stresses of their lives. These stresses make them more prone to health problems such as colds, flus, allergic episodes, indigestion, muscle and joint aches and pains, jet lag, sleeplessness, and even more serious illnesses. These as well as other common ailments significantly affect one's capacity to perform successfully in all tasks or endeavors.

THE CHEMISTRY OF SUCCESS CAN BENEFIT EVERYONE

We have written this book for the millions of people—men, women, and children of all ages—searching for resources that will help them improve their health and attain their success goals. You can use this book to improve your ability to perform in virtually any area of your life, including your career, creative endeavors, athletic performance, and personal relationships. Even if you have never considered yourself a peak performer, you can use the techniques described in this book to increase your level of energy, improve your ability to achieve your goals, and create a much improved level of health.

The baby boomers—those individuals born between 1946 and 1964—are concerned about maintaining their vitality and quality of life. (This is also more generally true of many individuals between the ages of thirty and sixty-five—and older.) Most of the baby boomers, who are now in their mid-thirties to mid-fifties, are beginning to experience the negative effects that a decline in their chemical functions has on both their level of performance and their health. None of the baby boomers want to experience the normal age-related changes in their physical appearance, vitality, sexual performance, athletic ability, or earning power. As a group, they want to maintain the same level of energy and performance capability that they had in their twenties and thirties. This book provides the tools necessary for them to achieve that goal well into old age.

Many of us, especially those of us above the age of forty, are also concerned about economic survival in today's competitive workplace. As we reach midlife and older, symptoms connected to the weakening of the six chemical functions needed for success and health begin to take their toll on our job performance and productivity. These symptoms include fatigue, loss of mental acuity and memory, aches and pains in our joints, and the inability to recover rapidly from colds, flus, allergies, bronchitis, surgery, and dental work.

The weakening of our crucial chemical functions can be a source of real distress in terms of our economic well-being. Many of us live from paycheck to paycheck. We worry about having enough money to cover such basic expenses as our mortgage or rent, car payments, food bills, and taxes. Parents often have to budget carefully to pay for their children's dental and medical bills and, even more significantly, their college education. All of us need to maintain our energy and stamina as well as remain in excellent health if we are to meet our financial obligations.

In addition, the effects of age-related declines in productivity are now a reality in the workplace. About 60 million workers in the United States are now forty years of age or older. They comprise about 45 percent of the total workforce, according to the Bureau of Labor Statistics. Increasingly, companies are replacing their over forty-year-old employees with workers in their twenties and thirties, who are considered more energetic and flexible. Older workers are perceived by their employers as less energetic, more fixed in their ways, and shopworn. A February 1997 article in the *Washington Post* discussed this trend in detail, citing the thousands of age-discrimination complaints now being brought against employers. Even more recently, this topic was the cover story of *Fortune's* February 1, 1999, issue. Yet, there is no need to experience age-related changes that significantly reduce your productivity in the workplace. By restoring the six chemical functions described in this book, you will go a long way toward staying vital and competitive in today's economy.

Peak performers who are currently enjoying excellent health and are at the height of their career and financial success can also benefit from the techniques described in this book, if they wish to continue to make incremental gains in their fields of endeavor. These people are often more in need of chemical fine-tuning than a total physical overhaul. The programs described in this book will help anyone maintain their ability to perform at peak levels for decades.

Even many highly successful peak performers begin to show a decline in one or more of their essential chemical functions by midlife. However, while these chemical weaknesses may show up in laboratory testing, and even some early physical symptoms, many of these individuals continue to maintain a strong level of energy and vitality. Their overall biochemical makeup is still so strong and resilient that their ability to function is often unaffected at this stage. These people can still run circles around everyone else. Like twenty-year-olds, many of these superachievers continue to behave as if they were immortal. We have seen this pattern repeatedly in highly successful people in their fifties and sixties.

However, ignoring the early-warning signs of age-related decline is a risky strategy. Many of these individuals do not make the necessary changes in their lifestyle and nutritional habits until they are forced to, usually when a health catastrophe, such as a heart attack or a diagnosis of cancer, occurs. There are millions of people like this in the United States today, including many highly successful people that we know personally. If you fit this profile, a more sensible strategy is to work to restore the functions that are showing early signs of decline. For individuals who want to maintain their vigor and health well into old age, prevention is truly the best medicine.

The strongest and most resilient natural peak performers also finally run out of gas as they reach their seventies, eighties, and nineties. Because of the inevitability of the aging process, no one remains a peak performer forever (though peak performers do tend to age much more slowly than their peers). Even these seemingly supermen and superwomen finally lose the peak-performance capabilities that they have enjoyed for decades.

Peak performers, who have been used to functioning effectively throughout their entire lives, are often frustrated by this loss of energy and vitality and are distressed by the decline in their health. No matter how many years of vital functioning a person may have had, for most of us it is never enough—we yearn for more. The information in this book can help restore these lost capabilities in individuals of any age.

Finally, be sure to share the information and techniques that you learn from this book with friends and family members, including your children, so that they can benefit, too. Many children and teenagers are not able to perform to their own expectations or to those of their family and teachers. In addition, many children suffer from a substandard level of health. Millions of children suffer from too many colds, flus, and episodes of bronchitis and asthma, as well as allergies, fatigue, difficulty concentrating in school, emotional ups and downs, social problems, and addictions. Many of these problems originate in chemical imbalances, particularly in the six functions described in this book. If you are a parent, you will find many useful tips in this book for improving the health and performance of your children.

HOW THE CHEMISTRY OF SUCCESS RESTORED OUR OWN PEAK-PERFORMANCE CAPABILITIES

Like millions of other people, both of us lost our ability to perform at peak levels relatively early in life, Susan in her late thirties and Jim in his early forties. We are telling our stories now to show you what you can accomplish with the restorative techniques described in this book. By using these techniques ourselves, we have not only regained our active and productive lifestyles, but enjoy an exceptional level of health and vitality in our fifties and are able to fully pursue and attain our goals and aspirations.

Jim's story

Even though I was very active in sports and outdoor activities and did well in school during my youth, I was not born with a superfunctioning physical system. In retrospect, there were signs all during my childhood and teenage years that my body was not in balance and did not have enough firepower in certain functions. For example, I had frequent colds, sore throats, and upper respiratory infections. Often, after consuming soft drinks or a lot of highly sugared processed foods, I would develop canker sores or an extremely sore and tender mouth. Also, when I came down with a cold or sore throat, I would not recover as quickly as many of my friends did. My body lacked the ability to resolve these minor illnesses that others seemed to have. At the time, I had no idea what these functions were or what could be done to strengthen them or bring them into balance so that I, too, could recover quickly from minor illnesses. But I was determined to find out how to create the necessary strength so that I would not continue to come down with these illnesses or, if I did, so that I could recover quickly.

My search for ways to restore my body's balance accelerated when I went away to college. I attended Yale University and subsequently received an MBA from Stanford University Graduate School of Business. The programs at both of these schools were difficult and demanding, and I could not afford to become ill with colds and flus, which would cause me to miss classes and assignments. My search led me to health food stores, where I began to learn about vitamins, minerals, herbs, and other supplements that could assist my body in warding off or recovering from these minor illnesses. Taking large doses of vitamin C allowed me to get through college and graduate school with many fewer illnesses than when I was a teenager.

During my thirties, I lived and worked in San Francisco. My work required me to be up at 5:00 A.M. so that I could begin to work with our East Coast headquarters when the stock markets opened. Work was busy, fast paced, and stressful, often continuing into the late evening courtesy of my expense account. All of this intense business and social activity caused a significant amount of wear and tear on my body.

By my early forties, supplementation with vitamins no longer prevented me from coming down with frequent respiratory infections. I was constantly plagued with nasal congestion, coughing, and painful sinuses, often to the point of being unable to work for sustained periods of time. These recurrent respiratory infections hampered my effectiveness, as I could not make a simple one-week business trip without coming down with some nasal problem. Finally, it got so bad that any unusual stress or several days of rich food or drink would trigger a cold or runny nose. After several years of this pattern, I resolved to find out what parts of my body were not functioning and to completely restore them so that I would never again have to limit my activities or operate in fear of coming down with a respiratory infection at an inopportune time.

By this time, I had married Susan. I now had a partner who was also vitally interested in this subject. With her medical background, she provided me with the technical knowledge and insights to fully understand these problems.

Today, by using the information set forth in the following chapters, I am healthier than I have ever been in my life. I have restored and strengthened the functions that had become so weakened by overwork and stress more than fifteen years ago. Now, if I feel myself coming down with a cold or flu, I restore balance to my body by using the techniques discussed in this book and am back fully functioning in twelve to twenty-four hours. Only a small number of peak performers are able to do this naturally. My recent medical tests are consistent with an excellent health profile and indicate that I am now at very low risk of developing such common illnesses as hypertension, heart disease, and prostate cancer, problems that begin to be relevant for men in their late fifties like myself. I have now built myself up to the point that I almost never get sick, and I am able to pursue my goals and aspirations with abundant energy and stamina.

While writing this book, I have often worked seven days a week, often putting in sixty- to eighty-hour workweeks. In addition to working on the book, I have also closed several other business deals and done a fair amount of business travel at the same time. By following the techniques described in this book, I have maintained tremendous energy, not been sick, worked out four to five times per week, and recovered from such exertions as a transcontinental flight after only one night's sleep, in the same way a natural-born peak performer is able to do.

The exciting implications for the readers of this book are that you, too, can restore the physical and chemical functions necessary to be able to perform at your best, regardless of your age. This is extremely important in today's competitive business and professional environment, especially if you are over forty. At that age, the many stress factors that we all have to deal with in our busy lives, and the inevitable effects of the aging process itself, are beginning to have a significant impact on our performance and enjoyment of life. This book will give you the guidance you need to restore your own functions and begin to have the drive, energy, and stamina to pursue your goals and dreams with the gusto of a peak performer.

Susan's story

I have always had plenty of energy and a sturdy constitution. Except for PMS and menstrual cramps during my teens and twenties, I was rarely ill. I almost never got colds or flus, and never suffered from the allergies or other health problems that seemed to plague some of my friends.

Unfortunately, by my mid-thirties, the stresses of my personal and professional life finally began to wear me down. I had spent years working hard as a busy physician. I spent long hours each day tending to the needs of my patients, having built a large and successful practice. In addition, as an instructor at Stanford University Medical School, I had teaching responsibilities to junior and senior medical students. During a three-year period, I went through a divorce, married Jim, and then gave birth to our daughter. To cap it off, our daughter was born somewhat prematurely and was frail and sick during her first year of life.

Given my busy schedule, I chose not to breast-feed, preferring instead to bottle-feed our daughter. To my dismay, she could not handle any of the formulas that we tried to feed her and threw them all up. In addition, she suffered from respiratory problems. Although she is now a strong and healthy teenager, her first year was very much touch and go. For six months, I had to secure donor breast milk from all over the San Francisco area as well as contributions collected by a local hospital. To say that I was frazzled and overwhelmed as a new mother is an understatement.

For the first time in my life, my body could not handle all the stresses I was loading on it. After the birth of our daughter, I became exhausted and ill. Several years earlier, I had begun to show signs that stress and overwork were taking their toll on my body, but I had ignored them. Now I had feelings of tension in the pit of my stomach, was not sleeping well, and noticed swollen glands in my neck. When my energy finally collapsed, I had a full-fledged health breakdown. For a year, I was constantly fatigued, had frequent sore throats and respiratory infections, and could not digest my food. For one bleak period, all I could digest were boiled potatoes and steamed vegetables. I also developed an extreme sensitivity to environmental pollutants, which had never bothered me before. I would become dizzy and practically faint if I was exposed to chemicals used to treat lawns and gardens as well as common household cleaning agents. I had to come to grips with the fact that in my late thirties I had gone from being an energetic peak performer to being an exhausted, worn-out person, barely able to function.

After years of hearing my patients complain about their inability to perform to their own expectations as their health deteriorated, this issue suddenly became an intensely personal one for me. I now had to turn my focus away from my practice and find solutions for myself to problems that I had been dealing with for years in my patients. During this period, I continued to work, and to take care of our daughter and household, but I was functioning inefficiently at best: Some days I felt like a six-cylinder engine with four dead spark plugs. All of the activities I enjoyed, like my art lessons, painting sessions, and our previously active social life, fell by the wayside as I struggled to regain my health.

However, I was determined to regain my strength and become a peak performer again. Life was too exciting and I was too young to be relegated to the sidelines. Since I was a trained physician, it was relatively easy for me to take stock of which physical and chemical functions were not working up to par. After a year of intensive work on my health, I was back on my feet again. Over time, using many of the techniques described in this book, I have restored my health and energy to their former levels and am committed to maintaining them for decades to come. I have restored the physical and chemical functions that became devitalized in my thirties, so that my body could once again perform at peak levels. To this day, I still work to maintain my body chemistry so that I can continue to achieve my goals and enjoy life to the fullest. As a woman over fifty, I now have to deal with the aging process that millions of other baby boomers are starting to experience.

The results of my work have produced remarkable benefits. Even though I am just turning fifty-four, I am not yet in menopause and continue to have regular, healthy menstrual cycles. As a result, my own production of hormones continues to help maintain my level of performance by supporting the health of my bones and tissues, my level of energy, and even my moods. It has been years since I have had a cold, flu, or allergic symptoms from pollutants. If I begin to feel a respiratory infection coming on, I nip it in the bud by improving my chemical balance and am normally symptom free within twelve to twenty-four hours. While the peak performers I know are able to do this naturally, I do it through the nutritional programs that I have developed. Unlike the average American, whose respiratory infections can linger on for as long as three to six weeks,

I am back at work and free of symptoms within a day or so. I am able to be productive and enjoy my life. My energy and vitality are tremendous and allow me to continue to work and play with vigor. I follow a careful program of nutritional supplements that I have put together for myself and modify periodically when any signs of impaired physical and chemical function begin to arise. I am very careful about what I eat. As you will learn in this book, it is important to eat to your body's chemical needs if you want to remain a healthy and vital peak performer.

I am not, however, one of those astonishing and relatively rare natural peak performers, who make it into their eighties and nineties on their own firepower, competing in marathons and triathlons, running their own businesses, and remaining socially active and involved in life well into old age. Like millions of other people, my body began to run out of steam at a much younger age than that. Instead, I provide myself with the nutritional support that I need on an ongoing basis so that I can continue to be a peak performer.

HOW TO USE THIS BOOK

By the time you have finished reading this book, you will understand each of the chemical functions needed for peak performance and health. You will also understand that peak performance and general health are intimately related, and that robust health is essential if you want to meet your goals in life. You will also find checklists that will help you evaluate how well your own chemical functions are operating. Each chapter on a chemical function (odd-numbered) is followed by a chapter with a highly effective program that you can use to restore that function (even-numbered).

One of the more helpful aspects of this book is that you can selectively use the information and techniques to restore those of your own physiological functions that are showing the most signs of decline. This approach will support many of the performance traits needed to attain your own personal goals. Some people want to perform in the broadest possible sense, enjoying and participating in all of life's activities: career success, sports and physical activities, social and family life, an active sex life, and enjoyment of food and drink. These individuals may want to maintain or strengthen, where necessary, all six of the chemical functions so that they can continue to enjoy a rich and varied life. However, not everyone has or needs such broad aspirations; many people are satisfied with a much more narrow focus. They prefer to direct their energies much more intensely in one or two areas of strong interest. Whether your interests are broad or narrow, it is the ability to participate, and even excel, in the areas that interest you the most, that gives meaning, excitement, and texture to life. When the physiological functions necessary to fully participate in these treasured activities begin to diminish, much of the joy and fun of life is lost.

While working to improve or restore the chemical functions discussed in this book, do not ignore the benefits that positive mental programming can confer. In other words, be sure to pay attention to your emotional and spiritual needs and development as well as your physical and biochemical ones. It helps mind as well as body to practice stress reduction techniques like meditation, yoga, and regular exercise. Should you find it helpful, seek emotional and spiritual counseling. Having both healthy chemical functions and positive mental programming provides the foundation upon which success and peak performance are built.

You can use this book in one of two ways to discover which of your functions are most in need of support: You can read through the entire book to gain an overview of all six of the chemical functions needed for success and optimal health. Or you can scan the bulleted items at the beginning of each introductory chapter for the six chemical functions (the odd-numbered chapters). We begin each introductory chapter by summarizing in a chart the peak-performance traits that each function supports. The traits are numbered ◀1 through ◀8, just as they are here in the introduction. Trait ◀1 is physical vitality and stamina; trait ◀2 is mental clarity and acuity; and so on. These charts also summarize the health benefits that each function supports. Scanning these charts will help you pinpoint which of your chemical functions are most in need of support and restoration. You may then choose to focus your attention on the chapters that are most relevant to your needs. (Some individuals may prefer to use the index at the back of the book for the same purpose.) Near the beginning of each odd-numbered chapter, there is also a paragraph we call a "roadmap" (indicated by this symbol 🅒); this will guide you to the part or parts of the text that you most want to read. For instance, you may be interested in learning more about the chemistry of each function; or you may want to read in more depth about the ways a function affects peak performance or health; or you may want to go directly to the practical advice on restoring each function. The roadmap will guide you to any of these. Finally, you can use the appendix to find some of the many helpful resources discussed in the book.

Not only does this book provide you with programs needed for restoring the essential chemical functions necessary for peak performance and optimal health, but it also includes tips on how to quickly restore the chemical balance of the body during times of acute stress. Grueling work demands and deadlines, excessive social commitments, travel, and emotional stress can lower resistance and make one more prone to acute problems such as colds, flus, allergic episodes, indigestion, jet lag, hangovers, sleeplessness, and fatigue. This book will provide you with dozens of Peak-Performance Tips (indicated by this symbol ▲▲) that will enable you to rapidly restore your own chemical balance and eliminate these "success saboteurs" in the shortest possible time.

You will be amazed at how easy these programs are to use. Once you begin your own peak-performance program, you should begin to notice positive changes rapidly. Over time, these changes can be dramatic and have the potential to enhance performance in every area that you desire.

How to Develop Your Own Peak-Performance Program

When the physiological functions necessary for peak performance and optimal health are working effectively, you are more likely to be able to achieve all of your goals and aspirations in life. It is important to remember that optimal health and peak performance go hand in hand. However, between the ages of thirty and sixty, at least several of these vital chemical functions begin to work less effectively in many people due to the cumulative effects of the normal wear and tear of life and the natural aging process. Susan has found that it is very rare for her patients to have only one function showing significant stress; it is much more common for them to complain about a wide variety of symptoms, indicating a breakdown in several functions.

For example, a fifty-year-old man may be concerned about his high blood pressure, his increased frequency of allergic symptoms, and the decline in his libido. Similarly, a fifty-year-old woman may complain about the difficulty she has digesting her food, her overly acid stomach, and her increasing fatigue, as well as the hot flashes and other symptoms that are occurring with her transition into menopause. The combinations of symptoms that patients can experience are limitless.

Susan usually finds it necessary to develop nutritional and lifestyle modification programs to support and help restore multiple functions simultaneously. None of her patients want her to alleviate only one or a few symptoms, leaving the rest for a later date. They want to begin to see relief of all the physical, mental, and emotional symptoms that are interfering with their ability to perform their day-to-day responsibilities as well as participate in the social activities that provide great joy and pleasure in their lives.

Putting together a program that restores one or more chemical functions at the same time is not as difficult as it might sound. Anyone reading this book should be able to do it without too much effort. Also, the benefits are much greater and occur much more rapidly than by trying to restore individual functions on a sequential basis.

Here are some guidelines on how to choose the best possible program to restore your own peak-performance capability and health.

Step one: Determine which functions are most in need of strengthening

To assist you in this regard, go to the beginning of the introductory chapters on each of the six chemical functions (the odd-numbered chapters). There you will find a chart summarizing the peak-performance health benefits that that particular chemical function helps to support or restore. Begin to look up the performance traits and health issues that are of greatest concern to you. You will then be able to determine which of your chemical functions are most in need of strengthening. (Alternatively, you may prefer to look up specific health issues and performance traits in the index.)

Step two: Use your own physician as an important resource

The diagnostic techniques of Western medicine are truly awesome. Both men and women should have complete physical exams or, at the least, standard blood chemistry tests and urinalysis performed every few years. Many physicians will also order diagnostic tests if they want to further evaluate your risk of specific diseases. The results of these tests can give you clues about the status of your own physiological functions. For example, the bone density studies that physicians may order on women entering menopause can provide valuable information about both hormonal status and acid/alkaline balance. Or, if liver function tests are elevated on a routine chemistry panel, reflecting stress or disease within the liver, detoxification capabilities are probably impaired.

More specialized tests of physiological functions—such as hair analysis to determine mineral levels within the body, salivary testing of hormone levels, detoxification panels, and testing of various parameters of digestive function—are more likely to be done by physicians practicing *complementary medicine*. (This catchall term describes the use of nondrug methods to treat and prevent disease, such as nutritional counseling, stress management, and acupuncture, to name but a few modalities. If you are interested in working with such a physician, the appendix contains a list of professional societies to which many of them belong. Contact these organizations to find such a physician working in your area.) What you learn from the self-quizzes contained within this book and from data provided to you by your physician can give you much valuable information as to which physiological functions need support and restoration.

Step three: Go to the therapy chapters of the book (the even-numbered chapters) for each function that you wish to restore

Many different treatment options are discussed within each chapter. If you know that you respond better to certain types of therapies, it obviously makes more sense to use those. You may also want to avoid therapies that have caused unpleasant side effects or adverse reactions in the past. For example, if herbs cause you to experience nausea or diarrhea, it is best to avoid them in favor of the vitamins, minerals, essential fatty acids, and amino acids listed in the particular chapter you are reading. If you find that you are particularly attracted to some of the treatment options discussed in the book, such as HeartMath stress reduction tapes or full-spectrum or SAD lights, it is worth investigating their use. Sources for obtaining these therapies are listed in the appendix.

Step four: Begin your new program slowly and cautiously

Starting slowly will help you to avoid many pitfalls, including adverse reactions to dietary changes or the use of new supplements. Because people have such widely differing biochemical makeups, it is important to use a trial-and-error approach to find your most effective dosages and frequency of use. For example, if you decide to put together a program containing ten different nutrients but have never used any of them before, begin by using just a single nutrient at a very low dose for a few days. If it is well tolerated, you can increase the dose over a few weeks' time to the therapeutic levels mentioned in the book.* Then, every few days, add a new nutrient to your program, until you are taking all ten. If any nutrient should cause distress, stop using it immediately and replace it with a different treatment option.

Step five: Take a periodic vacation from all your supplements

All of us have days when we simply cannot face all of those little brown supplement bottles lining our kitchen counters. Everyone needs an occasional break from taking their vitamins, including your authors. A program can still be effective if you take your supplements 80 to 90 percent of the time. Some practitioners even recommend that you take a break from your supplement use, from one day a week to several days per month. You will probably find that, over time, as your ability to handle stress becomes stronger, certain nutrients are no longer necessary and can be dropped from your regimen.

---

* Anyone beginning a nutritional supplement program should begin at one-quarter to one-half the recommended dosages given in this book. They can then increase their dosages slowly over the course of several weeks until they have reached either the full recommended dosage or a dosage that is therapeutic for them—whichever level comes first. Some individuals will experience therapeutic benefits at doses that are well below the doses recommended in this book. Also, while the dosages provided in this book are appropriate for most people, there are certain groups who should continue to use less than the recommended dosages. Children, the elderly, and individuals with a frail constitution or who are extremely sensitive to drugs and nutritional supplements usually do best at therapeutic dosages of no more than half the recommended levels. Consult your physician or nutritional consultant if you have any questions about the advisability of using a particular nutritional supplement or to determine the dosage most appropriate for you.

Step six: You may want to explore other restorative techniques besides dietary and nutritional therapies

We describe a number of lifestyle modifications, including various exercise programs as well as stress reduction and relaxation techniques. You can benefit greatly by integrating these into your daily routine. In addition, you may want to use such powerful healing tools as the microwater device, biofeedback equipment, and ozone air and water purification devices. These devices can greatly assist in restoring and supporting crucial chemical and physiological functions such as acid/alkaline balance, the ability to oxygenate to peak-performance levels, and the ability to modulate stress.

A FINAL WORD

Our goal is to assist you in becoming a peak performer in your own life. Optimal performance in every area of your life and a significant improvement in your health can be accomplished through the techniques and therapies described in this book. Most people will begin to notice an improvement in how they feel in as quickly as one to two days. However, the actual restoration of these functions to peak-performance levels will take some time. Remember, it took years for you to weaken these functions to the point where they are no longer working effectively. However, once you start a restoration program, you will be amazed by how much better you feel in a short period of time. Your levels of physical energy and mental alertness will improve. You will begin to notice such indicators of better health as improved digestion, greater resistance to colds, flus, and allergies, fewer aches and pains, and an increased feeling of serenity. These are but a few of the benefits you can achieve through the treatments contained in this book.

1

How Acid/Alkaline Balance Benefits Peak Performance and Health

In its natural, healthy state, the human body is slightly alkaline. Virtually all of our cells and tissues contain significant amounts of alkaline substances, such as minerals, oxygen, and bicarbonate. Our blood must maintain a state of slight alkalinity for our very survival. Almost all of our crucial physiological functions—including immunity, digestion, and cardiovascular function—as well as most of our metabolic processes and enzyme reactions require a slightly alkaline internal environment. It follows, then, that both peak performance and optimal health depend on the body's ability to maintain a slightly alkaline state in virtually all of our cells and tissues. The benefits of maintaining this healthful state of slight alkalinity are summarized in the chart on page 28.

Most peak performers are readily able to maintain a healthful state of slight alkalinity, which allows them to live life to the fullest and provides them with tremendous energy and stamina. Since peak performers experience very little downtime, they epitomize Woody Allen's observation that 80 percent of success is "just showing up." They are able to persevere and meet their goals when everyone else has dropped by the wayside. A slightly alkaline state is also necessary if one is to maintain the ability to solve complex mental problems or sustain the creativity needed to make breakthroughs in any field. It also supports our ability to socialize and create strong personal relationships. Finally, when our cells and tissues are slightly alkaline, we are better able to ward off or quickly recover from minor illnesses such as colds, flus, sinusitis, and allergies. We are also able to recover rapidly from injuries, minor surgery, and the effects of vigorous physical activity.

In contrast, when your cells and tissues are overly acidic, you tire easily and are often fatigued. It becomes more difficult to think clearly. You are more likely to develop a pessimistic outlook on life. Even if you have

Benefits of Acid/Alkaline Balance

Peak-Performance Benefits

 Increased physical vitality and stamina

Enhanced mental clarity and acuity

 Increased ability to get along with other people

Increased optimism and vision

Hastened recovery from illness, injury, and exertion (including colds, flus, sinusitis, bronchitis, pneumonia, allergies, and traumatic injury or surgery)

 Increased resistance to illness (includes colds, flus, sinusitis, bronchitis, and pneumonia)

Health Benefits

- Reduces incidence of digestive problems such as heartburn, irritable colon, Crohn's disease, and colitis
- Reduces the risk of and increases relief from urinary-tract conditions such as bacterial cystitis, interstitial cystitis, and uric-acid kidney stones
- Reduces the risk of gout
- Reduces the risk of and helps in the treatment of rheumatoid arthritis and other autoimmune diseases
- Lowers the risk of osteoporosis and promotes bone growth
- Aids in the prevention and treatment of diabetes
- Reduces hypertension
- May reduce the risk of cancer

high goals and aspirations in life, you will lack the energy and vital spark to carry them out to their fullest extent. Overacidity decreases your resistance to colds and flus. You are more likely to suffer from allergies that leave you bleary-eyed and tired at work or sleepy from the drugs you take to suppress the symptoms. Frequent episodes of these minor respiratory illnesses cause millions of Americans to miss work, athletic events, and social engagements. Overacidity also contributes to conditions like arthritis, which can interfere with the ability to succeed in our information economy. It can cause your fingers to become stiff and sore so that you are unable to use a computer, or it can cause hip pain that makes it difficult to sit at a desk for any length of time. Eventually, this inability to neutralize acids in the body causes the slow movements and stiffness of the elderly and contributes to chronic, long-term medical problems like high blood pressure, autoimmune diseases, cancer, and, finally, death itself.

Various physical traits, abilities, and health conditions can serve as helpful indicators of whether your body is fundamentally acid or alkaline. Work through the following checklists (photocopy them if you don't want to write in the book), and refer to them as you read through the chapter. Doing so will give you a better general idea of whether your own system tends toward acidity or alkalinity. For a simple self-test to further assess your acid/alkaline balance, see page 32. There are also tests that your doctor can order that will give you an indirect indication of your acid/alkaline balance; for descriptions of these, see page 96. Knowing whether you tend to be more acidic or more alkaline can help guide your choices in the foods you eat, the way you work, and how you spend your leisure time, and can help you to better manage your health.

CHECKLIST: ARE YOU OVERLY ACIDIC?

Put a check mark beside those statements that are true for you.

Lifestyle factors

❏ I do not feel my best when I eat fast foods, fried foods, colas, and desserts.

❏ I do not feel my best when I eat red meat or red meat dishes.

❏ I do not tolerate acidic condiments like vinegar and lemon juice.

❏ I regularly consume processed and refined foods that contain chemical additives.

❏ I regularly consume breads and baked goods made with white flour and sugar.

❏ I eat few fruits and vegetables.

❑ I drink more than one cup of coffee or tea each day.

❑ I frequently take ascorbic acid (vitamin C), aspirin, or antibiotics.

❑ I do not tolerate alcohol.

❑ I have a history of cigarette smoking.

❑ I frequently travel by plane.

Performance indicators

❑ I often feel exhausted after vigorous exercise or very physical work.

❑ I often experience fatigue and lack of stamina.

❑ I run out of breath running up stairs or walking briskly.

❑ I am physically and mentally tired after an hour of desk work.

❑ I have a tendency to be pessimistic, with little energy to begin new projects.

Physical indicators

❑ I have thin, porous bones.

❑ I have poorly developed muscles.

❑ I often experience muscle stiffness and soreness.

❑ I am over fifty years of age.

Medical history

❑ I catch colds or flus frequently.

❑ I am susceptible to heartburn, canker sores, food or environmental allergies, and sore throat.

❑ I have a history of osteoporosis, arthritis, gout, lung disease, or kidney disease.

CHECKLIST: ARE YOU A HIGH-ALKALINE PRODUCER?

Performance indicators

- ❏ I am able to sprint up stairs.
- ❏ I have great physical endurance.
- ❏ I am always on the go and full of energy.
- ❏ I need only a few hours of sleep each night.
- ❏ I am in a position of leadership at work or in the community.
- ❏ I prefer highly active sports and gravitate toward high-stress activities.
- ❏ I feel bright and energized after a steak dinner.
- ❏ I am able to digest a wide variety of foods.
- ❏ I feel de-energized after a vegetarian meal.
- ❏ I feel relaxed and healthy while leading a full life.
- ❏ I typically have lots of energy in the midst of intense emotions and high drama.
- ❏ I am able to do desk work for long hours at a time without becoming tired or losing mental clarity.
- ❏ I have an optimistic nature and am always ready to begin something new.
- ❏ I easily maintain an active social life.
- ❏ I rarely get a cold or the flu.
- ❏ I am free of allergies.

Physical indicators

- ❏ I have a stocky build and a large frame.
- ❏ I am strong and large-boned.
- ❏ I have well-developed muscles.

SELF-TEST: YOUR ACID/ALKALINE BALANCE

A pH test of your saliva or urine may be used in addition to the check-lists to help assess your relative acidity or alkalinity. You can buy pH Hydrion test paper at your local pharmacy and use it to test the acidity of your saliva or urine. This product consists of a roll of pH paper to test your body fluids and a color-graded pH chart. When the pH test paper is saturated with saliva or urine, it develops a color. The paper is then held next to the color chart to find the matching color, which indicates the pH. The spectrum of colors moves from yellow (acid) to dark blue (alkaline). Inexpensive pH meters are also available commercially and can be used to test body fluids as well as water and beverages.

While any particular spot test of the pH of your saliva or urine is not particularly helpful, measuring them periodically over a six- to twelve-month period may help you assess the effectiveness of an alkalin-izing program. To assess the pH of your saliva, a saliva sample should be taken one hour either before or after a meal. An average saliva pH can be obtained by taking a sample twice a day, at the same times, for seven days. This will give fourteen values, which are added and then divided by 14 to give an average reading. This series of tests can then be repeated in four to six weeks. The normal pH of the saliva is 6.0 to 7.5, which is needed to begin the digestion of starches in the mouth. To assess the pH of your urine, sample the first urine you void in the morning.

However, pH tests of urine and saliva need to be interpreted cau-tiously and only in concert with other medical testing and your medical history. This is because these tests do not simply reflect your internal acid/alkaline milieu but can also vary greatly in response to changes in your diet, levels of stress and exercise, and even exposure to environmen-tal toxins. For example, a highly acidic meal, a stressful situation, or vig-orous physical exertion can cause a rapid acidification of the body, which must be immediately corrected through the buffer systems described in this chapter. In contrast, the excessive use of alkalinizing agents (which are also described in this chapter) also has to be corrected through these buffer systems. These fluctuations can cause shifts in the pH of the saliva and urine. Jim's dentist routinely tests the pH of his patients' saliva to help him determine the appropriate type of filling material to use.

There is another very simple test that you can perform to get an idea of whether you tend to be overly acidic or are a high-alkaline producer. At least two hours before or after a meal, take $1/8$ to $1/4$ teaspoon of sodium bicarbonate (baking soda) dissolved in water. Overly acidic people will not feel any adverse reaction to the sodium bicarbonate—indeed, they may feel better in general. However, high-alkaline producers may not respond well. They may experience an unpleasant change in their energy level; they may begin to feel somewhat hyper or anxious. They may even suffer a mild digestive upset. However, high-alkaline producers will be able to tolerate highly acidic foods like vinegar or lemon juice without ill effect, while overly acidic people may find that eating these same foods causes canker sores, heartburn, bladder pain, or sore throats, to name but a few symptoms. People with healthy, well-balanced buffering capabilities can usually tolerate both sodium bicarbonate and vinegar or lemon juice. This is most commonly seen in healthy children, teens, and healthy adults in their twenties, thirties, and forties (as well as a much smaller part of the adult population who are in the midlife or older age groups).

C Now that you have a preliminary understanding of the importance of acid/alkaline balance to peak performance and optimal health, as well as some idea from the checklists of your own functioning in this area, you are ready to decide what to read next. To learn more about the chemistry of acid and alkaline and how the body regulates them, read the following section. To learn how diet, lifestyle, and aging affect acid/alkaline balance, read section 2, on page 43. For a detailed discussion of how acid/alkaline balance affects peak performance, read section 3, on page 55. For a detailed discussion of how acid/alkaline balance affects general health, including information on specific health issues related to acid/alkaline balance, read section 4, on page 77. (Ideally, these latter two sections should be read consecutively, as the effects of acid/alkaline balance on peak performance and health are intricately intertwined.) Finally, for information on how to restore your acid/alkaline balance, read chapter 2.

SECTION 1:
THE CHEMISTRY OF ACID AND ALKALINE

ALL SUBSTANCES IN nature can be classified according to their relative acidity or alkalinity. The origin of the word *acid* is the Latin word "acidus," which means sour or tart. These qualities characterize many of the common acidic substances that we come in contact with, such as the vinegar used in salad dressings, which contains acetic acid; soft drinks, which contain phosphoric acid and carbon dioxide; and black tea, which contains tannic acid. Citric acid is found in grapefruits, oranges, lemons, and limes; and tartaric acid comes from grapes. In contrast, alkaline substances have a bitter taste and feel slippery or smooth on the tongue. A good example is sodium bicarbonate, also known as baking soda, which is used as an antacid.

Several theories were proposed in the late 1800s and early 1900s to explain the chemistry of acid and alkaline substances. While a detailed discussion of these concepts is beyond the scope of this book, it is worth mentioning that the earliest of these theories was developed in 1884, by the Swedish scientist Savant Arrhenius. He limited his theory to water-based solutions and explained that when a substance releases positively charged hydrogen ions (H^+) into a solution, an acid is formed. The more hydrogen ions a solution contains, the more acidic it is. The hydrogen atom (the smallest atom found on Earth) is composed of a nucleus that contains a single positively charged particle called a proton. Outside of the nucleus, the hydrogen atom contains a single negatively charged particle called an electron. (Larger atoms contain more protons and electrons.) The hydrogen ion (H^+) consists of only the positively charged nucleus. In contrast, when hydroxide ions (OH^-), which are negatively charged molecules of oxygen and hydrogen bonded together, are released into water, they form an alkaline solution. Thus, an alkaline solution contains an excess of electrons.

A second theory of acidity and alkalinity, developed in 1923 by the Danish chemist J. N. Bronsted and the English chemist T. M. Lowry, expanded the concept to include not only water-based solutions but also solids and gases. In doing so, they broadened the definition of acid and alkaline substances beyond hydrogen and hydroxide ions to include many other substances. In their theory, an acid was defined more generally as a proton donor, and an alkaline substance as a proton acceptor.

HOW ACIDITY AND ALKALINITY ARE MEASURED

We have all heard the term *pH*. It literally refers to the "potential of hydrogen," which is the concentration of hydrogen ions in a given solution. The potential of hydrogen is measured on a scale from 0.00 to 14.00. A ranking above 7.00 indicates that a substance is alkaline, and below 7.00, that it is acid. Pure water has a pH close to neutral, or 7.00. The pH measurement is an extremely sensitive calibration, with an increase or decrease from one whole number to another indicating a tenfold increase or decrease in hydrogen ion concentration. Thus, seemingly small shifts in the pH value of a substance can reflect significant changes in its relative acidity or alkalinity.

How Acidity and Alkalinity Are Neutralized

When acidic and alkaline substances are combined, they neutralize each other. This means that the resulting compound will have a pH closer to the neutral pH of 7.0 than either of the original two substances. A simple example of this occurs when positively charged hydrogen ions (H^+) combine with negatively charged hydroxide ions (OH^-) to form water (H_2O), a neutral, stable compound. You can also find the end products of acid/alkaline reactions in baked goods, which rise during baking when alkaline ingredients like baking soda are combined with acidic ingredients like lemon juice or sweeteners.

How Acidity and Alkalinity Function Within the Human Body

Our bodies contain trillions of cells, fluid-filled structures that contain many alkaline substances: minerals such as calcium, magnesium, potassium, and sodium, as well as oxygen and bicarbonate. The combination of all of these substances within the cell produces a slightly alkaline intracellular pH of just above 7.00. The cells are also surrounded by fluids that contain alkaline minerals.

All of the metabolic and enzymatic reactions of the body function most efficiently in an alkaline environment. These include energy production, immunity, digestion, and the repair of the body, all of which are necessary for our survival. For example, to produce energy from the nutrients that we ingest in food, a healthy cell requires abundant oxygen, a highly alkaline element. In the presence of oxygen, a series of chemical reactions occurs within the mitochondria or energy-producing factories of the cell: Glucose and other nutrient substances are broken down and converted to adenosine triphosphate (ATP), the universal energy currency of the body. For the body to be able to extract the maximum amount of energy from the food we eat, an abundance of oxygen must be present. Energy production proceeds best, therefore, in a richly alkaline environment.

Not only are the cells of the body alkaline, but the blood that circulates throughout the body must maintain a very narrow range of slightly alkaline pH, 7.35 to 7.45. The constancy of the blood pH is fundamental to the body's ability to maintain a relatively unchanging internal environment. The blood is constantly exposed to a variety of mostly acidic substances (alkaline substances, such as baking soda and a few of the foods we eat, are much less frequently encountered by the body). Various things, from the foods we eat to the stresses in our lives, from the sports we participate in to the pollutants we are exposed to—as well as our own metabolic processes—produce chemicals within the body that are often more acidic than our own slightly alkaline pH. All of these substances are carried within the blood, which transports them to the cells for use as nutrients or carries them away from the cells as waste products. All of these substances potentially disrupt the healthy pH of the blood. As a result, the body has to have a mechanism to both neutralize and eliminate these substances in order to keep the pH of the blood constant. This is the pH-regulating system. Its importance is illustrated by the fact that a person cannot live more than a few hours if the blood's pH goes below 7.00 or above 8.00. For example, blood with a pH of 6.95, which is only slightly acidic, can lead to coma and even death.

A few compartments of the body, primarily those of the digestive tract, have a pH range that differs from that of the blood. For example, the pH of saliva is 6.0 to 7.5, which is needed to begin the digestion of starches in the mouth. Proteins are much harder to break down than carbohydrates and require an acid environment for their digestion—found in the stomach, which secretes hydrochloric acid. This brings the pH of the stomach down to a highly acidic 1.0 to 3.5.

Once the food leaves the stomach, it must be brought up to an alkaline pH so that the enzymes necessary for further digestion can be activated within the small intestine. The breakdown of nutrients into small particles as well as their absorption occurs in the small intestine. These processes also require an alkaline environment to proceed efficiently. Digestive juices containing sodium and potassium bicarbonate that are secreted by the pancreas into the small intestine have an alkaline pH varying from 8.0 to 9.0. Bile produced by the liver and secreted into the upper part of the small intestine also helps in the process of digestion by breaking down fats. Bile has a pH of 7.8, which is also slightly alkaline. Finally, the intestinal glands, which are located over virtually the entire surface of the small intestine, produce intestinal secretions that have a pH of 7.5 to 8.0.

How the Body Regulates Acid/Alkaline Balance

The pH-regulating system of the body is very complex and is made up of many parts. Within the body, the various parts of our pH-regulating system are carefully orchestrated to work well together. The system includes the alkaline minerals contained both inside and outside the cells, as well as the mineral reserves stored within our bones. We also have three buffer systems in the blood that help to keep its pH constant. In addition, the lungs help to regulate pH by breathing in alkaline oxygen and eliminating acidic waste products in the form of carbon dioxide. The role of oxygen in regulating pH will be discussed in chapters 7 and 8, which cover the subject of oxygenation and its effect on peak performance and health. Finally, the kidneys eliminate excessive amounts of either acid or alkaline substances from the body through the urine.

The pH-regulating system tends to be healthy and to work efficiently in children and young adults. There are, however, children who have weak buffer systems and tend to become overly acidic early in life as well as some youngsters who are high-alkaline producers and maintain this tendency throughout life. The healthy buffering capability of most young people is due to the robust mineral reserves stored in their bones, healthy buffer systems, and strong lung and kidney function. However, as people age and experience the mostly acidifying stresses of modern life, the pH-regulating system begins to decline in its efficiency. This decline is a part of the normal aging process and can be accelerated by such factors as strenuous athletic activity or years of acidifying stress or of eating the standard Western diet. As a result, with age, more and more individuals who formerly had good pH balance tend to become overly acidic.

Let's now look briefly at each component of the pH regulating system.

The mineral balance inside and outside the cells helps to maintain their alkaline pH

The minerals that are contained both within the cells and the fluids that surround the cells help to regulate the pH of this microenvironment. These minerals also help to maintain the fluid balance both inside and outside the cells. Minerals, such as sodium, potassium, magnesium, and calcium, are taken into our bodies through the foods we eat and the beverages we drink. Within the body, these minerals take the form of electrolytes, which are mineral salts that dissolve in water and carry an electrical charge. As these minerals move in and out of the cells, they draw fluids with them. Optimal electrolyte and fluid balance allows the cell to absorb nutrients and discharge waste products, as well as maintain its energy level.

Healthy cell membrane function plays an important role in controlling this flow of electrolytes. When the cell membrane is intact, it protects the alkaline pH within the cell. Good digestion also contributes to this process because the breakdown and absorption of food supplies all the cells and their surrounding fluids with the electrolyte minerals and other nutrients required for the buffering process.

The mineral reserves within the bones help to maintain the alkaline pH of the blood

Bones are composed of at least eighteen nutrients, many of which are minerals. These include magnesium, manganese, sodium, potassium, zinc, boron, copper, strontium, and calcium, the most publicized of the bone minerals. The bones contain as much as 85 percent of all the phosphorus, 60 percent of the magnesium reserves, and 99 percent of the calcium contained within the body. Most people assume that bone has a solid mineral structure throughout. In actuality, bone is made up of two distinctly different materials: (1) a flexible protein matrix (2) into which are deposited a variety of minerals such as calcium and phosphorus. These minerals provide the bone with tensile strength and rigidity. Thus, its unique structure allows bone to be both flexible and rigid.

Many of the minerals found within the bone are alkaline. While they give bones their strength, they also serve as a reservoir of highly important alkaline minerals, which are capable of buffering acids. Bones are constantly releasing their alkaline minerals to neutralize the acids that we are constantly producing within the body or ingesting in food. Special cells in the bone, called osteoclasts, break down bones, allowing their minerals to be released into the blood as needed for buffering. The greater the acidity of the body and the weaker the other buffer systems are, the more the bones will be called upon to donate their minerals to keep the body's pH slightly alkaline. When depletion of the bone's mineral reserves occurs over many decades, the result can be osteoporosis, a common disease of the elderly. People who have a tendency toward overacidity may so weaken the structure of their bones, through the loss of alkaline minerals such as calcium, that they begin to experience bone fractures by their sixties and seventies.

Three buffer systems maintain the slightly alkaline pH of the blood

The body also regulates pH through its acid/alkaline buffer systems. An acid/alkaline buffer is a solution that contains two or more chemical compounds with the unique ability to prevent radical changes in pH. A buffer limits how much the concentration of hydrogen ions in a solution can increase or decrease when an acid or an alkaline substance is added. For example, if a few drops of lemon juice are added to a glass of water, the pH of the water drops. However, if the water contains an alkaline compound like sodium bicarbonate, the citric acid in the lemon juice will instantly combine with it, thereby minimizing or preventing any lowering of the pH caused by the addition of the acidic lemon juice. Common buffering compounds used to treat health problems or in the preparation of food include calcium carbonate, sodium bicarbonate, and potassium citrate.

Not surprisingly, the blood contains three different buffer systems. Their complementary action enables the blood to maintain its tightly regulated, slightly alkaline pH of 7.35 to 7.45. These systems are the bicarbonate buffer system, the phosphate buffer system, and the protein buffer system. For example, a highly acidic meal, such as a cheeseburger, French fries, and a cola drink, can cause a surge of acid in the blood, which the body must neutralize. The buffer systems within the blood work very quickly, within one second, to reestablish the blood's normal pH.

The bicarbonate buffer system. Bicarbonate is the body's most important buffering substance and is present in large quantities. The bicarbonate buffer system consists of an acid and an alkaline compound, both of which can be used as buffering agents. The alkaline compound is sodium bicarbonate, while the acid compound is carbonic acid. Working together, they help to neutralize strong acid or alkaline substances that are released into the bloodstream, thereby preventing either a marked rise or fall in the pH of the blood. This system comes into play rapidly as the body is challenged by either acid or alkaline substances, providing a response that can occur within a fraction of a second.

Bicarbonate is also found within the cells of the body and helps to keep both the cells and the extracellular fluids slightly alkaline. Finally, particularly high concentrations of bicarbonate are also produced by the pancreas and secreted as part of the pancreatic digestive juices, whose concentration of bicarbonate is five times greater than that of the blood. As a result, the pancreatic digestive juices have a pH of 8.0. The secretion of these juices is stimulated by the presence of chyme (the mixture of partially digested food and stomach acids) in the small intestine. The pancreas secretes water and bicarbonate, which neutralizes the chyme. When this bicarbonate comes in contact with the hydrochloric acid in the chyme, the resulting reaction produces sodium chloride (table salt) and carbonic acid, which is much weaker than hydrochloric acid. Carbonic acid immediately breaks down into carbon dioxide and water. Carbon dioxide is eventually eliminated from the body by the lungs during exhalation.

This neutralization of the acidic gastric juice produced by the stomach is very important because otherwise the strong acids coming in contact with the surface tissues of the intestine would erode these tissues and could eventually cause ulcers. The bicarbonate excreted by the pancreas also plays another role in digestion, helping to provide the slightly alkaline pH at which pancreatic digestive enzymes are activated.

The phosphate buffer system. The phosphate buffer system acts in a similar manner to the bicarbonate buffer system, containing both acid and alkaline compounds that help to keep the pH of the blood close to neutral. This system also plays a role in helping the kidneys to regulate pH through the excretion of acidic hydrogen ions (H^+). The kidneys play an important role in maintaining the pH of the body by eliminating excessive amounts of acidic or alkaline substances through the urine. In addition, the phosphate buffer system also helps to regulate the pH of intracellular fluids, where it is found in high concentrations.

The protein buffer system. The proteins found within the bloodstream and cells are among the most abundant buffering agents found within the body. It is estimated that about 75 percent of all the chemical buffering power of the body fluids resides within the cells because the intracellular proteins act as weak acid buffers. The proteins contained within the cells also provide an important source of buffering for the extracellular fluids. This system acts more slowly since substances must move through the cell membrane in order to be buffered by the proteins contained within the cells. Thus, this system does not provide an immediate response to changes in pH but comes into play after several hours.

Within the bloodstream, hemoglobin, the protein portion of the red blood cell, transports oxygen, an alkaline element, to the tissues. Besides its responsibility as a transport protein, hemoglobin also has a buffering function since it controls the amount of oxygen released into the tissues. For example, during heavy exercise hemoglobin releases larger amounts of oxygen to the tissues. This helps to raise the pH of the tissues since heavy exertion produces acidic waste products that must be buffered; otherwise, these waste products would lower the pH to unhealthy levels.

The organs of elimination help to return pH to the normal range

The lungs and kidneys also play an important role in the regulation of pH. When acid levels rise too high, both of these organs help both to eliminate acid substances from the body and preserve alkaline substances within the body. The reverse occurs if the body becomes too alkaline.

The lungs: Respiratory regulation of acid/alkaline balance. As our organs of respiration, the lungs play a major role in maintaining the normal pH of the blood and tissues. When we breathe in, we inhale the surrounding air, which contains approximately 20 percent oxygen. Oxygen is an alkaline gas that is vital for life since it is used in all the energy-producing chemical reactions of the cells. When we exhale, we breathe out carbon dioxide, an acidic compound that is a waste product produced by all the cells of the body. The lungs help to regulate pH by bringing air and blood into contact so that the acidic carbon dioxide circulating in the blood can be expelled and the alkaline oxygen absorbed by the body. The structure of the lungs allows for maximum exchange of these gases. This exchange of oxygen for carbon dioxide occurs deep within the lungs where the alveoli, or microscopic air sacs, come into contact with tiny blood vessels called capillaries from the pulmonary arteries. Here, the blood and air are separated by only the thinnest of tissues.

When there is a change in pH, the respiratory system is capable of providing a fairly rapid response. While the buffer systems of the blood act within one second, the lungs help to correct pH imbalances within one to two minutes. When the body becomes too acidic, positively charged hydrogen ions have a direct effect on the respiratory center of the brain. This in turn causes ventilation within the lungs to increase four- to fivefold, allowing for more rapid discharge of acidic carbon dioxide, which helps to maintain the slightly alkaline pH of the blood. Conversely, when the body becomes too alkaline, ventilation decreases, and more carbon dioxide is retained within the body. This causes the pH to drop slightly and, thereby, remain in the normal range. While the lungs cannot completely correct the pH imbalances that occur within the body, they are 50 to 70 percent effective in achieving this goal.

The kidneys: A slow and powerful acid/alkaline regulator. The kidneys' response to changes in pH is the most powerful of all the regulatory systems. Their unique structure allows them to perform the final step in the buffering of excess acidity or alkalinity within the body. The two kidneys sit at the back of the abdominal cavity near the waist. Each kidney contains over 1 million microscopic structural units called nephrons. Each nephron contains tubules (the site of urine formation) and glomeruli (a network of capillaries that filters the blood circulating through the kidneys).

The many waste products of the cells filter from the glomeruli into the tubules, where the regulation of pH takes place. It is via this filtrate that hydrogen ions and organic acids can be excreted from the body through the urine in order to reduce overacidity. The kidneys also retain bicarbonate to help raise the pH. Conversely, it is also the kidneys' job to excrete excessive amounts of alkaline substances when the pH rises too high. The end result is that the kidneys respond to changes of pH within the body by excreting either an acid or alkaline urine. In the process of responding to pH imbalances, urine may have a pH as low as 4.5 or as high as 8.0.

While the kidneys provide a slow correction to pH disturbances, they continue to act until the pH of the body is restored nearly to normal. As a result, the kidneys' correction of acid/alkaline imbalances is total rather than partial and takes from several hours to as long as six days to restore balance. While the kidneys can normally handle a significant amount of acid or alkaline waste products, the production or ingestion of too much acid or alkaline substance can overburden their ability to regulate pH. Serious pH imbalances can then occur.

SUMMARY

All substances can be classified as either acid or alkaline. The human body is slightly alkaline, and has a complex system that works to maintain that balance. All parts of the system, including the mineral balance inside and outside the cells, the mineral reserves within the bones, and three buffer systems in the blood, work together, along with the lungs and the kidneys, to prevent the body from becoming overly acidic. However, some outside factors can alter this favorable balance.

SECTION 2:
HOW DIET, LIFESTYLE, AND
AGING AFFECT ACID/ALKALINE BALANCE

SUBSTANCES THAT ARE too acidic or too alkaline are constantly being produced within the body as a result of the many thousands of chemical reactions that occur on a continual basis. If our buffer systems are working efficiently, these substances are neutralized by our pH-regulating system almost as quickly as they are formed. Unfortunately, most of us begin to experience a decline in the efficient functioning of our pH-regulating system by the time we reach our forties or fifties. This process is accelerated in many individuals by overexposure to a wide variety of environmental stresses, which tend to expose our bodies to substances that either are highly acidic or create an excessive acid load within the body. With proper education and information, however, we can learn to avoid many of these environmental stresses.

For example, most of the foods in the standard American diet are either highly acidic or acid-forming. In addition, emotional stress, strenuous exercise, long airplane flights, medications, infectious diseases, and certain illnesses as well as the production of our normal metabolic waste products all contribute to acid buildup within the body. This excessive acid load will, over time, deplete the alkaline reserves of most individuals at a much younger age than what we would expect given a normal aging process. For example, constant overacidity depletes the stores of alkaline minerals contained within the bones as well as the ability of the pancreas to produce sufficient bicarbonate-rich digestive juices.

These stresses can lead to a wide range of symptoms due to chronic overacidity. One sign of acidity is feeling noticeably stiff upon arising. Another is feeling either extremely tired or energized after a day of physical exercise. You may find that having red wine with dinner gives you a runny nose or a headache the next day. At least once a month, you have a sore throat. Overacidity also dramatically increases the frequency of colds, flulike symptoms, allergies, canker sores, heartburn, alternating constipation and diarrhea, insomnia, inflammatory conditions, parasites, fungal conditions, and bone loss. You may also find yourself recovering more slowly from illnesses, cuts, minor surgery, or even normal physical exertion.

THE HIGHLY ACIDIC STANDARD AMERICAN DIET

The typical American diet is composed mainly of foods that are either highly acidic in their chemical makeup or, once eaten, cause an acidic reaction within the body. These foods include red meat, poultry, dairy products, most fruits, nuts, refined sugar, corn sweeteners, chocolate, refined flour products, soft drinks, beer, wine, coffee, and black tea. There are many reasons why these foods tend to be acidic. Many of them contain large amounts of acidic minerals such as sulfur, phosphorus, chlorine, and iodine. Some of these foods also contain acids such as the carbon dioxide used to create the carbonation in soft drinks and beer, the tannic acid found in black tea, and the acetic acid found in vinegar. Examples of acids found in fruits are the malic acid in apples and citric acid contained in oranges, lemons, limes, and grapefruits.

Some of these foods also cause an acidic reaction within the body. For example, red meat, dairy products, and wheat all contain tough and difficult-to-digest proteins such as the casein found in milk and the gluten found in wheat. When these foods are ingested, the stomach must secrete large amounts of hydrochloric acid in order to begin the breakdown of these proteins. This puts a significant stress on the pancreas, liver, and small intestine, which must then produce copious amounts of highly alkaline digestive juices and bile to neutralize the excess acid produced by the stomach. Other foods, such as coffee and alcohol, also trigger excessive acid production by the stomach.

In addition, as food is metabolized within the body, it is converted into a number of acidic waste products such as uric acid, lactic acid, and acetic acid. These acids will lower the pH of body fluids and must be neutralized by the buffer systems contained within the blood; their residues must then be eliminated from the body. Furthermore, acidic by-products derived from the sulfur, chlorine, and phosphorus in foods produce toxic acids such as sulfuric, phosphoric, and hydrochloric acid, which must also be neutralized to avoid damaging the kidneys and other organs of the body. When the liver's ability to detoxify is impaired, many toxic and highly acidic by-products are formed. These acidic by-products must also be neutralized and eliminated from the body.

Finally, many people are allergic to the proteins found in a variety of foods, including dairy products, wheat, peanuts, corn, soybeans, and the milk and nuts used in the preparation of certain chocolate products. Food allergies cause an acidic, inflammatory reaction in sensitive individuals. Some individuals are also sensitive or intolerant to various foods. Common examples are the sugars found in milk (lactose) or fruit (fructose) and the amines found in tomatoes, oranges, wine, chocolate, and Parmesan cheese. Individuals with these sensitivities either find these foods irritating to their systems or lack the enzymes to digest them, thereby leading to overacidity. Many of these same foods also tend to aggravate autoimmune conditions such as rheumatoid arthritis. The inflammation that results from these conditions causes the production of acidic chemicals within the body that must be constantly buffered if the blood is to remain at a slightly alkaline pH.

In summary, overacidity caused by the normal ingestion and breakdown of foods as well as toxic by-products caused by foods can greatly stress our buffering capability. Whether these foods are highly acidic or cause an acid reaction within the body, they must all be neutralized and any acid residues from the food eliminated from the body to keep the pH of the blood slightly alkaline.

Unfortunately, most people eat almost exclusively these highly acidic or acid-forming foods and skimp on foods that are less acidic and more alkaline such as vegetables, starches, whole-grain products (non-gluten-containing), beans and peas, seafood, eggs, and a few fruits like melons and papayas (a chart listing the exact pH of various foods can be found in chapter 2; see page 102). These foods are strikingly similar to those found in the Mediterranean diet, which medical authorities currently consider one of the most healthful diets on the planet. The Mediterranean diet has been linked to a lower incidence of such life-threatening illnesses as heart disease and cancer. It is worth noting that this diet is much less acidic than the standard American one.

The prevalence of highly acidic foods in the typical American diet is so overwhelming that our children begin to experience wear and tear on their buffering capability practically at birth. It is common to see very young children sucking on a bottle filled with highly acidic fruit juice. Three- and four-year-olds can commonly be seen drinking highly acidic cola drinks and eating hamburgers. If you look inside the lunch box of any American child or teenager, you are likely to see many different types of highly acidic processed foods like pizza, candy bars, cookies, potato chips, and sandwiches made from white bread and processed meats. What is lacking in our children's meals are enough of the highly nutritious, less acidic, more alkaline foods like fresh vegetables, legumes, starches, and fish. This dietary pattern has been confirmed in a number of research studies. One such study, published in the *Journal of the American Dietetic Association*, examined the diet during a twenty-four-hour period of nearly 1800 second- and fifth-graders in New York State. On the day they were surveyed, it was found that 40 percent did not eat vegetables except for potatoes or tomato sauce, and 36 percent ate at least four different types of snack foods. The study also found that 16 percent of the fifth-graders did not eat breakfast. Another study, reported in the same journal, found that children who did not eat breakfast had a lower intake of many essential vitamins and minerals, including alkaline minerals like calcium and magnesium. In other words, the children who skipped breakfast did not make up their nutritional deficiencies at other meals.

Adults in our society do not fare much better, given the enormous quantities of highly acidic coffee, beer, wine, fruit juice, fast foods, processed food, frozen entrées, and convenience foods that many of us eat. Many people consume highly acidic coffee and cola drinks for their caffeine content, to energize them and keep them awake. Most of us eat fast foods and convenience foods to help us manage our busy lives, and drink alcoholic beverages at night to help us relax. It is, therefore, no surprise that by midlife most of us have begun to wear out our buffering capability and are beginning to suffer the ill effects of overacidity on our performance and health. Only the peak performers who are high-alkaline producers can survive and even thrive on the standard American diet.

The 1995 statistics supplied by the Economic Research Service of the USDA confirm this imbalance in the American diet. We added up the number of pounds of highly acidic or acid-forming foods that the average American eats per year, and compared this with the average yearly intake of less acid, more alkaline foods. The ratio was an astonishing 17:3 in favor of acidic or acid-forming foods. This predominance of acid-forming foods in the American diet puts an enormous stress on the buffering capability of many Americans to neutralize all of this acid.

One reason for this imbalance in our diet is that highly acidic foods are far more available and much more highly promoted through advertising than more alkaline foods. The majority of space in the supermarket is devoted to highly acidic foods because these foods tend to have long shelf lives while many of the more alkaline foods are highly perishable. The mainstays of fast food—hamburgers, pizza, fried chicken, prepackaged wedges of apple pie, and colas—are primarily composed of highly acidic ingredients. American corporations involved in producing packaged foods that have long shelf lives or in selling fast foods are among the largest advertisers in the United States. Thus, while we are deluged with ads for highly acidic food products, we rarely see a promotional campaign for more alkaline foods like melons or papayas.

The following subsections describe the main categories of common foods and their general acid content.

Protein

The Western diet is relatively high in protein, ranging from 50 to 100 grams (g) per day (about 2 to 3½ oz.). Of this amount, the body can comfortably process only 40 to 60 g. You can see how easy it is to reach this amount when you look at the protein content of various foods. For example, an 8 oz. sirloin steak or serving of lamb or pork contains between 35 and 40 g of protein. A similar sized serving of chicken or turkey contains between 15 and 20 g of protein, while 8 oz. of fish contains an amazing 40 to 50 g. In addition, dairy products, eggs, and even vegetarian sources of protein such as beans, peas, seeds, nuts, and whole grains can greatly add to our daily protein intake.

While the body needs an adequate intake of protein each day to build and repair tissue, any excess must be broken down and then excreted. By-products of this process are sulfuric acid and phosphoric acid. Protein is eventually converted to uric acid, which is eliminated in the urine.

The amount of protein a person consumes can significantly affect acid/alkaline balance. This was demonstrated in a 1994 study, published in the *American Journal of Clinical Nutrition*. Volunteers were fed various protein-based diets consisting of either 49, 95, or 120 g of protein per day. The researchers measured hydrogen ion excretion in the urine to study the effect of protein intake on acidity. While the low-protein diet caused only a small increase in hydrogen ions in the urine, the hydrogen ion content increased thirtyfold with the high-protein diet. This increase reflected the body's need to eliminate the excessive amount of acid generated by the protein consumed to enable the pH of the blood to remain slightly alkaline.

A high intake of protein can further stress our acid/alkaline balance by accelerating the loss of alkaline minerals such as calcium from the body. There are many studies in the medical literature documenting this effect. For example, in a 1981 study published in the *Journal of Nutrition*, women were given a diet of either 46 or 123 g of protein a day for sixty days. The higher protein diet resulted in a doubling of calcium lost in the urine.

Refined flour and sugar

Another major source of dietary acid is refined flour products like white bread, pasta, crackers, cookies, donuts, and other pastries that are eaten by the great majority of us throughout the day. Many of these foods are also highly sugared, which further adds to their acid content. White flour is a simple carbohydrate. During the refining process, a significant portion of the vitamins, minerals, and fiber are lost; what remains is predominantly starch. When sugar is processed, all vitamins and minerals are removed; what remains is the simple sugar molecule, glucose. Refined flour and sugar enter the system rapidly and break down quickly, producing acids. Lactic acid is one highly acidic end product of glucose metabolism, occurring particularly during periods when oxygen levels are reduced within the body. Lactic acid must be buffered to keep the pH of the blood slightly alkaline. Furthermore, these foods do not provide the alkaline minerals necessary to buffer the acids that they generate.

Fats

For most Americans, fat composes 30 to 40 percent of their dietary intake. While the pH of fats cannot be measured because they do not go into an aqueous solution, fats are metabolized into acidic breakdown products. In addition, certain fats, such as those found in red meat and dairy products, contain arachidonic acid. Arachidonic acid is converted within the body to a variety of inflammatory substances such as leukotrienes and prostaglandins, which are powerful triggers of inflammation within various tissues. For example, leukotrienes can trigger asthmatic episodes, while prostaglandin production can worsen inflammatory-like rheumatoid arthritis and endometriosis. These inflammatory reactions cause acidic reactions within the affected tissues. Those suffering from diabetes are particularly prone to acidosis since they experience the breakdown of fats into substances called ketones that have an acidifying effect on the body.

Beverages

Many popular beverages including coffee, colas, wine, beer, and virtually all fruit juices are quite acidic. Coffee has a pH that varies from 4.9 to 5.2, beer has a pH ranging between 4.0 and 5.0, diet soft drinks are around 3.0, and colas, 2.6. Since Americans drink more soft drinks than water, these drinks contribute significantly to the high level of acidity in the American diet. The acidity is partly due to the carbon dioxide content of these beverages, which gives them their bubbles. Soft drinks also contain such acidic ingredients as sugar and flavoring and coloring agents. Fruit juices tend to be as acidic as soft drinks. For example, apple juice has a pH of 3.4, grapefruit juice has a pH of 2.9 to 3.4, and lime and lemon juice are very acidic, with a pH range of 1.8 to 2.6. On the positive side, some fruit juices like orange juice and apple juice are excellent sources of alkaline minerals like potassium. However, these fruit juices may be poorly tolerated by overly acidic individuals, who are sensitive to the low pH of these drinks. Such people may be able to enjoy these fruit juices when they are consumed in combination with foods having a higher pH that are also rich sources of alkaline minerals, such as many vegetables, grains, beans, and peas.

Flavoring agents and additives

Vinegar, a common flavoring agent in salad dressings, mustards, mayonnaise, and marinades, contains acetic acid. The acid content of commercial vinegars is clearly marked on the bottle at 5 percent, and these products have a pH ranging from 2.4 to 3.5. Acetic acid gives vinegar its tart and sour taste. The majority of processed and packaged foods usually contain added salt and sugar, which are both acidifying substances. If marketed as sugar-free, processed foods probably contain artificial sweeteners such as aspartame or saccharin, which are also acidic.

LIFESTYLE AND ACID/ALKALINE BALANCE

Many of the standard components of modern life act to increase the acid level of the body. These include stress, exercise, airplane travel, and the use of medications.

The acidifying effect of stress

When we are under physical and mental stress, we use more nutrients and generate more acidic waste products than the body can process and dispose of rapidly. Strong emotions of any kind increase acidity: Anger, fear, hostility, and even excitement generate acids within the body because they reduce oxygenation and blood flow to the tissues and increase muscle tension. People who are experiencing stress and are overly acidic may also be more prone to infections. Research conducted at Carnegie-Mellon University studied the relationship between emotions and depressed immunity. The researchers found that people who were currently involved in stressful personal relationships or experiencing problems with their job had a higher risk of developing the common cold, a condition related to overacidity.

Exercise

As a person exercises, oxygen is consumed, and lactic acid and carbon dioxide, among other waste products, are created. Studies have shown that the more vigorous the exercise, the more these acids accumulate, which results in a decrease in the pH of the muscles. This hampers energy production within muscle tissue and can significantly limit athletic endurance and performance. In extreme cases of acid buildup, the muscle, finally, can no longer function. We have all seen an athlete unable to continue sprinting or lifting a weight due to muscle failure caused by the buildup of excess acids.

Frequent airplane travel

Most people are unaware that spending hours in an airplane increases acidity within the body. This is because the stale, recirculated air in the passenger compartment of a commercial plane has a lower concentration of oxygen. At the same time, the confinement of several hundred people in a small area causes the level of carbon dioxide in the air to increase. In addition, international flights still permit cigarette smoking, which further depletes the oxygen content of the plane's cabin as well as adding many acidic chemicals to the recirculating air.

Medications

Many over-the-counter medications are acidifying, including aspirin (acetylsalicylic acid) and the sweet-tasting cough syrups that millions of Americans use to treat colds, flus, and bronchitis. Even an important nutritional supplement like vitamin C (ascorbic acid) is acidic. There have also been documented cases in the medical literature of acidic reactions to antibiotics.

Medical conditions

Some medical conditions also increase the acid level of the body. Most of these are chronic or traumatic, but it is important to know how they affect acid/alkaline balance, so that steps can be taken to correct imbalances.

Respiratory acidosis. Diseases such as emphysema and chronic bronchitis can lead, over time, to severe lung damage, which can impair one's ability to fully oxygenate the body through respiration. At the same time, the lungs are unable to efficiently eliminate carbon dioxide, which normally occurs during exhalation. This can cause a dangerous condition called respiratory acidosis in which the blood pH begins to drop. If not corrected, this condition can lead to significant impairment and death. Acute respiratory infections, like severe pneumonia, can also lead to respiratory acidosis and must be aggressively treated.

Metabolic acidosis. Many chronic health conditions can eventually lead to a condition called metabolic acidosis in which acidic waste products accumulate in the body. For example, with chronic kidney disease, the ability to eliminate waste products through the urine is impaired. Acute adrenal insufficiency is associated with severe electrolyte and fluid imbalances. Large amounts of hydrogen and potassium are lost in the urine, resulting in metabolic acidosis. Metabolic acidosis can also occur in severe liver disease since the liver is no longer able to perform its detoxifying function efficiently. This leads to the accumulation of highly acidic and toxic byproducts of metabolism. In diabetic ketoacidosis, the cells are not able to utilize glucose in the blood to produce energy. In this state of starvation, fat and protein are broken down to meet the body's energy needs. However, this breakdown can occur faster than the body is able to use these fuels, and their acidic residues build up in the blood, causing its pH to drop. This condition can also occur with severe diarrhea from any cause when alkaline minerals are lost through the digestive tract.

Burns and surgery. Burns and surgery cause physical damage to tissues, resulting in decreased blood flow and oxygenation to the affected areas. In severe cases, metabolic acidosis can develop. Acidosis may be aggravated in burn patients who have suffered from smoke inhalation, resulting in impaired lung function. The ability of surgical patients to regulate pH may be further compromised if they are prescribed diuretics, enemas, or laxatives, all of which accelerate the loss of alkaline minerals from the body.

The Ability to Regulate pH Diminishes with Age

The aging of the lungs, kidneys, and pancreas affects our ability to maintain acid/alkaline balance as we grow older. Children and young adults tend to have excellent functional capability of these vital organs. However, between the ages of thirty-five and sixty, the ability to buffer begins to decline in most people. While this is due, in part, to the normal aging process, the decline in our buffering capability is accelerated by the constant wear and tear caused by the standard American diet, stress, exposure to pollutants, and a variety of other factors.

With advancing age, our lungs' ability to take in oxygen declines significantly. The intake of oxygen with each breath declines by about 1 percent a year on average. Oxygen intake in men peaks at about age twenty-five and in women at age twenty. By age seventy, oxygen intake may be reduced by half. This is due to the loss of elasticity of the lung tissue and, even, reduced mobility of the rib cage, which can make breathing more of an effort. The result of these changes is that the body receives less alkalinizing oxygen and expels less acidifying carbon dioxide. Chronic exposure to pollutants such as formaldehyde, ammonia, and other toxic chemicals may cause lung irritation and asthma. Cigarette smoking increases the risk of serious lung diseases such as bronchitis and emphysema, which further reduce the pH-regulating function of the lungs and accelerate their aging.

The kidney's ability to regulate pH also declines with age. After the age of forty, the ability of the kidneys to filter waste from the blood diminishes by about 1 percent per year. After midlife, the ability of the pancreas to secrete bicarbonate begins to decline. There is also a drop in production of secretin, the hormone that stimulates the pancreas to release bicarbonate.

High-Alkaline Producers: The Exceptions to the Rule

Approximately 6 to 8 percent of the population tend to be high-alkaline producers. In contrast to the majority, these people often maintain excellent buffering capability well into old age. They usually have excellent lung capacity and digestive function as well as large reserves of alkaline minerals within their bones, which they can draw on for decades longer than the average person. The ability of these individuals to remain slightly alkaline allows them to outperform all of their more acidic peers. In fact, these people actually thrive on the acidic stresses of our modern world. High-alkaline producers are the only group who can withstand the effects of the highly acidic standard American diet, the environmental pollutants, and the level of physical and emotional stress that most of us are subjected to in our daily lives. They require hard endurance exercise nearly every day to create lactic acid and burn off some energy. They will also gravitate to a personal and professional lifestyle filled with excitement and even danger. These people do not usually start their day by meditating.

Most of the role models of our society, including top athletes, celebrities, business people, and politicians, tend to be high-alkaline producers. Their strong and resilient physiologies allow them to excel and outperform their peers in almost any activity or endeavor. They rarely get ill since the ability to maintain an alkaline pH within the body is necessary for immunity, structural repair, digestive function, and healthy metabolic function in general. Because they age more slowly, many of these individuals look younger than their age. In their later years, they tend to lead far more active lives than their more acidic contemporaries. Senior citizens who remain highly alkaline are able to lift weights, climb mountains, and run marathons at age eighty with a body that looks decades younger. Photographs of naturally alkaline older men and women sometimes appear in fitness and health magazines. These magazines are read by much younger individuals who see these elders as role models and hope to emulate them when they reach the same age. When these hearty individuals do seek medical help, it is usually not for problems related to overacidity.

Older individuals with alkaline constitutions are able to stay independent and engaged in life. Unlike their more acidic peers, who are unable to live without assistance, either in nursing and retirement homes or from their children, they are more likely to maintain their own homes in their seventies, eighties, and even nineties. Advertisements for cruise ships often feature pictures of these energetic oldsters, dancing aboard ship after having consumed a gigantic buffet dinner of rich foods that people with weaker buffering capabilities could not even conceive of eating. Many high-alkaline producers often continue to work to an advanced age and continue to pursue all their interests and hobbies, stay up on world events, and enjoy a wide circle of friends. These people defy the law of diminishing expectations. This is not to say that people with alkaline constitutions are immortal, but they are able to retain a tremendous edge in their performance capabilities.

SUMMARY

As we age, our ability to maintain a slightly alkaline balance in our cells and tissues diminishes. All too many factors in modern life, including the standard American diet, also affect acid/alkaline balance in the body. Our diet is high in acidic and acid-creating foods, and the fast pace of life today also increases acidity. Some people are naturally high-alkaline producers, and this characteristic helps them to maintain the peak-performance traits described in the next section.

SECTION 3:
ACID/ALKALINE BALANCE AND PEAK PERFORMANCE

THE ABILITY TO maintain acid/alkaline balance has an amazing effect on six of the eight peak-performance traits: physical vitality and stamina; mental clarity and acuity; the ability to get along with other people; optimism and vision; speedy recovery from illness, injury, and exertion; and resistance to illness. This section will explain how performing at your best is related to your body's ability to maintain a healthy, slightly alkaline state.

1 PHYSICAL VITALITY AND STAMINA

Some people have jobs that require muscular exertion. To be able to perform their work in a competent manner, they need physical energy, strength, and stamina. We see people performing these jobs on a daily basis: gas and electric repair crews, phone line repair crews, fire fighters and police officers rushing to an emergency, gardeners, farmers, construction workers, and road maintenance crews. Professional dancers and athletes must also be exceptionally physically fit to do their work. None of these people can sustain their careers over a long period of time without being able to maintain their body's slightly alkaline pH.

For example, professional dancers routinely engage in an activity that produces a great deal of acid. Rigorous daily practice and frequent performances constantly produce lactic acid within the muscles. While dancers in their twenties and thirties have the buffering capability to handle this acidic load, the capability to keep the body slightly alkaline in the face of this physical exertion diminishes with age. It is rare to see a dancer perform beyond the age of fifty, when most dancers can no longer keep up with the physical demands of their profession and have sustained too many injuries to continue. One exception to this rule was Fred Astaire, who continued to dance professionally until his mid-seventies. He retired from his dancing career, not for any physical reason, but because he felt that it was no longer appropriate for a man his age to be actively dancing and playing romantic leads. But even after that, he continued to be physically active. Biographies of Astaire describe him skateboarding well into his eighties. This level of physical exertion in individuals past the age of fifty is only possible if one maintains excellent buffering capability.

Similarly, professional and other highly trained athletes must have the strong buffering capability necessary to prevent muscle fatigue and maintain the stamina and endurance needed for endless practice sessions and frequent competitive events or regular season games and playoffs. The extraordinary level of performance of a great athlete like Michael Jordan has to be supported, in part, by world class buffer systems.

Another individual who has apparently exemplified excellent buffering capability is Katharine Hepburn. Ms. Hepburn has spent her life participating in strenuous, acid-producing physical activities, which is typical of a high-alkaline producer. In her youth, she was physically strong and robust, and she has continued to be so as she has aged. She has been an accomplished golfer and avid tennis player, and, as an adult, she has been photographed skateboarding, surfing, and swimming in the ocean, in midwinter, near her Connecticut home. Ms. Hepburn has also publicly expressed her enjoyment of foods that are highly acidic, declaring she eats chocolate pecan turtles every day. Her vigor has been apparent in many of her best movie roles, where she has played assertive, alkaline-type women who are full of energy and who automatically take charge of the circumstances that they find themselves embroiled in.

Most individuals whose jobs require them to do physical work are unable to maintain their physical prowess well into old age. This is because they lose their ability to regulate pH efficiently beginning in midlife or even younger. At this point, physical symptoms of overacidity—such as muscular fatigue, reduced endurance, stiffness, joint pain, and slower recovery from injury or exertion—begin to take their toll, causing many individuals to retire or change their careers to one that is less physically demanding.

The same phenomenon often happens to individuals who have spent years participating in vigorous physical activities such as bodybuilding, jogging, downhill skiing, handball, racquetball, and squash. Most of these sports are pursued by young, vigorous, alkaline individuals. As people begin to reach their forties and fifties, the dropout rate from these sports becomes significant, often for the same reasons that people leave physically demanding jobs. The accumulation of acids within the muscles and joints begins to cause too much physical discomfort and muscular fatigue for them to continue participating. Most people as they age switch to less physically demanding sports like golf, walking, and relaxed swimming, which are slower paced, more aerobic, and, therefore, less acid producing.

How overacidity restricts physical energy and stamina

Let's look at the mechanism of how overacidity restricts physical energy and stamina. Muscle tissue contains several specific buffer systems, including the proteins carnosine and anserine. In resting muscle tissue, these two proteins act as powerful buffering agents. At a neutral pH of 7, they contribute as much as 20 to 30 percent of the buffering action, according to a study published in 1960 in the *Archives of Biochemistry and Biophysics*. Phosphate contained within the muscle tissue is also an effective buffer. Finally, sodium bicarbonate provides only about 5 to 10 percent of the muscle's buffering capability.

When a person exercises vigorously, glycogen (a form of stored glucose or sugar in the muscles) is burned for energy. By-products of this process are lactic acid and pyruvic acid. As these acids accumulate, the pH of the muscle tissue drops, which begins to hinder muscular activity since these tissues function best, like the rest of the body, with a slightly alkaline pH.

Overacidity causes muscles to become fatigued. One reason this occurs was discussed in a research article published in 1989 in the *British Journal of Sports Medicine*. This study found that the accumulation of acids within the muscle limits production of the energy molecule ATP (adenosine triphosphate). It also inhibits the activity of muscle fibers, which impairs the mechanisms by which muscles contract. The body does this to protect the muscles from further physical activity, which would cause the muscles to become even more acidic.

Other studies have confirmed these findings. For example, a study conducted at the Institute of Work Physiology in Oslo, Norway, and published in 1972 in the *Journal of Applied Physiology* had volunteers exercise repeatedly for periods of one minute on a treadmill or stationary bicycle. The pH of their blood and muscles became significantly more acidic with this exertion. Another study, conducted at Children's Hospital of San Francisco and published in 1988 in the *Journal of Clinical Investigation*, showed that with both intermittent and sustained exercise, the more intense the activity, the faster acid accumulates.

Using alkalinizing agents to enhance physical performance

The role that buffering plays in supporting physical energy has primarily been studied in the area of sports performance. Researchers have focused on the use of alkalinizing agents as ergogenic aids, substances that increase the potential for accomplishing a given task and improving performance. In these studies, volunteers are given an alkaline substance such as sodium bicarbonate and then asked to perform an intense physical exercise for a short duration of time, such as sprinting or cycling for two or three minutes. Researchers then measure the degree to which a reduction in acidity will increase the time it takes for muscle exhaustion to occur.

The interest in alkalinizing agents to enhance sports performance goes back many decades. One early study, published in 1937 in the *German Weekly Medical Journal*, found that when runners were given an acidifying agent, they became exhausted more quickly than those who were not. In contrast, giving athletes an alkalinizing agent before endurance running or bicycling extended their performance by 30 to 100 percent and reduced their recovery time after physical exhaustion had occurred.

Three different alkalinizing agents have been researched for their beneficial effect on athletic performance: sodium bicarbonate, sodium citrate, and sodium phosphate. While not all of the studies have been positive in their results, most of them suggest that alkalinization is a very powerful tool in enhancing athletic performance.

Sodium bicarbonate. Researchers have learned that sodium bicarbonate buffers muscular acidity indirectly. A study published in the *Canadian Journal of Pharmacology* in 1980 found that sodium bicarbonate works by increasing the alkalinity of the blood, rather than entering the muscle cells and directly buffering the acid contained within the muscle tissue. The increased alkalinity of the blood creates a pH gradient between the blood and the more acidic muscle tissue. This gradient causes the acids to be drawn out of the muscle, which then allows them to be neutralized. Another study, published in 1981 in *Clinical Science*, reported that muscle biopsies done on athletes also found that pH changes in the blood with alkalinization reflected changes occurring within the muscle.

Subsequent research focused on the potential benefits that sodium bicarbonate loading could produce on extending performance time before muscles reach exhaustion. All of these studies tested athletic performance over a relatively short period of time. While some of these studies have shown that alkalinizing with sodium bicarbonate significantly improved performance, others found this effect to be limited. Studies published in the *British Journal of Sports Medicine* and *Medicine and Science in Sports and Exercise* found bicarbonate loading to be beneficial. The first study used twenty-three volunteers to participate in six trials on a cycle ergometer. Each trial consisted of ten 10-second sprints with a 50-second recovery time allowed between each sprint. A prior pilot study had established that these 10-second sprints would result in fatigue as well as a decline in "peak power." The six trials were double-blind, with the participants ingesting either sodium bicarbonate or a placebo prior to beginning each trial. The trials using sodium bicarbonate produced a higher level of exertional output than those using the placebo.

The second study examined the benefits of sodium bicarbonate loading on the racing times of six male varsity middle-distance runners at a university in Canada. These runners participated in an 800-meter race, an event in which fatigue normally results from the accumulation of lactic acid within the muscles. Sodium bicarbonate loading enabled five of the six participants to improve their running time by an average of 2.9 seconds. This represented a distance of 19 meters, which, the authors noted, in an 800-meter race could be the difference between first and last place.

A further study, published in 1984 in the *International Journal of Sports Medicine*, studied the effect that alkalinizing with sodium bicarbonate had on eleven volunteers both before, during, and after five 1-minute sprints on a stationary bicycle. While the volunteers were allowed to take a 1-minute rest between the first four bouts, the final sprint was performed until the subjects became fatigued to the point that they could not maintain their cycling rate. The use of sodium bicarbonate improved the performance time during the final bout by 42 percent in comparison to the same bout done using a placebo.

Finally, in a study published in 1988 in the journal *Ergonomics*, seven healthy males ran to exhaustion on a treadmill. Treatment with sodium bicarbonate postponed time to exhaustion by 17 percent, while the acidic compound ammonium chloride shortened the time it took volunteers to become exhausted by 19 percent.

One drawback in applying these findings to everyday exercise and sports routines is that most of the studies used very high doses of sodium bicarbonate to optimize athletic performance. Volunteers were usually given a single dose of sodium bicarbonate at the level of 300 mg/kg of body weight. In a 150-pound man, this would be nearly four teaspoons of sodium bicarbonate. Given that the normal dosage is one-quarter to one-half teaspoon repeated two to four times over a twenty-four-hour period, it is no surprise that many of these individuals suffered from intestinal upset and diarrhea.

Sodium citrate. Sodium citrate is a buffering agent that is sometimes used in place of sodium bicarbonate since it has the same buffering capacity but does not cause diarrhea, a common side effect of sodium bicarbonate. Historically, certain fruit juices, which are high in potassium citrate and alkaline salts of citric acid, have been used to raise blood pH. Studies done in the 1930s found that these drinks improved performance in events ranging from 100- to 400-meter swimming sprints to endurance cycling and running. However, results of more recent studies using sodium citrate have been mixed. One study, published in 1989 in the *European Journal of Applied Physiology*, examined the effect of sodium citrate when volunteers cycled for twenty minutes on a stationary bicycle. While there was a measurable increase in blood pH, the sodium citrate did not improve performance during this strenuous exercise.

Sodium phosphate. The mineral phosphorus helps to buffer acids that accumulate within muscle tissue during heavy exercise. Phosphorus produces its beneficial effect in several ways. It is needed for the production of an enzyme called 2,3-diphosphoglycerate (2,3-DPG), which is found in red blood cells. Red blood cells transport oxygen in the blood to the tissues, and 2,3-DPG insures that oxygen, an important alkalinizing agent, is delivered to the muscles. It reduces the affinity that hemoglobin, the carrier molecule in red blood cells, has for oxygen, so oxygen is more available to the tissues. Phosphorus promotes energy production within the cells, functioning together with the B vitamins. It also improves the production and use of glycogen, a sugar that is a ready source of energy in the muscles.

Because the standard American diet contains plentiful amounts of meat and dairy products, which contain large amounts of phosphorus, most people are far from deficient. However, athletes may need especially high amounts of this mineral, since studies have shown that muscles lose phosphorus into the bloodstream during periods of intense physical exertion. The more a person exercises, the more phosphorus is needed by the body. Endurance athletes, such as marathon runners, will have low levels of phosphorus immediately after participating in an athletic event. One study, published in 1987 in the *British Medical Journal*, found that sixteen of the thirty-eight men who collapsed during the 1981 to 1986 Great North Runs had significantly lower phosphate levels than those individuals who successfully completed those races. Another study, published in 1988 in *Muscle and Nerve*, found that weight training also causes the loss of phosphorus from muscle tissues. Loss of phosphorus can impair buffering within the muscle tissue and limit the amount of oxygen delivered to the muscle cells.

Phosphorus is given to athletes in a buffered form, sodium phosphate. The sports performance benefits of phosphate loading have been studied, with mixed results. In one study, published in 1984 in the *Journal of Laboratory and Clinical Medicine*, six volunteers received infusions of a phosphate-based drug (Didronel) plus fructose-phosphate as well as fructose-phosphate infusions alone. The researchers measured levels of 2,3-DPG and cardiopulmonary (heart-lung) function at three 5-minute intervals as the participants exercised on a stationary bicycle. They found that with either treatment, 2,3-DPG levels increased and the volunteers were able to perform a comparable workload and use the same amount of oxygen without the heart having to work as hard.

However, a later study, conducted at the Human Performance Laboratory at Old Dominion University and published in 1990 in *Medicine and Science in Sports and Exercise*, gave volunteers 1000 mg of tribasic sodium phosphate four times daily for six days. This resulted in increased blood levels of phosphate and increased oxygen uptake; however, it did not improve their performance when they competed in a five-mile run.

Alkalinizing agents and recreational sports

While buffering agents have been researched to help serious athletes gain a competitive edge in their field, no one has focused on the benefit that buffering can produce when used in much smaller doses for individuals engaged in everyday sports and athletic activities. We have found alkalinizing agents like sodium and potassium bicarbonate to be tremendously helpful in reducing fatigue, muscle stiffness, and achiness when taken either during or after a long hike, bicycling, playing tennis, or a day on the golf course (carrying your bag, not using a cart). The use of alkalinizing agents may be particularly beneficial to weekend warriors, especially those in the baby-boomer age group. They often tend to balance their intense work schedules with aggressive, acid-producing exercise. Recovery from such hard exertion can sometimes be slow, due to the production of acid within the muscles. Instead of the ergogenic use of sodium bicarbonate, which entails using a single and very substantial dose for a quick performance boost, most of us would benefit from taking more moderate doses periodically during an athletic event or on a day of strenuous physical activity.

▲▲ You may find it useful to take moderate amounts of an alkalinizing agent before, during, and after an athletic event to reduce or prevent soreness and to increase endurance and stamina. Jim takes a container full of an alkalinizing agent to sip on periodically during an event or outing. The constant intake of small amounts of alkaline liquid, such as a dilute solution of sodium and potassium bicarbonate (ranging from a 4:1 to an 8:1 ratio of sodium to potassium, depending on your tolerance for potassium), helps ward off fatigue caused by acid buildup due to the physical exertion. This will help you remain much more energized during an event than eating an acidic energy bar or consuming highly acidic soft drinks, both of which add to the acid load and can subject you to a significant energy letdown. In addition, anti-inflammatory digestive enzymes should also be taken prior to and/or following strenuous physical exertion to prevent stiffness and soreness from occurring. See chapter 4 for specific recommendations.

Stressful careers and the alkaline constitution

The necessity of maintaining an alkaline pH is important not just for sports performance but also for many other careers and endeavors that involve arduous schedules, stressful work conditions, long hours, and frequent travel demands. Examples of such careers include emergency room physicians and nurses, upper- and middle-managers of corporations, salespeople, investment bankers and brokers, and management consultants as well as touring entertainers and musicians. These professions do not necessarily demand muscular strength, but they do require a high level of physical energy and stamina. High-alkaline producers have the edge here, just as they do in sports performance. Let's look at a few exceptional examples of individuals in unusually high-profile careers for which being a high alkaline producer is a virtual necessity.

Queen Victoria had the longest reign of any monarch in English history. She exemplified the physical stamina typical of high-alkaline producers. Victoria survived tremendous political upheavals and setbacks, including being the target of seven assassination attempts. She outlived her husband by several decades, and, by the time she died in 1901 and left the throne to her son, Edward VIII, he was already fifty-nine. In addition to her obvious physical stamina and fortitude in the face of adversity, Queen Victoria also demonstrated her alkaline constitution by giving birth to nine children, a process that puts tremendous stress on the alkaline mineral reserves of the mother. Not only does a fetus grow and develop from the nourishment it derives from its mother's diet, but it also will draw down on the alkaline mineral reserves contained within the mother's bones if her dietary intake is inadequate. This is one reason why women often feel depleted after pregnancy. Only strong alkaline women like Queen Victoria can sustain nine full-term pregnancies without impairing their vitality and exhausting their reserves.

Similarly, great physical stamina is required to hold many of the highest posts in government. The president of the United States has a job that is arduous, stressful, and physically demanding at a level that few people can even comprehend. Presidents have to be high-alkaline producers to maintain the energy, resistance to disease, and ability to recover from injury needed to handle the stresses and physical demands inherent in this job. Another job that requires an alkaline constitution is secretary of state. Individuals holding this position must constantly participate in many acid-producing activities. In our era of shuttle diplomacy, they are required to travel frequently, often facing a grueling work and social schedule upon arrival at their destination. The secretary of state is required to attend formal state dinners and cocktail parties, which usually serve only rich, acid-producing foods and beverages. Their high-stress work involves daily meetings with various heads of state and other decision makers, each dealing with difficult international issues and tense diplomatic situations. Without superb buffering capability, the people in these positions could not function effectively.

Like U.S. presidents, CEOs are the lords of their own fiefdoms, the American corporation. Their job may be almost as stressful and demanding as that of our political president. This is particularly true for entrepreneurs who have grown their companies from scratch. High-alkaline producers make the best entrepreneurs, since this job requires staying power, stamina, and most importantly, physical endurance. With no guaranteed paycheck, entrepreneurs must be able to withstand the risks and frustrations that occur when one is trying to build an enterprise. There is perhaps no better example of such a personality type than Richard Branson, founder of a business empire that includes Virgin Atlantic Records and Virgin Airways. Having achieved enormous success in the business world, he still chooses pastimes full of acid-generating risk and excitement, such as skiing across ravines and attempting to circumnavigate the globe in a balloon.

At the local level, alkaline individuals can be found heading up community boards and spearheading fund-raising campaigns. We know women in these positions who have the energy to run a major corporation, often juggling their civic duties with a full-time career, managing a home and even raising a family at the same time. Our research assistant recounted a story about a friend of hers whose mother had had a stroke in her seventies. The grandmother, at age ninety-eight, stepped in to nurse her daughter. This is a feat that only an alkaline and unusually hearty oldster could do.

While few individuals have the alkaline constitution necessary to be president of the United States, secretary of state, or the CEO of their company, most of us would like to have, and in fact need, more physical energy and stamina to perform at an optimal level in our careers and in other areas of our lives. Unfortunately, as overacidity becomes a sad fact of life, usually between our thirties and sixties, fatigue, lack of stamina, and even physical exhaustion can occur. Overacidity can result from long hours of immobility spent working at one's desk or in front of a computer, overly acidic meals eaten hastily on the job, job-related stresses, and frequent travel. Luckily, we can once again enjoy a high level of physical energy as we improve our buffering capability and restore the body to its slightly alkaline pH.

▲▲ The millions of overly acidic people in our society can improve their performance on the job and in their personal lives by restoring their buffering capability. This can be done through the use of a less acidic, more alkaline diet, alkaline minerals, and alkalinizing agents such as sodium and potassium bicarbonate (particularly helpful for prolonged periods of desk work and travel). Reducing one's level of stress and exposure to pollutants will also help to restore the body to a more healthful, slightly alkaline state. Techniques to accomplish this are covered in the following chapter.

2 MENTAL CLARITY AND ACUITY

Individuals whose work requires intense mental activity and concentration will generate a great deal of acid in the process. Doing intellectual work for many hours at a time can greatly overburden the body's ability to buffer acids. This occurs, in part, because the brain consumes oxygen at a much faster rate when doing strenuous mental work, so reserves of this alkalinizing substance are diminished. There is also a tendency during mental activities to take shallow breaths, so that less oxygen is inhaled and more acidic carbon dioxide is retained. People often become so involved in mental work that they will sit in a cramped position for hours without getting up to stretch or move around. This can result in the accumulation of acidic waste products in the tissues. After intense periods of mental work, most of us become tired as acidic wastes accumulate within the body. We may have to stop working for a short period of time until our pH balance has been restored and our mental energy returns.

High-alkaline producers, however, are able to do mental work for long periods of time without becoming fatigued. A good example of an individual with this trait is Margaret Thatcher, the former prime minister of Great Britain. While in office, she routinely needed little sleep, and she used her extra waking hours to study papers and reports in preparation for meetings. Even though her first appointment often took place as early as 6:00 A.M., she would be fully prepared to discuss the topics at hand with her advisors. Amazingly, she scheduled these meetings at fifteen-minute intervals. Such mental clarity is only possible in a person with an alkaline constitution.

▲▲ If your job requires long periods of sitting at a desk or computer, it is important to take frequent, short, alkalinizing breaks away from your desk. Get up every fifteen or thirty minutes to stretch or walk around your office or up and down stairs. Breathe deeply and slowly to begin to reexpand your lungs and reoxygenate your body. Frequent breaks combined with physical activity will held reestablish your alkaline pH and allow you to maintain your mental sharpness. During particularly strenuous periods of mental exertion, make sure you are taking alkaline mineral supplements on a daily basis as well as one to five grams of buffered vitamin C and one-quarter to one-half teaspoon of sodium and potassium bicarbonate (ranging from a 4:1 to an 8:1 ratio of sodium to potassium, depending on your tolerance for potassium) two to four times a day. Vitamin C (ascorbic acid) loses its natural acidity when buffered with alkaline minerals.

Preventing work-induced overacidity can help prevent job burnout. While Susan's natural tendency is to be overly acidic, her care in restoring her own alkaline reserves has allowed her to function as well as a naturally alkaline peak performer. Over the past seven years, she has written eight books, each requiring intense mental work sustained over a period of months. This was certainly the case while writing this book. While she normally follows her own advice by taking frequent alkalinizing breaks, she occasionally gets so wrapped up in her projects that she will work fourteen- to sixteen-hour days, often as late as 2:00 or 3:00 A.M. Such intense periods of work can cause her to go well beyond her normal pH tolerances and become overly acidic. When mental fatigue sets in, she knows she has reached this point. When she realizes that this has happened, she will stop working and will begin alkalinizing her system by drinking a dosage of bicarbonate in water every hour or two. Invariably, within a half-hour or so, her mental energy will be restored.

4 THE ABILITY TO GET ALONG WITH OTHER PEOPLE

Many alkaline types channel their prodigious energy into socially beneficial activities. They are the leaders of their communities, businesses, and church groups. They are the organizers and doers. These individuals occupy the seats on the town councils and are the tireless fund-raisers who support every charitable cause that comes along. These people are intensely social, always at meetings, parties, and events.

In contrast, overly acidic individuals tend to lack the energy for intense social interactions and may even be withdrawn and introverted. The effect of pH on mental health is well demonstrated in the work of William H. Philpott, MD, an environmental psychiatrist who spent many years researching the links between food allergies, overacidity, and mood. In treating mental illness over a twenty-five-year period, he frequently observed that these conditions were often not emotional in origin but rather were due to chemical imbalances. Dr. Philpott prescribed a combination of enzyme therapy and alkalinizing agents for patients who had severe psychological reactions to certain foods that they ate, and observed that their mental problems rapidly disappeared. Dr. Philpott described the case of a man who had suffered from autism as a child and schizophrenia in his teenage years. He discovered that this young man was severely overacidic. By restoring the patient to a normal alkaline pH through a variety of alkalinizing therapies, Dr. Philpott was able to get someone who had been fully dependent on his parents' care to drive a car and attend a university, where he studied art. The young man was eventually able to move out of his parents' house, live independently, and sell his artwork.

◀6 OPTIMISM AND VISION

There are many people who work in careers that require great optimism and vision. An example would be successful salespeople, who are able to envision the opportunity that they are offering a potential customer strongly enough for that person to see it, too—and then buy the product or service. To be successful, a salesperson must be able to sustain a positive outlook. In cold-call marketing, the difference between a salesperson who can't close deals and one who does is that the successful salesperson has the emotional stamina to keep making phone calls. Only an alkaline individual has the energy and tenacity required to maintain their optimism and enthusiasm in the face of frequent rejection.

Charitable fund-raisers also tend to be alkaline since they, too, need to maintain their enthusiasm and optimism in order to raise money for deserving causes. They must remain optimistic, with a can-do attitude, so that they can inspire people about the worthiness of the projects for which they are soliciting funds.

Artists, authors, and playwrights also have to maintain a positive frame of mind in order to gather their creative energies and produce works of art, often in the face of criticism and poor reviews if not outright rejection. Even if the statement an artist makes is full of doom and gloom, the very act of creating it requires an outgoing energy and the ability to stay focused on a goal. Overacidity can undermine creative work and silence the muses.

One physiological reason for the link between alkalinity and optimism is that overacidity acts as a depressant to the central nervous system, whereas alkalinity acts as a natural mood elevator. When acids accumulate in tissues throughout the body, they can directly affect the mental energy underlying our ability to create and maintain a positive outlook as much as our sex and stress hormones can affect mood.

◀7 SPEEDY RECOVERY FROM ILLNESS, INJURY, AND EXERTION

◀8 RESISTANCE TO ILLNESS

Peak performance and optimum health are intricately intertwined, for the ability to resist common illnesses and the ability to recover quickly from illness, injury, exertion, allergy symptoms, and minor surgery are fundamental to feeling and performing at your best at all times.

Respiratory illnesses

The most common health-related success saboteurs in our society today are minor respiratory illnesses. When the body is overly acidic, a person is more susceptible to such ailments as colds, flus, bronchitis, sinusitis, and even pneumonia. The bacteria and viruses that cause these infections thrive in low-oxygen, acidic environments. Overacidity, due to a highly acidic diet, emotional stress, or poor oxygenation, makes a person more susceptible to respiratory infections. The symptoms of respiratory illnesses—sneezing, sore throats, runny noses, and coughing—worsen as an individual becomes increasingly more acidic. In the more serious cases of respiratory infection, such as severe pneumonia, affected individuals can even develop respiratory acidosis, a potentially life-threatening condition in which the pH of the blood drops to dangerously low levels, and the lungs are no longer able to ventilate properly and make the necessary pH corrections by eliminating carbon dioxide from the body.

The statistics on the prevalence of respiratory ailments reflect how common overacidity is in the United States. The National Health Interview Survey estimated that in 1994 there were 66 million cases of the common cold that resulted in either medical treatment or at least one day of restricted activity. This figure represents approximately 25 percent of the U.S. population. Given that most people do not go to a doctor when they develop a cold, the number of reported cases is all the more impressive. In the same year, 90 million people, or 45 percent of the population, were treated for the flu or had at least one day of downtime. In addition, there were nearly 35 million cases of chronic sinusitis, 26 million cases of hay fever and allergy, 14 million cases of chronic bronchitis, and 14.5 million cases of asthma. Millions of children and adults suffer from middle-ear infections, which are triggered, in part, by overacidity due to allergy or sensitivity to dairy products. The prevalence of respiratory infections triggered by overacidity translates into an enormous drain on both individual and corporate resources as well as huge outlays of money spent on treating these conditions.

To counteract these ailments, Americans spend billions of dollars on over-the-counter remedies. Unfortunately, these products are relatively ineffective and have unpleasant side effects. They only provide symptom relief and do not help to restore the slightly alkaline pH of the body that is needed to recover rapidly from these conditions. Ironically, the medications themselves often increase acidity, retriggering the symptoms. No matter what medications respiratory illness sufferers use, recovery can be prolonged if the underlying overacidity of the system is not corrected.

Minor respiratory illnesses are success saboteurs because most people are often incapacitated by these episodes of colds, flus, bronchitis, and sinus infections. These conditions can persist for as long as one to six weeks, and many Americans, both adults and children, suffer from as many as four to six episodes each year. In fact, nasal conditions are one of the leading causes of lost productivity at school and work. All of these conditions drastically reduce people's energy, create sleep disturbances, and impair concentration. They also greatly hamper socializing and make travel unpleasant. Their symptoms often occur at inopportune times and hinder consistent performance, causing sufferers to make uncharacteristic mistakes on the job, or even preventing them from showing up for work or social engagements. In addition, individuals with minor illnesses often feel miserable and tend to isolate themselves from coworkers, friends, and family members.

▲▲ Traditional home remedies for colds and flus include drinking a glass of orange juice or ginger ale to settle the stomach, or eating a bowl of Jell-O. While these might seem like comfort foods, they are highly acidic and will actually prolong recovery time. Instead, you should drink herbal teas (ginger tea is particularly good for the treatment of colds and flus) or vegetable or chicken broths. For the first twelve to twenty-four hours after the onset of symptoms, fasting on these liquids and avoiding solid food will help to bring the pH back into balance more rapidly. Remember, all food is eventually converted within the body to the acidic products of metabolism.

▲▲ To rapidly suppress a respiratory infection, begin an alkalinization program immediately at the first sign of symptoms. Use one-quarter to one-half teaspoon of sodium and potassium bicarbonate, taken in from a 4:1 to an 8:1 ratio, depending on your tolerance for potassium. Sodium bicarbonate may also be used alone if the mixture causes intestinal discomfort. Take the alkalinizing agent every one to two hours in the acute phase and then decrease to three to four times per day until the condition has been resolved for at least two days. Do not stop alkalinizing prematurely since the overacid condition may not have been completely neutralized and symptoms may recur. You should also take vitamin C buffered with alkaline minerals.

A Caution on Taking Bicarbonate of Soda

Very occasionally, a person will use too much bicarbonate and become overly alkaline. If this occurs, you may experience any of several symptoms, including a tingling sensation in the extremities, feeling overenergized, being unable to sleep, and, rarely, muscle spasms. If you should experience any of these symptoms, immediately discontinue use of the bicarbonate. Acidifying the system with a teaspoon or two of cider vinegar or the juice of half a lemon in water will help to neutralize the excess alkalinity. You can try instituting treatment again the following day, but at a lower dosage and at less frequent intervals. If symptoms are severe, you may want to consult with your physician as to the advisability of using bicarbonate therapy at all for your particular case.

▲▲ Individuals who are prone to frequent respiratory infections should also consider using the remedies discussed in the chapters on digestive enzymes (chapter 4), liver detoxification (chapter 6), oxygenation (chapter 8), and stress hormones (chapter 10). These therapies can also be very useful in building up your resistance and making your susceptibility to these infections a thing of the past.

High-alkaline producers and respiratory illnesses

In contrast to the rest of us, individuals who are high-alkaline producers tend to be more resistant to respiratory illnesses. If they do come down with a cold or flu, overacidity is usually not the trigger. Often, other factors such as liver toxicity or diminished production of anti-inflammatory digestive enzymes or stress hormones may increase their susceptibility.

If these naturally alkaline individuals do come down with a cold or flu, they tend to recover quickly. They will leave work for a half day or a day, take a nap, eat lightly, and bounce right back. Interestingly, people with superfunctioning systems have no idea why they are this way. A good example of these disease-resistant types are physicians. Most family-practice doctors and pediatricians are exposed to respiratory infections from their patients on a regular basis. However, physicians tend to have hearty, alkaline constitutions—a prerequisite if a young doctor is to survive the rigors of the medical training process.

Occasionally, Susan sees patients who have many of the signs of good buffering capability yet are poor oxygenators. This seemingly contradictory situation can occur in high-alkaline producers who have suffered lung damage, either due to environmental exposure or a prior lung infection. These individuals may maintain their naturally alkaline constitutions, yet they may still be prone to respiratory illnesses.

If you are a high-alkaline producer and develop a respiratory condition, then the old-fashioned remedy of orange juice and Jell-O *is* just what you need. Do not use alkalinizing agents since they will tend to overalkalinize you and will probably worsen your symptoms. Your condition is probably due to a chemical imbalance other than pH. In your case, the anti-inflammatory therapies, oxygen therapies, and detoxification therapies described later in this book would probably be most helpful in aborting a respiratory infection.

Two success stories

Each of us has a story of how rapid treatment of respiratory infections with alkalinizing agents saved the day for us. The use of alkalinizing agents allowed us to resume our normal schedules very rapidly, despite the onset of severe respiratory symptoms. These infections would normally have caused us to be ill and functioning inefficiently for as long as two to three weeks.

Jim's story. Since learning how to restore my acid/alkaline balance in my forties, I have been able to prevent the onset of or easily contain the symptoms of colds, flus, sinusitis, and bronchitis. As I mentioned in the introduction, these problems had plagued me since my early-childhood days. I am now able to eliminate these success saboteurs the way all naturally alkaline peak performers do. However, since I am not one of those individuals, I must always be ready to counter any tendency toward overacidity that can occur if I overstress my body beyond its normal pH tolerances. If you are like me and tend toward overacidity, the following story will show you the importance of always having a fully stocked alkalinizing kit available when traveling.

Several years ago, I scheduled a multicity cross-country trip, in mid-summer, to close a business deal that I had been working on for many months. Halfway into the scheduled ten-day trip, I realized it would have to be extended for at least another week. This meant more hotel living, airplane flights, and entertaining the potential business partners with rich foods and, often, too many cocktails and wine with dinner. The last city on the itinerary was New Orleans. Due to a shortage of rooms, I was given a room reserved for smokers (I have never smoked) that had been treated with toxic chemicals in an attempt to remove the smell of cigarette smoke. On top of that, the air conditioner's thermostat was set very low to combat the New Orleans summer heat and could not be adjusted by the hotel engineer.

The unhealthy conditions at the hotel plus the stress of travel, too much work, and all the rich food and drink sent me into a violently overacidic state. As I got on the plane to return to San Francisco, I knew I was coming down with something. Due to the length of the trip, I had used up my alkalinizing travel kit and sat on the six-hour flight without any emergency supplies. During the flight, I developed a sore throat, and my nose began to run. When I arrived home, I felt weak and was sneezing, coughing, and shaking with the chills, even though it was July. I immediately began an accelerated alkalinizing program, rested, and dramatically reduced my food intake. Within a few days, I was well on the road to recovery.

Susan's Story. Several years ago, I pushed myself beyond my limits when I accepted numerous teaching engagements all over the state of California and was also completing several professional projects. I worked almost two months without a break, with relatively little sleep each night. Toward the end of the second month, Jim and I were driving to a weekend seminar where I was the featured lecturer. En route to the seminar, we stopped at a deli where I ate an extremely acidic meal consisting of salads and vegetables that seemed to be marinated in pure vinegar. The acidity of the meal coupled with my high level of work-related stress finally threw me into a state of extreme overacidity. As soon as we left the deli, I began to have a runny nose and couldn't stop sneezing. This occurred six hours before I was due to give my first lecture. Fortunately, I had brought my buffering agents and supplements with me, as I usually do in case of an emergency. I started taking sodium and potassium bicarbonate every half hour for the first several hours, and then continued this regimen every hour. I also began to take digestive enzymes and buffered vitamin C to reduce the inflammation. After five hours of alkalinizing myself, I had restored my pH balance. My sneezing stopped, and the congestion cleared up almost entirely. I was able to meet my responsibilities and teach for the entire weekend, but I continued to use these alkalinizing agents to avoid a relapse. Given how tired and stressed I was, there is no question that without these lifesavers I would have begun a downward spiral and spent a number of days in bed. By restoring my pH balance, however, I was able to get through a very busy weekend and continue with my normal schedule on Monday.

Business travel and lavish vacations create the perfect conditions for becoming overly acidic. Unless you are a high-alkaline producer, you should always take an emergency alkalinizing kit to ward off colds and flus when traveling for business or pleasure. The kit should contain an alkalinizing agent, buffered vitamin C, alkaline minerals, herbs such as ginger or curcumin with aspirin-like properties, and anti-inflammatory digestive enzymes. See chapters 2 and 4 for more information on these remedies.

Allergies and sensitivities

Millions of Americans suffer from runny noses, sneezing, itching and tearing of the eyes, wheezing, abdominal pain, bloating, diarrhea, skin rash, and a propensity to middle-ear infections due to environmental or food allergies as well as food sensitivities. A wide variety of substances can trigger an allergic reaction, including pollens, molds, trees, and animal hairs as well as foods such as dairy products, wheat, corn, peanuts, and soy. Many individuals have sensitivities to foods such as wine, chocolate, tomatoes, oranges, and mushrooms as well as milk and fruit sugars either because of chemicals, such as amines, found in these foods or because they lack the enzymes needed to digest these foods.

The allergic response is triggered by mast cells. These are large cells found in connective tissue, particularly in the linings of the nose and lungs, as well as in the skin, the gastrointestinal tract, and reproductive organs. When an allergen is present, the mast cells release histamines and other chemicals that initiate the allergic response. This is actually the body's attempt to heal from the effects of the allergen. Histamines cause fluid to enter tissues of the affected areas, causing redness, swelling, and constriction of the smooth muscles.

The specific symptoms of an allergic reaction depend on where histamines are released. In the intestines, the result can be diarrhea. In the chest, histamines can cause coughing and asthmalike symptoms (asthma is an extreme allergic reaction in which there is partial obstruction of the air passage to the lung as the muscles in these ducts contract). However, the severity of these symptoms depends on the degree of acidity of the internal environment. When the body is overly acidic, and mast cells are activated by an allergen, they will tend to break down more quickly and are more likely to generate histamines and other inflammatory chemicals. Chronic inflammation can, in turn, damage cells and tissues, causing them to become even more acidic, thereby sending the body into a destructive downward spiral.

Overacidity can both trigger the symptoms of and lengthen the period of convalescence in allergic individuals. Unfortunately, the underlying cause is often overacidity, which is rarely treated. Obviously, environmental and food allergens and sensitizing agents should be avoided as much as possible. However, when a person is exposed to these substances, they should begin an aggressive alkalinizing program (along with taking the anti-inflammatory enzymes described in chapters 3 and 4). Allergic or sensitivity reactions can often be contained very quickly. Many people are unaware of the role that overacidity plays in their reactivity to allergens. Consider the following three cases:

1. Steven is a thirty-nine-year-old man who has suffered from allergies since childhood. With testing, he was found to be allergic to a wide variety of environmental allergens, including pollens, trees, and cat and dog hair. He was also sensitive to acid-forming foods

such as dairy products and wheat, which his doctor had told him to avoid but which he ate anyway. His stressful job as a stockbroker also worsened his tendency toward overacidity.

2. Louise is a forty-eight-year-old woman who has suffered from recurrent episodes of bronchitis two or three times a year. These episodes were so disabling that she routinely missed a week to ten days of work each time she became ill. She was particularly prone to these episodes in the spring rainy season, when mold invaded her home. Allergy testing confirmed a mold allergy.

3. Laura is a fifteen-year-old high school sophomore with severe allergies to wheat, dairy products, and the milk and nuts contained within chocolate. Unfortunately, she had intense cravings for these foods, which she periodically binged on despite her mother's admonitions. These bingeing episodes were always followed by fatigue, sneezing, sore throats, and earaches, which caused her to be absent from school.

Avoiding the offending substances and following alkalinizing programs helped all of these individuals stop the downward cycle of allergic reactions that was undermining their health and well-being. Instituting a less acidic, more alkaline diet and using buffering agents and other supplements to reduce inflammation and build up their immunity has greatly improved their resistance to many allergens.

Traumatic injury and surgery

The use of alkalinizing agents can be helpful in healing any type of acute injury, whether traumatic or surgical. Any bodily injury will cause the injured tissue to become overly acidic. Individuals who are overly acidic and sustain a significant injury cause an added stress on their buffering capability. Injured tissue becomes relatively acidic because the swelling, hemorrhage, and other physical changes that occur within an injured area will impair oxygenation to these tissues. Diminished blood flow and the accumulation of waste products within the area also increase acidity. At the same time, there is an increase in metabolic activity and protein synthesis as the body's healing processes are activated. The effect of injury on metabolism was discussed in a study published in 1988 in the journal

Muscle and Nerve. Volunteers who performed arm and leg exercises designed to cause mild muscle injury had elevated levels of inorganic phosphate in their muscle tissue for three to ten days. Since the processes of repair function best in an alkaline environment, supplementing with alkalinizing agents promotes healing within the injured area.

▲▲ If you are overly acidic and tend to recover slowly from injuries, begin an alkalinizing program immediately following an acute injury. This should be done whether the injury is incurred taking part in strenuous physical activity or is due to trauma or surgery. Because injuries are always accompanied by inflammation, see chapter 4 for information on the anti-inflammatory benefits of digestive enzymes. Be sure to ask your physician about the advisability of following such a program if you have any specific questions.

SUMMARY

A healthy alkaline balance enhances six of the eight peak-performance traits, which shows how very important this function is in achieving success in all our endeavors. Two of the most significant traits are speedy recovery from illness, injury, and exertion and resistance to illness, a clear indication of the close relationship between peak performance and general health.

SECTION 4:
ACID/ALKALINE IMBALANCE AND HEALTH

PHYSICIANS NORMALLY DEAL with acid/alkaline-related problems in hospitalized patients who have fluid and electrolyte imbalances. These imbalances are usually the result of the underlying disease process itself or occur as an undesirable side effect of medical therapy. As a result, much of the work done on acid/alkaline imbalances usually occurs on a crisis management basis. Many of these patients may have even lost their ability to buffer acid/alkaline imbalances adequately on their own.

However, the regulation of pH can be an important factor in the treatment of many diseases. This has been confirmed by hundreds of research studies. Once a decline in the efficiency of our pH-regulating system begins to occur, usually between our thirties and our sixties, many health problems begin to become more prevalent, in part because of overacidity. This is certainly the case with such common success saboteurs as the common cold, flus, sinusitis, bronchitis, middle-ear infections, allergies, and traumatic injuries. Other common health issues such as digestive overacidity, bladder infections, kidney stones, rheumatoid arthritis, hypertension, and even cancer are also linked to overacidity. All of these conditions can be improved by restoring the body to its normal, slightly alkaline state.

Just as restoring alkalinity supports many peak-performance traits, it can also go a long way toward improving resistance to and preventing recurrences of many other common health conditions. These health conditions, in their turn, tend to compromise people's ability to perform at high levels in all aspects of their lives. Disease and chronic illness very understandably lead to absenteeism, reduced energy levels, and inability to perform job and personal responsibilities. Medical conditions of all kinds have a direct impact on peak performance, illustrating the interconnectedness of peak performance and overall health.

How Overacidity Affects Health

Many degenerative diseases are the result of the body becoming overly acidic. As mentioned earlier in this chapter, the cell, the basic unit of life, is alkaline. A healthy cell contains large amounts of alkaline substances like oxygen, bicarbonate, and alkaline minerals. All of our metabolic processes and the enzymes that initiate chemical reactions function their best in a slightly alkaline environment. However, the wear and tear of daily life and the aging process itself gradually cause our cells to lose their healthy alkalinity and become more acid over time, thereby making us more prone to disease. This can occur as a result of poor dietary habits, nutritional deficiencies, exposure to chemical pollutants, and emotional stress.

As mineral imbalances, a decrease in the level of oxygenation, and damage to our cells accumulate, the cells become too acidic. Depending on which tissues of the body become damaged and overly acidic, a variety of medical conditions can begin to develop. It is important to mention that the overacidity that occurs in many medical conditions is initially more of a localized phenomenon rather than a systemic problem, since the pH of the blood remains stable except in conditions of severe and even life-threatening illnesses. However, as health continues to decline with age, acidosis becomes more prevalent throughout the body. Thus acid-related conditions like digestive problems, allergies, gout, chronic fatigue, joint pains, and interstitial cystitis can coexist within the same individual. We describe some of these health conditions in this section.

Digestive problems

Gastric overacidity is considered one of the most common digestive problems in the Western world. Pharmacies and supermarkets have shelves full of products designed to reduce the overacidity that occurs after a person has eaten something they cannot digest. Overacidity can stem from various causes. The stomach may secrete too much hydrochloric acid, even when there is no food in the stomach to be digested. At the same time, the pancreas may not be producing enough alkaline digestive juices to adequately buffer the acidic contents of the stomach as they move into the small intestines. When the pancreas produces insufficient amounts of bicarbonate, the enzymes necessary for digestion within the small intestines are unable to be activated. Overacidity can also result from injury to the mucosa of the small intestine, leading to damage and acidosis of the underlying tissues. Crohn's disease, an inflammatory condition of the small intestine, or colitis due to acid stools can result from this overacidity. Susan sees this problem frequently in midlife patients who suddenly find that they begin to have heartburn or digestive distress after eating highly acidic foods like pizza, steak, and orange juice.

However, heartburn may sometimes mask a more serious underlying condition. In a 1999 study done at the University of Oklahoma Medical Center, researchers assessed 178 patients with a long-term history of heartburn. Many of these patients reported using antacids for more than ten years. The study confirmed that almost all of them were sensitive to acid. However, over half also suffered from underlying conditions such as hiatus hernia (a condition in which stomach acid refluxes or backs up into the esophagus), and 40 percent suffered from an inflammatory condition called erosive esophagitis. Of greatest concern was that 7 percent were found to have serious underlying medical conditions like peptic ulcer disease, esophageal spasm, and cancer.

Sometimes people with symptoms of heartburn and gastric distress are actually underproducing hydrochloric acid in the stomach. Physicians practicing complementary medicine may find that patients who have weak pancreatic function (producing insufficient digestive enzymes and alkaline digestive juices) also produce insufficient amounts of stomach acid. These people tend to have poor digestive function at all levels of the digestive tract. They may suffer from food allergies as well as food intolerances. These individuals could actually benefit from hydrochloric acid supplementation to assist in the digestion of protein. Unfortunately, however, because of their poor buffering capability, they may be unable to tolerate the supplemental hydrochloric acid. In such individuals, hydrochloric acid capsules or drops may actually cause stomach burning and discomfort. Some physicians find the use of Swedish bitters, artichoke bitters, and ginger tea to be effective substitutes for hydrochloric acid supplementation for patients who are both low acid producers in the stomach and low alkaline producers from the pancreas. (These individuals may also have reduced secretion of bile—which is also an alkalinizing substance needed to emulsify fats.) In addition, the amino acid glycine may also enhance gastric acid secretion (take 500 mg per day apart from meals).

▲▲ Individuals with chronic, long-term symptoms of heartburn should have their symptoms evaluated by a physician to rule out a more serious condition.

Doctors usually recommend countering digestive overacidity with antacids or drugs that decrease the production of hydrochloric acid. Popular brands of antacids include Maalox, Mylanta, and Tums. These antacids tend to contain various types of alkaline mineral substances such as magnesium oxide or hydroxide, aluminum hydroxide, magnesium trisilicate, and calcium carbonate.

Alka-Seltzer is another short-term remedy for indigestion used by millions of people. This product is simply sodium bicarbonate combined with citric acid. When water is added to this mixture, an effervescent gas is released, turning the Alka-Seltzer powder into a bubbling drink.

Both calcium citrate and sodium citrate are also useful as buffering agents for counteracting digestive overacidity. A study published in 1978 in the *South African Medical Journal* found that in thirty healthy volunteers, a sodium citrate preparation raised the pH level of the stomach significantly. The researchers measured gastric acid output after a single 12 g dose and found that the stomach pH rose to 3.0. (The stomach normally has a pH of 1.5 to 2.5.) Similar results were achieved after three to six days of continuous therapy, using 4 g and 12 g dosages. In addition, calcium citrate has been shown to be an effective antacid for patients with kidney disease who can no longer regulate their pH effectively.

The alternative to the above remedies is to take a medication that suppresses acid production completely. Many foods and caffeine stimulate receptors within the stomach to secrete stomach acid, and a class of drugs has been developed to block this action. Many are sold without prescription, such as Zantac, Pepcid, Axid, and Tagamet. All these treatments are meant to reduce the annoying symptoms of overacidity such as gas, bloating, nausea, constipation, and diarrhea.

Although taking antacids can be very effective in relieving digestive symptoms, the timing of their use is very important. If antacids are taken with meals, or right after eating, they can interfere with the digestion of food. Antacids neutralize the hydrochloric acid produced by the stomach, which in turn inactivates the enzymes that are essential for the breakdown of protein. This makes it difficult for the body to effectively digest foods such as meat, milk, wheat, and nuts and beans (all of which contain hard-to-digest protein), and to efficiently extract the minerals that these foods contain.

A Caution on Using Antacids

In rare cases, the use of antacids can also lead to systemic alkalosis, raising pH throughout the body. Symptoms of alkalosis include tingling in the lips or extremities, tense muscles, anxiety, or an unusually strong surge of energy after taking an alkalinizing agent. If you experience these symptoms, stop taking the antacid, and restart at a much smaller dose taken at greater intervals. If symptoms are severe, you may want to consult with your physician as to the advisability of using antacids. The next chapter provides more specific information on how to best use these various products to counteract overacidity.

▲▲ It is helpful to wait one to one and one-half hours after a heavy protein meal before taking the antacid. Some people, however, produce such large amounts of acid that they begin to feel discomfort immediately upon eating. These people may need to use antacids with the meal.

Cystitis or bladder infections

Several research studies confirm the usefulness of alkalinizing therapies for cystitis, an inflammatory condition of the bladder caused by bacterial infection. Cystitis is a very common ailment, with millions of cases being treated by physicians each year. Women tend to be infected more readily than men, due to their short urethra, which allows for easier bacterial contamination of the bladder. While cystitis can occur in women of all ages, it is particularly prevalent in postmenopausal women, due to age-related changes in which the walls of the urethra thin out and become drier. It is estimated that 10 to 15 percent of women over age sixty have frequent bladder infections.

Bacteria can thrive and multiply in the warm, wet urine within the bladder. As the bacteria attack the lining of the bladder, superficial erosion of the lining can occur, which exposes this sensitive tissue to the irritating effects of urine. Individuals with cystitis frequently experience a burning sensation or a feeling of pressure in the bladder area, as well as the need to urinate frequently.

Antibiotics are prescribed as the usual treatment for this condition. However, with the increasing resistance of the bacteria causing these infections to a number of antibiotics, alternative therapies may be quite helpful in eradicating infection and reducing symptoms. Drinking cranberry juice, which acts as an acidifying agent, has traditionally been recommended as a home treatment under the rationale that chemicals contained in cranberries prevent the bacteria within the bladder from adhering to its lining. However, the form of cranberry juice readily available in the supermarket is loaded with sugar because the pure juice is so tart. By adding sugar to the bladder, the juice may actually promote the growth of bacteria. In addition, the pure juice is so acidic that it is best used only by high-alkaline producers.

In contrast, both the clinical experience of some physicians and several research studies support the use of two alkalinizing agents, sodium citrate and potassium citrate, for the treatment of bladder infections. The use of alkalinizing agents may actually be more useful for overly acidic individuals who tend to have bladder infections. Because potassium citrate tends to be unpalatable, the much blander sodium citrate preparations are preferable. In a 1984 study published in the *Journal of International Medical Research*, 205 women between the ages of eighteen and sixty with typical symptoms of cystitis, but only 20 percent of whom showed large amounts of bacteria in the urine, were treated with sodium citrate. (This is not unusual since clinical symptoms and urine culture results do not always correlate well.) Each volunteer was asked to take 4 g of sodium citrate in a glass of water three times a day for forty-eight hours (4 g is equal to $^1/_7$ oz.). At the conclusion of the treatment period, 80 percent of the women without bacteria in their urine reported significant relief of symptoms; about 50 percent of the women whose initial urine cultures showed evidence of a bacterial infection also experienced symptom relief as well as a clearing of the urine.

In a further study, sixty-four women were also given sodium citrate every eight hours for two days. Eighty percent of these women noted relief of their symptoms, while 12 percent found that their symptoms became worse. These results were similar to the earlier study in that women with symptoms but no evidence of bacteria in the urine had more uniform results than those women with proven bacterial infections. A 1993 study published in the *European Journal of Microbiology and Infectious Disease* found that alkalinizing the urine improved the ability of the body to destroy and eliminate the bacteria.

▲▲ The following simple steps will help both to eradicate bladder infections and to prevent their recurrence: (1) Take 5 to 10 g of buffered vitamin C each day (that's 5000 to 10,000 mg), divided into four dosages; and (2) avoid acidic foods such as coffee, soft drinks, sugar, and alcoholic beverages.

Interstitial cystitis

Interstitial cystitis is another type of bladder disease; it is frequently mistaken for bacterial cystitis. This condition occurs when there is inflammation between the bladder lining and the bladder muscles. This is a chronic condition that can be far more painful and debilitating than ordinary bacterial cystitis. While the great majority of patients are women, men sometimes develop this ailment.

Interstitial cystitis occurs when the lining of the bladder becomes chronically irritated. The frequent use of antibiotics, hormones, exposure to viruses, and a history of prior bladder infections can damage the bladder lining and increase the risk of developing this condition. In a healthy bladder, the tissues lining it secrete a mucuslike substance that forms a protective barrier. This barrier consists of sugar, an amino acid, and sulfur, and is called the GAG layer. The GAG layer protects the underlying tissue from being colonized by bacteria. It also helps to maintain the integrity of the bladder lining, which is constantly exposed to acidic urine, food, pollutants, and chemicals. If the protective GAG layer is damaged or destroyed, the cells of the bladder can become damaged. As a result, the cells begin to lose their normal state of healthy alkalinity as they lose bicarbonate. At the same time, they gain hydrogen ions (protons), causing them to become more acidic.

In the early stages of the disease, when urine begins to erode through the tissues of the bladder lining, individuals affected will experience a feeling of urgency to urinate. With further erosion of the GAG layer, these symptoms begin to worsen as the bladder becomes scarred and ulcerated. There may be a nearly constant sensation of pressure and burning in the bladder, pain during intercourse, and fatigue, as well as such diverse symptoms as sore throat, headache, diarrhea, bowel problems, joint pains, and asthmalike symptoms. The bladder may also shrink to hold only one or two ounces of urine. The consumption of acidic foods can immediately trigger symptoms. Patients with interstitial cystitis frequently complain of pain and burning after ingesting foods with an acidic pH or foods that are highly acid-forming or inflammatory, like citrus fruits and juices, chocolate, spicy foods, coffee, black tea, soft drinks, and alcoholic beverages. Acidic vitamin C (ascorbic acid) also increases symptoms. Painful symptoms can occur almost immediately after ingesting the offending food or substance. Symptoms can also be triggered by emotional stress.

To test for interstitial cystitis, a urine sample is normally analyzed for the presence of bacteria. The urine should show no sign of bacterial infection and often has an alkaline pH. As mentioned above, when bladder cells are damaged, they become more acidic. They leak their contents into the urine, losing their alkaline minerals while, at the same time, gaining acidic hydrogen ions from the surrounding environment. Thus the cells become more acidic while the urine pH begins to rise. The overacidity of the cells makes it more difficult for the bladder tissue to repair itself.

▲▲ Several alkalinizing agents can be very useful in treating interstitial cystitis. Sodium bicarbonate can provide almost instantaneous relief of symptoms by helping the bladder tissue become more alkaline. Calcium carbonate or sodium citrate can be taken several times per day to slowly release bicarbonate into the bladder tissues (sodium citrate has been found to partially convert to carbonate within the bladder). Anti-inflammatory agents such as digestive enzymes and MSM (methylsulfonylmethane) are also helpful in treating interstitial cystitis. These remedies are discussed in chapter 4.

Kidney stones

Kidney stones are very common in our society, affecting about 10 percent of the population. They occur more frequently in men than women. The recurrence rate is high, with 20 to 50 percent of the individuals affected forming new stones. Kidney stones are also an expensive problem to treat, with $2 billion spent annually on medical therapy.

5 to 10 percent of them are uric-acid stones. Individuals with gout or who have an elevated uric-acid level in the blood are at higher risk of forming these stones. Alkalinizing the urine helps to make the uric acid more soluble so that stones are less likely to form. Alkalinizing agents such as sodium and potassium citrate are also used in the treatment of kidney stones, both to dissolve the stones and to prevent their recurrence. One study, published in 1985 in *Drug Intelligence and Clinical Pharmacology*, reported that fifty-three patients with uric-acid stones who were treated with potassium citrate had a reduction in the number of stones formed and less likelihood of recurrence. During the period of treatment, which lasted from one to one and one-half years, between 75 and 92 percent of the patients went into remission.

Individuals who tend to form uric-acid kidney stones should limit their intake of foods such as meat that contain purines, which convert to uric acid as they are metabolized. Instead they should follow a more vegetarian-based, less acid, more alkaline diet. Vitamin C should be taken in a buffered form rather than as ascorbic acid. Aspirin, another acidic compound, should be avoided. Drinking plenty of water on a daily basis is also recommended to help maintain a dilute urine.

Magnesium has also been added to preparations of potassium citrate. This combination has been found to be very effective in reducing the recurrence of stones. Researchers at a Kaiser Permanente Medical Care Program in Oakland, California, gave this compound to sixty-four patients who had a tendency to form kidney stones on a recurrent basis, over a three-year period. According to their study, published in 1997 in the *Journal of Urology*, the researchers found that while untreated patients had a 69 percent recurrence rate, only 13 percent of those receiving the magnesium and potassium citrate subsequently developed kidney stones. Another benefit to adding magnesium to this regimen was that it reduced the unpalatability of the potassium citrate.

Rheumatoid arthritis and other autoimmune diseases

Rheumatoid arthritis is a disabling and crippling inflammatory disease of the joints. It chiefly affects the synovial membrane (a thick tissue covering the joints) of the small joints of the body. Symptoms include joint stiffness, especially in the morning, tenderness, warmth, and pain, most often in the joints of the fingers, wrists, toes, ankles, and knees. Other symptoms include fever, fatigue, loss of appetite and weight, and depression. As the disease progresses, the joints thin out and become deformed. Cartilage, bone, ligaments, and tendons in and around the joints are weakened or destroyed, which can lead to muscle atrophy and imbalances of opposing groups of muscles.

While rheumatoid arthritis can occur anytime in life, 70 percent of the cases are diagnosed between the ages of thirty and seventy with the peak incidence in the fourth decade. It is estimated that approximately 10 percent of all people sixty-five years of age and older suffer from this condition. Women with this disease outnumber men by a ratio of almost 3:1.

Many research studies have implicated diet as a major risk factor in the development of rheumatoid arthritis. All of the foods that have been found to worsen the symptoms of this disease are either highly acidic or produce an acid response within the body. When volunteers with this disease were taken off these foods and either fasted for a period of time or were placed on more alkaline vegetarian diets, they experienced a notable improvement in their symptoms. One such study, published in 1980 in

Clinical Allergy, placed twenty-two patients on an elimination diet in which highly acidic and allergenic foods were excluded from their daily intake. Twenty out of the twenty-two patients noted an improvement in their symptoms.

In another study, published in 1996 in the *Scandinavian Journal of Rheumatology*, twenty-seven patients with rheumatoid arthritis were taken off their customary highly acidic diet, fasted for seven to ten days, and were then placed sequentially on a wheat-free vegan diet for three and one-half months followed by a lacto-vegetarian diet for nine months. Twenty-six rheumatoid sufferers in a control group continued to eat their normal, highly acidic, meat-based diet. Twelve of the twenty-seven patients on the more alkaline vegetarian diet noted an improvement in their symptoms, whereas only two people in the control group noted similar relief during the study period.

Although vegetarian diets have been found to promote symptom relief in individuals with rheumatoid arthritis, including fish in the diet also appears to be beneficial. This is because the polyunsaturated fatty acids contained in fish like salmon, tuna, trout, and halibut are converted within the body to very potent, hormonelike, anti-inflammatory chemicals called series III prostaglandins. Several studies, including a 1986 study published in *Clinical Allergy*, a 1985 study published in *Lancet*, and a 1988 study published in the *Annals of the Rheumatic Diseases*, found that fish-based diets reduced morning stiffness and the number of tender joints that volunteers complained of as well as laboratory indicators of inflammation. In contrast, volunteers who ate diets high in saturated fats had no improvement in their symptoms. A 1994 study published in the *American Journal of Clinical Nutrition* suggested that flax seed oil, another series III prostaglandin precursor, could be substituted for fish oil as a potent anti-inflammatory substance. Thus, fish and flax seed oil decrease the production of highly acidic inflammatory chemicals within the body, which can greatly benefit arthritis sufferers. Susan has found one to two tablespoons of flax seed oil to be highly effective in treating her arthritis patients.

Rheumatoid arthritis is a significant problem for people who work with their hands, such as computer programmers, physical therapists, people involved in assembly work, illustrators, and artists. Because these individuals are involved in precision work, this disease can significantly affect their ability to earn a living. Susan has treated many such patients over the years. In most cases, her patients ate a very acidic diet and were unaware of the effect that their food choices were having on their disease. Many of these individuals improved significantly after modifying their eating habits, using alkalinizing agents, and following a number of other therapies described in this book. The following case exemplifies the usefulness of an alkalinizing program.

Dorothy is a fifty-one-year-old executive secretary whose work requires that she spend many hours a day doing word processing on a computer. When she first consulted Susan, she was suffering from severe pain and stiffness in her fingers. Upon examination, Susan found that Dorothy's joints were already moderately deformed and swollen. After taking a dietary history, she found that Dorothy's favorite foods, such as red meat, wheat pasta, dairy products, and sugary desserts, were highly acidic or acid forming. Dorothy was initially unhappy at the idea of giving up so many of her preferred foods but was highly motivated to do anything that would reduce her symptoms. As a self-supporting single woman, she did not relish the idea of quitting an excellent job that she truly enjoyed. She made a number of dietary changes over a three-month period, eliminating the highly acidic foods from her diet and finding more alkaline substitutions that satisfied her tastes. She also started an alkalinizing program as well as a strong program of nutritional supplements designed to help support and rebuild her joints. She made steady progress during this period and was pleased to report significant decreases in her joint stiffness and discomfort.

Besides rheumatoid arthritis, many other autoimmune diseases—such as thyroiditis, Crohn's disease, colitis, and systemic lupus erythematosus—are worsened by highly acidic diets. A less acidic, more alkaline diet should be used by individuals suffering from any of these conditions.

▲▲ Besides taking alkalinizing agents and eating a more alkaline diet, you may find that anti-inflammatory supplements such as digestive enzymes, curcumin, and MSM (methylsulfonylmethane) can be very useful in the treatment of arthritis and other inflammatory conditions. See chapters 3 and 4 for more information on these remedies.

Gout. While not as prevalent as rheumatoid arthritis, gout is another disabling joint disease. Gout occurs when there is an excess of uric acid in the blood, causing crystals of uric acid to be deposited in the tissues surrounding the joints. Gout can affect many different joints, including the big toe. (Prints done in the eighteenth century often portray gout suffers sitting in large, overstuffed chairs, with their red and throbbing foot propped on a hassock.) Acute attacks of gout are particularly painful, causing severe, viselike pain that can last for two to ten days. Attacks will often occur early in the morning upon awakening if a person has eaten a dinner of highly acidic foods, such as meat and alcohol, the night before. Symptoms of gout may also occur after surgery and as a side effect of taking certain medications. As men age, they are more likely to have gout than women, but after menopause, the risk for females increases also.

Gout is linked to high levels of purines produced by the body and consumed in the diet. Purines are found in foods such as red meat, whole grains, and legumes. The body converts purines to uric acid, which circulates in the blood. The uric acid is then excreted in the urine or via the digestive tract. Individuals with gout should avoid highly acidic foods and instead eat a more alkaline, vegetarian-based diet.

Since individuals with gout are more likely to form uric-acid stones than the rest of the population, the use of alkalinizing agents may also be helpful in individuals who have both conditions.

Osteoporosis. Osteoporosis is one of the most common diseases of old age. It occurs when the bones lose their alkaline mineral reserves and become thin, porous, and progressively weaker. Osteoporosis is most prevalent among postmenopausal women, affecting nearly one-third of all women. The incidence of fractures of the hip, wrist, and spine due to osteoporosis increases significantly by the sixth and seventh decades. About 10 to 15 percent of all men also develop osteoporosis.

While doctors normally treat osteoporosis with hormone replacement therapy, vitamin D, and calcium supplements, they often do not address the underlying overacidity that causes the demineralization of the bone. The bones contain one of our major reserves of alkaline minerals such as calcium. Ninety-nine percent of the calcium in our bodies is in the bones. If the body becomes overly acidic, and the other buffer systems are inadequate, calcium and other alkaline minerals are released from the bones to keep the pH of the blood stable.

Any successful treatment of osteoporosis should address the acidity of the diet. One of the major sources of acid in the diet is meat. Not only is meat high in acid, but its tough fibrous protein causes the stomach to secrete large amounts of hydrochloric acid, which is necessary to begin the breakdown of this protein into its constituent amino acids. Processed foods also contain many phosphate food additives. Coffee is another highly acidic substance that is widely consumed in our culture. According to a 1994 study published in the *American Journal of Clinical Nutrition*, women with calcium intake lower than 750 mg a day who drink more than two or three cups of coffee on a daily basis showed an increased loss of bone mass.

Another study, published in 1984 in the *American Journal of Clinical Nutrition*, found that an increase in protein intake from 44 g to 102 g resulted in a significant increase in the urinary excretion of calcium and a lowering of the pH of the urine. Treatment with a small amount of sodium bicarbonate reversed this effect by alkalinizing the urine and reducing calcium excretion.

Researchers also compared the effect of a meat-based diet to that of a lacto-vegetarian diet on bone mass in elderly white women. Interestingly, they found that a diet high in animal protein led to more loss of bone mass than a vegetarian diet, even if both diets provided ample protein. Their study, which was published in 1980 in the *Journal of the American Dietetic Association*, found that women who followed a lacto-vegetarian diet had an 18 percent decrease in their bone mass, while the women who included meat in their diet lost 35 percent of their bone mass, nearly double that of the other group.

While a less acid, more alkaline diet slows the loss of bone mass in postmenopausal women, adding a buffering agent to the treatment program can significantly reduce bone demineralization. An interesting study documenting the benefits of potassium bicarbonate was published in 1994 in the *New England Journal of Medicine*. Eighteen healthy postmenopausal women were given potassium bicarbonate coupled with a diet that provided 80 g of protein per day, an amount typically found in the standard American diet. Potassium bicarbonate therapy reduced the excretion of both acid and calcium in the urine. It also promoted new bone growth and caused a decrease in bone loss. A separate study, using sodium bicarbonate, found that alkalinization reduced calcium loss and improved calcium balance within the body.

Diabetes. In insulin-dependent diabetes, the pancreas no longer produces sufficient insulin. (Insulin is the hormone that allows sugar or glucose to be transported across the cell membrane so that it can be used by the cell as its major source of energy.) As a result, glucose levels rise in the blood after ingesting a meal. Elevated blood sugar levels can have an acidifying effect on the blood and the tissues throughout the body, since sugar is acidic.

Many treatments to reduce the stress on the pancreas include using insulin as a replacement therapy and taking nutritional supplements such as chromium, manganese, zinc, B vitamins, and digestive enzymes to facilitate glucose metabolism. In insulin-dependent diabetes, pancreatic production of alkalinizing bicarbonate may also be impaired. In such cases, eating a less acidic, more alkaline diet that emphasizes vegetables, fruits such as papayas and melons, and certain grains and legumes is also highly recommended.

Hypertension. Hypertension, or high blood pressure, is a condition in which the blood pressure is elevated above 140/90 mm Hg. In this condition, the muscular layer of the blood vessels constricts. There may also be an accumulation of plaque on the walls of the blood vessels. As a result, the passageway through which the blood must flow narrows. The heart must then pump harder to circulate blood to the tissues. Approximately 60 percent of Americans over the age of sixty have high blood pressure. Blacks, people who are overweight, diabetics, or individuals who have a family history of high blood pressure are more likely to develop this condition. Hypertension increases the risk of heart attacks and strokes as well as kidney and eye problems.

Various medications have proven effective in the treatment of high blood pressure. However, all medications have negative side effects such as loss of essential minerals, impotence, or elevation of the blood sugar level. Many people are able to manage mild to moderate high blood pressure simply through lifestyle changes. These include weight loss, following a low-fat and low-salt diet, and stress reduction techniques such as biofeedback. Alkalinizing the body can also reduce high blood pressure. For many years, the standard treatment was the use of potassium chloride. However, recent studies suggest that the acidic chloride component of this compound may actually raise blood pressure. In a 1997 animal study, Dr. Curtis Morris and his colleagues at the University of California, San Francisco, compared the effect of different salts on blood pressure. They tested table salt (sodium chloride), potassium chloride, and two nonchloride, alkaline forms of salts found in plants, potassium bicarbonate and potassium citrate. The researchers found that potassium bicarbonate and potassium citrate actually lowered blood pressure and reduced the incidence of stroke. Their work also suggested that the chloride in table salt or combined with other minerals as a salt may trigger high blood pressure.

Cancer. Many factors are known to increase the risk of cancer in susceptible individuals. These include genetic factors, familial predisposition, dietary factors, and exposure to toxic chemicals. Some studies have also suggested that an acidic cellular environment seems to be a predisposing factor for the development of certain cancers. This connection was first discussed in a landmark paper by Otto Warburg, MD, who received two Nobel prizes for his work. His paper, entitled "On the Origin of Cancer Cells," was published in 1952 in the journal *Science*. Dr. Warburg was the first to propose that a deficiency of oxygen (a highly alkaline element) within the cells caused changes in the cellular metabolism leading to the development of cancer.

Dr. Warburg found that normal, healthy cells depend on an adequate supply of oxygen along with glucose (sugar) for the production of their energy needs. When deprived of oxygen, cells revert to a more primitive, fermentative metabolism, which is typical of cancer cells as well as disease-causing bacteria and fungi. The end product of fermentation is lactic acid, a substance that causes cells to have a lower pH. The amount of energy that can be produced by fermentation is eighteen times less than the amount that can be optimally produced by cells that are well oxygenated. The lack of oxygen thereby limits the amount of energy available to the cell to carry out its normal metabolic functions.

Although Dr. Warburg's original work has been modified by subsequent research, many studies have found that certain types of cancers can be treated effectively with oxygen therapies, because of their alkalinizing and tumor-destroying effects, as well as a less acidic, more alkaline diet. Oxygen therapies are discussed in detail in chapters 7 and 8. Many other factors thought to promote cancer also produce overacidity within the body. These include free radicals, food allergies, aberrant electromagnetic energy, industrial chemicals, and other environmental toxins. However, highly alkaline individuals who develop cancer should not be treated with alkalinizing agents since they can create severe imbalances in these individuals. Other types of cancer treatments, such as enzyme and detoxification therapies and many other treatment options, would be more appropriate and more beneficial, depending on the type of tumor.

High-Alkaline Producers and Health

While individuals who are high-alkaline producers represent only a small fraction of the population, their strong constitutions provide them with remarkable resistance to disease. They often have great reservoirs of alkaline minerals contained within their cells, tissues, and bones that give them ample buffering capability well into old age. Even in their eighties and nineties, they do not tend to develop many of the common diseases related to overacidity, such as osteoporosis, kidney, or lung failure—provided, of course, that their other physiological functions remain strong.

High-alkaline producers need to constantly create acid within their bodies to stay in balance, through a highly acidic diet, physical exertion, and a fast-paced, busy life. While naturally alkaline individuals thrive on the types of diets, activities, and stresses that are toxic to almost everyone else, the converse is also true: They need to avoid the types of lifestyle choices that are most beneficial to their more acidic peers. For example, their dietary needs run counter to the current recommendation of a less acidic, more alkaline, vegetarian-based regimen espoused by Dean Ornish, MD, the Pritikin Institute, and even the American Cancer Society. When these people do try to follow the trends and adopt a low-fat, low-protein, and high-complex carbohydrate diet with a more vegetarian emphasis, they feel weak, devitalized, and mentally foggy. Eating this way will cause them to lose their natural robust energy and stamina, and their performance in many areas will begin to suffer. Some of Susan's patients who are high-alkaline producers have felt terrible when they have tried to eliminate meat from their diet. Naturally alkaline people instinctively gravitate to a highly acidic diet of red meat, soft drinks, sugar, white-flour products, beer, wine, caffeinated beverages, and fruit juices in order to maintain their pH within the normal range.

A patient that Susan saw some years ago exemplifies this issue. Joseph was a forty-seven-year-old businessman who was raised in an eastern European family that continued to eat their traditional diet, which was high in meat protein and saturated fat, long after they resettled in the United States. Joseph continued to eat this way throughout his entire adult life. A physically strong and highly energetic individual, he was concerned about his elevated cholesterol level because of a strong family history of heart disease. After reading several books on cardiovascular health, he tried to become a vegetarian. After a week of eating mostly grains, beans, raw salads, and steamed vegetables, he no longer felt like himself and complained of feeling tired and listless. He quickly went back to his old dietary habits.

While alkaline individuals are not prone to diseases related to overacidity, they may have a higher risk of heart attacks, strokes, and cancer of the prostate and colon than their peers who follow a more vegetarian-based diet. Since the digestive function of most high-alkaline producers is so strong, they typically eat a diet high in animal protein and saturated fat. This may result in elevated blood lipids and the buildup of plaque within the arteries, thereby increasing their risk of cardiovascular disease. This is a common scenario among hard-driving, typically alkaline CEOs, who run their companies with enormous energy and staying power right up to the time that they have their first heart attack, in their fifties or sixties.

Although many of these individuals need the acidity of meat to remain healthy, they would do better to eliminate red meat and dairy products and eat fish instead. For while fish provides needed protein, it also provides healthy polyunsaturated oils, which lower cholesterol, prevent clotting, and promote cardiovascular health. However, we should clarify that although these individuals can handle the acidity of the standard American diet, this diet in no way provides the essential nutrients that all individuals, whether naturally alkaline or overly acidic, need to maintain their health and well-being. High-alkaline producers are better served by following a diet that is both highly acidic and nutrient rich. This type of diet includes seafood, poultry, vegetables, fruits, legumes, whole grains, and condiments like vinegar—basically, a more highly acidic version of the Mediterranean diet. However, while naturally alkaline people can eat more of the meat, fruit, and vinegar-doused antipasti, vegetables, and salads, overly acidic people should emphasize more of the vegetables, whole grains, and legumes of this regimen. In addition, these individuals should significantly decrease their intake of highly acidic foods and beverages that have a deleterious effect on health. This category includes alcohol, coffee, tea, soft drinks, and rich, sugary desserts.

On Susan's recommendation, Joseph began to substitute fish and range-fed poultry for the fatty red meat that was his chief source of protein. He also began to supplement his diet with various types of fiber to help promote the elimination of cholesterol from his body. Within six months, his cholesterol level had dropped significantly.

The fatty foods that alkaline types tend to eat can also lead to weight gain. This is particularly true if these individuals are older and have begun to lose their oxygenating ability. As oxygen intake begins to decline, people burn calories less efficiently. Since fat has more than twice the number of calories of protein and starch, eating a high-fat diet can easily lead to weight gain. It is very common in our country to see a stockily built, middle-aged man with a noticeable belly. To counteract this tendency, alkaline individuals need to reduce their fat intake by eating leaner cuts of meat, more salads and steamed vegetables, and the healthier fats and oils, such as extra-virgin olive oil, rather than butter.

Naturally alkaline peak performers also have a need for constant excitement, activity, hard physical exertion, and even stress, which runs counter to the current advice promoting the health benefits of stress management and a relaxed and moderate lifestyle. Remember, these people are continually producing large amounts of alkaline buffers, so they need to generate acid through their lifestyles to stay within a normal pH range.

Finally, these individuals should avoid antacids such as baking soda (sodium bicarbonate) and Tums. Although these remedies help tens of millions of Americans counter the ill effects of gastric overacidity, canker sores, and other minor ailments related to overacidity, Susan has seen them produce toxic effects in her naturally alkaline patients. These people tend to become bloated, gassy, fatigued, and even panicky when using these remedies since they tend to push these individuals' pH even further toward the alkaline side (of course, overly acidic individuals should avoid the overuse of antacids also).

Finally, severe diarrhea can cause the body to lose a significant amount of acid minerals in a short period of time, thereby causing overalkalinity in anyone, of either acid or alkaline constitution. This type of diarrhea is often associated with eating contaminated foods either while camping, eating at a restaurant or social gathering, or visiting a foreign country. To resolve this condition and restore a normal pH balance, drink a sugar and salt solution, which will replace the lost electrolytes, including the acid minerals. These solutions are readily available in pharmacies and health food stores. If you do a lot of camping, you may wish to keep some electrolyte solutions at your base camp.

LABORATORY TESTS TO ASSESS ACID/ALKALINE BALANCE

In addition to the self-administered pH tests described on page 32, there are several laboratory tests your doctor can order that will provide an indirect indication of your own acid/alkaline balance. These include hair mineral analyses and bone density studies.

Hair mineral analysis

Traditionally, hair mineral analysis has been used primarily to assess exposure to toxic minerals such as mercury, lead, and arsenic. For example, the technique was employed in 1961 to analyze a sample of Napoleon's hair, which was found to contain at least 100 times the usual level of arsenic considered normal, suggesting that arsenic poisoning led to his death. Today, hair analysis is a diagnostic method used by many complementary physicians. A small sample of the newest hair growth is taken from the first inch to inch and one-half of hair starting at the scalp. This sample is then sent to a commercial lab to assess its mineral content. While mineral levels in the blood may not be representative of the amount stored in the tissues, the hair is extremely sensitive to changes in mineral reserves in the body. Another advantage to analyzing hair rather than blood is that while the blood only contains very small amounts of minerals, making measurement more difficult, the hair contains ten to fifty times higher amounts of minerals than either blood or urine. As hair grows, minerals become part of the evolving hair protein. Several dozen trace minerals have been found in hair, including aluminum, arsenic, bromine, calcium, chlorine, cobalt, copper, iron, manganese, nickel, phosphorus, lead, sulfur, uranium, and zinc.

Bone density tests

Bone density scans test for osteoporosis. How porous the bones are directly reflects the decline in the reservoir of alkalinizing minerals contained within the bone to buffer excessive acids. The technology involved is similar to conventional X-rays but far more sophisticated and capable of detecting very small changes in bone density.

There are two different types of scans, single photon absorptiometry and dual-photon absorptiometry (DPA), plus an upgraded version of DPA, dual X-ray absorptiometry (DEXA). Each technique assesses different bones within the body. Single-photon absorptiometry is used to measure the density of the wrist and heel, whereas DPA and DEXA are used to assess the density of the spine and hip.

Monitoring bone density is especially important for woman as they age, as the risk of osteoporosis increases dramatically after menopause. Older men are also at greater risk of developing this condition than younger men. However, men lose bone mass much more slowly than women due to the protective benefits of testosterone.

SUMMARY

Overacidity affects health in a wide variety of ways, from digestive problems, infectious diseases, and arthritis to such diseases as high blood pressure, osteoporosis, and cancer. Fortunately, each condition can be treated to some extent by correcting the acid/alkaline balance of the body through a combination of dietary changes and the use of alkalinizing agents.

2

RESTORING YOUR ACID/ALKALINE BALANCE

THIS CHAPTER CONTAINS a very effective and powerful four-part plan that will enable you to restore your body to its healthy, slightly alkaline state. As you begin to reduce the acid load of your body and restore your mineral reserves and buffer systems and reduce the stress on your organs of elimination, you will begin to see astonishing results in your level of performance in many crucial areas. You will also begin to experience a significant improvement in your health. Your level of physical energy, mental clarity, emotional well-being, and even optimism and creativity will be enhanced as your body regains its healthful alkalinity. The frequency of respiratory illnesses like colds, flus, and sinusitis should begin to drop dramatically. Aches and pains, heartburn, allergies, and many other chronic ailments should also begin to diminish in intensity and, finally, disappear.

The four parts of this program are as follows:*

1. Following the alkaline power diet.

2. Restoring the alkaline mineral reserves of your cells, tissues, and bones.

---

* Several components of this program include recommendations for nutritional supplementation. Anyone beginning a nutritional supplement program should begin at one-quarter to one-half the recommended dosages given in this book. They can then increase their dosages slowly over the course of several weeks until they have reached either the full recommended dosage or a dosage that is therapeutic for them—whichever level comes first. Some individuals will experience therapeutic benefits at doses that are well below the doses recommended in this book. Also, while the dosages provided in this chapter are appropriate for most people, there are certain groups who should continue to use less than the recommended dosages. Children, the elderly, and individuals with a frail constitution or who are extremely sensitive to drugs and nutritional supplements usually do best at therapeutic dosages of no more than half the recommended levels. Consult your physician or nutritional consultant if you have any questions about the advisability of using a particular nutritional supplement or to determine the dosage most appropriate for you.

3. Using alkalinizing agents for quick symptom relief.

4. Initiating healthy lifestyle changes to reduce the stress on your buffer systems and organs of elimination.

If you follow this program carefully, symptoms of overacidity should begin to diminish quickly. Even long-standing health conditions, including chronic problems that have been present for decades, will begin to improve. If you maintain this program over time, you will rebuild your mineral reserves and restore your buffering capability. This is particularly important once you reach midlife, since most of us become progressively more acidic as part of the normal aging process. Restoring your body to its healthy, slightly alkaline pH will help you to maintain vitality and good health well into old age.

At the end of the chapter, we also provide a number of very important peak-performance tips for individuals who are high-alkaline producers. Unlike most of the population, these individuals actually need a diet that is both highly acidic and very nutritious. They also need acidifying nutritional supplements and medications as well as plenty of strenuous physical exercise and a fast paced, busy life to maintain a healthy pH.

PART 1:
FOLLOWING THE ALKALINE POWER DIET

THE ALKALINE POWER diet will help to restore you to a naturally healthy state of slight alkalinity. By avoiding highly acidic foods and eating foods that are neutral to slightly alkaline in their pH, you will restore your reserves of alkaline minerals and other important nutrients. Equally important, this diet will decrease the wear and tear on your buffer systems and organs of elimination by reducing the acid load of the body. This diet comprises four simple steps: (1) selecting more alkaline foods, (2) using delicious and readily available substitutions for highly acidic foods, (3) planning more alkaline meals, and (4) rotating foods for greater variety of nutrients. This diet will also cause fewer inflammatory reactions, which are extremely acidifying to the cells and tissues.

We have also included information on how to survive a binge on acidic foods, as well as guidelines on how to meet the special dietary needs of overly acidic individuals in various special groups, including athletes, corporate employees, and children and teenagers. In this section we provide much valuable information and advice that Susan has developed over the past two and a half decades and found to be effective for her own patients. This information will allow you to implement the alkaline power diet much more easily on your own.

STEP 1: SELECTING THE PROPER FOODS FOR THE ALKALINE POWER DIET

First, look at the chart on pages 102–108 showing the pH values of dozens of common foods and beverages. This chart will help you to learn the relative acidity or alkalinity of the foods that most of us eat on a daily basis. (You may be surprised at how acidic many of the foods you currently eat are.) It gives the pH of foods prior to being consumed and does not reflect the substantial acid production that some of these foods can trigger within the body. (This information is also provided in this section.) There is a lot of misinformation about the relative acidity and alkalinity of foods. Many other books have acid/alkaline food charts; however, these charts tend to contradict one another. One chart will list a food as being highly acidic, while another chart will state that the same food is highly alkaline. This can be very confusing to the reader who is trying to use this information to make intelligent choices.

Our chart is based on scientific research done at major universities. This information was obtained from technical sources compiled at the University of California, Davis, Department of Food Science and Technology, and Cornell University, Department of Food Science. In addition, we obtained the pH value of certain foods from their appropriate professional associations such as the National Coffee Association. You will notice that while most food groups are listed, oils are not. Oils do not have a pH since they cannot be mixed with water, which is necessary for taking pH measurements.

The chart will help you to plan a diet best suited to your pH needs, depending on whether you tend toward overacidity or are a naturally alkaline person. Overly acidic individuals can restore their bodies to a healthier, more alkaline state by using this chart to select foods that are less acidic and more alkaline. The chart will also indicate which foods have the highest level of acidity and should be avoided.

pH of Common Foods and Beverages
Prior to Being Consumed

Highly Acidic Foods (pH between 1 and 4.6)	pH Range Prior to Being Consumed
Beverages	
Ginger ale	2.0–4.0
Lime juice	2.2–2.4
Lemon juice	2.2–2.6
Wines	2.3–3.8
Cranberry juice	2.5–2.7
Cider	2.9–3.3
Grapefruit juice	2.9–3.4
Currant juice	3.0
Orange juice	3.0–4.0
Apple juice	3.3–3.5
Pineapple juice	3.4–3.7
Prune juice	3.7–4.3
Tomato juice	3.9–4.3
Fruit	
Lime	1.8–2.0
Lemon	2.2–2.4
Cranberry sauce	2.3
Gooseberries	2.8–3.1
Loquats	2.8–4.0
Orange	2.8–4.2
Plum	2.8–4.6
Rhubarb	2.9–3.4
Apple	2.9–3.5
Raspberries	2.9–3.7
Grapefruit	2.9–4.0
Boysenberries	3.0–3.3
Grapefruit sections	3.0–3.5

Highly Acidic Foods (pH between 1 and 4.6)	pH Range Prior to Being Consumed
Fruit, continued	
Strawberries	3.0–4.2
Blackberries	3.0–4.2
Kumquat	3.1–3.5
Quince	3.2
Blueberries	3.2–3.6
Pineapple, crushed	3.2–4.0
Crab apples, spiced	3.3–3.7
Kiwi	3.3–3.8
Apple sauce	3.4–3.5
Apricots	3.5–4.0
Pineapple, sliced	3.5–4.1
Fruit cocktail	3.6–4.0
Raisins	3.6–4.2
Vegetables	
Sauerkraut	3.1–3.7
Cucumber	3.1–3.8
Tomatillo	3.9–4.1
Dairy Products	
Yogurt	3.8–4.2
Sweeteners	
Fruit jellies	3.0–3.5
Fruit jams	3.5–4.0
Condiments and Seasonings	
Vinegar	2.4–3.4
Pickles, sweet	2.5–3.0
Pickles, dill	2.6–3.8
Pickles, sour	3.0–3.5
Fermented olives	3.5
Mayonnaise	3.8–4.0

Moderately Acidic Foods (pH between 3.1 and 5.6)	pH Range Prior to Being Consumed
Beverages	
Beer	4.0–5.0
Fruit	
Peach	3.1–4.7
Cherries	3.2–4.7
Pear	3.4–4.7
Mango	3.9–4.6
Asian pear	4.2–4.6
Guava	4.3–4.7
Banana	4.5–5.2
Vegetables	
Tomato	3.7–4.9
Potato salad	3.9–4.6
Eggplant	4.5–4.7
String beans	4.6
Red Meat	
Dry sausage	4.4–5.6
Dairy Products	
Cottage cheese	4.1–5.4
Condiments and Seasonings	
Fermented vegetables	3.9–5.1
Red pimento	4.3–5.2

Low Acid to Alkaline Foods (pH between 4.6 and 9.5)	pH Range Prior to Being Consumed
Beverages	
Coffee	4.9–5.2
Mineral water	6.2–9.4
Distilled water	6.8–7.0

Low Acid to Alkaline Foods (pH between 4.6 and 9.5)	pH Range Prior to Being Consumed
Fruit	
Figs	4.6–5.0
Papaya	5.2–5.7
Persimmon	5.4–5.8
Avocado	5.5–6.0
Dates	6.2–6.4
Cantaloupe	6.2–6.5
Melon	6.3–6.7
Vegetables	
Pumpkin	4.8–5.5
Sweet pepper	4.8–6.0
Spinach	4.8–6.8
Carrot	4.9–6.3
Squash	5.0–5.4
Asparagus	5.0–6.1
Turnip	5.2–5.6
Cabbage	5.2–6.3
Broccoli	5.2–6.5
Parsnip	5.3
Sweet potato	5.3–5.6
Onion	5.3–5.8
Peas	5.3–6.8
Turnip greens	5.4–5.6
White potato	5.4–6.3
Artichoke	5.6
Cauliflower	5.6–6.7
Parsley	5.7–6.0
Celery	5.7–6.1
Alfalfa tops	5.9
Corn	5.9–7.3
Lettuce	6.0–6.4
Mushrooms	6.0–6.5
Brussels sprout	6.3–6.6

Low Acid to Alkaline Foods (pH between 4.6 and 9.5)	pH Range Prior to Being Consumed
Beans	
Baked beans	4.8–5.5
Dried beans	4.9–5.5
Kidney	5.2–5.4
Lima	5.4–6.5
Soybeans	6.0–6.6
Nuts and Seeds	
Walnuts	5.4–5.5
Almonds	> 6.0
Flax seeds	> 6.0
Hazelnuts	> 6.0
Pecans	> 6.0
Poppy seeds	> 6.0
Pumpkin seeds	> 6.0
Sesame seeds	> 6.0
Sunflower seeds	> 6.0
Fish and Shellfish	
Halibut	5.5–5.8
Sardines	5.7–6.6
Tuna	5.9–6.1
Mackerel	5.9–6.2
Oysters	5.9–6.7
Clams	5.9–7.1
Codfish (canned)	6.0–6.1
Salmon	6.1–6.5
Haddock	6.2–6.7
Whiting	6.2–7.1
Catfish	6.6–7.0
Scallops	6.8–7.1
Crab	6.8–8.0
Shrimp	6.8–8.2

Low Acid to Alkaline Foods (pH between 4.6 and 9.5)	pH Range Prior to Being Consumed
Poultry	
Chicken	5.5–6.4
Duck	6.0–6.1
Egg yolk	6.0–6.3
Egg white	7.9–9.5
Red Meat	
Beef	5.3–6.2
Pork	5.3–6.4
Corned-beef hash	5.5–6.0
Spiced ham	6.0–6.3
Hot dogs	6.2
Dairy Products	
Roquefort cheese	4.7–4.8
Most cheeses	5.0–6.1
Parmesan cheese	5.2–5.3
Evaporated milk	5.9–6.3
Whole cow's milk	6.0–6.8
Butter	6.1–6.4
Camembert	6.1–7.0
Grains	
Wheat	> 6.0
Rice	> 6.0
Barley	> 6.0
Oats	> 6.0
Rye	> 6.0
Millet	> 6.0
Quinoa	> 6.0
Amaranth	> 6.0
Hominy	6.9–7.9
Baked Goods	
White bread	5.0–6.0
Date-nut bread	5.1–6.0
Soda crackers	6.5–8.5

Low Acid to Alkaline Foods (pH between 4.6 and 9.5)	pH Range Prior to Being Consumed
Sweeteners	
Molasses	5.0–5.4
Glucose syrup	5.2
Honey	6.0–6.8
Brown-rice syrup	6.1–6.4
Maple syrup	6.5–7.0
Condiments and Seasonings	
Hot peppers	4.8–6.0
Garlic	5.3–6.3
Cocoa	5.5–6.0
Ripe, canned olives	5.9–7.3
Dutch processed chocolate	7.0–8.0

Eat a more alkaline diet

If you have symptoms of overacidity, it is important to eat foods listed in the "Low Acid to Alkaline" section of the chart. Eating foods such as vegetables, grains, beans, small amounts of raw seeds and nuts, and fish and shellfish will help to lessen the acid load of the body and reduce the wear and tear on the pH-regulating systems as well as the organs of elimination. Ground, raw flax meal deserves a special mention as a rich source of both alkaline minerals and anti-inflammatory polyunsaturated oils. Flax meal can be used in blender drinks and as a cereal (see chapter 6 for specific recipes).

If you are overly acidic, eating these foods will begin to enhance your performance in many areas of your life as well as increase your physical energy, stamina, and resistance to disease. The more alkaline foods are higher in nutrients and are full of the alkaline minerals needed to restore the alkaline reserves in your cells, tissues, and bones. These foods also tend to be less allergenic and less likely to cause inflammatory reactions, which acidify your cells.

The alkaline power diet has enormous variety and includes a tremendous range of flavors. Its major food groups include vegetables, starches, nongluten-containing grains, legumes (beans and peas), seeds, nuts, fish, sea vegetables, and fruits like papaya and melons. Besides helping to restore your performance capability, the alkaline power diet provides many health benefits such as reducing the risk of heart attacks and strokes, cancer, and crippling, inflammatory conditions like arthritis.

Your diet and food selection should concentrate on foods that have a pH above 5.0. This will create a diet that has a vegetarian emphasis but includes rich sources of proteins like legumes, whole grains, raw seeds and nuts, and fish and shellfish. Fish and shellfish do not have the tough, fibrous protein found in red meat. As a result, the stomach produces less hydrochloric acid to digest these foods than is necessary for the breakdown of red meat. Fish such as salmon, mackerel, trout, and tuna also contain anti-inflammatory polyunsaturated oils rather than the inflammatory saturated fats found in red meat and dairy products.

▲▲ Most people eat seeds and nuts salted, fried in oil, or coated with sugar. These are popular snack foods while watching TV or movies, sitting in airplanes, or socializing in cocktail lounges. Instead of partaking of these snacks, bring your own raw organic seeds and nuts as highly nutritious, low-acid alternatives.

Avoid highly acidic foods and acid-forming foods

More than 90 percent of Americans become overly acidic during their lifetime due, in part, to the foods they eat. The amount of overly acidic foods consumed each day in the United States is staggering, especially when you consider that a person needs a slightly alkaline pH to be able to perform to their best and remain in optimal health. The damage that these highly acidic foods inflict on the body is often demonstrated in high-school experiments in which a tooth is placed in a glass of cola and allowed to remain there for several weeks or months. Within a relatively short period of time, the tooth begins to dissolve. Jim's high-school chemistry teacher would perform this ritual yearly. When taken into our bodies, these same cola drinks would inflict similar damage if they were not neutralized by our pH-regulating systems. While colas are a synthetic creation, there are many extremely popular natural foods that we eat that have pHs that are similar to or even lower than cola drinks, including limes, lemons, orange juice, most berries, cranberry sauce, vinegar, dill and sweet pickles, jams and jellies, and wine.

If you have an overly acidic constitution, the constant consumption of highly acidic food will, over time, rob you of your energy and vitality, reduce your mental clarity, and even dampen your optimism and enthusiasm for life. You may experience a slowdown in your ability to recover from injuries, surgery, and strenuous physical activities. The overconsumption of acidic foods can also cause you to become more prone to infections, runny noses, and allergic reactions. You may also notice an increase in aches and pains. Susan has had many overly acidic patients tell her that drinking a glass of orange juice triggered heartburn, drinking a cup of coffee caused bladder discomfort, and eating dairy products triggered nasal congestion.

As you look at the chart showing the pH values of common foods and beverages, you will probably be surprised at how many commonly eaten foods are highly acidic. Examples of the various acids contained within our daily fare include acetic acid, which gives vinegar its tartness, and citric acid, found in oranges, lemons, and limes. Carbonated soft drinks bubble because they are infused with carbon dioxide, a highly acidic substance that is actually a waste product of our own metabolism. A major component of tea is tannic acid. Caffeinated coffee contains many volatile acids, which are particularly abundant in gourmet blends and provide coffee with its desirable rich flavor. Red meat, dairy products, and soft drinks are high in acidic minerals like sulfur and phosphorus (which are converted to sulfuric acid and phosphoric acid).

Many of these foods are not necessarily "bad." For example, citrus fruits contain vitamin C in the juice and bioflavonoids, which are beneficial antioxidants, in the pulp. They also contain small amounts of alkaline minerals such as potassium (unlike the juices of the other, more tart citrus fruits, orange and tangerine juices are actually rich sources of the alkaline mineral potassium, despite their low pH). In fact, in traditional folk medicine, lemon juice and vinegar (particularly cider vinegar) are frequently prescribed for detoxification and purification of the body. They have even been recommended as alkalinizing agents, in part because of their purported high content of alkaline minerals. However, the actual alkaline mineral content of lemon juice and cider vinegar is very low and does not counter their intrinsic acid content. In addition, the low pH of these two delicious and useful condiments indicates that they are actually highly acidic and, like all acidic foods, must be buffered when eaten to neutralize their low pH. As a result, lemon juice and cider vinegar are best used as detoxification or purification remedies only by high-alkaline producers or individuals with healthy buffering capabilities (usually younger adults in their twenties, thirties, and forties), for whom frequent doses or large quantities may be prescribed and well tolerated. If you need to increase your intake of alkaline minerals, you are better off using more-alkaline, high-pH condiments or even multimineral supplements. The accompanying chart compares the pH and mineral content of lemon juice and cider vinegar with other, more-alkaline condiments and flavoring agents.

pH and Alkaline Mineral Content of Common Flavoring Agents and Condiments (per tablespoon)

Food	pH	Calcium	Magnesium	Potassium	Sodium
Lemon juice	2.2–2.6	2 mg	1 mg	15 mg	3 mg
Lime juice	2.2–2.4	1 mg	1 mg	17 mg	0 mg
Cider vinegar	2.4–3.4	0.8 mg	3 mg	14 mg	trace
Blackstrap molasses	5.0–5.4	137 mg	52 mg	585 mg	19 mg
Tahini (sesame paste)	> 6.0	64 mg	14 mg	110 mg	17 mg
Flax meal	> 6.0	35 mg	63 mg	120 mg	7 mg
Kelp	not available	156 mg	104 mg	753 mg	42 mg

In her clinical practice, Susan has found that the ingestion of more-acidic, low-pH foods such as citrus fruits and juices and different types of vinegars can be incredibly stressful to overly acidic persons despite these foods' potential nutritional benefits. The reason for this is that their highly acidic pH can trigger either immediate or slower-acting stress responses within the body. For example, many of Susan's overly acidic patients have frequently complained about citrus fruits and vinegar causing unpleasant reactions like canker sores, heartburn, bladder pain, and joint discomfort. Other potentially nutritious but highly acidic foods like tomatoes, pineapple, raspberries, and wine can also cause similar symptoms. Repeated consumption of these low-pH foods tends to trigger chronic damage, inflammation, and overacidity in the affected tissues of sensitive people.

Interestingly, these symptoms can occur in some individuals even before the food has left the stomach. This suggests that a nonchemical process may be taking place since the pH-regulating systems of the body cannot work this rapidly. To explain this phenomenon, some researchers have suggested that certain stress factors, like the overacidity of foods, may cause an immediate electrical imbalance within the body, which is then followed by the actual chemical responses to the stressor agent.

In contrast, high-alkaline producers or younger individuals with healthy and intact buffering capability may actually benefit from the wide variety of beneficial nutrients contained within highly acidic foods. Such individuals can handle these foods' low pH without their causing negative side effects. For example, certain fruit juices that are high in potassium citrate and alkaline salts of citric acid can be used to maintain energy and stamina while participating in athletic activities. Such drinks are best used by high-alkaline producers who can tolerate their high content of simple sugar and do not develop tissue reactions such as canker sores, heartburn, and other types of irritation from the use of these drinks.

Whether acid or alkaline in their pH prior to ingestion, many foods can also generate a tremendous amount of acid within the body once they are eaten. For example, protein-rich foods of animal origin, like red meat and dairy products, or tough plant protein like the gluten contained in wheat, rye, barley, and oats can stimulate the stomach to produce large amounts of hydrochloric acid, which is needed to begin the breakdown of these proteins. In addition, coffee, alcohol, and fast foods like pizza can also trigger significant hydrochloric-acid production.

Many foods also cause overacidity, because they trigger either food allergies or specific sensitivities in susceptible individuals (see the chart on page 113). Milk products, wheat, soy, peanuts, and eggs are examples of common foods that contain proteins to which the body can mount an exaggerated immune response in susceptible people. Many individuals are also allergic to sulfites (see the chart on page 113). These are chemicals used as preservatives in canned, frozen, and otherwise processed foods. Other foods like tomatoes, oranges, wine, and chocolate as well as the sugars found in milk (lactose) or fruits (fructose) can trigger symptoms of overacidity in individuals who have sensitivities to these foods or lack the enzymes needed to digest them. Finally, many foods—such as red meat (including hamburgers and hot dogs), dairy products, margarine, coconut oil, and palm kernel oil—contain saturated fats, which can cause highly acidic, inflammatory reactions within the body. Foods that trigger allergies, sensitivities, or inflammation within the body can damage tissue far from the site of ingestion. The joints, skin, bladder, reproductive organs, and thyroid are but a few of the organs and tissues that can incur injury due to improper food selection. Over time, chronic damage to and injury of the affected cells and tissues can lead to reduced energy production, a decrease in oxygen levels, and a loss of alkaline substances and minerals—all of which can contribute to overacidity and, ultimately, disease.

Foods That Commonly Cause Allergies

Wheat	Citrus fruits
Dairy products (milk, cheese, etc.)	Strawberries
Rye	Pork
Corn	Nuts
Soybeans	Shellfish
Chocolate	Eggs
Tomatoes	

Foods That Tend to Contain Sulfites*

Potato chips	Carrots
Soups (canned or dry)	Tomatoes
Mushrooms (canned or fresh)	Peppers
Pickles	Potatoes
French fries (frozen)	Scallops
Coleslaw	Shrimp
Beer	Oysters
Wine	Clams
Cider	Lobster
Lettuce	

*Sulfites are used as preservatives and sanitizing agents in food processing. Many individuals have adverse reactions to sulfites.

If liver function is impaired and the liver is unable to fully detoxify certain components of our diet, acidic by-products will accumulate. Alcohol, red meat, dairy products, pizza, peanuts, and cashews, among other foods, are hard for the liver to process. Finally, most foods are broken down into acidic waste products, which must be neutralized and then eliminated from the body. Not surprisingly, all of these by-products and waste products can greatly add to the acid load of the body and produce a constant and ongoing stress on our buffer systems and organs of elimination. As a result, everyone except high-alkaline producers has the deck stacked against them when eating the standard American diet.

How to modify common acidic foods and dishes

We have included the following tips to enable you to still enjoy some of the highly acidic but nutritious foods that you may currently be eating. While high-alkaline producers can eat these foods as a regular part of their diet, overly acidic individuals cannot.

Fruit drinks. Many overly acidic people would like to enjoy blenderized fruit drinks and smoothies because of their delicious taste and high nutrient content. Unfortunately, the high level of acidity of many fruits can cause canker sores, heartburn, abdominal discomfort, and even a drop in energy in overly acidic people. To neutralize the acidity of the fruit, add sodium bicarbonate to your fruit drinks: one-half to one teaspoon (or less if you are sensitive to supplements) per quart, depending on the acidity of the fruit used to make the drink. The addition of the bicarbonate will make the drink taste smoother and richer as well as increase the pH. For best digestibility, these drinks should be consumed by themselves on an empty stomach, preferably in the morning. If you wish to add protein powder to this drink, use vegetable protein derived from rice or legumes, which are less acidic than animal protein. In addition, do not consume this drink with a protein-rich meal containing meat or milk, since these proteins require more acid production within the stomach for their digestion.

Wine. Many overly acidic individuals would love to drink an occasional glass of wine but find that it causes heartburn and other digestive symptoms. This is because wine has an acidic pH. The alcohol contained within wine also triggers the production of hydrochloric acid within the stomach. For special social occasions, take a sodium and potassium bicarbonate mixture right after drinking an alcoholic beverage to blunt its acidic effect on the body. Bicarbonate can also be used to help neutralize the uncomfortable symptoms of an alcohol-induced hangover.

Coffee and tea. If you feel you cannot live without your daily cup of coffee or black tea, no-acid versions are available from Coffee Bean and Tea Leaf Company (800-TEA-LEAF).

Sparkling water. If you are at a bar or restaurant and want to drink mineral water but only bubbling varieties are available, you can get rid of the carbonation by adding a pinch of table salt. This will allow the water to go flat, leaving you with a more alkaline drink.

Salad dressings. You can substitute Bragg Liquid Aminos for vinegar when making salad dressings. Bragg Liquid Aminos is a delicious flavoring agent that can be purchased in most health food stores. Combine it with olive oil and herbs for a delicious dressing. Alternatively, you can prepare a salad dressing by decreasing the amount of vinegar by half and increasing the amount of water and oil, as well as by adding extra flavoring agents such as herbs.

Marinated vegetables. Avoid vegetables marinated in vinegar. These are highly acidic and are commonly served in Italian and Spanish restaurants and occasionally in American ones. Many restaurants offer alternative vegetable appetizers such as steamed artichokes or asparagus. You can also order small side dishes of whatever cooked vegetables are being served that day.

Salt. Sea vegetables are rich in minerals and can be used to replace the more acidic table salt as a flavoring agent. Sea vegetables are now available in shakers to be used as a condiment in natural-food stores.

STEP 2: MAKING SUBSTITUTIONS IN YOUR DIET

Once you know which foods are either high in acid or become so after being eaten, and which foods are more alkaline, you can begin to substitute the more alkaline foods for the ones that are causing you to become acidic.

Replace acid foods with less acidic/more alkaline ones

One of the most difficult obstacles we all face when making dietary changes is the prospect of giving up foods we really love. In fact, the inability to give up things we find enjoyable is often the biggest barrier to making changes that can lead to long-term improvements in health and performance. Now that you have had a chance to review the pH values of many common foods, you may find that some of your most enjoyable and "can't live without" foods are in the highly acidic category. These are foods that either contain high levels of acid before we ingest them, like lemon juice and vinegar, or cause acid to be produced in the body after we eat them, like red meat, dairy products, and wheat. Many of these are probably foods that you have eaten all your life, and you may be reluctant to give them up because you enjoy their flavor, taste, or texture.

Fortunately, you can replace a highly acidic food or beverage with a similar one that is more alkaline. The trick is to do this with a substitution that retains a similarly pleasurable flavor yet is also high in nutrients. For example, you can use soy- or rice-based frozen desserts instead of ice cream, or vegetarian patties instead of hamburgers. To help familiarize you with the substitution options that are available, we have developed the chart on page 118, which lists many highly acidic foods as well as their less acidic, more alkaline substitutes.

Over the past twenty years there have been incredible improvements in the quality, taste, and appearance of food substitutes. This has primarily occurred as the demand for low-fat food substitutes has increased. More recently, foods have been developed to meet the demand for alternatives to foods that are known to be highly allergenic, such as wheat and dairy products. While none of these substitutes was originally developed to restore pH balance, you can use many of them for this purpose because they also happen to be much less acidic than the foods they replace (soy is a notable exception: many individuals are soy intolerant and should avoid soy-containing foods). The market for these substitutes is growing rapidly, with many companies now competing for shelf space. Therefore, the quality is continuing to improve as food technologists are continually making refinements in taste and texture.

Twenty years ago, these products were of very poor quality, with the carton often tasting better than the product inside. Today, however, there are substitutes for cheese that both taste and melt the way real cheese does. There are substitutes for wheat pasta (such as rice, corn, and quinoa) that taste like the pasta you grew up with. There are also substitutes for meat and dairy products that are hard to tell from the originals. In fact, our daughter has made nachos for her teenage friends with nondairy cheese that are so tasty that they had no idea they weren't eating real cheese. If these foods can pass the "kid test," then you can feel comfortable giving them a try.

These substitutes are now easy to find in health food stores, many supermarkets, and a surprising number of restaurants. Gardenburgers are now being served in many restaurants, and you can order pizzas made with vegetarian-based soy and rice cheeses. Given the improvement in flavor and texture, any overly acidic person can enjoy these substitutes whether they are cooking for themselves, dining out, or preparing meals for an entire family. Susan has been recommending these food substitutes to her patients for years and has seen excellent results. With the many different brands available, you should be able to find substitutes that appeal to your taste.

Use substitutes in cooking

You can reinvent an old-favorite recipe with new, more alkalinizing ingredients. Check the chart on page 118 and see where you can make some of these substitutions and have a favorite recipe become a much less acidic dish. You can also start with one of the appetizing new food products, such as mozzarella-like cheese substitutes made with soy, and create a homemade pizza that is far more alkalinizing and healthful than the dairy-based version. Pancakes, cheesecake, and fettuccine Alfredo can also be made with substitute ingredients and are quite delicious and more healthful since they are not as acid forming within the body. Review the chart and purchase one of the substitutes each time you shop. Try them in your favorite recipes, and you will soon have a number of less acidic food substitutes to choose from.

Make substitutions at your own speed

As with any habit or pattern, one's personal preference for how best to initiate a change will vary from person to person. Some people prefer to make changes all at once and will immediately adopt a completely non-meat, nondairy, vegetarian diet. Others prefer to ease themselves slowly into dietary changes and will begin to add new foods and substitutions gradually, while reducing the frequency and portion size of many of their favorite and highly acidic foods. Choose the method that suits you best. Even after a healthier, more alkaline pH has been restored to the cells and tissues, a person who tends to have an acidic constitution will probably have to continue a more alkaline diet for the rest of their lives. However, as with most things, you will become accustomed to the new way of eating, enjoying the many benefits of increased energy and stamina. Before long, highly acidic foods such as greasy French fries or pizza with extra cheese and meat toppings will no longer seem as appealing.

A Warning on Substituting Foods

If you know you are allergic or find that you are sensitive to any of the food substitutes listed, do not use them as they will cause an acidic inflammatory reaction in your body and defeat their purpose. This situation is seen most often in individuals who are allergic to soy products, as mentioned above.

Food Substitutes for Highly Acidic or Acid-Forming Foods

Natural-food stores carry many of the following substitute foods, and even supermarkets carry some of these products.

Highly Acidic or Acid-Forming Foods	Less Acidic, More Alkaline Substitutes
Wheat Products	
Wheat bread	Bread made with rice, millet, amaranth, quinoa, soy*, and oat flours
Wheat crackers	Rice- and potato-based crackers
Wheat pasta	Rice, corn, quinoa, and buckwheat pasta
Wheat waffles	Rice and oat waffles
Wheat cookies	Rice, oat, barley, and millet flour cookies

Dairy Products

Cow's milk	Soy*, rice, nut, and multiple-grain milks made from oats, barley, amaranth, and rice
Cheese	Soy*, rice, and almond cheeses
Ice cream	Frozen desserts made with rice or soy milk*

Meat Products

Beef, veal, lamb, and pork	Fish, shellfish, and range-fed poultry, soy-based chicken substitutes*, and occasional range-fed red meat and game
Hamburger	Tofu, soy*, and multigrain gardenburgers
Hot dogs, breakfast sausage	Tofu, soy hot dogs and sausages*
Meat loaf	Multigrain and legume loaves

Fried and Fatty Foods

Deep-fried corn chips and potato chips	Baked corn chips and potato chips
Pizza made with a wheat crust	Pizza made with a rice flour crust and nondairy cheese

Beverages

Coffee	Grain-based coffee substitutes
Black tea, green tea	Herbal teas such as peppermint, chamomile, and rose hips
Soft drinks and fruit juices	Mineral water

Sweeteners

Refined white sugar	Maple syrup, brown-rice syrup, barley malt, honey

Condiments and Flavorings

Vinegar	Bragg Liquid Aminos**
Mayonnaise	Safflower oil–based mayonnaise
Ketchup	Sugar-free ketchup
Salt	Garlic, fresh herbs, sea vegetables, lemon rind, Bragg Liquid Aminos**

*Soy products such as tofu, soy milk, and soy flour can be acid-forming for individuals with soy allergy.
**Bragg Liquid Aminos is a seasoning agent available in health food stores.

Alkalinizing food supplements

Spirulina and other green foods are nutrient rich and promote alkalinity within the body. They are an excellent source of many easily absorbable, alkaline minerals as well as amino acids, vitamins, enzymes, and chlorophyll, and can be used to supplement your regular meals. The following is a list of green foods commonly found on the market:

Spirulina and chlorella are microalgae that provide a concentrated source of protein containing all the amino acids and are a good source of minerals as well.

Green magma, made from young barley leaves, supplies amino acids and minerals.

Kyo-green, a combination of barley, wheatgrass, kelp, and chlorella, provides amino acids and many nutrients.

Alfalfa is a source of abundant calcium, magnesium, phosphorus, and potassium in a balanced ratio that promotes absorption.

Barley grass is an excellent source of all the amino acids, calcium, and iron.

STEP 3: MEAL PLANNING

While you are following a program to restore your body to a more alkaline pH, proper food selection is critical to avoid putting undue wear and tear on your already stressed buffer systems. See the chart below for sample menus that you can use as a model for meal planning at home.

Typical Alkalinizing Meals

Breakfast

Puffed-rice cereal

Soy or other nondairy milk

Papaya slices

Pancakes made with rice and soy flour, topped with maple syrup

Melon

Peppermint tea

Breakfast (cont.)

 Soft-boiled egg

 Rice toast with honey

 Vegetable juice

 Tofu scramble with onions, mushrooms, and green peppers

 Soy/millet or rice bread toast with a canola oil spread
  (nonhydrogenated)

Lunch

 Lentil soup

 Grilled soy cheddar cheese sandwich on rice bread toast

 Coleslaw with carrots

 Noncarbonated mineral water

 Gardenburger (or other soy-based meat substitute), lettuce,
  and onion

 Coleslaw

 Potato salad

 Chef's salad with mixed greens, tuna, kidney beans, and
  hard-boiled egg

 Corn muffin

 Split-pea soup

 Rice pasta

 Baked yam

 Steamed carrots

Dinner

 Vegetable soup with a tofu meatball

 Tostada made with a corn tortilla, red kidney beans, rice,
  avocado, grilled Spanish onions, and cilantro

 Grain-based coffee substitute

 Hummus

 Rice tabbouleh

 Caesar salad with romaine lettuce

Dinner (cont.)

Broiled tuna

Lightly steamed broccoli seasoned with Bragg Liquid Aminos*
and flaxseed oil

Coleslaw

Broiled salmon

Baked potato

Steamed kale seasoned with Bragg Liquid Aminos* and
olive oil

*Bragg Liquid Aminos is a seasoning agent available in health food stores.

Choosing less acidic/more alkaline meals in restaurants

Traditionally, people have chosen mostly highly acidic dishes and entrées when eating in restaurants. Luckily, all-American fare such as the 16 oz. porterhouse steak, French fries, and rich, sugary deserts, and French cuisine with its heavy butter- and cream-based sauces have been replaced or supplemented in many restaurants by lighter, healthier, and less acidic, more alkaline dishes. This is true both in American restaurants and in those serving ethnic cuisines. The important thing is to know which dishes on the menu represent the less acidic, more alkaline options and to select a variety of such dishes when dining out.

We have prepared the following list to assist you in making intelligent menu selections, particularly if you are working hard to restore your body to a healthier, more alkaline state. In general, you will want to order salads, nondairy soups, vegetable or bean appetizers and side dishes, and vegetarian or fish entrées. Remember, most restaurants are willing to make up vegetarian entrées and platters at your request, even if they are not on the menu.

American cuisine: salad or salad bars, bean or vegetable soups, baked potatoes, rice, vegetable side dishes or platters, fish or shellfish entrées.

Italian cuisine: escarole soup, bean or minestrone soup, white bean salad, Caesar salad, risotto, polenta (cornmeal) with a mushroom sauce, grilled eggplant entrée, fish or shellfish entrées.

French cuisine: vegetable or seafood salads, nondairy soups, vegetable side dishes, stewed beans, fish or shellfish entrées.

Indian cuisine: lentils, rice pilafs, cucumber salad, curried vegetable or shellfish dishes.

Chinese cuisine: stir-fried vegetables, sizzling rice soup, tofu or bean curd dishes, steamed rice, shrimp and mixed vegetable entrées.

Japanese cuisine: Japanese salads, miso soup, sticky rice, sushi, side dishes and soups made with vegetables and tofu.

Mexican cuisine: mixed vegetable salads, tostada salad, bean and rice side dishes, bean or shrimp burritos, bean or seafood tacos.

How overly acidic and naturally alkaline people can dine well together

Married couples and members of the same family can have different acid/alkaline constitutions and may require different food choices. One spouse may be overly acidic while the other is a high-alkaline producer. Children's acid/alkaline balance may differ from that of their parents. This same issue can also arise when socializing with friends or business associates. Since the standard American diet is so prevalent, overly acidic people will often try to keep up with their more alkaline spouse or friend, much to their detriment. It is important to eat according to the needs of your basic constitution: You will feel better and maintain your health more readily if you stick to the diet best suited to your pH needs.

This is not as difficult as you might expect. When cooking at home, overly acidic and more alkaline individuals can share soups, salads, vegetable dishes, and starches. Their entrées, however, may differ. A more alkaline individual may choose to eat meat as an entrée much more frequently and often in larger portions. Remember, high-alkaline producers need to do this to maintain their level of energy. Overly acidic people should choose grain- and legume-based entrées instead with occasional servings of fish and poultry eaten in smaller amounts. Susan's overly acidic patients have reported that customizing entrées while keeping all of the side dishes the same is really not too difficult. Sometimes, they will even prepare food for the whole family—like spaghetti and meatballs, tacos, and casseroles—and simply not add the red meat to their portions. In addition, overly acidic people may want to skip the vinegar marinades and dressings, wheat bread, wine, coffee, and dessert that their naturally alkaline dining partner(s) can enjoy in moderation. Luckily, these individuals can enjoy the many substitutions that are now available and not feel deprived. For example, slices of very tasty rice bread can be served alongside the wheat bread. Or gardenburgers can be prepared on the grill right next to the all-beef hamburgers.

Restaurant dining is somewhat easier when people with different acid/alkaline constitutions eat together, because a restaurant menu normally contains many more dishes than are prepared for one meal at home. On the negative side, diners have no control over the ingredients used to prepare a dish or the types of dishes offered. While your naturally alkaline dining partner may choose to order a highly vinegary antipasti followed by steak with a glass of red wine and an apple tart for dessert, an overly acidic person can put together a tasty and varied meal by ordering a vegetable soup, salad, and several vegetable side dishes or rice-based dishes or fish as an entrée. This allows for great flexibility in both ordering and eating. And if you and your dining partner are willing to share your dishes, all the better. When you order a broccoli and beef dish in a Chinese restaurant, for example, the acidic diner can eat most of the broccoli while the alkaline one eats most of the beef.

STEP 4: ROTATE YOUR FOODS

Food allergies and food sensitivities are frequently seen in many overly acidic individuals. Food allergies occur when an individual has an exaggerated immune-system response to specific proteins found in various foods. The body's immune system reacts to these foods as if they were foreign invaders, much like the viruses and bacteria that can cause disease. The allergic reaction will trigger an outpouring of inflammatory substances that cause cells and tissues to become overly acidic. This can cause a runny nose, itching and tearing of the eyes, swelling of the sinuses, tightness in the throat, coughing, wheezing, skin rashes, fatigue, anxiety, and a host of other symptoms. Approximately 25 percent of the population is estimated to have wheat and dairy allergies. Millions of other individuals have specific intolerances to these same foods, due to enzyme deficiencies and the inability to properly digest them. Other foods such as peanuts, corn, soy, eggs, and chocolate can also trigger an allergic reaction in sensitive individuals. In addition, the milk or nuts used in preparing chocolate products can also cause the sensitivity reaction. While fish and shellfish are highly recommended as primary sources of protein in the alkaline power diet, they should be avoided in individuals with sensitivities to these foods. When an allergic reaction to any food occurs, the cells become more acidic.

Many other foods also cause overacidity in the body because individuals lack the enzymes needed to digest them. The best example of this is lactose intolerance. Lactose is a sugar found in milk that cannot be digested by 70 to 100 percent of blacks, Asians, and Native Americans and 60 to 90 percent of Mediterranean populations. Many individuals are also sensitive to fructose, or fruit sugar, which is found in thousands of food products. Finally, foods that contain amines (monosodium glutamate, or MSG, being the best known) are also irritating to the body. Amines are found in tomatoes, bananas, oranges, wine, chocolate, mushrooms, and Parmesan cheese.

Unfortunately, most overly acidic individuals tend to crave the foods that they are allergic to or have specific intolerances for. They will often eat these foods on a repetitive basis, sometimes consuming them every day for months or even years. This type of eating stresses the immune system and constantly triggers an allergic or sensitivity reaction within the body, leading to symptoms that are both uncomfortable and chronic.

To break this pattern and reduce the amount of overacidity being constantly created within the body, try rotating your foods so that they are eaten, at most, once every four days. A four-day rotational diet will greatly reduce your sensitivity to foods that you may be allergic to, thereby reducing acidic, inflammatory reactions within the body. For example, a typical rotation might alternate beans, fish, and eggs, with grain- and vegetable-based burgers, casseroles, and loaves as primary sources of protein.

All foods should be rotated on this program, including your beverages, condiments, and oils. People who eat a rotational diet tend to eat fresh, unprocessed foods, which change seasonally as different crops are planted and harvested. This type of eating provides a much greater variety of alkaline nutrients and essential nutrients than eating the same thing every day. Some individuals choose to eat the same foods day after day simply because they do not like to cook or feel that they do not have time to prepare food due to a very busy work and social schedule. Fortunately, health food stores, delis, and supermarkets often serve less acidic food options like falafel, hummus, gardenburgers, broiled salmon, grilled shrimp, and a wide variety of salads and even vegan mashed potatoes, grilled vegetables, and vegetable purees, all of which can be taken home and eaten. Gardenburgers can be put in a toaster at home and are ready to eat in one to two minutes. Similarly, fish can be simply broiled or grilled with no more preparation involved than sprinkling on a few herbs.

SURVIVING AN OCCASIONAL BINGE OF HIGHLY ACIDIC FOODS

All of us are occasionally invited to birthday parties, weddings, bar mitzvahs, Christmas parties, and Thanksgiving dinners, where virtually every food served is highly acidic and tempting to the eye and taste buds. Such festivities and holiday celebrations tend to include champagne, canapés, roast beef, ham, and beautifully prepared desserts. On these occasions, even the most overly acidic person will want to throw caution to the wind and eat, drink, and be merry. However, no one likes to wake up the next morning with an acid stomach, hangover, brain fog, or even a runny nose and aching joints from seriously overindulging on these highly acidic foods.

To minimize the deleterious effects that an occasional binge on highly acidic foods can cause, you can pursue the following program before, during, and after the binge itself. A half hour before you plan to eat, take the following nutritional supplements: 1 to 3 g of buffered vitamin C, one to two pancreatic digestive enzyme tablets, 500 mg of bromelain, a plant-based digestive enzyme (see chapters 3 and 4 for more detailed information on digestive enzymes), and 50 to 100 mg of vitamin B complex. With the meal, take one or two more pancreatic enzymes tablets and an additional bromelain tablet. One hour to one and one-half hour after eating, take one-quarter to one-half teaspoon of sodium and potassium bicarbonate (in either a 4:1 or 8:1 ratio, depending on your tolerance for potassium) in 4 to 8 oz. of water. Continue taking the alkalinizing agents every hour or two until all the symptoms of overacidity have disappeared. If bingeing on highly acidic foods or beverages tends to trigger respiratory infections, also consider taking one to two dosages of colloidal silver immediately following and two hours after the binge (see chapter 4, page 240, for more information on colloidal silver).

DIETARY NEEDS FOR SPECIAL GROUPS

Specific groups such as overly acidic athletes, corporate employees and businesspeople, and children and teenagers, are at particular risk of impaired performance in their jobs or activities if particular attention is not paid to the acid/alkaline makeup of their diet. This is discussed in this section.

Athletes with overly acidic constitutions

Most professional athletes must be high-alkaline producers to survive and excel in their competitive environment. However, many dedicated amateurs and weekend warriors do not have the professional athlete's buffering capability. Given the millions of Americans who regularly jog, bike, play tennis, life weights, and even compete in very strenuous events such as marathons, triathlons, and bodybuilding contests, a knowledge of your own buffering capability can give you a real edge in both enjoying and performing well in sports or athletic events.

Obviously, amateur athletes who are high-alkaline producers and have larger mineral reserves have a physiological edge on their more acidic peers. This is particularly true for those athletes who participate in strenuous anaerobic exercise, which tends to generate large amounts of lactic acid while, at the same time, depleting oxygen and the reserves of buffering substances contained within the muscles. In addition, alkaline minerals can be lost in the perspiration generated by exercise. A study published in the *Annals of the New York Academy of Sciences* examining mineral loss during marathon running found that athletes lost significant amounts of sodium, potassium, magnesium, and chloride; even small amounts of calcium may be lost in perspiration.

As a result, not all amateur athletes have the healthy alkaline constitution necessary to benefit from (and, in some cases, properly digest) the many protein powders, bars, and high-protein regimens that are recommended for athletic performance. In addition, overly acidic athletes may not perform as well on the highly acidic meat-based diet that is often recommended for those doing strenuous activities such as weight lifting or playing football. Athletes who are overly acidic will probably find that they have much more energy and perform better when they eat a less acidic, more alkaline diet. They may feel better consuming vegetable-based sources of protein or fish instead of red meat. They can also benefit from the use of alkaline mineral supplements and alkalinizing agents, particularly if they are using the highly acidic glucose and protein-based powders to gain weight and/or muscle mass or are eating protein bars for additional calories and energy. In such cases, the use of alkalinizing agents one hour after ingesting these foods will help to neutralize the acid load that they produce within the body.

Corporate America

Corporate employees will enjoy better health and greater productivity if they eat according to their pH needs. Most corporations are constantly looking for ways in which they can boost productivity and limit absenteeism. Most of the solutions have focused on improving morale, creating better mental programming, and enhancing physical fitness through corporate trainings, pep talks, and elaborate corporate fitness centers. However, the importance of meal planning, based on the relative alkalinity or acidity of the employees, has been totally ignored. Many corporations now provide meals for their employees through corporate kitchens. Corporate chefs can greatly benefit the employees of the companies they work for by incorporating the principles of acid and alkaline foods into their menu planning. Awareness of these principles can provide management with a powerful tool to greatly improve the health and productivity at all levels of the organization. The more education management can provide to all employees regarding the performance and health benefits of maintaining a slightly alkaline pH, the more the company will benefit from reduced health care costs and absenteeism. The result will be a more energetic, effective, enthusiastic, and productive workforce.

Both of us have frequently observed the detrimental effects on energy and productivity that highly acidic food, served in corporate settings, can have on tired, overworked, and highly stressed businesspeople. Several years ago, we did a consulting job for a West Coast corporation. We were closeted, off-site, for three days of meetings with the executives of the company. Many of the participants had been traveling extensively for the previous month. They were constantly drinking highly acidic beverages laden with caffeine, such as coffee and colas, to try to boost their flagging energy.

At the meetings we were served a series of highly acidic meals and snacks. For example, at the end of one long work session, we were given Chinese takeout food for lunch, including fried pork, egg rolls, and oil-drenched noodles and rice dishes. Bowls of M&M's and chocolate cake for dessert were then left out for us to snack on for the rest of the afternoon—along with other acidic snacks such as chocolate bars, licorice sticks, cookies, and soft drinks. We did not eat most of these dishes, preferring to eat the less acidic salad and only the cooked vegetables from the pork dish. By midafternoon, the sales manager, who had been downing coffee and chocolate candies since he had arrived the day before, turned to Jim and confided, "It's only two in the afternoon, and I feel horrible." This basically healthy man in his mid-forties further confided that these energy drops happened to him frequently and he had no idea why.

At another all-day strategy meeting that we attended, twelve people from various parts of the country gathered in a small conference room of a downtown hotel. Everyone began the day bright-eyed, energetic, and full of ideas. Our hosts then served us a highly acidic breakfast consisting of orange juice, ham-and-cheese omelettes, hash brown potatoes, buttered toast, and a basket of sweet rolls, with plenty of strong coffee. After a lunch of equally acidic foods, we could not help but notice that everyone's energy dropped immediately. Their formerly bright eyes became dull and glazed over. Several of the participants even developed runny noses. When the waiters offered more coffee during a midafternoon break, virtually everyone accepted this further assault on their pH-regulating systems in an effort to boost their declining energy. We have seen this same sequence of events occur countless times after corporate lunches and dinners. Only the naturally alkaline peak performers can maintain their enthusiasm and vitality at these meetings after days of eating highly acidic corporate fare.

If you are a corporate employee or business consultant and are frequently expected to attend meetings, seminars, trade shows, and conventions, you may find that eating highly acidic business fare is causing a drop in your energy and vitality. Neutralize these ill effects with a corporate survival kit. Instead of heading for the coffee, colas, and M&M's, use alkalinizing agents like sodium and potassium bicarbonate to neutralize excess acidity and restore your energy levels. In addition, taking digestive enzymes both during and after corporate meals will also help to maintain your energy level (see chapters 3 and 4 for further details on digestive enzymes). This same tip applies to anyone who is frequently faced with eating highly acidic food at civic-related or social events.

Children and teenagers

The consumption of an overly acidic diet by children and teenagers should be of great concern to all parents. Children and teenagers are in a crucial phase of physical growth: Their bones are still growing, and their organs are still increasing in size. Even maturation of the sexual organs does not begin until the early teens. Children need an abundant intake of alkaline minerals and other nutrients in order to develop strong muscles and bones and create the alkaline mineral reserves within their cells and tissues. For example, teenagers need 1500 mg of calcium a day to support their bone growth. This is the same amount of calcium needed by a postmenopausal woman experiencing a significant amount of bone loss who is at risk for osteoporosis.

However, a 1994 Gallup study indicated that although most children try to eat a balanced diet, few do. Half of all children do not meet the RDA for vitamin B_6, calcium, and zinc (calcium is one of the critical alkaline reserve minerals). The study also found that a child who is deficient in one nutrient is probably deficient in others. The poor nutritional status of many children has been confirmed in a number of research studies. For example, one study, published in 1993 in the *Journal of the American Dietetics Association*, examined the diet of schoolchildren in New York State. On the day they were surveyed, 40 percent of the students did not eat vegetables, except for potatoes or tomato sauce, while 36 percent ate at least four different types of snack foods. Children of lower socioeconomic status were found to have less diversity in their diets than children of more affluent families. However, the children from more affluent families were found to eat more snack foods—snack foods in our society are invariably highly acidic.

The diet of many children and teenagers in this country is highly acidic, mainly through ignorance. Even more than adults, children tend to eat heavily promoted, low-nutrient, and highly acidic foods. The staples of the diet for many children tend to be soft drinks, candy bars, cookies, hamburgers, hot dogs, pizza, chips, French fries, milkshakes, and ice cream. Many children begin their day with a highly sugared refined-grain cereal, white toast and butter, fruit drinks, and frozen pastries or waffles. This is followed by a lunch of processed meat on white bread, potato chips, and cookies, all washed down with a highly acidic soft drink. And dinners often consist of highly acidic fast food.

This acid assault depletes the mineral reserves of children and teenagers and puts an enormous stress on their acid-buffering systems and organs of elimination even before their growth and development has been completed. As a result, there is an epidemic of illnesses related to overacidity in children and teenagers. Many children suffer from four to six respiratory ailments per year, such as colds, flus, middle-ear infections, and bronchitis. Moreover, the incidences of childhood allergies and asthma have increased dramatically over the past few decades. The incidence of asthma has doubled since 1980, making it the leading chronic disorder in children under seventeen years of age. There are now between 5 and 6 million children diagnosed with asthma. Furthermore, diabetes and cancer are seen more frequently in younger individuals.

Symptoms of overacidity are now affecting the performance of children and teenagers as well as their health. Many children find it difficult to concentrate in the classroom or while doing their homework. Attention deficit disorder is estimated to occur in 3 to 6 percent of American children. There is more violent behavior in the schools and on the streets. Children continue to succumb to cigarettes, recreational drugs, and alcohol, all of which are highly acidic substances. Parents need to educate themselves about the short- and long-term deleterious effects of children and teenagers consuming large amounts of overly acidic foods and beverages. Children have no idea about the negative consequences that eating these highly acidic foods will have on their performance capability and health once they enter adulthood.

▲▲ Virtually all of the food packed into children's lunch boxes and all of the treats they are given, both at school and at home, are highly acidic. Avoid giving your children lunches consisting of highly acidic pizza, hamburgers, potato chips, soft drinks, brownies, and chocolate chip cookies. Instead, provide them with gardenburgers, tofu hot dogs, tuna sandwiches, baked chips, air-popped popcorn, carrot and celery sticks, and nondairy beverages or water.

▲▲ Do not reward your children with candy bars, cookies, and cakes made with refined white sugar and flour. Instead, give them cookies and cakes made with whole-grain flours and sweeteners such as rice bran syrup and molasses that are less acid-forming. Molasses, in particular, is a very rich source of many alkaline minerals, especially potassium.

▲▲ Children with allergies should have pastries made with non-wheat flours such as rice, oat, millet, and tapioca flours. A wide variety of these products are readily available in health food stores, and they tend to be as delicious as their less healthy counterparts.

▲▲ Children and teenagers whose performance and health are suffering because of overacidity should follow the same alkaline power diet as their parents. Overly acidic children can also benefit from the use of a vitamin and mineral supplement. Parents may also want to give their children one-quarter to one-half the normal adult dose of an alkalinizing agent such as sodium and potassium bicarbonate when they come down with common respiratory conditions. (Many teenagers are big enough to take a full adult dose.) Consult with your pediatrician or family physician if you have any questions on the advisability of doing this.

PART 2:
RESTORING YOUR ALKALINE MINERAL RESERVES

ONE OF THE MOST important ways to restore buffering capability is to replenish the body's mineral reserves. The larger the reserves of alkaline minerals contained within the body, the greater the capability a person has to neutralize the acids that result from eating acidic foods or doing strenuous exercise or that are the waste products of the body's ongoing metabolic processes. The mineral content of our cells and extracellular fluids must be maintained to enable the body to remain slightly alkaline. Our reserves of bone minerals, in particular, need to be constantly replenished since the bones provide an important reservoir of alkaline minerals that help to keep the pH of our blood stable when our other buffer systems are no longer functioning as well.

It is difficult if not impossible to replenish our mineral reserves through diet alone. The use of mineral supplements to rebuild our reserves is essential once we reach our forties and fifties. The use of supplemental minerals will allow overly acidic individuals to build up their reserves much more rapidly. In addition, our modern diet is so deficient in many of the essential major and trace minerals that it is virtually impossible to take in adequate amounts of them through food alone. This is particularly true in overly acidic individuals whose cells, tissues, and bones may be lacking many of the minerals needed for optimal health and performance.

HOW THE MODERN DIET BECAME DEFICIENT IN ALKALINE MINERALS

The alkaline mineral deficit of our modern diet is a problem of relatively recent origin. In late Paleolithic times, 35,000 to 20,000 years ago, our hunter-gatherer ancestors ate a highly varied diet that supplied all of the major minerals and most of the trace minerals. These people ate greater amounts of food than we consume today, yet their food contained more nutrients and fiber and fewer calories than the diets of most people in Western societies. Moreover, their main beverage was water, not highly acidic beverages like our soft drinks, coffee, tea, wine, and beer.

How the development of agriculture changed the food supply

Agriculture began in various parts of the world 10,000 to 5,000 years ago as the Paleolithic hunter-gatherers made the transition to farming. While cultivation of crops is usually thought of as an advancement in human development, it actually caused the nutritional value of the human diet to decline. With the advent of farming, only certain crops were cultivated to the exclusion of others, and only certain strains within each crop were selected to be cultivated from year to year. The human diet consequently became much more limited. A person was less likely to consume a broad range of minerals as well as other nutrients. However, in these early days, vegetables and fruits still had significant nutritional value since they were raised in naturally organic, mineral-rich soil, and according to farming practices that returned minerals to the earth. Up to the days of our grandparents and great-grandparents, most people still lived on farms and ate fresh seasonal produce. If they lived in cities, they still ate fruits and vegetables grown locally and sold in season. These foods were still grown using farming practices that included time-tested methods such as crop rotation, mulching, and manure fertilization, which helped insure high mineral content in the crops.

How modern food production affects the mineral content of foods

As the Industrial Revolution introduced mass production to agriculture, methods to refine grains and sugar were developed, and the processing of oils was soon to follow. New food products were created at the expense of nutrition, as minerals and other nutrients were removed during the manufacturing process. After World War II, farming itself changed radically. Manufacturers of chemicals, such as the phosphates and nitrates used in wartime to produce explosives, needed new markets for their products. These chemicals became the raw materials for producing fertilizers. By 1960, 97 percent of all crops were treated with chemical fertilizers that used salt-based nitrogen, phosphorus, and potassium (NPK fertilizers). This method of growing food produced fruits and vegetables that were full of color and perfectly shaped. However, these new farming techniques sacrificed mineral content. For the last fifty years, America's farmland has been progressively stripped of minerals, notably selenium, zinc, and a variety of trace minerals.

In response to this potentially devastating loss, some farmers who are aware of the deterioration of the soil have turned to organic farming to restore their land and have produced crops of higher nutritional value. The production of organic foods is accelerating each year, far beyond early expectations; organic foods are even starting to be sold in supermarkets. A study published in 1993 in the *Journal of Applied Nutrition* reported on over two years of research in which the nutrient content of organic produce, including potatoes, apples, peas, and corn, was measured. The results showed that the organic produce had twice the nutrient content of regular supermarket produce. Another comparison of the nutrient content of organic produce with regular supermarket produce appeared as a review article in 1997 in the *Townsend Letter for Doctors & Patients*. Lab tests again found that organic produce contained double the amount of vitamins and minerals as standard produce. At the same time, the organic foods also contained lower amounts of toxic heavy metal residues including lead, aluminum, and mercury.

The problem with the standard American diet

With the depletion of soil minerals, on the one hand, and the processing and refining of foods, on the other, the American diet is highly acidic and at the same time does not supply sufficient minerals to buffer these acids. As we discussed in chapter 1, the great majority of foods commonly eaten in our country are highly acidic—red meat, dairy products, refined flour and sugar, coffee, and soft drinks—while only a scant portion of meals are comprised of less acid, more alkaline vegetables, whole grains, legumes, starches, fish, and certain fresh fruits like papaya and melons. As mentioned in chapter 1, a comparison of the foods eaten per person each year shows 2143 pounds of acid or acid-forming foods versus only 380 pounds of alkaline foods.

Our plant foods today have been grown in depleted and exhausted soils. In addition, many of the foods we eat have been refined and are thus stripped of their mineral content. Therefore, the alkaline minerals contained within the foods we eat are inadequate to buffer our heavy intake of protein. For example, the amounts of minerals lost when whole wheat is refined are 67 percent of the calcium, 77 percent of the magnesium, 79 percent of the potassium, 44 percent of the iron, and 62 percent of the zinc. The baked goods and fast foods we eat in great quantity also rely on processed and refined ingredients that are low in minerals.

For health, the balance between minerals such as sodium and potassium is also important. Today's methods of food processing and cooking add acidic table salt to foods and remove alkaline potassium. As a result, we consume about one and a half times more sodium chloride than potassium, with our average daily intake of sodium ranging from 2300 mg to 6900 mg. Take a look at how today's foods compare with those of our Paleolithic ancestors. An apple contains 1 mg of sodium and 301 mg of potassium, whereas a piece of apple pie contains 110 mg of sodium and

80 mg of potassium. A portion of venison, one of the game meats eaten by our early ancestors, contains 65 mg of sodium, whereas today's hot dog contains 1100 mg of sodium.

Our calcium intake has also declined. The Paleolithic diet provided 1500 to 2000 mg of calcium a day, contributed by wild plant foods, meat, and the bones of small animals and fowl. There is more calcium in wild fruits and vegetables than in cultivated hybrids. Early humans took in more than enough calcium (and iron) by modern standards. The average daily intake of calcium for Americans today is only 400 to 500 mg.

Yet while agriculture and our food supply have changed, our genes have not. Ninety-nine percent of our genes are ancient in origin, dating from our earliest prehistoric ancestors. Of the remaining 1 percent, 99 percent of these originate prior to the time that systematic growing of crops began. Thus, most of our physiology and biochemistry were adapted to dietary conditions that existed prior to 10,000 years ago—which is astounding to consider, given the way we eat today.

The dietary content of alkaline minerals and bone structure

The decline in the minerals and other nutrient content of the diet occurred once humans switched from the Paleolithic mode of hunter-gatherer to farming. This is quite apparent when scientists examine the skeletal remains of ancient humans. Paleolithic men and women had a body structure similar to that of modern athletes. Skeletal remains show that these people had large, dense bones and strong teeth, reflecting the huge mineral reserves they had that could be used for buffering acids in the diet. There are no structural signs of overacidity, such as osteoporosis. The hunter-gatherers were also tall. Preagricultural humans were our height or slightly taller for over a million years. Men grew to be, on average, five feet ten inches to six feet two inches, and the average height of women was five feet five.

We tend to think of our ancient ancestors as being shorter than we are. However, it was only after the advent of agriculture, 10,000 to 5,000 years ago, and the more limited array of foods that domestication of crops provided, that height declined. Our immediate historic ancestors of the past five to ten millennia were shorter than modern human beings. This point is strikingly illustrated if you visit a museum exhibiting clothes that human beings wore 500 years ago: You're likely to see small mannequins, wearing clothes that would nearly fit a child today. When people of today visit the birthplaces of great artists and historic villages, they usually have to stoop to walk through the doors that were high enough for the people of Mozart's or Shakespeare's day and for our colonial ancestors.

It is only in the last hundred years that human beings began to regain stature because of the higher fat and protein content of our diets and our higher caloric intake. Modern Americans tend to be taller and more muscular and to carry more weight than previous generations. However, because our mineral intake is so low, we have regained our former height but not the former mineral content of our bones. Unlike the dense bones of our Paleolithic ancestors, the bones of many Americans are porous and even osteoporotic. Our teeth are also weaker, resulting in widespread tooth decay and gum recession. The only exceptions tend to be the small minority of individuals who have a naturally alkaline constitution or other individuals who have made the effort to consume a mineral-rich diet.

THE ACID/ALKALINE MINERAL NEEDS OF MODERN HUMANS

Human tissue contains all ninety-two elements that naturally occur on Earth. We require sodium, potassium, calcium, and phosphorus in relatively large quantities, in dosages of hundreds to thousands of milligrams per day. We also require trace amounts of many other minerals on a daily basis, such as chromium, copper, iodine, iron, selenium, and zinc. The average amounts of minerals in a 154-pound man are as follows:

Acid-Forming Elements		Alkaline-Forming Elements	
Chlorine	85 g	Sodium	63 g
Phosphorus	670 g	Potassium	150 g
Sulfur	112 g	Calcium	1160 g
Iodine	0.014 g	Magnesium	21 g
		Iron	3 g

Source: Guyton, A. O., *Textbook of Physiology* (Philadelphia: Saunders, 1981).

Many people are not consuming the quantity of minerals needed to maintain these mineral reserves and normal body composition. The consequences of such deficiency are well documented. Studies of people of the South Pacific done in the 1930s found that once these people changed from their traditional diet to one that emphasized refined flour and sugar, they developed many diseases commonly found in industrialized cultures, such as diabetes, tooth decay, and even deformity of the jawbones, in just one or two generations. In our own culture, the prevalence of osteoporosis is a telling sign of just how widespread mineral depletion has become. One-third of American women will develop some form of osteoporosis, as will 10 to 15 percent of American men.

Taking a mineral supplement

To counteract the lack of minerals in the food we eat, most people need to supplement their diet with a variety of minerals. The optimal dose of minerals varies by individual, depending on whether the minerals are needed for maintenance or to correct a deficiency. The chart on page 139 lists alkalinizing minerals and dosages that are appropriate for a person who has a tendency to be acidic or is overly acidic. These minerals can correct a pH imbalance directly; some will also promote the chemical pathway necessary for a healthy pH. For example, chromium and manganese are necessary for the healthy metabolism of sugar, a substance that can potentially be highly acidifying to the system. Calcium can be taken in either an acid or an alkaline form: Calcium carbonate is alkaline, derived from limestone. Calcium lactate and calcium citrate are acidifying forms.

Not only will mineral supplements restore the alkaline reserves of the body, thereby improving our buffering capability, but they are also needed for the activation of hundreds of essential enzyme reactions needed for healthy metabolism, digestion, and immunity, as well as other vital functions. Having sufficient levels of minerals within the body helps support our physical energy and stamina and helps us to recover rapidly from physical and mental exertion.

Mineral Supplement Dosage per Day

Mineral	Daily Dose
Calcium	800–1500 mg
Magnesium	400–800 mg
Potassium	99–300 mg
Zinc	15–60 mg
Manganese	10–30 mg
Chromium	200–1000 mcg
Iron*	10–18 mg
Selenium	50–200 mcg
Copper	1–2 mg
Iodine	150–225 mcg
Boron	3 mg

*Men should consider taking multimineral formulas without added iron because of possible toxicity since men do not lose iron, as women do, through menstruation. Many postmenopausal women may have low iron stores, particularly if they suffer from iron-deficiency anemia during their active reproductive years. These women may benefit from continued moderate iron supplementation until the deficiency is corrected, at which point they should switch to an iron-free supplement.

It is important to read the label carefully before buying a mineral product for use in an alkalinity restoration program. Many products that are labeled high-potency vitamin and mineral combinations tend to have higher dosages of vitamins than minerals. This is particularly true of formulations of one to two tablets or capsules per day. It is very difficult to incorporate the amount of supplemental minerals that an overly acidic person needs in so few tablets or capsules. We instead recommend buying separate vitamin and high-potency mineral supplements to insure that dosage levels of the minerals are in the therapeutic ranges. Individual minerals can also be purchased separately.

PART 3:
USING ALKALINIZING AGENTS FOR
QUICK SYMPTOM RELIEF

ALKALINIZING AGENTS CAN be tremendously beneficial in assisting the body to rapidly neutralize overacidity. Alkalinizing agents such as sodium and potassium bicarbonate, sodium and potassium citrate, and sodium phosphate can relieve the symptoms of overacidity within a very short time. Alkalinizing agents can rapidly catalyze a shift from overacidity to a more healthy, alkaline state. The almost immediate relief that these agents can provide makes them an extremely powerful part of any program in which an individual needs to restore their buffering capability for both peak performance and optimal health. Two other alkalinizing agents, buffered vitamin C and alkaline water, are also tremendously beneficial and should and can be used daily as part of an alkalinity restoration program. They are not only powerful buffering agents, but will also help to build up your mineral reserves. In addition, they both have powerful antioxidant effects, helping to protect the body from heart attacks, strokes, and immune-system problems. While a less acid, more alkaline diet and the use of supplemental alkaline minerals will begin to restore our buffering capability, these remedies tend to work slowly and will not provide the quick symptom relief seen with the use of alkalinizing agents. In this section we also discuss two other alkalinizing treatments: alkaline water and magnetic therapy. Supplemental oxygen therapy, which is an extremely powerful alkalinizing therapy, is covered in depth in chapters 7 and 8.

It is important to realize that the need for alkalinizing agents can vary greatly with one's level of health, as well as one's current levels of environmental, dietary, and emotional stress. For example, when one is trying to recover from an acute illness or is eating a highly acidic diet, the need for alkalinizing agents is much greater and dosages may be larger and taken more frequently. In contrast, during periods of good health, relative lack of emotional stress, or eating a more alkaline diet, the need for alkalinizing agents may decline to smaller dosages taken once or twice a day for maintenance purposes. For example, when you have a severe cold, you might need as much as one-half to one full teaspoon of a sodium and potassium bicarbonate combination, taken four to six times a day, to effectively reduce symptoms. However, when you are symptom-free and feeling well, you may only need half a teaspoon once or twice a day. (These dosages, of course, may vary according to the needs of each individual.)

SODIUM BICARBONATE

Sodium bicarbonate is a nontoxic, white crystalline powder that has a mild, neutral taste. It is also referred to as baking soda and bicarbonate of soda. As a buffering agent, sodium bicarbonate easily reacts with other compounds, making acidic substances more alkaline and alkaline substances more acidic. Sodium bicarbonate produces a significantly alkaline end product with a pH of 8.1.

Not only is sodium bicarbonate an essential part of the buffer system of our body, it is also active in the natural ecology of the Earth. Sodium bicarbonate plays a role in maintaining the pH balance in all living things. It is found in lake sediments, mineral deposits, groundwater, and even the ocean, where it helps stabilize the amount of carbon dioxide in the atmosphere.

Because of sodium bicarbonate's ability to buffer a wide variety of substances, it has many common uses within the home. People often store an opened box of sodium bicarbonate in the refrigerator as a deodorant, because it chemically neutralizes unpleasant odors which are usually caused by a strong acid, such as sour milk, or a strong alkaline food, such as spoiled fish. Sodium bicarbonate also works as a cleanser, alkalinizing the fatty acids in dirt and grease so that they become water soluble and can be washed away. And as a leavening agent, sodium bicarbonate, or baking soda, causes baked goods to rise. It is added to dough, along with an acid such as lemon juice, and when the dough is baked, heated bubbles of carbon dioxide are released. The bubbles, trapped inside the dough, cause it to stretch and rise. Baking powder, which is also used for leavening, is a mixture of sodium bicarbonate and an acid, such as cream of tartar.

POTASSIUM BICARBONATE

Unlike sodium bicarbonate, potassium bicarbonate is only available from a chemical supply house; it is also occasionally found in nutritional supplement products. A pharmacist can also prepare a mixture of sodium bicarbonate and potassium bicarbonate, or an individual can make his or her own mixture. Like sodium bicarbonate, potassium bicarbonate is a white, crystalline, nontoxic powder. Both substances will last indefinitely if stored in a cool, dry place. However, while sodium bicarbonate has a mild, pleasant taste, potassium bicarbonate is somewhat sharp and chalky on the tongue. Potassium bicarbonate is rarely taken alone because of its unpalatable taste. It can also be irritating to the digestive tract in individuals with intestinal conditions like inflammatory small bowel disease. Furthermore, if taken alone in a high dosage for prolonged periods of time, it may cause an irregular heartbeat.

SODIUM AND POTASSIUM BICARBONATE COMBINATIONS

It is preferable to use sodium and potassium in combination in a ratio of 4:1 to 8:1 sodium to potassium (depending on your tolerance for potassium) rather than using sodium bicarbonate alone. First of all, the digestive juices produced by the pancreas contain both sodium and potassium. In addition, many individuals do not eat enough potassium-rich foods in their diet. There are also other health benefits to supplementing with both buffering agents since this helps to maintain the sodium-potassium balance of the cells. For a cell to be healthy, there must be a predominance of potassium inside the cell and sodium outside it. This condition generates an electrical charge that allows the cell wall to control which substances enter the cell and to discharge toxins from the cell. Since the standard American diet contains an overabundance of sodium and is low in potassium (commonly supplied by fresh plant foods), our diet itself can potentially disturb the important balance of these intracellular and extracellular minerals.

Using large amounts of sodium bicarbonate alone as a buffering agent is not recommended for people on a low-sodium diet, such as individuals with severe hypertension or congestive heart failure, persons taking certain heart medications, and women who are pregnant. However, there are individuals who do find potassium bicarbonate irritating to their digestive tract or have a preexisting health condition for which the use of a potassium-based supplement is contraindicated. Such individuals can use sodium bicarbonate alone as an alkalinizing agent. See your physician if you have any specific questions.

Sodium and Potassium Bicarbonate Treatments for Performance and Health

Individuals who use sodium and potassium bicarbonate for a variety of performance- or health-related reasons will vary greatly in both the dosage and the frequency with which these alkalinizing agents should be used. For instance, a person with a severe allergic reaction or an intense bout of the flu may need to use an alkalinizing agent every one to two hours for a short period of time until their symptoms start to diminish. At this point, dosages can be spread out to every three to four hours while the person is still in the acute phase of the illness. In contrast, an individual with mild sinusitis may find that using bicarbonate once or twice a day on a daily basis provides enough buffering to prevent their symptoms from occurring. However, a generally recommended dosage is one-quarter to one-half teaspoon of a mixture of sodium bicarbonate and potassium bicarbonate in a 4:1 or 8:1 ratio (depending on how well the individual tolerates potassium). Sodium bicarbonate may be used by itself in individuals with digestive problems who find potassium supplements irritating to the intestinal tract.

Occasionally, an individual will find that he or she needs to go as high as a one-teaspoon dosage for a very short period of time in order to relieve their symptoms. Conversely, very sensitive individuals may find that a tiny dose, such as one-eighth teaspoon, is sufficient.

Physicians who work with nutritional programs to restore acid/alkaline balance often find that highly acidic people may need to use sodium and potassium bicarbonate on a regular basis, for as long as several years. Higher dosages may be necessary during the first four to six months of treatment to counteract their overacidity. The dosages can gradually be reduced, except during periods of great physical or emotional stress, when higher dosages may be necessary. At the same time, however, these physicians will place their patients on more alkalinizing diets and mineral supplementation, both of which are needed to build up the alkaline reserves of the body and counteract overacidity. The use of alkalinizing agents alone on a long-term basis will not produce maximum therapeutic benefits unless these other restorative steps are followed so that the healthful, slightly alkaline pH of the body can be restored. However, in order to restore major body systems that are greatly overly acidic and to offset the overacidity that develops as part of the normal aging process, an individual (particularly if past midlife) may have to continue a maintenance program for a prolonged period of time or even indefinitely.

It is always helpful to begin any program to restore your acid/alkaline balance with the help of either a physician who is knowledgeable about nutritional medicine or a well-trained nutritionist.

Work-related physical and mental fatigue

Strenuous work demands and long hours can significantly increase the production of acidic waste products within the body. Using alkalinizing agents can neutralize these waste products and restore one's energy and stamina.

SUGGESTED DOSAGE: To treat physical and mental strain and fatigue, take one-quarter to one-half teaspoon of sodium bicarbonate, or a mixture of sodium bicarbonate and potassium bicarbonate in a ratio of 4:1 to 8:1 (less potassium if you tolerate it poorly), every two to four hours.

Athletic activity

Weekend warriors and individuals who frequently participate in sports and athletic activities can also benefit from supplementing their diet with sodium bicarbonate. It can be used prophylactically to prevent muscle fatigue and to promote the healing of most athletic injuries once they have occurred. Sodium bicarbonate is also beneficial in reducing nasal congestion and a runny nose, which can result when a person has overtrained or pushed their limits of endurance in such sports as long-distance running or cycling.

SUGGESTED DOSAGE: To counteract these symptoms, take one-quarter to one-half teaspoon of sodium bicarbonate, or a mixture of sodium bicarbonate and potassium bicarbonate in a ratio of 4:1 to 8:1 (less potassium if you tolerate it poorly), as often as necessary to eliminate symptoms. Cases of severe muscle spasm or an acute condition of nasal congestion may require a dose every hour, but a more general recommendation is sodium bicarbonate every two to three hours. Some individuals who are extremely overly acidic may find that they need a dose of up to one teaspoon during the acute phase.

Colds, flus, sore throats, bronchitis, middle-ear infections, sinusitis, and allergies

Most individuals who develop minor respiratory illnesses tend to be overly acidic (except for a small minority of the population who develop respiratory symptoms because of low enzyme production, poor detoxification, or poor oxygenation). For most people with these symptoms, restoring your body rapidly to a more healthful, slightly alkaline state is one of the most important steps that you can take to recover rapidly.

SUGGESTED DOSAGE: To treat a respiratory ailment in the acute stage (from the first sign or symptom), take one-quarter to one teaspoon of sodium bicarbonate, or a mixture of sodium bicarbonate and potassium bicarbonate in a ratio of 4:1 to 8:1 (less potassium if you tolerate it poorly), every one to two hours, until symptoms begin to abate. One dose should be taken before bed and another on rising in the morning. During the acute phase, you may even take the bicarbonate mixture every one to two hours during the night. Acids tend to accumulate during the night, and a person with relatively few symptoms the night before may wake the next day with a return of their congestion. Also see chapters 3 and 4 for additional anti-inflammatory support.

▲▲▲ In the acute stages of a respiratory infection, it's a good idea to prepare a solution of sodium bicarbonate and water in a closed container and keep it next to the bed so that you can sip on it whenever you wake up or go to the bathroom. This constant drinking of the mixture will allow for the continuous alkalinizing of the body that is necessary to restore the environment needed for the body to control and eliminate the bacteria or viruses that are causing the symptoms. Also, be sure to continue the alkalinizing process for several days after the acute symptoms have subsided to prevent a recurrence of your symptoms.

Digestive problems

Sodium bicarbonate is an effective buffering agent, alleviating acid indigestion, sour stomach, and heartburn. It also aids digestion by raising the pH necessary to activate the pancreatic enzymes responsible for breaking down protein. Bicarbonate can be combined with enzyme therapy to enhance the digestive process. Many people who are experiencing digestive problems have a pancreas that is producing only low amounts of bicarbonate and pancreatic enzymes. This use of digestive enzymes is discussed in detail in chapters 3 and 4.

When combining enzymes and sodium bicarbonate, take the enzymes with the meal or immediately following it. However, sodium bicarbonate should not be taken at this time as it will interfere with the acid stage of digestion. Take sodium bicarbonate either one-half hour before a meal or one to one and one-half hours after eating, especially following a large meal. Enzymes can again be taken at this time.

SUGGESTED DOSAGE: For indigestion, take one-quarter to one-half teaspoon sodium bicarbonate in a half glass of water every two hours until symptoms are relieved. Usually one or two doses will be sufficient. Sodium citrate is also effective as an antacid for indigestion (see page 150).

Inflammatory conditions

People with chronic inflammatory conditions such as food allergies, arthritis, colitis, and thyroiditis can benefit from alkalinizing with sodium bicarbonate, as it can have an anti-inflammatory effect when used over a long period of time.

SUGGESTED DOSAGE: Take one-quarter to one-half teaspoon three to four times per day, preferably one-half hour before a meal or two hours after a meal.

Steroid medications like prednisone are used to treat various acute and chronic inflammatory conditions. Steroid medication can only remain active in an alkaline pH. Individuals who are being treated with any cortisonelike drugs might want to consider using sodium and potassium bicarbonate to create an internal environment in which these drugs can provide the most efficacious results. Of course, consult with your own physician to discuss the advisability of doing this in your own personal case.

Cancer

Certain cancer treatment regimens also factor in a person's chemical makeup and pH. To pursue this approach to cancer treatment, it is important that a patient be assessed by a physician skilled in identifying these metabolic types and designing a corresponding regimen. Many people with cancer tend to be overly acidic and can benefit from an alkalinizing program. Such programs can include oxygen therapies and bicarbonate, both of which are potent alkalinizing agents, as well as the use of digestive enzymes. See the chapters on oxygen therapies (chapters 7 and 8) and digestive enzymes (chapters 3 and 4) in regard to the treatment of cancer.

Osteoporosis

Sodium and potassium bicarbonate can also be used in the treatment of osteoporosis, a condition in which loss of bone density can lead to hip, vertebral, and wrist fractures. Osteoporosis is commonly seen in postmenopausal women and, less frequently, in older men. Since it is due, in part, to overacidity of the body, the use of alkalinizing agents can be an important part of the treatment program (as well as following a less acidic, more alkaline diet and supplementing with alkaline minerals like calcium and magnesium as well as vitamin D).

SUGGESTED DOSAGE: For long-term prevention and treatment, take from one-quarter to one-half teaspoon of a mixture of sodium bicarbonate and potassium bicarbonate in a ratio of 4:1 to 8:1 (depending on your tolerance for potassium) or sodium bicarbonate twice a day, in the morning on rising and before bedtime.

Skin conditions

Many skin conditions, such as poison oak, poison ivy, and skin abrasions, can be ameliorated through the use of sodium bicarbonate. Fill a bathtub with tepid water and add one cup of baking soda. Take a bath in this water for as long as it is comfortable to do so. The same treatment can be used for insect bites: The alkalinizing action of the bicarbonate neutralizes the venom from the bites, reducing redness and itching.

First aid for burns. To help prevent blisters, use a cloth dipped in a solution of baking soda and ice water and apply this to the skin until all heat has gone from the burn area.

First aid for sunburn. Combine one-quarter cup baking soda with one-half cup cornstarch and add this mixture to a bath of tepid water. Soak in this as long and as often as possible.

Dental problems

Tooth decay occurs when bacteria in the mouth digest sugars consumed in food. The end product is an acid that can begin to erode the protective outer enamel layer of the teeth. When baking soda is used to clean the teeth, it neutralizes the acid and prevents decay. The slightly abrasive texture of sodium bicarbonate also removes plaque. And when baking soda is combined with hydrogen peroxide, which has an effervescence, the bubbles also help float away food particles as well as kill bacteria in the mouth. To clean the teeth in this fashion, first dip a toothbrush in hydrogen peroxide and then in sodium bicarbonate.

Overdosing with Sodium or Potassium Bicarbonate

Overdosing with sodium and potassium bicarbonate can cause an individual to become too alkaline, a condition called alkalosis. Alkalosis can result in symptoms like tingling in the extremities and lips, as well as feeling anxious or panicked. In cases of severe overdosing, the nerves becoming overexcited, firing automatically and repeatedly. This can result in muscle spasms (tetany), which usually start in the forearms and can spread throughout the body. Tetany of the muscles involved in breathing can be fatal. In some people, bicarbonate can also cause digestive symptoms such as bloating or gas. If any of these problems arise, immediately reduce the dosage and frequency of use. Drinking black coffee, black tea, the juice of a half lemon diluted in water, or cola drinks or taking vigorous exercise will all cause the body to become more acidic and help restore the pH to normal. Above all, be aware of which dosage regimen works best for you. If you are extremely sensitive, start with a lower dose than recommended. If you are highly acidic, you may have to use a higher dosage to obtain symptom relief.

Six to eight percent of the population is naturally alkaline and should avoid the use of alkalinizing agents altogether. If you fit this profile, the use of bicarbonate can cause you to become even more alkaline. This can result in fatigue, feelings of anxiety or panic, digestive symptoms such as gas and bloating, or tingling of the extremities, or even the more severe symptoms of alkalosis.

SODIUM AND POTASSIUM CITRATE

Both sodium citrate and potassium citrate are used in the treatment of a variety of kidney and bladder diseases. Sodium citrate helps relieve bacterial cystitis and interstitial (inflammatory) cystitis, while potassium citrate is especially useful for treating kidney stones. Sodium and potassium citrate alkalinize the urine and help to maintain a higher urinary pH over the long term, without alkalinizing the entire body. Sodium citrate is more often prescribed for indigestion. Sodium citrate is mild and pleasant tasting and much more easily tolerated than potassium citrate, which can sometimes cause digestive upset.

Both sodium citrate and potassium citrate can be ordered from health food stores. They are also prescribed by physicians treating kidney and bladder-related problems. Citrate is combined in nutritional products to produce magnesium citrate, calcium citrate, and various other mineral combinations.

Bacterial cystitis

While bacterial cystitis is normally treated by antibiotics, the use of alkalinizing agents, like sodium citrate, may be helpful in reducing the symptoms of this condition.

SUGGESTED DOSAGE: 4 g of sodium citrate, taken three times a day, for at least two days to one week (4 g is the equivalent of $^1/_7$ oz.).

Interstitial cystitis

The symptoms of this painful and chronic inflammatory condition can be greatly improved by the use of alkalinizing agents. Sodium citrate can be used to treat interstitial cystitis in combination with sodium bicarbonate.

SUGGESTED DOSAGE: Sodium bicarbonate can be used to provide rapid relief during the acute, symptomatic phase in dosages of one-quarter to one-half teaspoon every hour or two until symptoms abate. Symptom relief can then be sustained with the use of the slower-acting sodium citrate in a dosage of one-half to three-quarters teaspoon twice a day.

Kidney stones

To prevent the recurrence of acidic types of kidney stones, physicians will use potassium citrate alone or in combination with magnesium. Magnesium is added to some regimens to reduce the gastrointestinal distress caused by the use of potassium citrate alone. This regimen should be done only under a physician's care. Potassium citrate is also used in certain protocols for treating gout and more serious kidney diseases.

Digestion

Sodium citrate is effective as an antacid for indigestion. Take 4 to 8 g of sodium citrate as a single dose (this is equivalent to $1/7$ to $2/7$ oz.). It is important to wait at least one to one and one-half hours after eating before treatment to allow the acid phase of digestion to proceed normally.

Side Effects and Cautions When Using Sodium and Potassium Citrate

Sodium citrate is not recommended for people on a sodium-restricted diet or for those taking aluminum-based antacids. Side effects of overdosing with sodium citrate are nausea, vomiting, diarrhea, and convulsions.

Potassium citrate should be avoided by individuals with certain health problems such as urinary-tract infection, diabetes mellitus, kidney failure, adrenal insufficiency, and acute dehydration. High levels of potassium can cause tingling in the hands and feet and, in extreme cases, mental confusion, paralysis, and even cardiac arrest. Potassium citrate is also not recommended for pregnant women and nursing mothers.

Potassium citrate is generally well tolerated, although it can cause digestive symptoms such as diarrhea, abdominal discomfort, nausea, and vomiting.

SODIUM PHOSPHATE

Phosphorus is the second most abundant mineral in the body and is found in every cell. It is an easily absorbed mineral. The phosphorus compound sodium phosphate is an effective buffering agent used as an aid to improve sports performance. A typical dosage used in studies is 4 g a day for three days prior to an event. This has been found to improve both anaerobic and endurance exercise. Sodium phosphate is nontoxic in normal amounts. However, taking large doses can lead to calcium loss as phosphorus interacts with calcium during metabolism.

BUFFERED VITAMIN C

Almost all animals are able to produce vitamin C within their own bodies, primarily in the liver. Exceptions include guinea pigs, monkeys, and human beings. Human beings lack the enzyme necessary for the conversion of glucose to vitamin C. It is estimated that if our body were able to manufacture vitamin C, we would produce as much as 10 g a day. However, the current RDA for vitamin C is a modest 60 mg.

As we are unable to produce vitamin C, we must depend on food and nutritional supplements for our supply. Many fruits and vegetables are rich sources of natural vitamin C including citrus fruits, strawberries, papayas, red and green peppers, broccoli, Brussels sprouts, tomatoes, asparagus, parsley, dark leafy greens, and cabbage. There is almost no vitamin C in meats, seeds, grains, and beans. However, when seeds, grains, and beans are sprouted, they become an excellent source of vitamin C. Unfortunately, many people eat diets that are very low in this important nutrient due to a high intake of fast and processed food.

Vitamin C is crucial for the maintenance of optimal health. While most people think of taking vitamin C when they have a cold, this remarkable vitamin has great value far beyond its use as a home remedy for nasal congestion. It has been studied for its usefulness as an antioxidant in the prevention of heart disease. Researchers have also investigated how vitamin C bolsters immune function. It has been found to activate neutrophils, which are part of the immune system's first line of defense. Vitamin C may also increase production of lymphocytes. These white cells are important in the production of antibodies and help coordinate the body's immune response to bacteria and viruses. Vitamin C may also decrease histamine production, thereby reducing the likelihood of an allergic reaction.

Millions of people use vitamin C on a daily basis for its health benefits. However, in choosing a vitamin C supplement, you must consider its effect on pH, especially when using it in high dosages, more than 1 to 2 g a day. Such dosages are commonly taken by many individuals for both treatment and prevention of many diseases. Dosages as high as 3 to 10 g per day are often used when fighting acute illnesses. Vitamin C in its natural form, ascorbic acid, is actually a mild acid. In addition, most of the vitamin C products on the market are acid-based. This acidic form of vitamin C is fine for people who are fundamentally alkaline or have good buffering capability. However, the people who can benefit most from vitamin C tend to be overly acidic. These people need to take vitamin C in its buffered form, which is combined with alkaline minerals that increase its pH, creating a more alkaline and better tolerated form of this vitamin. Overly acidic individuals do not usually have the buffering capability to neutralize large amounts of ascorbic acid. Another benefit of using buffered vitamin C is that it is less likely to cause diarrhea or intestinal irritation, which can occur with ascorbic acid.

With buffered vitamin C, ascorbic acid is usually combined with minerals such as calcium, magnesium, potassium, and zinc. Taking calcium ascorbate alone requires supplementing with additional magnesium to keep these two minerals in balance within the body. For persons predisposed to kidney stones, taking magnesium also helps to keep the calcium soluble, so that it does not form calcium oxalate stones.

Ascorbic acid is also helpful for people who are naturally alkaline. They are able to buffer its acidity without any problem, and may even need it to balance their pH. Vitamin C is as effective at lowering pH as a cola or a cup of coffee but without the harmful effects of the caffeine or other chemicals in these beverages. Alkaline individuals often need the antioxidant effects that this vitamin provides. Since alkaline types can easily digest rich meals full of fat and protein, they also run the risk of developing heart disease caused by this diet. As an antioxidant, vitamin C can help reduce the amount of oxidized low-density lipoprotein (LDL) cholesterol in the arteries, the type of cholesterol most associated with the development of heart disease.

ALKALINE WATER

Several devices use an innovative technology to convert ordinary tap water, through filtration and electrolysis, into an alkaline water that has extraordinary health benefits. The technology was developed in Japan in the early 1950s; commercial devices have been available there since 1958.

The equipment is extremely popular in Japan, where it has received governmental approval and sells over a million units a year.

The commercial alkaline water device fits on the countertop near the sink so it can use tap water as its source. The unit, which is slightly taller and thicker than a large dictionary on end, is an electrical appliance connected to the kitchen faucet to perform electrolysis on tap water before you drink it or use it for cooking or cleaning. When the tap water enters the unit, it is first filtered to remove all chlorine, impurities, odors, and tastes. Next, the water passes into an electrolysis chamber equipped with positive and negative electrodes. Positive ions are attracted to negative electrodes, which creates water with an excess amount of electrons, thereby raising the pH of the water to levels as high as 9 to 11. This highly alkaline water is diverted into a stream that comes out the faucet to be used for drinking and cooking.

In contrast, negative ions are attracted to the positive electrode in the chamber. Through electrolysis, this water gains a positive charge and becomes more acidic, with its pH decreasing to 4 or less. This acid water is diverted into a separate hose that sits in the sink and can be used for washing hands, cleaning fruits and vegetables, sterilizing cutting boards or kitchen utensils, skin care, and treating minor wounds.

The benefits of the alkaline water created through electrolysis far exceed just its ability to gently raise the pH of the cells and tissues of the body and to neutralize acids. Because the alkaline water has gained a significant number of free electrons through the electrolysis process, it is able to donate these electrons to active oxygen radicals in the body, thereby becoming a super antioxidant. By donating its excess free electrons, alkaline water is able to block the oxidation of normal tissue by free oxygen radicals. Another significant benefit of the electrolysis process is that the cluster size of the alkaline water is reduced by about 50 percent from the cluster size of tap water. This allows the ionized alkaline water to be much more readily absorbed by the body, thereby increasing the water's hydrating ability and its ability to carry its negative ions and alkalinizing effect to all the cells and tissues of the body. If you are overly acidic, an alkaline water device can provide a safe, gentle, and effective way of restoring the pH balance of all the cells in your body as well as providing excess free electrons to act as super antioxidants. For more information on alkaline water devices, see the appendix.

▲▲ Drinking four to six glasses of alkaline water a day will help to neutralize overacidity and over time will help to restore your buffering capability. Alkaline water should also be used when conditions of overacidity develop, such as a cold, the flu or bronchitis. Like vitamins C, E, and beta-carotene, the alkaline water acts as an antioxidant because of its excess supply of free electrons. This can help to protect the body against the development of heart disease, strokes, immune dysfunctions, and other common ailments.

▲▲ Because acid water is mildly astringent, it can be used to restore the protective mantle of the skin, which is naturally acid. Over time, washing the skin with acid water has cosmetic benefits, improving the texture and quality of the skin. Because of the small cluster size of the water molecules, the water is able to hydrate the outer layer of the skin much more effectively than ordinary tap or bottled water. CAUTION: Acid water is intended for external use only and it should never be ingested.

MAGNETS

Modern research has found that magnetic therapy has a profound healing effect on a variety of medical conditions including pain, spasms, bone fractures, neurological conditions, and depression. Therapeutic magnets create these benefits, in part, by producing alkalinizing effects on cells and tissues.

Magnets come in two types, the static or permanent magnet, such as the ones found sticking to many household refrigerators, and electromagnets, whose field is created by running an electrical current through a coil. Magnetic field strength is measured in gauss. The Earth has its own magnetic field, measuring less than 10 gauss, while magnets used for recreational and therapeutic use will have gauss ranging from 300 to 4000. Magnetic fields used for medical diagnostic procedures such as magnetic resonance imaging (MRI) will have gauss in excess of 10,000. Magnets used in therapeutic applications come in various shapes and sizes from as small as one-half inch in diameter to six-inch squares. When larger areas of the body require treatment, smaller magnets are often sewn into a fabric, thereby creating a seat cushion or full-body mattress. While magnets were originally made from iron ore, most of today's commercially available magnets are ceramic. They are permanent and hold their gauss for decades.

Magnets have been used for many medical applications. The primary uses have been to relieve pain from soft-tissue injuries such as sprains, strains, bruises, bursitis, tendonitis, arthritis, and lower back pain, and to facilitate wound healing. Magnets have also been used for treating depression and migraine headaches and for shortening recovery times from physical exertion. Interestingly, the FDA has approved the application of electromagnetic fields to broken bones that have failed to heal. The electrical coil is placed around the break and left on for up to two to three months. This treatment has proved quite successful in uniting and healing broken bones.

Recently, interest in the therapeutic use of magnetic fields has increased dramatically because of their use in sports medicine and through newly released double-blind research studies. For the past several years, Jim Colbert has been one of the leading money winners on the Professional Senior Golf Tour. However, a few years ago Colbert thought his golf-playing days were over. He suffered from chronic back pain that forced him to stop playing professionally. A friend suggested that he try magnets to treat the pain. He began sleeping on a magnetic mattress pad and strapping magnets against his lower back during and after playing a round of golf. The dramatic effect that the magnets have had for Colbert has influenced many golfers who suffer lower back and shoulder injuries to try magnets. Magnets are now available for soft-tissue injuries of the ankle, knee, wrist, elbow, and shoulders. Other well-known athletes who have had success using magnets for pain relief and to speed recovery from exertion are two NFL quarterbacks, Dan Marino of the Miami Dolphins and Dan Pastorini, who retired after a successful career with the Houston Oilers.

Several recently released scientific studies are confirming anecdotal evidence about the therapeutic benefits of magnetic field stimulation and prompting a number of new studies. The first study, reported in November 1997 in the *Archives of Physical Medicine and Rehabilitation*, was a double-blind study designed to test the effect of magnets on fifty patients suffering from pain associated with postpolio syndrome. All patients were told to hold the active magnets or inactive devices over the area of most intense pain for forty-five minutes. Prior to the treatment, the patients were asked to rate their pain on a scale of 1 (no pain) to 10 (extreme pain). After the treatment, the patients were again asked to rate their pain. The twenty-nine who used active magnets reported a reduction in pain from 9.6 to 4.4; the twenty-one who used the placebo device reported a much smaller decline, from 9.5 to 8.4.

The second study, reported in the April 1997 issue of the *Australia New Zealand Journal of Psychiatry*, exposed seventeen patients suffering from depression to an electromagnetic field for five daily sessions. Eleven of the seventeen patients showed a marked improvement that lasted for two weeks after the treatments, with no reported adverse effects.

A third double-blind study, published in the January 1999 issue of the *American Journal of Pain Management*, reported that the wearing of magnet-laden socks seemed to reduce or eliminate the pain associated with a foot disorder common in diabetics. The constant wearing of magnetic devices dramatically suppressed the neuropathic symptoms of burning pain, numbness, and tingling in diabetic patients' feet. Diabetic peripheral neuropathy is a progressive deterioration of nerve function in the extremities that can trigger pain in the feet. It is notoriously difficult to treat, and often the patient becomes disabled. The study involved nineteen patients suffering from foot pain, ten of whom were diabetic. All participants wore special "magnet socks" for four months. Real magnets were sewn into one foot of each of the pair of socks, while the other foot contained a fake magnet (the placebo). Patients were not told which sock contained the real magnet, and socks were switched from one foot to the other after the first month of the study. At the end of four months, 90 percent of the diabetic subjects reported a dramatic reduction in foot pain. In contrast, just one third of the nondiabetic patients reported symptom reduction after magnetic therapy. The results of this study show the effects of the magnetic therapy to be palliative but not curative, since symptoms recur when the magnet is removed.

The results of these and other studies have prompted numerous new studies to begin. For example, the Center for the Study of Complementary and Alternative Therapies in Virginia will study the effects of static magnetic fields on 100 patients suffering from fibromyalgia.

The exact mechanism of action for the therapeutic use of magnetic fields is unknown. There are, however, several theories of how magnets may provide therapeutic benefits, and it is possible that two or more of the suspected mechanisms may be operating simultaneously. The first theory is that magnetic fields increase blood flow to the area exposed to the field. This allows for increased oxygen and nutrients to enter the area and for waste products to be removed more rapidly, thus decreasing inflammation and relieving pain. A second theory is that the magnetic field may affect pain receptors. It produces a slight anesthetic effect by altering neuro-chemical levels in the brain, including dopamine, monamines, and sero-tonin. These are the same neurochemicals that are related to depression and chronic pain when their production is diminished. This theory also suggests that magnetic fields may actually increase the production of endorphins, chemicals that act as natural pain relievers. A third theory is that the negative, or north pole, of a static magnetic field increases the level of alkalinity in the cells and thereby reduces the level of cellular acid-ity, inflammation, and pain. Thus the use of the negative pole of a magnet helps to restore the body's naturally slightly alkaline state.

The major proponent of the alkalinizing effect of the negative pole of a magnetic field is William H. Philpott, MD, a psychiatrist who has researched and written extensively on this subject. Philpott, who won the Linus Pauling Award from the Orthomolecular Health Society in 1998, has spent years researching and observing the beneficial effects of the neg-ative pole of a magnetic field on various medical conditions. Philpott con-cludes that the negative or north pole of a magnetic field is life enhancing and promotes health. He states that the magnetic field generated by the north magnetic pole increases cellular alkalinity, activates the enzymes that process free radicals, and frees oxygen from its bound state in free radicals, thereby increasing the production of ATP in cells. As a result of these biochemical changes, the negative magnetic field speeds healing, reduces cellular stress, increases the production of melatonin (thereby aid-ing sleep), and assists in fighting bacteria, viruses, and even cancer. Philpott has found these negative-pole magnets effective for such varied conditions as chronic pain, inflammation, arthritis, diabetes, depression and other mental conditions, addictions, movement disorders, pelvic and intestinal disorders, and eye problems. For people who are overly acidic, these negative-pole magnets may assist in restoring and maintaining the natural slightly alkaline balance the body needs for optimal performance and health.

Magnets with a negative pole on one side are available in a variety of sizes, shapes, and gauss strengths, and as mattress pads and seat cushions. (See the appendix for further information on where to find various types of magnets.)

OXYGEN THERAPIES

Oxygen is the most abundant element found within our bodies and has a profound effect upon our body chemistry. Individuals who develop health conditions like respiratory illnesses, hardening of the arteries, and iron deficiency anemia may become overly acidic because of decreased oxygenation of their cells and tissues. The use of oxygen therapies can help to reduce acidosis and promotes a more healthy alkaline state within the body. See chapters 7 and 8 for more information.

PART 4:
THE ROLE OF A HEALTHY LIFESTYLE

OVERLY ACIDIC INDIVIDUALS need to carefully assess their habits when undertaking a program to restore their body to a more naturally healthy alkaline pH. Emotional and mental stress, a hectic, fast-paced lifestyle, and hard physical exercise will tend to generate acidic waste products within the body. All of these factors increase the wear and tear on our buffer systems as well as the lungs and kidneys, our main organs of elimination. Many studies have confirmed that stress does, indeed, accelerate the aging of the body and plays a significant role in the development of disease. In contrast, by practicing stress modification through leading a calmer and more peaceful life and engaging in moderate aerobic physical activity, you can actually improve circulation and oxygenation to all of the tissues and organs within the body. Over time, our buffering capability and the health of our organs of elimination can actually improve with these healthful practices.

PHYSICAL EXERCISE

Overly acidic people tend to feel their best when engaged in aerobic activity that is moderately strenuous and can be done in a relaxed and leisurely way. Activities in this category include golf, swimming, walking, and bicycling at a leisurely pace. With these types of exercise, a person will tend to breathe more deeply and slowly. Over time, this helps to improve the elasticity of our lungs and relaxes the diaphragm and chest muscles, thereby allowing us to inhale more oxygen. Moderate aerobic exercise also relaxes, dilates, and expands the network of blood vessels in the body, and enables the heart to work more efficiently. With improved circulation, the alkalinizing oxygen that we breathe in is better able to reach all of our tissues and organs, promoting a more alkaline pH throughout the body. Better circulation and oxygenation improve the health of all our organs, including our pH-regulating organs such as the lungs and kidneys. Acidic waste products such as carbon dioxide are more effectively removed from the cells via exhalation and through the urinary tract. Moderate aerobic exercise also produces less lactic acid and is less likely to deplete the level of oxygen and buffering substances within the muscles than more strenuous physical activities like long-distance running or weight lifting.

STRESS MANAGEMENT

Emotional and mental stress generate acidic waste products within the body that can put undue wear and tear on our pH-regulating systems. This is particularly true once we pass through our young-adult years. By our thirties, forties and fifties, excessive levels of stress within our lives can predispose us to chronic health problems triggered, in part, by overacidity. Practicing stress reduction techniques can help stress-prone people control their tendency toward overacidity and enable them to remain more healthfully alkaline.

Overly acidic individuals can benefit by finding a balance between the excitement and challenges of life and sufficient periods of rest and relaxation. Peaceful, calming activities such as meditation, yoga, listening to relaxing classical music, or taking quiet walks alone or with friends and family can help to promote a more alkaline pH within the body. In addition, taking frequent hot baths or saunas or even treating oneself to a massage periodically will have similar pH-normalizing benefits.

One easy way to alkalinize the body is by breathing deeply. The practice of yoga and meditation promotes deep, slow breathing. Deep inhalation oxygenates the tissues, while deep exhalation helps to remove carbon dioxide from the body. Deep breathing also promotes relaxation of the muscles and blood vessels. In addition, the normal outpouring of stress chemicals caused by the fight-or-flight response can be interrupted. Taking a short holiday from worry and stress by calmly breathing deeply can facilitate the restoration of our buffering capability.

Another way to promote the removal of acidic waste products from the body is by warming the interior tissues with hot baths, saunas, and massage. Once the internal temperature of the body is raised, the small blood vessels dilate, and circulation throughout the body is improved. An alkalinizing bath can be particularly beneficial for conditions such as stiffness and muscle tension, both of which are worsened by the accumulation of acids within the body. To take an alkalinizing bath, run a tub of hot water, add one cup of bicarbonate of soda, and soak for twenty minutes. You will feel very relaxed and sleepy after this bath, so it is best to enjoy it at night before going to sleep. You will probably wake up feeling refreshed and energized the following day. Many harried and busy people have also learned that a weekly professional massage can greatly help to reduce their level of stress and thereby help to normalize the pH of the body. The areas of the body where a person is massaged are warmed as blood circulation is stimulated. This enables stored acids to enter the circulation and be eliminated.

DIET AND LIFESTYLE TIPS FOR HIGH-ALKALINE PRODUCERS

The following tips will help naturally high alkaline individuals maintain their tremendous physical energy, stamina, and resistance to disease.

EAT A HIGHLY ACIDIC AND NUTRIENT-RICH DIET

Naturally alkaline people are the only ones who can thrive on the dozens of acidic foods that make up the backbone of the standard American diet. Their alkaline mineral reserves and their production of alkaline buffers like bicarbonate are so great that a nutrient-rich, highly acidic diet will help them stay in balance and allow them to maintain their ability to perform at peak levels and remain in excellent health for decades longer than most other people, provided that their other chemical functions remain intact.

These individuals should emphasize nutritious foods that are higher in acid content. Unless they have a particular food sensitivity, they can eat all of the following highly acidic fruits and their juices: citrus fruits, berries, apples, apricots, grapes, pineapples, and tomatoes. Not only are these fruits acidic, but they are rich sources of important nutrients like vitamin C, bioflavonoids, and potassium. Most vegetables tend to be either moderately or low acid in their content. Alkaline individuals can enjoy and even thrive on beans and peas, asparagus, artichoke, eggplant, lettuce, cabbage, broccoli, and many other highly nutritious vegetables. They can also benefit by dressing or marinating vegetables in vinegar. This popular condiment has a beneficial acidifying effect since it lowers the pH of the vegetables. Antipasti, cured olives, dill and sweet pickles, marinated bean salads, coleslaw, potato salads, and green salads are all normally flavored with vinegar-based dressings. In contrast, overly acidic people may find that the use of vinegar can produce heartburn, abdominal discomfort, and other acid-related symptoms.

Naturally alkaline individuals will feel their best on an acidic, meat-based diet. They tend to need several servings of meat per day. They can enjoy range-fed beef, lamb, and veal, as well as game meat, which contains a much lower content of saturated fat than most meat found in supermarkets. They can also benefit from fish and free-range poultry. While fish and poultry are neutral to slightly alkaline when first eaten, their high protein content requires significant amounts of hydrochloric-acid production within the stomach—and results in significant amounts of acid-breakdown products. Fish, poultry, and organically raised red meat should be chosen over the cuts of red meat found in most supermarkets, which are typically very high in saturated fat. The higher polyunsaturated fat content of fish, poultry, and organically raised red-meat products will help to protect naturally alkaline individuals from the heart attacks and strokes that they are prone to. In addition the total fat content of organically raised animals is usually lower than that of animals raised by conventional methods.

This does not mean that these individuals should eat the standard American diet with its high saturated-fat and refined-sugar content as well as its notoriously low nutrient content. Like the rest of the population, naturally alkaline people should avoid fatty cuts of red meat, dairy products, rich, sugary desserts, and the overconsumption of caffeinated beverages, alcohol, and soft drinks. Overconsumption of these foods will increase the risk of heart attacks, strokes, adult-onset diabetes, arthritis, and cancer of the prostate, colon, and breast as well as other common diseases even in these inherently strong and sturdy individuals. At the same time, these individuals should ignore the current belief that vegetarian-based diets should be eaten by everyone to insure optimal health. An exclusively vegetarian-based diet will make these individuals feel tired, edgy, and enervated. People with naturally alkaline constitutions are at their best eating a high-protein diet with two to three servings of meat per day.

USE ACIDIFYING THERAPIES

A variety of nutrients and medications not only have beneficial therapeutic effects but are also highly acidic. As a result, these substances can be used to great benefit by naturally alkaline individuals. Several examples of commonly used acidic substances include vitamin C (ascorbic acid), acidic forms of calcium, and aspirin (acetylsalicylic acid). Other standard over-the-counter drugs like cough syrups and expectorants, which are usually manufactured as highly acidic, sweet-tasting products, are also better tolerated by high-alkaline producers or younger individuals with healthy buffering. Naturally alkaline individuals should avoid the buffered forms of these substances, as well as other substances used to treat various health problems. They should take ascorbic acid instead of buffered vitamin C, calcium citrate instead of the more alkaline calcium carbonate, and regular aspirin instead of the buffered form. Thus, it is important to read labels and buy the proper acidifying substances and medications whenever possible.

PARTICIPATE IN VIGOROUS PHYSICAL ACTIVITIES

High-alkaline producers tend to be drawn to strenuous types of exercise that are more likely to deplete both the oxygen content and the natural buffering agents contained within the muscles as well as to generate lactic acid. Physical activities such as jogging, weight lifting, competing in triathlons, competitive cycling, and mountain climbing will generate the acid waste products that help to maintain the pH balance of high-alkaline producers. These individuals also tend to do very well in rigorous team sports such as football, rugby, ice hockey, soccer, and basketball.

Many naturally alkaline people can maintain this level of intense physical activity well into their later years, provided that their other chemical functions remain reasonably intact. It is not unusual to see vigorous and naturally alkaline oldsters participating in triathlons and doing bodybuilding and long-distance swimming well into their eighties and nineties. Many of these individuals will also play golf frequently in their older years, populating the ranks of the many senior golf tournaments that are enjoying popularity all over the country. Walking a five-mile golf course several times a week is tremendously healthful for these vital seniors.

Former U.S. president George Bush is an excellent example of an individual who has very likely possessed tremendous buffering capability throughout his life. During his entire four-year term as president of the United States, he was known for his enjoyment of often fast-paced physical activity such as jogging, driving a speedboat, and golfing. He often would talk to reporters while playing a game such as horseshoes, and ask them to join in. At the age of seventy-two, he kept a longtime promise made during World War II and successfully parachuted out of an airplane from 12,500 feet. He repeated this feat in June of 1999 to celebrate his seventy-fifth birthday, and plans to do it again to celebrate his eightieth.

LEAD AN ACTIVE LIFE

High-alkaline producers thrive on fast-paced, busy schedules. They prefer to pack their social and business calendars with many activities. They do not tend to participate in the more alkalinizing pastimes such as meditation and yoga, which tend to be quieter and more contemplative. High-alkaline producers also tend to avoid low-stress, undemanding jobs. They prefer work and social activities that provide the level of excitement and even stress needed to generate sufficient acid within the body to counter their naturally alkaline constitutions.

Like everyone else, they do enjoy having time away from work and responsibilities. However, high-alkaline producers are never away from the action for very long since they thrive on excitement and stress. Their idea of leisure is to attend a boisterous boxing match or to go whitewater rafting. While these types certainly do attend ballets and operas, they are often happier doing action-based activities. They may also prefer to listen to a heated debate or an emotional inspirational lecture rather than a dry academic class. Whatever activities they choose to participate in, high-alkaline producers will maintain a higher degree of physical and mental health if they remain busy and actively engaged in every aspect of their life.

SUMMARY OF TREATMENT OPTIONS
FOR RESTORING YOUR ACID/ALKALINE BALANCE

A. Overly acidic individuals

The alkaline power diet

Restore your alkaline mineral reserves through sufficient intake of calcium, magnesium, potassium, and other alkaline minerals

Use alkalinizing agents and therapies for quick symptom relief
Sodium and potassium bicarbonate
Sodium and potassium citrate
Sodium phosphate
Buffered vitamin C
Alkaline water
Magnets
Oxygen therapies

Alkaline-enhancing habits
Moderate aerobic exercise
Stress management techniques like meditation and yoga

B. High-alkaline producers

Diet: more acidic and nutrient-rich foods

Better tolerance of acidic minerals like phosphorus and sulfur

Use acidifying agents and therapies
Vitamin C (ascorbic acid)
Acidic nutritional supplements like hydrochloric acid and cider vinegar
Aspirin and other acid-forming drugs

Acid-enhancing habits
Vigorous physical activities
Active, fast-paced life

3

HOW DIGESTIVE ENZYMES BENEFIT
PEAK PERFORMANCE AND HEALTH

ABUNDANT DIGESTIVE-ENZYME production is crucial for more than just processing the food we eat. In fact, digestive enzymes are essential prerequisites for peak performance. Peak performers derive their physical energy, stamina, mental clarity, and the ability to recover rapidly from illness and injuries, in part, from the abundant levels of digestive enzymes that they produce. Healthy digestive function also contributes to one of the great pleasures of life—enjoying a wide variety of cuisines in both social and business settings. When digestive-enzyme production is diminished, much of this pleasure is lost because we are severely limited in the types and amounts of foods we can eat. The important benefits of digestive enzymes in supporting peak performance and maintaining optimal health are listed in the chart on page 166.

In this chapter, we will discuss the important role that digestive enzymes play in supporting peak performance and health. We begin with the stories of two individuals whom we know personally to illustrate the dramatic effect that the production of digestive enzymes can have on a person's life. Both of these individuals are likable, responsible, and well educated. However, they differ greatly in their level of digestive health, which has had a dramatic effect on their ability to attain not only career success but a richly textured life. Both of these individuals are middle-aged men. One of them has all the strengths and attributes commonly seen with abundant pancreatic-enzyme production. In contrast, our other friend has been hampered, in both his professional and his social life, by a long history of digestive complaints. Their differing innate ability to produce pancreative digestive enzymes has, in part, affected their degree of success in their careers as well as their ability to derive personal enjoyment from their activities and relationships.

Benefits of Healthy Digestive-Enzyme Production

Peak-Performance Benefits

 Increased physical vitality and stamina (helps improve work productivity)

 Enhanced mental clarity and acuity

 Increased ability to get along with other people (permits enjoyment of extensive social and business entertaining)

Hastened recovery from illness, injury, and exertion (includes inflammation from colds, flus, sinusitis, bronchitis, and allergies; athletic and repetitive-stress injuries; minor surgery; and dental procedures)

Health Benefits

- Optimizes digestion

- Improves absorption of nutrients and medications, thereby increasing their effectiveness

- Lowers the risk of inflammatory diseases such as rheumatoid arthritis, colitis, endometriosis, prostatitis, and thyroiditis

- Reduces menstrual cramping

- Decreases the risk of and accelerates healing from heart disease, stroke, and blood clots

- Is used as a complementary therapy for the treatment of cancer

---

Our friend Tom is a natural digestive peak performer. Currently in his mid fifties, he is an international management consultant. He has many of the traits common to high-digestive-enzyme producers: the ability to eat a wide variety of foods from virtually any cuisine (a real benefit when traveling for business or pleasure), tremendous levels of energy, the ability to work, when necessary, sixty to eighty hours per week without tiring, and the stamina to travel internationally, often on short notice. For example, not long ago, Tom received a call from a Scandinavian company to meet with them in Stockholm in just two days. He flew from San Francisco to Stockholm to attend the meeting, spent three days there, and then continued on to the Far East for more meetings. He was back in San Francisco the following week, having traveled virtually around the world in seven days.

Tom has no problem eating and digesting a multiple-course dinner in China, a fat-laden dish in an eastern-European city, and a fiery meal made with chilies in Thailand. His healthy digestive function allows him to consume the local foods and beverages wherever he goes. Tom's ability to socialize in settings where food and drink are a focal point has played a major role in the success he has enjoyed in his professional life. Of course, his affable personality and good sense of humor have also contributed to his success.

Tom is also able to recover rapidly from physical stresses and illness. He can sit in the usually cramped accommodations of an airplane, traveling internationally for as long as fifteen to twenty hours without feeling much stiffness or achiness after the trip. If he goes skiing and strains his muscles a bit, he recovers very quickly. If he comes down with a cold, he either works through it or takes a half day off from work to sleep and is fine the next day. Because Tom can recover so quickly, and has so much energy, he is incredibly productive in his work and also finds the time to enjoy his favorite leisure activities, golfing and hiking.

In contrast, our friend Michael is a perfect example of how the inability to produce adequate pancreatic enzymes can radically curtail one's scope of activities and enjoyment of life. Michael is a small-business owner in his late forties. Several decades ago, he served as an officer in the Vietnam War, where he began to suffer from digestive symptoms that persisted for many years. Michael found himself unable to tolerate the standard military rations without considerable digestive distress, such as bloating, gas, abdominal cramping, and occasional bouts of diarrhea, as well as fullness and discomfort in the region of the pancreas. In the years following his military discharge, Michael became more limited in his food choices and was tired much of the time. Although he has had several offers from potential business partners that would have allowed him to greatly expand his business, he has passed on these opportunities, not wanting to overcommit himself beyond his capabilities.

While Michael enjoys golf and swimming, he basically lives a low-key, quiet life. As a single male, he enjoys the company of women but doesn't date often because he feels he lacks the necessary energy it would take to initiate and sustain an intimate relationship. Unlike Tom's life, Michael's has been bounded by his physiological limitations. He has had to make his food selections carefully so as not to overtax his digestive capability, and has limited his activities so he doesn't exceed his energy reserves.

Over the years, doctors have prescribed a variety of drugs for Michael, which have been only mildly helpful. At our prodding, he finally consulted a physician, who decided that an in-depth diagnostic evaluation was warranted, given the chronic nature of his symptoms. The tests found that Michael was neither producing sufficient pancreatic enzymes nor absorbing his food properly.

There are millions of individuals in the United States today who, like Michael, lack both the digestive firepower and the energy to perform to their own goals and expectations and live life to the fullest. However, even if an individual does not possess a peak performer's digestive capability, the ability to restore this function is within everyone's grasp.

To see if you have the kind of digestive enzyme production needed for peak performance and optimal health, work through the following checklist (photocopy it if you don't want to write in the book), and refer to it as you read through the chapter. Doing so will give you a better idea of how well this function operates in your body.

CHECKLIST: DO YOU HAVE GOOD DIGESTIVE-ENZYME PRODUCTION?

While the diagnosis of pancreatic insufficiency or disease requires medical testing (see page 206), the occurrence of the following symptoms on a chronic basis suggests that your enzyme production may be deficient. You can use the following checklist as a tool to help you assess whether you need to begin to make some dietary changes and take digestive-enzyme supplements as recommended in the next chapter. This checklist can also help you decide whether you should be evaluated by your doctor to determine if you have undetected disease. Your responses to this checklist can provide your physician with a useful tool for diagnosis and a starting point for your medical care. While there is no quantitative grading for this questionnaire, any of the symptoms listed below could be an indicator of pancreatic disease or other digestive problems. If a number of these items apply, you should consult a health care professional and begin to implement a program to restore your digestive health.

Lifestyle/environmental factors

Put a check mark beside those statements that are true for you.

❑ I have a history of excessive alcohol intake.

❑ I feel poorly on a diet high in fats, animal protein, and sugars.

Performance indicators

❑ I feel I am restricted in my ability to eat a wide variety of foods, either in business or social settings.

❑ I experience a low level of energy despite eating adequate amounts of food.

❑ I am slow to recover from injury.

❑ I experience excessive stiffness and/or soreness the day after heavy exercise.

❑ I tire easily from work or play.

❑ I am unable to travel without great fatigue.

❑ I have difficulty thinking clearly and quickly.

Physical indicators

❑ I often suffer from indigestion.

❑ I frequently have abdominal bloating and discomfort after meals, a condition unrelieved by antacids.

❑ I often experience intestinal cramps after eating.

❑ I often experience flatulence after meals.

❑ My food appears relatively undigested and greasy in the stools.

❑ I suffer from chronic diarrhea.

❑ I am frequently constipated, particularly after eating certain foods.

☐ I have difficulty digesting highly spiced and unfamiliar foreign foods.

☐ I often feel tired after a meal.

Medical history

☐ I have a history of chronic pancreatitis.

☐ I have a history of Crohn's disease, ulcerative colitis, or irritable-bowel syndrome.

☐ I have had gallstones.

☐ I suffer from rheumatoid arthritis.

☐ I have a history of vasculitis.

☐ I have a history of endometriosis.

☐ I have food and environmental allergies.

 Now that you have a preliminary understanding of the importance of digestive-enzyme production to peak performance and optimal health, as well as some idea from the checklist of your own functioning in this area, you are ready to decide what to read next. To learn more about the chemistry of digestive enzymes and how they are produced, read the following section. To learn how diet and lifestyle affect digestive-enzyme production, read section 2, on page 176. For a detailed discussion of how digestive-enzyme production affects peak performance, read section 3, on page 187. For a detailed discussion on how digestive-enzyme production affects general health, including specific conditions caused or exacerbated by inadequate digestive-enzyme production, read section 4, on page 200. (Ideally, these latter two sections should be read consecutively, as the effects of digestive-enzyme production on peak performance and health are intricately intertwined.) Finally, for information on how to restore your digestive-enzyme production and how to support healthy digestive function, read chapter 4.

Section 1:
The Chemistry of Enzyme Production

Our bodies produce thousands of different enzymes, all catalyzing different chemical reactions that are crucial to health and survival. These reactions regulate functions as diverse as the production of energy, digestion, the repair of cells, and the elimination of waste products. Thus, enzymes allow us to breathe, digest, grow, heal, perceive with our senses, and reproduce.

Enzymes affect chemical reactions in the following manner: An enzyme acts on another substance, called a substrate, grasping, holding, and binding the substrate with other molecules to help trigger a chemical reaction. Enzymes allow these reactions to proceed more efficiently, making it possible for them to occur with less expenditure of energy. Thus, an enzyme is a catalyst. Relative to the substances they are acting on, enzymes are present only in small amounts; moreover, enzymes are not changed by the biochemical process they help to initiate. Because each enzyme has a unique shape that only fits with a certain substance, the various enzymes have very specific functions. For example, pancreatic enzymes, which are discussed in detail in this chapter, break down very specific types of food. Pancreatic protease enzymes digest only proteins, whereas pancreatic lipase is necessary for the proper digestion of fats, and pancreatic amylase works only on starch molecules.

The Critical Digestive Enzymes

The process of digestion is dependent on several dozen digestive enzymes that are produced by the body at different sites along the digestive tract: in the mouth, stomach, and small intestine. The activation of a digestive enzyme is regulated through changes in the pH (see page 36). Each part of the digestive tract has an optimal range of pH in which the digestive enzymes produced within that site can be activated and will also work most efficiently.

These enzymes break down the foods we consume into particles small enough to pass through the intestinal wall and be absorbed by the cells. It is within the cells that the molecules of food are converted into usable energy. Within the bloodstream, microscopic particles of food are transported to cells throughout the body. The cells rely on a steady supply of nutrients from the blood to produce adenosine triphosphate (ATP), which is the main energy unit of the body. Our body uses ATP to fuel literally hundreds of thousands of chemical reactions. When the pancreas is producing adequate amounts of digestive enzymes, this process repeats itself meal after meal, providing the body with the nutrients needed to produce and sustain energy.

If digestive-enzyme production is diminished, none of the food that we eat can be properly absorbed and assimilated by the body. This concept is often a surprise to many Americans, who assume that if they eat a lot of food, they'll be well nourished and healthy. However, a full plate doesn't always translate into a healthy body and a vital life, particularly if the body is unable to properly use the food we eat due to a lack of adequate digestive enzymes.

THE STAGES OF DIGESTION

Ptyalin, a digestive enzyme found in saliva, begins starch and sugar digestion in the mouth. Sugar and starch break down relatively easily, compared with protein and fats, because of their simple structures. A molecule of table sugar is composed of just two molecules (glucose and fructose), and starch is composed of long chains of glucose connected together.

In comparison, proteins and fats have a more complex structure, and their digestion begins farther down in the digestive tract. Proteins are composed of various combinations of twenty-two amino acids. While the core structure of the amino acids is the same, they vary greatly in their chemical properties and in their effects on the body due to the varying side chains that branch off of every core chain. There are several different kinds of fats commonly found in the foods we eat. Much of our dietary intake of fat is in the form of triglycerides, which are composed of three fatty acids attached to a single molecule of glycerol (an organic alcohol). Phospholipids, an important component of cell membranes, differ from triglycerides in that they contain only two fatty acids and a phosphatidylcholine molecule attached to the glycerol (choline is a B vitamin). Cholesterol, a white, waxy, fatty material, is both found in our foods and produced within the body by the liver.

Most of the digestion occurring in the stomach relates to the breakdown of protein. Protein derived from meat and milk (casein) is particularly tough in texture and is either curdlike or fibrous. The digestion of protein in the stomach begins with the action of the enzyme pepsin. Pepsin is activated only in an acid environment. The necessary level of acidity is provided by the hydrochloric acid (HCl) secreted by the stomach, which allows digestion to proceed at an optimal pH of 1.8 to 3.5.

It is in the small intestine that the greatest amount of digestion of all types of foods occurs, whether carbohydrate, protein, or fat. The pancreas produces the digestive enzymes amylase, trypsin, and chymotrypsin, which further digest the molecules of protein and starch. Pancreatic lipases begin the digestion of fats. (These enzymes are discussed more fully in the next section.) The liver also secretes bile into the small intestines, which helps to emulsify or break up dietary fat. Water also plays an important role in the digestive process: Molecules of water in the gastrointestinal tract split large molecules of food into smaller, more absorbable units.

THE POWERFUL PANCREATIC ENZYMES

Of all the digestive enzymes, pancreatic enzymes are among the most critical for the absorption of food and maintenance of good health. Pancreatic enzymes are also the most well researched of all the digestive enzymes, showing a wide variety of benefits necessary for health and peak performance.

The pancreas is an organ that lies mostly under the stomach, except for one end, which is tucked into the curve of the upper intestine. Within the pancreas are special glands called acini that secrete digestive enzymes. These enzymes pass through a network of ducts that come together to form the main pancreatic duct and are then secreted into the small intestine. Stored within the pancreas, the digestive enzymes are in an inactive form, preventing them from digesting the organ itself. Once secreted into the intestine, the stored form of trypsin is then activated—which, in turn, activates the other digestive enzymes. Since pancreatic enzymes are activated only in an alkaline environment, pH plays an important role. As discussed in chapters 1 and 2, the necessary alkalinity is attained through the secretion of bicarbonate-rich digestive juices, also produced by the pancreas. The pancreas secretes about 2.5 quarts of pancreatic juice each day.

The pancreas also contains the islets of Langerhans, which secrete important hormones including insulin, which regulates the level of sugar in the blood. Insulin is a protein that binds with sugar molecules and allows them to pass from the blood, across the cell membrane, and into the cell, where the sugar is used as the main source of energy for the cell. When insulin production is insufficient to clear sugar from the bloodstream, hyperglycemia or diabetes mellitus can result.

PANCREATIC ENZYMES AND DIGESTION

Pancreatic digestive enzymes are capable of breaking down all types of food: carbohydrate, protein, and fat. The protein-digesting (proteolytic) pancreatic enzymes include trypsin, chymotrypsin, and carboxypeptidase. These enzymes can digest up to 300 g of protein per hour. In the final stages of digestion, pancreatic and other enzymes break protein down into approximately twenty amino acids, which can then be readily absorbed into the bloodstream through the small intestine. These amino acids are then recombined into the various proteins needed to maintain both the structure and health of the body. For example, proteins are an important structural component of tissues as diverse as hair, skin, blood, and bones. Important body chemicals such as antibodies, hormones, and all enzymes (not just digestive ones) are also composed of protein.

Pancreatic amylase digests starches, breaking them down into simple sugars. Starch-digesting enzymes can process up to 300 g of carbohydrate per hour. The pancreatic lipases help break down fats, oils, and cholesterol. Fat-digesting enzymes can digest up to 175 g of fat per hour. Fats are first emulsified (split into tiny particles) within the small intestine by the action of bile salts from the gallbladder. Bile is a thick, bitter fluid secreted by the liver and stored in the gallbladder. It is composed of lecithin, cholesterol, bile salts, and bile pigments. Pancreatic lipase also continues the digestion of fat within the small intestine. Lipases break down large fat globules, but this action is much more effective when the fat has been emulsified first.

Animal studies suggest that the amount of pancreatic enzymes varies in relation to the composition of the diet. For example, a study published in 1943 in the *American Journal of Physiology* found that laboratory animals produce a range of specific pancreatic digestive enzymes in response to eating certain foods. The researchers fed rats a constant diet high in carbohydrates and observed an increased production of amylase. Rats on a high-protein diet produced higher levels of trypsin. Similarly, when you drink a glass of orange juice, your body produces amylase to digest the sugars. And when you eat a shrimp cocktail, the pancreas produces proteolytic enzymes to break down the protein.

Research studies have confirmed that enzymes are absorbed from the intestinal tract into the circulation intact and still in active form. In one such study, reported in 1997 in *Clinical Pharmacology and Therapeutics*, twenty-one healthy volunteers were given preparations of the enzymes bromelain and trypsin four times a day for four days. Researchers found that the blood levels of the enzymes rose with the administration of the supplemental enzymes.

Not only can supplemental digestive enzymes be absorbed into the circulation, but the body has a method to recycle and even reuse its own pancreatic enzymes. A study published in 1975 in *Science* found that intact digestive-enzyme molecules, produced by the pancreas and excreted into the intestines, can be reabsorbed, stored within the body, and reused as needed. This is an excellent example of the economy with which the body functions by reducing the demand on the pancreas to constantly produce new enzymes. Thus, the use of supplemental digestive enzymes, over time, will actually help to restore pancreatic function by reducing the workload of the pancreas.

PANCREATIC ENZYMES AND INFLAMMATION

A second important function of pancreatic digestive enzymes is to facilitate recovery from tissue damage or injury. All traumatic injuries are characterized by an inflammatory response. Similarly, internal injury to tissues due to such stressors as infectious bacteria, viruses, allergens, and toxins can also cause inflammation. Inflammation of an injured area is characterized by swelling, heat, stiffness, a reduced range of motion, and pain on weight bearing or use of the extremity or joint. No matter where the site of the injury, the physical manifestations are the same.

When an area of the body becomes inflamed, the blood vessels and capillaries in the injured area begin to dilate (expand), allowing fluids carrying the body's own healing substances to reach the area quickly. At the same time, the capillary walls become more permeable, and fluids force their way into the surrounding tissue, causing congestion. Very quickly more fluid and waste accumulate than the area can handle. Helper cells seal off the damaged area, creating fibrin clots made of protein, to prevent the spread of bacteria and toxins to surrounding areas. The result is blockage of the blood and lymph vessels, leading to redness, swelling, heat, pain, and the formation of excess fluids in the tissue (edema).

The inflammatory process is controlled by numerous digestive enzymes, especially the body's own pancreatic protein-digesting (proteolytic) enzymes, which eliminate debris at the injury site and initiate the repair of tissue. These enzymes also break up the fibrin, which is made of protein, so that it can be excreted. Digestive enzymes keep the pathological process from spreading and considerably reduce the duration of the injury by speeding up the healing process. Thus, abundant production of digestive enzymes can greatly limit the severity and scope of inflammation diseases or external injuries.

SUMMARY

Digestive enzymes, particularly pancreatic enzymes, are catalysts that break down the foods we consume into molecules that can pass through the intestinal wall and be absorbed by our cells. The cells then convert these molecules into energy. Pancreatic enzymes are essential in the process of converting food into energy. A second important function of these enzymes is to break up inflammation caused by trauma, infections, allergens, and toxins and to initiate the repair of tissue; therefore, these enzymes help the body recover from injuries.

SECTION 2:
HOW DIET, THE AGING PROCESS, AND LIFESTYLE AFFECT DIGESTIVE-ENZYME PRODUCTION

MANY FACTORS CAN affect digestive function, causing it to become less efficient. The production of pancreatic enzymes, in particular, may decline as a consequence of the normal aging process, poor dietary habits, excessive alcohol intake, and pancreatic and gallbladder diseases. Each of these factors is discussed in detail in this section.

Diet and Eating Habits

The hard-to-digest standard American diet takes its toll on the digestive health of millions of individuals. As people change and adapt their eating habits to the reality of their stressful workload and family responsibilities, they are less likely to prepare the healthful meals, complete with enzyme-rich fresh fruits and vegetables, that medical groups like the American Heart Association and the American Cancer Society recommend. In her clinical practice, Susan has seen thousands of patients who do not have the digestive health of their own parents and grandparents, who were raised in an era when synthetic and fast foods were much less prevalent. Meals were still prepared from scratch at home, and much of the food purchased, from grocery stores or roadside stands, was fresh from the farm.

The foods in the standard American diet, which is high in saturated fats, sugars, and animal protein, place a great demand on the pancreas. Hard-to-digest foods force the pancreas to secrete higher levels of digestive enzymes in order to break them down into small enough units that they can be absorbed across the small-intestinal wall and used as fuel by the cells. Overworking the pancreas by eating pizza, cheeseburgers, bacon, French fries, donuts, and chocolate cake can compromise pancreatic digestive-enzyme function and accelerate the aging of this organ. These foods are laden with saturated fats, red-meat protein, and sugar, which is ubiquitous in commercially prepared foods. People assume that if they are avoiding desserts and sweet baked goods such as cakes, pies, Danish pastry, and cookies, they have eliminated sugar from their diet. But sugar and assorted sweeteners are also added to crackers, breakfast cereals, canned soups, ketchup, and pickles, among other dietary staples.

Digesting a meal high in fat, protein, and sugar requires a lot of energy, which is why people often feel tired after a heavy meal. Symptoms of indigestion can be an early sign that the pancreas is stressed and unable to meet the demands being placed on it. Over time, an improper diet can increase the risk of diseases such as diabetes and pancreatitis.

Furthermore, the time pressures on many Americans, both in the business world and in family life, result in many meals being eaten hastily. People eat on the run, grabbing a quick bite at their desk or between appointments in their car. The millions of people who frequent fast-food outlets are testament to the hurried pace of modern life. Between these less-than-ideal meals, people are constantly snacking on foods and bever-ages that contain refined sugar, white flour, trans fatty acids (partially hydrogenated oils found in almost all cookies, crackers, and energy and breakfast bars), and caffeine. Very little enzyme-rich, fresh food is con-sumed, creating stress on the pancreas, which leads to a reduction in its functional capability and premature aging. As a result, Americans in record numbers suffer from digestive complaints, low energy levels, and poor health. Look in any pharmacy or supermarket and you will be aston-ished to see all the products being sold to treat digestive complaints.

A lifetime of unhealthy eating habits can accelerate the normal aging of the pancreas as well as the rest of the digestive tract. The following story illustrates this point. Some years ago we became acquainted with an affluent retired couple, Charles and Marie. After spending many decades working hard at busy and successful careers, they embarked on a life of leisure and travel, taking four or five cruises a year. They both enjoyed the endless procession of meals on shipboard, starting with eggs Benedict and fresh-baked rolls and pastries for breakfast. This would be followed by lunches and dinners that included delicacies such as richly sauced red meat and seafood entrées, caviar and patés, cheese trays and decadent homemade desserts. They both particularly enjoyed the fine cuts of beef, and the delicious chocolate confections served at the end of the meals. Charles also frequently sampled the fine wines offered with the various courses. Finally, at tea time, there were trays of tarts and savory sand-wiches to snack on.

However, Marie and Charles differed significantly in their ability to handle such rich fare. Marie is a true digestive peak performer. She has always been able to eat these meals aboard the cruise ships without suf-fering any digestive discomfort, and without the typical ten- to twenty-pound weight gain that many people incur on cruises. Charles was not as fortunate. Although he endeavored to eat the same high-stress diet as his wife, his digestive function was not nearly as strong. He was constantly complaining about bloating, gas, and heartburn, which worsened over time. After several years of feasting aboard cruise ships, he was diagnosed with gallstones and deteriorating liver health, with an elevation noted in his liver enzymes. After undergoing gallbladder surgery, Charles was warned by his physician to change his eating habits by adopting a low-fat, vegetarian-emphasis diet. But Charles ignored his doctor's warning and continued his life of feasting and leisure. Several years after his gallbladder surgery, he was diagnosed with pancreatic cancer. He died within three months of diagnosis.

The story of Charles and Marie illustrates another important point: People who live together often have differing digestive capabilities. One of the partners in a relationship often has a much healthier digestive system than the other. Often, the person with the "less sturdy" digestive capability will try to keep up with the stronger partner, with disastrous consequences. This is a difficult situation for many people because eating together provides enjoyment and is the social focus of many people's lives. For busy working couples, eating out or bringing home a takeout meal may be the only time they spend together. Unfortunately, this can result in significant digestive stress for the person with the weaker digestive system and can eventually result in digestive problems as well as chronic fatigue and illness.

▲▲ If you lack the digestive stamina of your partner, always have dishes available that are easy for you to digest and do not put a strain on your digestive system.

LIFESTYLE

Several other lifestyle factors besides diet and eating habits affect digestive-enzyme production, including caffeine, drugs, alcohol, and stress, as well as pancreatic disease, which may be caused by these factors. We discuss these various lifestyle factors in this section.

Stimulants

As the production of pancreatic enzymes begins to diminish, people often compensate for the decline in their energy by increasing their use of stimulants such as caffeine. Chemicals like caffeine hype the system, usually by overstimulating the adrenals and the nervous system. However, these stimulants by themselves do not create or sustain long-term energy. Midlife and older people who are currently in the workforce often increase their use of stimulants to help them keep up with the demands of their jobs. The National Coffee Association, based in New York, stated in their 1997 Winter Coffee Highlights report that people between the ages of fifty and fifty-nine consume the most coffee, followed by those aged forty to forty-nine, and then by those aged sixty to sixty-nine. Most people aged forty to fifty-nine are performing in the workplace even if they are not producing adequate amounts of energy. Since digestive-enzyme production begins to diminish around the age of forty, stimulants such as caffeine are used to generate the energy needed by midlife people to compete with younger workers, who still have relatively intact pancreatic function and a high level of energy. Other stimulants like nicotine (found in cigarettes and drugs) may also be used by some individuals to bolster their level of energy. However, the use of stimulants to combat fatigue cannot sustain performance over time.

Jeff's and Helen's stories

Jeff typifies the digestive decline that can occur when a person is required to travel frequently for business. A sales manager in his early forties, Jeff traveled between one-third and one-half of the time. His preferred dinner on the road consisted of steaks or chops accompanied by a baked potato filled with butter and sour cream, finished off with pie and ice cream. Eventually, Jeff began to find that eating this customary meal triggered symptoms of heartburn, bloating, and abdominal cramps, and even more importantly, that his energy level was beginning to decline. Taking a red-eye flight for a breakfast meeting was becoming more difficult; energy would flag by midafternoon. It was also hard to maintain his energy and enthusiasm in business meetings that could last into the evening. Although Jeff enjoyed his work, he began to consider finding a less stressful position with lower pay and less responsibility.

Like Jeff, Helen's work required her to travel constantly. As a veteran flight attendant working on cross-country routes, she would eat the peanuts, pretzels, and cookies served to passengers as snack foods. The meals she ate on layovers were usually no more nutritious. She ate chocolate bars and drank caffeinated cola drinks each day for a quick energy boost and favored fast foods such as hamburgers and pizza. By her mid-thirties, she was beginning to suffer from digestive symptoms such as bloating, gas, and indigestion as well as PMS-related fluid retention and mood swings. Moreover, she was finding it increasingly difficult to sustain the energy necessary to perform her job well.

Both Jeff and Helen contacted Susan for a nutritional consultation to relieve their symptoms. Susan worked with each of them to develop dietary programs that would enable them to continue their rigorous travel schedules and still maintain the level of energy necessary to perform their jobs. Both Jeff and Helen began to order more wisely from restaurants, selecting more soups, salads, and vegetable side dishes. When Jeff felt the need for more protein, he ordered salmon or grilled chicken. Helen also began to carry her own snacks when flying, passing up the usual airline snacks in favor of fresh fruit, raw seeds and nuts, and rice crackers. Finally, they both began to take supplemental digestive enzymes with each meal. Within several months, both Jeff and Helen began to experience higher levels of energy, and they found that they were once again able to handle the demands of their work.

▲▲ Millions of people travel regularly as part of their work. Business travel presents its own nutritional challenges. One major problem is that all business activities are concentrated into as short a time as possible. This often means that one is either entertaining or being entertained for breakfast, lunch, drinks, and dinner. Often, this means eating rich meals with wine or other alcoholic beverages. In addition, when businesspeople are away from home with nothing to do after work, they tend to reward themselves with rich meals on their expense account. If you are required to travel frequently for work and are having a hard time handling the stress of eating on the road, always travel with supplemental digestive enzymes. If you tend to be overly acidic, you will also want to travel with alkalinizing agents (see chapters 1 and 2 for more details).

▲▲ If your job requires you to travel extensively, either by car or plane, be sure to bring enzyme-rich snacks like raw sprouted seeds and legumes, which are crunchy and tasteful. Other high-enzyme snacks include carrots and celery sticks, slices of green and red pepper, salads with fresh sprouts, or fresh fruit. These foods will help you maintain your energy much more effectively than the chips, candy bars, cola drinks, coffee, and fast foods that most people eat on the road or in airports.

Alcohol

The excessive use of alcohol stresses many vital organs of the body, including the liver, pancreas, and brain, causing inflammatory changes and destruction at the cellular level. Alcohol increases the risk of acute pancreatitis, a serious inflammatory condition that can become chronic and recurring if alcohol consumption is not curbed.

Because of the high rate of alcohol consumption throughout the world, the potential for disease of the pancreas is enormous. There are over 100 million regular drinkers in the United States alone. About 11 million Americans report heavy alcohol use, and more than half the population are social drinkers. An even more alarming statistic is that among children, alcohol consumption is on the rise. In 1992, an estimated 5 percent of children aged twelve to seventeen consumed alcohol more than fifty days during the year. Individuals with poor pancreatic function should avoid alcohol entirely or only use it on special occasions (birthdays, holidays, and other celebrations). A serving should be limited to one 4 oz. portion of wine.

Fasting

When a person fasts, there is no food in the stomach and therefore no need to produce pancreatic digestive enzymes. In the fasting state, the pancreas becomes relatively inactive, and many functions slow, including enzyme production. An animal research study on the effects of fasting, published in 1977 in the *Proceedings of the Society for Experimental Biology and Medicine*, documented a decline in such basic biochemical processes as the synthesis of pancreatic DNA (deoxyribonucleic acid). Fasting can also cause the pancreas to lose its ability to secrete adequate levels of amylase, a starch-digesting enzyme, and when an individual eats again, the individual may have digestive problems if there is a high amount of starch in the meal. Symptoms include excessive gas, intestinal discomfort, and bloating.

Gas is produced when undigested and unabsorbed nutrients travel to the colon, where the resident bacteria ferment them, producing gas as a by-product. The most common gases produced by bacteria in the intestines are odorless: methane and hydrogen. Poorly digested sulfur-rich proteins—found in beans, onions, garlic, eggs, and meat—produce the odoriferous gases. If soybeans are a regular food in your diet, it is important to make sure that they are thoroughly cooked before eating them. Uncooked soybeans contain a trypsin inhibitor that impedes the digestion of protein.

When a person ends a fast, or dramatically changes his or her diet, the pancreas must adapt to the new conditions by adjusting its secretion of digestive enzymes. For example, when a person eats a high-protein diet, the pancreas secretes up to seven times the normal amount of digestive enzymes capable of breaking down protein. Likewise, if the diet is exceptionally high in starch, the pancreas will secrete up to ten times the necessary amount of amylase. To minimize the stress of change, we recommend that a person alter their diet slowly, not overnight.

Stress

It is important to remember that the process of digestion begins even before we take our first bite of food. As we see and smell the food and think positive thoughts about it, digestive enzymes are already being secreted in the mouth and hydrochloric acid in the stomach. This is known as the cephalic phase of digestion, when the mind and senses trigger the body to prepare to receive food. However, when a person is stressed, these responses are inhibited. Someone who is upset at mealtime may not be able to secrete enough acid or digestive enzymes, and this negative cephalic response can cause poor digestion.

A study published in 1989 in *Digestive Diseases and Sciences* assessed the effect of acute mental stress on the secretion of pancreatic enzymes. Working with twelve healthy fasting volunteers, the researchers had each volunteer swallow tubing, which was then passed through the stomach and into the duodenum (upper intestine). The tubing allowed the researchers to monitor each volunteer's output of pancreatic chymotrypsin. In order to induce mental stress, the volunteers were asked to perform mental arithmetic and solve anagrams for one hour. During the first half hour, there was no significant change in the average chymotrypsin concentration in the duodenum. However, during the second half hour, the concentration of chymotrypsin increased by 74 percent. Then, in a thirty-minute period following the stressful activity, chymotrypsin concentration dropped precipitously, by 42 percent.

Managing stress can do much to improve digestive problems caused by low enzyme production. It is very important to take a moment before starting a meal to relax and prepare to enjoy the foods you are about to eat. When you are calm, you can better savor the flavors and textures of the foods being served as well as receive the health benefits that relaxed eating confers.

Pancreatic disease

The pancreas is very sensitive to the deleterious effects of certain drugs, alcohol, caffeine, and gallbladder disease. All of these factors can predispose an individual to pancreatitis, an inflammatory condition of the pancreas. Pancreatitis can manifest itself in two ways, depending on the speed and intensity of the disturbance. It can manifest in an acute form, known as acute pancreatitis, and in a slower, more insidious form, known as chronic pancreatitis. Both diseases impact pancreatic digestive-enzyme production.

Acute pancreatitis. The principal cause of acute pancreatitis in persons under fifty is alcoholism; but for older patients, the principal cause is cholelithiasis (gallstones). Younger patients tend to be men, whereas older patients are more likely to be women.

The acute form of pancreatitis is characterized by the sudden onset of severe episodes of abdominal pain. The pain is usually located in the region over the pit of the stomach (epigastrium) but may progress and involve the entire abdomen. It is almost invariably accompanied by nausea and vomiting, and fever is often also present.

Acute pancreatitis is characterized by inflammation. Normally, digestive enzymes in the pancreas are stored in a kind of protective shell, in an inactive form, and are only activated when needed in the intestinal tract. In acute pancreatitis, these digestive enzymes are suddenly activated and released within the pancreas itself. Trypsin (a protein-digesting enzyme) begins to break down the pancreas tissue, leading, over time, to the destruction of this organ.

Chronic pancreatitis. With some individuals, acute pancreatitis can progress to a chronic, recurring form. This is often seen in alcoholics. Individuals at high risk often have an intake of alcohol averaging thirteen ounces of liquor or two bottles or more of wine a day. Symptoms, which can last days to weeks, include unremitting abdominal pain with nausea and vomiting. The interval between attacks may progressively shorten until the pain becomes almost continuous. There may be mild jaundice, with dark urine, fat in the stool, or symptoms of diabetes. As the disease progresses, it causes irreversible damage to the pancreas with severe consequences to the health of individuals affected. Supplementation with pancreatic enzymes may be necessary in people with chronic pancreatic disease since their own production of enzymes is impaired with the destruction of the pancreatic tissue.

▲▲ Many people largely ignore digestive distress for years, often treating their symptoms with over-the-counter remedies. By the time they are finally uncomfortable enough to seek medical care, a serious condition like pancreatic insufficiency or even pancreatic cancer may have developed.

▲▲ When symptoms begin to occur and are not readily treatable with over-the-counter medication, or persist despite these medications, it is important to see your physician for a diagnostic evaluation. Be sure that your physician does a complete diagnostic workup including an assessment of pancreatic function. If pancreatic and other digestive functions are showing signs of impairment, it is crucial to begin a therapeutic program, implementing any needed dietary changes as well as the use of digestive enzymes and any nutritional supplements necessary to restore the health of your digestive tract.

THE AGING PROCESS

Pancreatic and other digestive-enzyme production is normally at its peak in children and young adults. But by the time most people reach their forties and fifties, the biochemical aging of the body begins to accelerate and the production of digestive enzymes diminishes. Such peak-performance attributes as the ability to absorb and assimilate food, the ability to suppress inflammation due to injury or disease, or even the ability to ward off the development of cancer begin to be compromised. Susan frequently hears from her patients that foods that were formerly easy to digest suddenly cause digestive distress.

Not only does digestive-enzyme production diminish with age, but all other digestive processes also become less efficient. There is reduced motility of the intestines, which hinders the ability to move food through the digestive tract, increasing transit time (the time it takes for a meal to be thoroughly digested and to pass from the body as feces) and making it more likely that a person will experience cramps, bloating, gas, constipation, diverticulosis (weakening of the intestinal wall), and perhaps even colon cancer.

With age, the stomach also produces less hydrochloric acid, which assists protein digestion by activating pepsin, a digestive enzyme necessary for the breakdown of protein. Hydrochloric acid encourages the flow of bile and pancreatic digestive enzymes and facilitates the absorption of a variety of nutrients, including folic acid, vitamin C, beta-carotene, iron, calcium, magnesium, and zinc. It also prevents bacterial and fungal overgrowth of the small intestine. Research studies have found that 30 percent of U.S. men and women over the age of sixty have atrophic gastritis, a condition in which little or no acid is secreted by the stomach, and that 40 percent of postmenopausal women have diminished gastric acid secretion.

There is, however, a great deal of variation as to the age at which symptoms of pancreatic—and, more generally, digestive—aging begin to manifest themselves. Symptoms of compromised digestive function can occur as early as the childhood or teen years or as late as the eighth or ninth decade of life—or even never, for digestive peak performers. Whenever the signs of diminished pancreatic function appear, it is crucial that the problem be identified and pancreatic function restored for the continued health and well-being of the individual. Even digestive peak performers can finally lose their ability to efficiently digest virtually anything they eat and convert their food into usable energy when they reach old age. Older people in their eighties, nineties, or even hundreds, who have always enjoyed robust health, excellent digestive function, and abundant energy, may find that even they must finally adopt an easier-to-digest diet.

When pancreatic-enzyme production diminishes to the point where individuals begin to experience symptoms that interfere with their ability to function adequately in important areas of their lives, they often seek medical help. These individuals often complain about a reduction in their energy level, decreased mental acuity, or painful inflammatory conditions.

Many of them are concerned that their symptoms will interfere with their ability to earn a living and lead a full and varied life. When Susan takes a health history from such individuals, she finds that they are often too tired to participate in many of their usual activities, such as their normal exercise routine or their usual round of social activities. They will spend more time at home and rest for longer periods of time. As their energy level diminishes, people begin to reduce their expectations of what they are capable of doing or achieving. Luckily, one's diet can be modified to include more enzyme-rich foods, and supplemental digestive enzymes available in health food stores and pharmacies can help to restore physical and mental energy by improving the absorption and assimilation of nutrients. These supplements are discussed in detail in the next chapter.

SUMMARY

The passage of time eventually affects the amount of pancreatic enzymes we produce, but diet and lifestyle are also important factors. The standard American diet, a high level of stress, and the overuse of alcohol, caffeine, and drugs all adversely affect the enzyme production of the pancreas.

SECTION 3:
PANCREATIC ENZYMES AND PEAK PERFORMANCE

ABUNDANT PANCREATIC DIGESTIVE-ENZYME production helps to maintain our physical and mental energy, as well as our productivity on the job. It also allows for varied and pleasurable social and business entertaining. Equally important, sufficient production of pancreatic enzymes is necessary for the prevention of and speedy recovery from minor illnesses, sprains, strains, and even injuries incurred in the workplace.

1 PHYSICAL VITALITY AND STAMINA

2 MENTAL CLARITY AND ACUITY

Abundant physical and mental energy are prerequisites for success in any endeavor. The production of adequate pancreatic enzymes is a crucial link in the production of energy within the body. The link between healthy digestive function and physical and mental energy is not simply a modern concept, originating in Western medicine. It has been recognized for thousands of years in traditional healing models such as Asian medicine and the ancient Indian healing system of Ayurvedic medicine. In these models, individuals with weak digestive function are much more likely to be devitalized and fatigued.

Success in any career depends on having a high level of either physical or mental energy, or both. Abundant pancreatic-enzyme production is needed to assist the body in producing the energy needed to perform at an optimal level at one's job. For example, most professional athletes eat enormous amounts of food in order to meet the energy demands of their nearly constant physical exertion. Abundant pancreatic-enzyme production is needed to convert the large amounts of calories that these individuals consume into usable energy, as well as to help maintain their body mass. Only digestive peak performers can eat steaks, pizza, or several chicken breasts on a daily basis and turn this food into the energy they need to compete in major athletic events. In contrast, people with low pancreatic-enzyme production would normally feel tired and even suffer from indigestion after eating such foods, much less be able to go out and play a professional football, basketball, or baseball game.

Because pancreatic enzymes are also among our body's most potent natural anti-inflammatory substances, they provide professional athletes with another benefit: the ability to recover quickly from traumatic injuries incurred during either practice sessions or competitive events or games. They also enable athletes to recover from periods of hard physical exertion and be able to compete effectively the following day.

Many nonathletic professions also require a high level of physical energy for success. For example, politicians, businesspeople who travel frequently, and entertainers on tour all require vitality, stamina, and the ability to convert the food eaten on airplanes and in hotel restaurants throughout the world into usable energy.

Mental acuity and sharpness depend as much as physical energy on adequate pancreatic-enzyme production. Our brains use 20 percent of our body's total energy. The millions of individuals who are engaged in careers requiring a high level of cognitive function depend, for their very livelihood, on a constant and abundant source of energy from the food that they ingest. Thus, peak performance in any intellectual endeavor is dependent on healthy digestive function as well as native intelligence.

Over the years, we have both known a number of scientists, researchers, authors, and physicians who have attained the highest levels of success in their fields. Like professional athletes, these individuals have very high energy requirements, which they are able to fulfill, in part, because of their healthy digestive function. Susan has found that a surprising number of these individuals eat what would be considered medically unhealthy diets. Yet, like professional athletes, they are able to digest and convert the food they eat into the high level of mental energy that their demanding careers require without any obvious signs of pancreatic weakness, such as indigestion or inflammatory diseases.

4 THE ABILITY TO GET ALONG WITH OTHER PEOPLE

Many of our social interactions involve the sharing of meals with our business associates, friends, and family. Sufficient digestive-enzyme production is necessary for successful participation in these gatherings. Diminished pancreatic-enzyme production can limit the range and types of social interactions in which you can participate and even reduce the number of people with whom you feel comfortable spending time. A person with weak digestive function may instinctively avoid unfamiliar settings and cuisines, limiting their travels and experience to more comfortable settings, which they can count on not to stress their limited digestive capabilities.

For example, the capacity to enjoy many different types of cuisine is almost a prerequisite for a political career. You shouldn't even think of going into politics if you don't have a cast-iron stomach and tremendous digestive capability. Every politician on the campaign trail has to eat the food of the constituency that he or she is wooing. This can mean eating knishes in the Jewish neighborhood, egg rolls in the Chinese section of town, and kielbasa in the Polish neighborhood. We still remember a photo of Bob Dole stuffing down a huge "Dagwood-style" sandwich with ease during the 1996 presidential campaign. This is a feat that many individuals half his age couldn't accomplish. Likewise, those individuals engaged in careers that require frequent socializing—such as public relations, sales, and even the diplomatic corps—face similar challenges as they attend endless rounds of cocktail parties, banquets, and other formal occasions where rich and hard-to-digest food is the staple.

Businesspeople whose work requires them to travel frequently often face the same challenges. Business travel often includes lavish meals given or sponsored by the visitor or host. It is not unusual to have business meetings preceded or followed by a large breakfast buffet, lunch at the country club, *and* dinner at the new restaurant in town—three large, hard-to-digest meals in one day.

Executives working abroad must adapt not only to foreign foods, but to different traditions surrounding meals. In Spain, little plates of hors d'oeuvres called tapas are served all evening, with dinner not served until eleven o'clock or midnight. In the Middle East, dinner is also eaten later in the evening. Eating late can be very stressful for someone with marginally functional digestive capability. The digestive organs need to rest at night, and going to bed on a full stomach can leave a person feeling exhausted the next morning. A patient of Susan's attended a Persian wedding at which only nuts and dried fruits were served during the hours before midnight. The actual wedding dinner, a lavish buffet with many highly spiced dishes, was served at 1:30 A.M. This heavy meal was a challenge to Susan's patient; she needed to get up early in the morning and be fresh and alert for her job.

▲▲ If your job or social life involves frequent attendance at events that include hard-to-digest food, be sure to load up on the enzyme-rich salads, fresh fruit, and vegetable side dishes. Avoid the heavy meat courses, butter, cheese, and desserts, which put excessive strain on the pancreas (leave those foods for the digestive peak performers). In addition, the regular consumption of supplemental digestive enzymes both before and during your meal when attending banquets, cocktail parties, and other festive events can help you to prevent indigestion and maintain your energy level, allowing you to enjoy these events more.

7 SPEEDY RECOVERY FROM ILLNESS, INJURY, AND EXERTION

One of the hallmarks of peak performance is the ability to recover rapidly from physical stresses of all sorts, whether due to illness, physical exertion, long periods of immobility, accidents, injury, or even surgical procedures. Abundant production of pancreatic enzymes helps the body to heal more rapidly from the inflammation caused by virtually any physical trauma, and reduces the stiffness and achiness that occur after exercise or even after long hours of sitting at a computer or in a car or airplane while traveling.

The important role that abundant pancreatic-enzyme production confers is dramatically illustrated by healthy children. Not only do children have the abundant digestive enzyme production that allows them to eat pizza, hamburgers, potato chips, ice cream, and cake, all at the same meal (a feat that few adults over the age of fifty can do without indigestion), but their strong pancreatic function also allows them to heal rapidly. They are able to recover quickly from the falls, spills, and tumbles that occur while playing games and participating in sports. Children also remain active all day, moving from one activity to another, and experience very little, if any, stiffness or soreness the following day.

Similarly, adults who maintain a high level of pancreatic digestive-enzyme production are more likely to be able to stay active and recover reasonably quickly from a weekend athletic event or from sitting in a cramped position on an airplane during a seventeen-hour international flight. Unfortunately, most people lose their rapid-recovery capability as their pancreatic digestive-enzyme production begins to diminish at midlife. In her practice, Susan hears a continuous litany of complaints about aches, pains, and stiffness from her middle-aged and older patients. Luckily, the use of supplemental digestive enzymes can shorten recovery time and help limit the effects of injuries incurred from athletic activities or other types of physical trauma in the many individuals who have lost this important peak-performance function. The use of digestive enzymes can also help to reduce joint and muscle stiffness and achiness during periods of prolonged travel.

Sports injuries

The benefits that supplemental pancreatic digestive enzymes provide in helping to limit the extent of traumatic injury and in promoting healing are so well known in sports medicine that they are routinely used in America and abroad by athletes at all levels of competition, both prophylactically and as part of treatment once a bruise or rupture of tissue has occurred.

Numerous studies confirm the effectiveness of pancreatic enzymes in treating sports injuries, regardless of the type of injury or its severity. In a study published in 1987 in the *South African Medical Journal*, twenty-three patients with soft-tissue damage from sports injuries were given proteolytic-enzyme treatment. Researchers noted that patients on enzymes, as compared with those not treated, experienced quicker recovery from bruising. Function of the injured site was restored more rapidly, and the athletes more quickly regained their fitness to resume play. The researchers suggested that the use of enzyme treatment to accelerate healing could be valuable in maintaining morale and personal fitness as well as performance skills.

In another study, appearing in the *British Journal of Clinical Practice*, 100 patients with fractures of the hand were divided into two groups, with one group receiving pancreatic-enzyme treatment and the other remaining untreated. The dosage was two tablets every four hours, taken half an hour before meals, for five days. Researchers measured the subjects' ability to move the affected fingers, since this reflected the degree of swelling, pain, and function of the joint and tendon. Over 80 percent of those patients receiving enzymes showed a significant improvement in mobility, as compared with only 50 percent in the untreated group.

Further, in a pair of studies conducted at a clinic in Wiesbaden, Germany, and presented at the FIMS World Congress of Sports Medicine in 1990, pancreatic enzymes were given to patients undergoing surgery for sports injuries. In the first study, 80 patients having knee surgery were divided into two groups, one treated with enzymes postoperatively. These patients experienced a significantly more rapid reduction in edema (retention of fluid in the tissues) and a more rapid return to complete mobility. In the second study, 120 patients who were undergoing surgical treatment of fractures were divided into two groups. The patients in one group received enzyme treatment, beginning five days before the operation. Treated patients had significantly less preoperative edema and notably less pain and edema on the day of the operation. In a comparison of the two studies, the researcher concluded that enzyme treatment was most beneficial when begun before admission to the hospital, as it reduces symptoms, better prepares the patient for surgery, and allows patients to leave the hospital earlier.

Many professional athletes use pancreatic enzymes prophylactically, anticipating that they will sustain physical wear and tear during a sporting event. They cannot afford to sustain an injury that would incapacitate them or force them to curtail their playing time. Periods of forced inactivity can mean large financial losses to highly paid athletes, their teams, and their sponsors if they miss tournaments, play-off games, or infrequent events like the Olympics.

In a clinical trial published in 1960 in the *Practitioner*, 494 boxers with cuts, hematomas (blood clots), bruising, superficial laceration, and sprains of the finger joints were given enzyme treatment. Half of the group took enzymes before boxing, while the rest were given a placebo. Prophylactic use of the enzyme preparation resulted in a 50 percent reduction in bruising and an 11 percent reduction in the incidence of hematomas. Boxers who received lacerations were able to return to the ring as soon as one to two weeks after injury, as opposed to the four weeks that it normally takes to recover from such trauma. Hematomas and bruises treated with enzymes resolved even more rapidly, clearing in just four to five days.

▲▲▲ The results of these studies suggest that taking enzymes prophylactically (before the event, as a preventive measure) or while engaging in an intense physical activity offers great benefit for those people who engage in sporadic intense physical exertion. Several days before engaging in competitive athletic activities that require maximum effort (like a fun run) or physical contact (like touch football or pickup basketball games) or that result in unavoidable falls (like skiing, skateboarding, or rollerblading), take supplemental digestive enzymes. The same advice holds for those who enjoy active vacations centered on skiing, bicycling, or hiking. Likewise, for those who engage in intense activities such as gardening, shoveling snow, or strenuous home repair, a routine program of using enzymes prophylactically or therapeutically can reduce or eliminate day-after stiffness or soreness.

▲▲▲ Baby boomers are particularly prone to accidents and injuries while engaging in strenuous physical activity. In fact, according to a May 24, 1999 article in *Newsweek* entitled "The Jock vs. the Clock," sports-related injuries in individuals between the ages of twenty-five and sixty-four have increased by 18 percent between 1990 and 1996. This is due in part to the tendency of baby boomers to resist the notion of their own physical aging. They often balance their intense work schedules with sporadic, aggressive physical exercise. If you do sustain an accident or injury, immediately begin an aggressive program of enzyme supplementation using a combination of bromelain, papain, and/or pancreatic enzymes (see chapter 4 for specific recommendations) to reduce the inflammation and facilitate the repair process. Continue this program until the inflammation is eliminated and the injury is healed. You will be back in action much sooner and have less downtime, especially as you get older.

Repetitive stress injuries

According to a statement by the administrator of the Occupational Safety and Health Administration that appeared in the May 26, 1995, issue of the OSHA Compliance News, the fastest-growing occupational health hazard in the United States is injury resulting from repetitive stress. The growth rate of these injuries is so rapid that the National Institute for Occupational Safety and Health predicts that approximately 50 percent of the workforce will suffer some form of cumulative trauma disorder (CTD) by the year 2000. CTD is an umbrella term that includes all types of work-related repetitive-stress injuries to the muscles, nerves, and tendons of the upper body. The medical conditions that develop from repetitive stress are chronic back pain, tendonitis, bursitis, frozen shoulder, epicondylitis (more commonly known as tennis or golfer's elbow), and carpal tunnel syndrome, the wrist disorder that can cause numbness, tingling, and severe, incapacitating pain. In addition, chronic conditions that typically impair performance on the job, such as osteoarthritis and rheumatoid arthritis, are also worsened by repetitive stress.

Repetitive-stress injuries are incurred in occupations or fields as diverse as computer programming or data entry, meat cutting and packing, assembly line work, grocery scanning, painting, telemarketing, and dental hygiene. The parts of the body affected by these conditions tend to become chronically inflamed, with pain and swelling at the primary location of the injury. Many hobbies, such as knitting and sewing, and sports activities, such as tennis and golf, require repetitive motions, so their practitioners may also be prone to these types of injuries. The economic costs of these CTDs are very high. BusinessWeek magazine reports that the lost earnings and medical costs of these injuries are in excess of $27 billion annually. For carpal tunnel syndrome alone, the costs of medical treat-ment, surgical procedures, lost time from work, and rehabilitation expenses are estimated to be $25,000 to $60,000 per incidence. For many people, the injuries are so debilitating that they are unable to continue with their current jobs or to participate in their favorite sports for pro-longed periods of time.

Unfortunately, very little emphasis has been placed on healing the damage caused by repetitive-stress injuries. Most people who alter or eliminate the repetitive motions that caused the injury are still unable to reduce or eliminate the pain, swelling, and discomfort in the affected area. In all of these cases, digestive enzymes can play a powerful healing role. Pancreatic enzymes and plant-based enzymes such as bromelain and papain, which are discussed in the following chapter, are very effective anti-inflammatory agents. Used aggressively, these enzymes can be very effective in reducing pain at the site of the injury and promoting healing and recovery of function.

The therapeutic benefit of enzymes was corroborated in an interest-ing medical study published in 1973 in *Clinical Medicine* of individuals suf-fering from tenosynovitis of their arms due to injury incurred in their work, which required repetitive motion for many hours each day. Symptoms resolved much more rapidly in workers who were treated with digestive enzymes than in untreated workers.

▲▲ Individuals with repetitive-stress injuries or joint or muscle con-ditions aggravated by repetitive stress will heal more readily if supplemental digestive enzymes are taken as often as four times per day until symptoms begin to resolve. See the next chapter for specific treatment regimens.

Minor surgery and dental procedures

Another area where enzymes can play a significant role in healing and recovery time is before and after minor outpatient surgeries and dental procedures, which have increased dramatically in recent years. According to the U.S. National Center for Health Statistics, there were over 28 million outpatient operations performed in 1994 in hospitals and free-standing surgical centers (not including dentistry, abortions, podiatry, birthing, family planning, pain blocks, or other small procedures). In addition, there were over 45 million dental surgeries and tooth extractions in 1990 (the last year for which data are available), according to the American Dental Association.

While considered minor, these operations and procedures can cause a great deal of pain, swelling, and discomfort, with recovery times lasting up to seven days. However, by using enzymes both pre- and postoperatively, the inflammatory response is significantly diminished, lessening pain and swelling and enhancing the body's ability to heal. Enzymes can be used in conjunction with any prescribed antibiotics, painkillers, or hot or cold compresses.

▲▲ Acute illnesses, repetitive-stress injuries incurred on the job or while participating in sports, or trauma from surgical procedures should be treated aggressively with digestive enzymes to limit inflammation and promote rapid and efficient healing. Begin enzyme therapy several days prior to surgery or immediately once an acute illness or repetitive-stress injury begins to become symptomatic. These conditions should never be allowed to proceed to a chronic state, where recovery is much more prolonged and difficult to achieve. The immediate therapeutic use of digestive enzymes can save people weeks or even months of disability and pain.

Colds, flus, bronchitis, sinusitis, and allergies

Peak performance—and even the ability to just show up at work or social engagements—is significantly hampered by common respiratory illnesses. Millions of Americans, both children and adults, suffer from as many as four to six colds per year, or have allergy symptoms to common triggers such as pollens, grasses, and mold that can drag on for months. The symptoms that accompany these conditions can seriously hamper a person's ability to fulfill their job or household and family responsibilities, much less perform at optimal levels. Although considered minor illnesses, colds, flus, bronchitis, and allergies often force those affected to take time off from work or abstain from athletics or social activities. Moreover, colds and flus are one of the most common reasons for children to miss school, and constant absenteeism due to these conditions can greatly hamper a child's ability to learn and keep up with the rest of the class.

In her practice, Susan often sees people who have had acute sinus conditions, colds, and flus that have taken anywhere from two to six weeks to be completely resolved, despite the use of prescription or over-the-counter drugs, which often simply substitute one set of lingering symptoms for another and do not cure the underlying causes. These conditions are truly major success saboteurs.

As mentioned in chapters 1 and 2, there are four functions necessary for combating colds, flus, bronchitis, sinusitis, middle-ear infections, and allergies: good buffering capability (the ability to alkalinize), the ability to suppress inflammation through the production of pancreatic enzymes, healthy detoxification, and the ability to keep our cells and tissues well oxygenated.

In chapters 1 and 2 we discussed the role of the highly acidic, inflammatory diet that most Americans eat in triggering respiratory infections and allergies. When respiratory tissues are inflamed from either infection or allergy, the result is nasal congestion, sore throat, swollen and painful sinuses, itching and tearing of the eyes, fluid in the middle ears, and excess bronchial secretions that lead to coughing. Unfortunately, while over-the-counter drugs can help to suppress coughs, reduce fever, and dry up nasal congestion, they often produce equally unpleasant side effects such as racing heart, drowsiness, and feeling light-headed or drugged.

One of the most effective ways to suppress respiratory inflammation is by taking supplemental pancreatic enzymes as well as other natural anti-inflammatory substances such as plant-based digestive enzymes like papain, which is derived from papayas, and bromelain, which is derived from pineapples. One study, published in *Drugs Under Experimental and Clinical Research*, examined the therapeutic effect of a plant-based digestive enzyme product used in combination with an antibiotic on patients with respiratory illnesses such as chronic bronchitis and pneumonia. The addition of the digestive enzyme to the treatment regimen improved the absorption of the antibiotics and increased their level in the lungs, thereby improving the efficacy of the antibiotics. In addition, more of the patients on enzyme therapy had total resolution of their symptoms. There were also far fewer patients who failed to respond to the combined therapy than to drug treatment alone. Enzyme therapy was found both to reduce the inflammation of the respiratory tissue and to help suppress coughing.

In a clinical study involving patients with chronic bronchitis, reduction of coughing was noted after ten days of enzyme therapy. Another research study found that 87 percent of patients undergoing treatment for sinusitis with digestive-enzyme therapy had a significant reduction of their symptoms. Susan has seen similar results in her own practice, with many patients experiencing dramatic relief from long-standing sinus conditions after using supplemental digestive enzymes.

A guide to rapid recovery from colds and flus

We know two digestive peak performers, both in their mid-fifties, who have described to us their amazingly quick recovery from colds, runny noses, and sore throats during the past year. At the first signs of a cold or flu, they leave the office and go home to take a rest or nap and eat lightly and go to bed early. They are normally able to resolve their symptoms rapidly and without the use of drugs and be back at the top of their game in one to two days rather than the two to six weeks that many other people require. Their instinctive, and obviously successful, strategy in dealing with these minor illnesses plays to their innate strength. They allow the digestive enzymes that they both abundantly produce to reduce the signs of respiratory inflammation. By immediately reducing their food intake, they can use their digestive enzymes to reduce inflammation instead of to digest a rich meal. These individuals also tend to be naturally alkaline; therefore, they have excellent buffering capability and are able to neutralize the excess acidity seen with infection and allergies, and their strong immune systems are able to overcome any exposure to bacteria or viruses.

If you tend to produce low levels of pancreatic enzymes and are prone to colds, flus, sinusitis, middle-ear infections, bronchitis, and allergies, it is very helpful to use supplemental digestive enzymes at the first sign of any of these conditions. To get the most benefit from these powerful anti-inflammatory enzymes, eat lightly for the first twelve to forty-eight hours after the onset of symptoms, mostly soups and steamed vegetables. In addition, be sure to reduce your level of activity and rest or nap. Finally, consume large amounts of water. These measures should help to significantly reduce your symptoms in one to two days. In addition, improving your acid/alkaline balance, promoting healthy detoxification, and following a program to increase the oxygen levels within your cells and tissues will help to improve your resistance to respiratory conditions.

▲▲ If you are prone to respiratory conditions and tend to travel frequently, or are involved in stressful work or recreational activities, be sure to always have an emergency kit with you that contains supplemental digestive enzymes as well as the other cold remedies described in this book, such as sodium and potassium bicarbonate, colloidal silver, and anti-inflammatory and anti-infectious herbs such as echinacea and ginger.

Food allergies

The allergic reactions that millions of people experience in response to certain foods as well as environmental allergens such as mold, dust, trees, and pollen can cause uncomfortable and even debilitating symptoms. Common foods such as milk, wheat, eggs, and peanuts can seriously impair the performance capability of affected individuals. Intestinal cramps, food intolerances, brain fog, fatigue, poor physical stamina and endurance, emotional and behavioral upsets, and a variety of other physical symptoms can occur in response to eating foods that one is allergic to.

Digestive enzymes can help to reduce the allergic reactions that some people have to certain foods. When a person lacks sufficient digestive enzymes, large molecules of incompletely digested protein can be absorbed through the small intestine and trigger an allergic reaction. The immune system is unable to respond appropriately and reacts to improperly digested food as a foreign substance, which can initiate an allergic, inflammatory reaction. This occurs either directly at the intestinal wall or creates a systemic reaction, resulting in fatigue, inflammation and swelling in various tissues like the joints or thyroid, headaches, or even psychiatric disturbances.

As we age, there is a greater likelihood of developing these allergic reactions to various foods as the production of our anti-inflammatory digestive enzymes diminishes. Susan often sees patients in their forties and fifties who had previously been able to eat wheat or dairy products (statistically, two of the most allergy-producing foods) suddenly become unable to tolerate them. While this is a reasonably common occurrence as people reach midlife, it can also occur in much younger individuals. Many young children, teenagers, and adults in their twenties and thirties have food allergies. Research studies have linked food allergies to conditions that typically affect younger individuals such as attention deficit disorder, chronic fatigue, behavioral disorders, and respiratory conditions. All of these conditions can impair the performance capability of younger individuals, affecting their ability to learn, enjoy good social relations, and even participate in the type of vigorous physical activity that healthy children and young adults normally participate in. Allergies can also be an underlying cause of chronic-fatigue symptoms. Psychiatrists who have done research in the area of nutrition and mental health have even suggested that food allergies may trigger schizophrenia and other mental aberrations. The use of supplemental digestive enzymes is a very important part of any treatment program for individuals with food allergies.

SUMMARY

Because of their role in helping to provide the body with energy, pancreatic enzymes are essential for anyone wanting to perform at the peak of their ability. Abundant enzyme production allows us to be at our best in the world of work and in social interactions, helps to lessen susceptibility to illness, and speeds recovery from physical trauma.

SECTION 4:
DIGESTIVE-ENZYME PRODUCTION AND HEALTH

WHILE PANCREATIC DIGESTIVE enzymes are very useful in maintaining many aspects of peak performance, they can also play an important role in the treatment of various health problems. The benefits of abundant digestive-enzyme production in assisting rapid recovery from accidents and injury as well as colds, flus, and allergies were discussed in the previous section; they are also useful in combating a variety of other inflammatory conditions, as we will discuss in this section.

INFLAMMATORY DISEASES

Inflammation and its accompanying pain are a major component of a number of diseases, including rheumatoid arthritis, interstitial cystitis, Crohn's disease, endometriosis, and colitis. Because pancreatic digestive enzymes help to reduce inflammation, they can be a useful part of the treatment program. While all inflammatory diseases are characterized clinically by pain, heat, swelling, and discomfort, the specific symptoms vary depending on the type of tissue affected.

Rheumatoid arthritis

Research on the benefits of enzymes for the treatment of rheumatoid arthritis has been done in Europe, particularly Germany, where enzymes have been found to be effective in reducing such common symptoms as stiffness, swelling, pain, and limited mobility. Rheumatic disease is characterized by increases in the presence of immune complexes. Circulating immune complexes form when bacteria, viruses, toxic chemicals, and overly large molecules of protein are absorbed into the systemic circulation. These foreign substances stimulate the immune system to produce antibodies, which act as the body's SWAT team. They are shaped like the letter Y and bind to substances they come into contact with. The resulting compounds are known as circulating immune complexes (CICs), large aggregates or clumps of foreign cells (antigens) and antibodies.

While CICs can be free-floating in the blood, sometimes they are deposited in tissue. Once in tissues, they can trigger an inflammatory response, leading to localized tissue destruction. Elevated levels of CICs have been reported in patients suffering from rheumatoid arthritis, Crohn's disease, lupus, and thyroiditis. A study published in 1988 in *Biomedicine & Pharmacotherapy* found that digestive-enzyme treatment can be used successfully to destroy these complexes, thereby neutralizing their detrimental effect on the various tissues of the body, including the joints.

Susan has worked with many arthritis patients, ranging from a preteen boy to a woman in her eighties. However, this condition is more common in women, particularly after midlife. Most of these patients have responded well to nutritional therapy. One such case was a fifty-three-year-old female technical writer who was diagnosed with rheumatoid arthritis two years after going through a difficult menopause. Her job, which required extensive use of a computer, had become extremely difficult due to the pain and swelling in the joints of her hands. She was concerned that her symptoms would make it impossible for her to continue a career that she was both proficient at and enjoyed. However, after several months of nutritional therapy, including dietary modification and the use of digestive enzymes, along with conventional therapy (which had been only moderately helpful on its own), she found that the swelling and pain in her hands greatly subsided.

Crohn's disease

Crohn's disease is another health condition for which the therapeutic use of pancreatic enzymes can produce significant benefits. Like those with rheumatoid arthritis, patients with Crohn's disease test positive for the presence of circulating immune complexes. The extent of the damage these CICs cause within tissue can be limited by the use of digestive enzymes. In Crohn's disease, the affected tissue is usually within the small intestine, primarily the terminal part called the ileum. These tissues can become chronically inflamed and irritated. As the inflamed tissues heal, they can form scar tissue that narrows the intestinal passageway. The onset of the disease is typically around the age of twenty; symptoms include diarrhea, periodic cramping, lower right abdominal pain, fever, malabsorption, possible anemia, a lack of energy, poor appetite, and weight loss.

Endometriosis

A relatively common problem, endometriosis affects 7 to 15 percent of the female population of the United States. Cells comprising the lining of the uterus, called the endometrium, break away and grow outside the uterine cavity, implanting themselves in many locations within the pelvis, including the ovaries, ligaments of the uterus, cervix, appendix, bowel, and bladder. Endometriosis causes inflammation and scarring in the pelvis, resulting in chronic pain and discomfort. Elevated estrogen levels in the body stimulate the growth of these implants with each menstrual cycle. Thus, lowering the level of estrogen within the body is needed to limit the growth and spread of this condition.

In addition, controlling the inflammation within the pelvis is equally important if a woman suffering from this condition is to achieve symptom relief. The use of natural anti-inflammatory agents like digestive enzymes can be quite helpful in this regard. A study published in 1957 in the *American Journal of Obstetrics and Gynecology* found that two plant-based digestive enzymes, papain and bromelain, were quite useful for the relief of menstrual pain. Another study, published in 1978 in *Drugs Under Experimental and Clinical Research*, examined the tissue penetration of several antibiotic drugs and indomethacin, an anti-inflammatory medication, in women with a variety of gynecological complaints, including fibroid tumors of the uterus and ovarian cysts. Some of the women were also given bromelain as part of a controlled study. After administration of the drugs with or without bromelain, all of the women underwent surgical removal of reproductive tissue to treat their primary conditions. The study found that when bromelain was administered concurrently with antibiotics, the absorption and tissue penetration of the antibiotics were significantly increased. This was found to be true in all of the reproductive tissue examined after surgery, including the uterus, fallopian tubes, and ovaries. Enzyme therapy can also benefit male reproductive function. Anti-inflammatory digestive enzymes can also be used to reduce the swelling and pain that occur with prostatitis.

VASCULAR DISEASE

Heart attacks and strokes are caused by obstruction in the arterial blood vessels due to atherosclerosis, which blocks the normal flow of blood to the heart and brain. Atherosclerosis is a condition characterized by deposits of cholesterol on the inner layer of the arterial walls, which results in the formation of fibrous, fatty plaques. Although most people are unaware that inflammation plays an important role in the development of these plaques, current medical research has found a strong association between the development of heart disease and inflammation. The use of pancreatic enzymes can help to limit the inflammatory damage occurring within the blood vessels and to reduce the tendency of platelets to clump or aggregate. Platelets are a component of the blood necessary for normal clotting. The risk of heart attacks and strokes is increased when platelets become abnormally sticky and impair normal blood flow through the blood vessels.

Another risk factor for strokes and heart attacks is elevated levels of cholesterol and triglycerides. Research studies have found that treatment with digestive enzymes can reduce levels of these blood lipids. A study published in 1982 in *Atherosclerosis* examined eighty-four female volunteers, aged sixty-three to ninety-five, in a geriatric ward in a hospital in Sheffield, England. During a twenty-five-day trial, half of the women received a daily enzyme preparation that included lipase, while the other volunteers were given a placebo. On the day after admission to the trial, the volunteers were fed a high-fat, high-cholesterol meal that included eggs and cream. The researchers then recorded the rise in the women's triglyceride and cholesterol levels following the fat-rich meal. This same procedure was repeated at the end of the trial, and changes in triglyceride levels and cholesterol were compared. Levels of triglycerides after meals at the end of the study, as compared with levels at the start, were only 1.25 percent lower in the untreated women, while levels dropped 14.4 percent in those volunteers receiving enzymes. At the end of the trial, researchers also observed lower levels of cholesterol in those women receiving enzymes if their initial levels were relatively high.

Enzyme therapy can also be useful in the treatment of venous thrombosis, a condition in which blood clots form most commonly within the veins of the legs, which can lead to a blockage or occlusion of the affected blood vessel. The greatest danger associated with these types of clots is that they can become detached and move through the circulatory system toward the heart or lungs and cause a life-threatening embolism.

Enzymes have also been found to be effective in treating postthrombotic leg ulcers. According to a study published in 1975 in the *British Journal of Clinical Practice*, ten patients out of a group of nineteen, aged thirty-two to eighty-seven, were treated with an ointment containing protein-digesting enzymes. The other patients in the group were treated with an ointment containing an antibiotic/steroid formulation without enzymes. After six weeks, ulcers receiving the enzyme treatment were more reduced in size and in two cases were completely healed. No comparable improvement was observed in the other group. Enzyme treatment has the further advantage of being relatively painless and requiring less nursing time.

CANCER

The antitumor effect of pancreatic enzymes was discovered at the turn of the century by John Beard, a highly respected embryologist at the University of Edinburgh Medical School. He reasoned that the placenta is, from one perspective, much like a cancer: It is foreign tissue that grows at a fast rate and is highly invasive. Theoretically, it should be rejected by the mother since half the genes in these cells are from the father, making the placenta genetically incompatible.

Then Beard made a remarkable discovery. He observed that in all mammals, the growth of the placenta stops on a certain day. This occurs in humans fifty-six days after conception. For decades, he searched for an explanation. What he found was that in both animals and humans, placental growth ceased when the fetal pancreas began to produce enzymes. Beard concluded that these enzymes were the trigger that stopped the growth.

Based on this conclusion, he then set up experiments to test if the pancreatic enzymes also had a more generalized role of limiting or stopping uncontrolled growth in other parts of the body. Beard injected pancreatic extracts containing high levels of enzymes directly into malignant tumors, treating a total of 170 cancer patients in this manner. Using the enzyme-rich pancreatic digestive juices of newborn lambs, pigs, and calves, Beard found that more than half the patients with advanced cancer survived longer than expected, and in some individuals, cancers disappeared completely.

Between 1902 and 1905, the use of enzymes in the treatment of cancer generated interest within the medical profession. But in 1905, Marie Curie was showing great progress in successfully shrinking tumors with radiation, and her work drew attention away from Beard's efforts. Enzyme therapy was eclipsed by this new work, and it wasn't until the 1960s that there was renewed interest in its benefits.

A current explanation of why pancreatic enzymes are able to reduce tumors is based on a particular defense mechanism of cancer cells. Cancer cells that escape initial attack and destruction by the immune system travel through the circulation and adhere to cell walls and multiply at various sites. In order to avoid detection, they coat themselves with an adhesive fibrin layer fifteen times thicker than that of normal cells. Pancreatic enzymes are able to break down this fibrin layer, reducing inflammation and exposing the cancer cells. This allows the cancer cells to be more easily detected and destroyed by the immune system.

Today, a small number of modern physicians in the United States and Europe follow Beard's theories, prescribing pancreatic enzymes for the treatment of cancer. Like Beard, some of these physicians claim to be able to produce unusually long survival times in their pancreatic cancer patients. In contrast, the cure rates for patients with pancreatic cancer undergoing conventional chemotherapy are abysmal. Most of these patients follow a very rapid downhill course, often dying within sixty to ninety days of diagnosis. (The use of enzymes in cancer treatment is discussed more fully in chapter 4.)

LABORATORY TESTS TO ASSESS PANCREATIC AND GENERAL DIGESTIVE FUNCTION

There are now stool tests that allow physicians to accurately assay pancreatic digestive-enzyme production by measuring levels of enzymes in the stool, as well as monitoring such crucial digestive functions as the digestion of animal proteins, vegetable matter, and starch. These tests also measure the presence of any excess fat in the stool (which is seen with weak pancreatic function), the maintenance of intestinal pH levels, and the adequacy of intestinal immune function. Culturing is also done to monitor the presence of mucus, blood, and both normal and abnormal bacteria, yeast, and fungi. Other tests measure the presence of enzymes in the urine and blood that can be elevated when there is inflammation of the pancreas. Pancreatitis and related gallbladder disease may also be assessed using ultrasound and X-rays.

Urinary analysis is helpful in assessing the health of the pancreas. With acute pancreatitis, there is increased urinary amylase, the result of spillage when the gland is damaged. Values exceeding five times the upper limit of normal are characteristic of acute pancreatitis. Because of intermittent elevations of amylase from hour to hour, a single specimen is inadequate; a two- or six-hour collection is more accurate.

Ultrasound testing, a method of imaging our internal organs, is a simple and noninvasive test to detect pancreatic disease. When pancreatitis is acute, an enlarged, inflamed pancreas is seen in 90 percent of cases. The pancreas will have an irregular shape, sometimes with a dilated pancreatic duct. In the case of acute pancreatitis caused by gallbladder disease, the physician may order an ultrasound of the upper abdomen, which is useful in visualizing the stones.

SUMMARY

The production of abundant pancreatic enzymes not only helps to hasten recovery from trauma, respiratory illnesses, and exertion, but can be useful in the treatment of a number of inflammatory diseases, vascular diseases, and possibly even cancer.

4

RESTORING YOUR DIGESTIVE ENZYMES

IN THIS CHAPTER we will provide you with a very effective and easy-to-follow four-part plan to both improve your digestive capability and help restore your own production of digestive enzymes. In part 1, you will learn which foods supply enzymes in their natural state and how to best prepare these foods for optimal absorption and assimilation. In part 2, we provide you with much valuable information on pancreatic and other digestive enzymes. The use of supplemental digestive enzymes will give you the immediate digestive firepower that you may have lost years ago or perhaps never had. You will also learn how to use these enzymes as powerful anti-inflammatory agents. Part 3 will provide you with information about other natural anti-inflammatory substances that can be used in combination with digestive enzymes to treat a variety of inflammatory conditions. Finally, part 4 provides information about additional digestive aids that can be used to support proper absorption and assimilation of foods and nutrients in individuals with weak digestive function.

PART 1:
THE ENZYME-RICH DIET

FOODS THAT ARE rich in their own natural enzymes provide you with natural digestants and anti-inflammatory chemicals. In this way, the foods themselves aid in the process of digestion and ease the work of the pancreas. There are four steps to eating an enzyme-rich diet:

1. Choose enzyme-rich foods.

2. Avoid foods that stress the pancreas.

3. Drink blenderized drinks if indicated.

4. Eat pureed foods if indicated.

We will now discuss each of these steps in detail.

STEP 1: CHOOSE ENZYME-RICH FOODS

The best foods for an enzyme-rich diet are fresh fruits (particularly ones with low acid content like melons and papayas, if you tend to be overly acidic) and vegetables, along with sprouted beans and seeds. These foods are easy to digest because they contain natural enzymes and, if well chewed, do not create stress on the pancreas; they should be included with many of your meals.

Various plant enzymes assist in the ripening and maturation process as well as the eventual breakdown and decay of the plant. When raw plant foods are consumed, their enzymes assist in the breakdown of food, beginning in the upper digestive tract. As the food passes through the digestive tract, these plant enzymes ease the workload of the digestive system and reduce the demand on the body's store of enzymes. Over time, this assistance can have a restorative effect on the body's digestive capability.

Fresh fruits and vegetables

All fresh fruits and vegetables contain natural digestive enzymes. Two fruits in particular, pineapple and papaya, contain some of the most potent protein-digesting enzymes. The proteolytic enzyme in pineapple is bromelain, and in papaya, papain. Of these two, papain is most useful as a digestive enzyme because of its soothing effect on the stomach. Bromelain is used as a potent anti-inflammatory. Susan may recommend to patients that they include papaya in their diet. However, many individuals with low enzyme production are also highly acidic, and pineapple and its juice are highly acidic and may cause canker sores and digestive upset in overly acidic individuals. Therefore, Susan does not recommend eating pineapple except on an infrequent basis. Luckily, the best delivery system for these enzymes is in supplemental form, which allows one to benefit from the enzymatic properties of both fruits. Supplementation with papain and bromelain is addressed in detail on pages 222–230.

Sprouted seeds, grains, and legumes

All sprouted seeds are exceptionally rich sources of natural enzymes. A seed that is in the process of sprouting is in a very active state of maturation, rich in enzymes and nutrients. When a seed sprouts, its nutrient value multiplies many times. Alfalfa sprouts contain as much beta-carotene as carrots, as well as high levels of calcium, iron, magnesium, potassium, phosphorus, sodium, sulfur, silicon, chlorine, cobalt, and zinc. Green peas, lentils, garbanzo beans, sunflower seeds, adzuki beans, and mung beans can all be sprouted. A wide variety of sprouts are available in local supermarkets as well as natural-food stores and farmers' markets.

While all raw foods including fish, meat, and poultry contain enzymes, eating raw flesh foods can be very hazardous due to bacteria and parasites. This is especially true when you do not personally know how the meat, fish, or poultry has been handled since it was slaughtered or caught. Therefore, the eating of raw flesh foods, even though they retain their natural enzymes, is not encouraged.

It is important to know that cooked foods do *not* contain active enzymes. When food is heated above 140°F, all its valuable enzymes are destroyed. All common cooking techniques such as sautéing, frying, boiling, and baking occur at temperatures that are well in excess of this threshold. Even such reputedly healthy cooking techniques as steaming and slow cooking in a Crock-Pot are commonly done at temperatures well above 140°F. All food that is canned or otherwise heat-processed has also lost all of its living enzymes and must rely on the enzymes created by the body for its digestion. The cooking process also destroys certain amounts of vitamins, minerals, and other phytonutrients. While such food may still have many healthy vitamins and minerals, all of its natural enzymes have been inactivated. Frozen foods, usually considered healthier than canned foods, also retain virtually none of their active enzymes. Almost all frozen foods have been blanched (placed in boiling water for two to six minutes, depending on the fruit or vegetable) prior to freezing with the express purpose of arresting the enzyme activity so as to not bring about other nutritional losses or create off flavors through the activity of the natural enzymes. Commercial fruit juices have been pasteurized, which also inactivates their enzymes. However, fresh juices made at home using a juicer retain the active enzymes found in the raw fruits and vegetables they are made from.

A Caution on Raw Seeds

All raw seeds, beans, and grains are rich in natural enzymes. However, these plants also contain enzyme inhibitors that prevent self-digestion. Without these inhibitors, the seeds, beans, and grains would ripen and decay before they could find the right location in which to germinate and grow. These foods have naturally extended shelf lives due to these inhibitors, but they can cause digestive difficulties when consumed because these inhibitors affect not only the enzymes contained in the plants, but also the enzymes produced by the digestive organs, thereby placing an extra burden on the pancreas. So if you eat raw seeds as snacks, be sure to take supplemental enzymes to reduce the stress on your digestive tract.

When seeds, beans and grains germinate, the inhibitors are deactivated. Cooking also deactivates many of the inhibitors, but experts differ as to whether it completely removes all of them.

▲▲ To significantly increase the level of nutrients and natural enzymes in your diet, add sprouted seeds and beans to your meals, for example, in salads or sandwiches. You may enjoy the taste of some sprouts more than others—so experiment. Try sprouted sunflower seeds, flax seeds, radish, broccoli, onions, adzuki beans, garbanzo beans, and lentils. You can find sprouts in natural-food stores and at farmers' markets.

▲▲ When traveling, always have access to fresh fruits or vegetables. However, try to avoid highly acidic fruits like citrus and berries if you are overly acidic. Stop at a local market to stock up on high-enzyme foods like sprouts, carrots, celery, or papaya to snack on. When eating in restaurants, concentrate on including as many salads, raw vegetables, and less acidic, more alkaline fruits such as melons and papayas. We also recommend traveling with a brown-bag meal, particularly when you fly across time zones. For example, if you are flying from New York to Los Angeles and you arrive at your hotel at 9:00 P.M. (which for you is actually midnight), you will probably be too tired to go out for dinner—even if you have skipped the dinner served on the airplane and feel hungry. Instead of raiding the room's refrigerator, which is filled with nutrient-poor, enzyme-deficient, highly acidic or acid-forming snacks like potato chips, peanuts, and colas, you'll have an energy-rich meal that you brought from home. Some raw, fresh vegetables, with a flavorful dressing or dip, a whole-grain muffin with some almond butter as a spread, and a piece of fruit (or a salad and fresh fruit ordered from room service) makes a great light supper that won't keep you up all night with indigestion. You'll wake up refreshed and ready to go in the morning.

Fermented foods

Fermented foods are staples in the traditional cuisines of Europe, throughout the Mediterranean and Middle East, and in Asia, where the fermented tea *kombucha* is a common drink and fermented soy products such as soy sauce, shoyu, tamari, and tempeh are eaten every day. These cultured foods all contain living microorganisms that enhance the food's flavor, digestibility, and nutritional value, as well as acting as a preservative.

Many fermented foods are also rich sources of enzymes that enhance digestive function. Fermented foods include yogurt, sauerkraut, kefir (a beverage made from cow's milk), olives, pickles, beer, wine, vinegar, cheese, cottage cheese, and buttermilk. However, when these foods are commercially processed so that they have a longer shelf life, the enzymes can be destroyed. For the enzyme-rich, homemade version, it's best to shop in natural-food stores, which sometimes carry items such as freshly made sauerkraut, cured olives, and natural yogurt.

Combining Raw and Cooked Foods

It is not necessary to eat only raw foods to receive the digestive benefits of plant enzymes. Raw and cooked foods can be eaten in combination. A bowl of lentil soup and a carrot slaw provide legumes that are cooked (the lentils), coupled with living enzymes in the raw carrots. Poached salmon salad made with sliced onions and served on romaine lettuce is also a mix of both cooked and enzyme-rich raw ingredients.

People with weak digestive function may find that eating mostly raw foods can cause digestion symptoms like gas and bloating. Raw vegetables are made up of nonnutritive cellulose, which is tough, fibrous, and difficult for some individuals to digest. To make fibrous foods more easily digestible, it is important to chew them thoroughly. For patients with sensitive digestive systems, Susan recommends lightly steamed foods, easy-to-digest dishes like soups, and well-cooked grains along with side dishes of raw foods like salads. (As digestive function improves, her patients are usually able to tolerate more raw foods in their diets.) If you do enjoy salads and raw vegetables, it is fine to include these more and more in your meals as you restore your digestive function with enzyme-rich foods. However, Susan recommends making the transition slowly so that your body can adapt.

STEP 2: AVOID FOODS THAT STRESS THE PANCREAS

As discussed in the previous chapter, certain foods should be consumed minimally or not at all by people who are trying to restore their ability to produce pancreatic enzymes. These include wheat, red meat, and dairy products, which are all very hard to break down and require the body to produce large amounts of enzymes and other digestants like pepsin and hydrochloric acid. Such foods are also often high in saturated fats, sugars, and animal protein. Some of these hard-to-digest foods are used in combinations to create dishes that are not only difficult to digest but may also be highly allergenic and acid-forming. The list includes mainstays of the standard American diet like pizza, barbecued ribs, cheese steaks, cheeseburgers, all fried foods including chicken, French fries and chips, donuts, pastries, ice cream, hot dogs, and chocolate.

For example, the pancreas must produce significant amounts of enzymes to digest a meal of steak, a fully dressed baked potato, buttered bread, wine, and chocolate cake for dessert. The meal is laden with saturated fats, red-meat protein, and sugar. Not only are the individual foods difficult to digest, but when mixed together they poise a formidable digestive task. The difficulty that many people have digesting these foods is the reason that you are often more tired after eating such a meal than you were before. In contrast, a light meal of bean soup, mixed green salad, and an undressed baked potato is full of vitamins, minerals, carbohydrates, and easy-to-digest vegetable-based protein. The pancreas is not overly stressed, and the digestive process proceeds efficiently, leaving you feeling energized and comfortable after eating.

STEP 3: DRINK BLENDERIZED DRINKS IF INDICATED

If you are a person with digestive problems or weak pancreatic function and suffer from a variety of inflammatory conditions, or even have a very serious health problem like cancer, one way to reduce the stress on the pancreas and help restore its functional capabilities is to drink blenderized meals. Processing ingredients in a blender liquefies food, breaking all of its components into extremely small particles, and enhances (or replaces) the mechanical digestive step of chewing. The surface area of the food is dramatically increased, thereby eliminating one of the functions of pancreatic enzymes in the breakdown process and hence requiring less enzyme production. This takes an enormous amount of stress off of the pancreas and other digestive organs. Liquefied food is partially predigested. It is absorbed and assimilated very easily, with minimal symptoms of incomplete or poor digestion such as bloating, gas, and food remaining in the digestive tract for long periods of time. The nutrients from the food are much more readily available when food is taken in blenderized form.

Foods such as vegetables, fruits, seeds, and nuts can be blenderized to make delicious shakes and drinks. Vegetables such as squash, turnips, yams, sweet potatoes, and potatoes can all be blenderized into purees. Thickened soups that are full of solids like beans and pieces of vegetables can be pureed and made more easy to digest. People with really weak digestive systems should consider blenderizing one to two meals per day, with the third meal consisting of easily digestible solid food such as cooked salads, steamed vegetables, cooked grains, and meats like salmon or trout that tend to be softer and easier to digest than more tough, fibrous meats like grilled steak. Susan has found that patients who substitute one or two blenderized meals per day have much more rapid healing and recovery times.

Blenderized drinks can be made from ingredients that are both enzyme-rich and more alkaline. Millions of Americans have both low digestive enzyme production and a tendency toward being overly acidic.

Drinks such as these can provide therapeutic benefits for both conditions. Liquefying the solid ingredients into a drink further reduces the workload of the pancreas and other digestive organs. These liquid meals can be tremendously beneficial for conditions related to either overacidity or low enzyme production such as fatigue, brain fog, inflammatory conditions, autoimmune problems, and even cancer.

Any commercially available blender or food processor can be used; however, we have found that the Vita Mix Total Nutrition Center (see the appendix for more information, as it is not available in stores) is a super-powerful blender that can pulverize virtually any whole food into a liquid (in contrast, juicers tend to extract the juice while discarding the nutrient-rich pulp). This blender can emulsify raw or cooked foods and can be used for any combination of fruits, vegetables, seeds, nuts, liquids, or oils.

Many athletes and others who require very high energy levels to perform in stressful or physically demanding jobs rely on one or two blenderized meals per day. Over the years, we have developed several drink recipes that provide protein, carbohydrates, and fats in an easily digestible form that can replace an entire solid meal. Use these recipes exactly as stated or modify them to your own tastes or specific food tolerances. Please refer to the chart listing the pH values of common foods (on page 102) to find other less acidic, more alkaline ingredients.

Fruit drinks

All of the ingredients in the following two recipes are readily available in health food stores, gourmet markets, and well-stocked supermarkets. We strongly recommend using organic ingredients whenever possible, since their nutrient content is higher than that of commercial-grade food. Although these delicious blenderized drinks can be used at any time of the day, many people prefer to have one for breakfast as these drinks can be made quickly and can easily be consumed in the car while commuting.

CANTALOUPE-BANANA DRINK

12 ounces rice milk	*1 tablespoon rice bran syrup*
2 tablespoons rice protein powder*	*¼ cantaloupe, seeded and peeled*
2 ounces raw almonds (shelled)	*½ banana, peeled*
1 tablespoon flax oil	

Combine all the ingredients in a blender or food processor and run it on high speed for 60 to 90 seconds or until the drink is totally liquefied. Add more rice milk if a thinner drink is desired. Drink immediately.

Provides a complete meal for 1 person.

*Vegetarian protein powders usually contain both legume- and grain-based protein sources.

PAPAYA-APPLE DRINK

12 ounces almond or oat milk	*1 teaspoon barley syrup*
1 organic egg	*½ papaya, peeled, seeded, and*
2 ounces shelled raw pumpkin seeds	*chopped*
1 tablespoon avocado oil	*½ apple, peeled, cored, and chopped*

Combine all the ingredients in a blender or food processor and run it on high speed for 60 to 90 seconds or until the drink is totally liquefied. Add more almond or oat milk if a thinner drink is desired. Drink immediately.

Provides a complete meal for 1 person.

Individuals who have weak liver function in addition to diminished enzyme production may not be able to tolerate seeds, nuts, and their oils. The amount of seeds and nuts in the above two recipes may be reduced to 1 or 2 tbsp. or eliminated entirely. Flax oil is actually beneficial for liver function but may be halved in quantity or even eliminated from the above recipes for people who have severely impaired liver function. The amount of flax oil used in these recipes may then be gradually increased as liver function improves. See chapters 5 and 6, on detoxification, for more information on restoring liver function.

Vegetable drinks

These three vegetable drinks are enzyme-rich "liquid salads," made by combining fresh vegetables and spring water in a blender or food processor that is capable of completely liquefying vegetables, such as a Vita Mix. (If you do not have such a powerful food processor, peel vegetables as directed; if you do, the peels can stay on if you like.) The vegetables should be cut up into large pieces before putting them in the food processor.

VEGETABLE DRINK No. 1

¹/₃ cucumber, peeled	1 to 2 tablespoons olive oil
2 to 4 peeled garlic cloves	1 tablespoon maple syrup or rice
10 to 12 sprigs parsley	bran syrup
¼ large red bell pepper, seeded	½ teaspoon Bragg Liquid Aminos
½ cooked beet, outer layer scrubbed off	2 cups spring or filtered water
½ carrot, peeled	4 or 5 ice cubes

Combine all the ingredients in a blender or food processor and run it on high speed for 60 to 90 seconds or until the drink is totally liquefied. Add more water if a thinner drink is desired. Drink immediately. You can use this recipe as a base for experimenting with your favorite seasonal vegetables.

Provides a complete meal for 1 person.

VEGETABLE DRINK No. 2

2 carrots, peeled	1 stalk celery
¹/₂ cup cooked beets	2 cups spring or filtered water
¹/₄ cup parsley	

Combine all the ingredients in a blender or food processor and run it on high speed for 60 to 90 seconds or until the drink is totally liquefied. Add more water if a thinner drink is desired. Drink immediately.

Serves 1.

VEGETABLE DRINK No. 3

2 carrots, peeled	1 stalk celery
¹/₂ cucumber, peeled	2 cups spring or filtered water
2 beet tops	

Combine all the ingredients in a blender or food processor and run it on high speed for 60 to 90 seconds or until the drink is totally liquefied. Add more water if a thinner drink is desired. Drink immediately.

Serves 1.

 If you suffer from overacidity or any inflammatory conditions, be sure to avoid adding such common hot, spicy, or acidic seasonings and flavorings as chili pepper, Tabasco sauce, black pepper, vinegar, citrus juices, Bloody Mary mix, and Worcestershire sauce, which can trigger symptoms of overacidity or inflammation. Many herbs can be safely used as flavoring agents. Naturally alkaline individuals can probably use most seasoning agents without ill effect unless they have a sensitivity to a particular one.

STEP 4: EAT PUREED FOODS IF INDICATED

Unlike blenderized drinks, pureed foods are usually cooked before being processed in a blender or food processor. While these are cooked foods and their enzymes have been deactivated, serving them in pureed form will significantly reduce stress on the digestive process, especially the pancreas. These recipes are especially helpful if you have digestive problems, weak pancreatic function, or a serious health problem.

SPLIT-PEA SOUP PUREE

1 cup dried split peas, picked over and rinsed	2 carrots
	4 cups spring or filtered water
1 onion, chopped	¹/₄ to ¹/₂ teaspoon sea salt or salt substitute

Combine the peas, onion, and carrots in a stockpot. Add water. Bring to a boil, then turn heat to low, and cover pot. Cook for 45 minutes. Add sea salt and continue cooking until peas are soft. Let soup cool, then puree in a blender or food processor until smooth.

Serves 2 to 4.

CARROT SOUP PUREE

4 cups peeled and sliced carrots	4 cups vegetable broth
2 cups diced onion	1 cup rice or soy milk
½ cup sweet red pepper	

Combine all the ingredients in a large stockpot. Cook for 30 minutes over medium heat or until carrots are tender. Let soup cool, then puree in a blender or food processor until smooth.

Serves 2 to 4.

BUTTERNUT SQUASH PUREE

1 large butternut squash,	1 tablespoon rice bran syrup
peeled and cubed	ground nutmeg, allspice, or
2 cups rice or soy milk	cinnamon to taste

Place the cut squash in a steamer and steam for 12 to 15 minutes or until very tender. While it is still hot, place the steamed squash in a blender or food processor. Add the nondairy milk and rice bran syrup and puree until smooth. Serve hot, with or without spices. This drink tastes like a rich dessert.

Serves 2 to 4.

PART 2:
TAKE SUPPLEMENTAL DIGESTIVE ENZYMES

THERE ARE A WIDE variety of plant- and animal-based digestive enzymes that can you take as supplements in addition to eating an enzyme-rich diet. In this section, we will discuss the two main types of supplemental enzymes available and how to use them for a number of conditions, such as digestive problems, sports injuries, surgical wounds, and respiratory infections.

It is important to remember that, when taken with a meal, supplemental enzymes will tend to be used in the digestive process. When taken between meals, on an empty stomach, the enzymes will instead be used by the body for their anti-inflammatory and cellular repair capabilities. For those individuals who have both weak digestive function and other health conditions, the use of supplemental enzymes both with and apart from meals may be most appropriate.

Various types of supplemental enzymes can be combined and taken simultaneously. Many commercial preparations are, in fact, combinations of various enzymes. For example, you may take pancreatic enzymes, bromelain, and papain at the same time to enhance their therapeutic benefits with no adverse effects.

When you are customizing your program, it is helpful to know if your constitution tends to be more alkaline or more acidic. As we stated in chapter 1, most people in the United States are overly acidic. Many of these individuals have low production of pancreatic enzymes. If you are overly acidic and enzyme deficient, avoid enzyme products that contain betaine or glutamic hydrochloric acid (HCl) as they may cause a burning sensation in the stomach or increase a tendency toward overacidity. If, on the other hand, you are one of the small number of individuals who have exceedingly good buffering capability, HCl supplementation combined with enzyme products may be beneficial.

The use of supplemental enzymes may cause side effects or detoxification symptoms because digestive enzymes, including pancreatic enzymes as well as bromelain and papain, are protein digestants. When taken supplementally, they will attack and begin to dissolve unhealthy tissue buildup in the body (which is their basis for use in alternative cancer treatments). When they are used in large amounts or to excess, the breakdown process initiated by supplemental digestive enzymes can, on occasion, overwhelm the body's ability to remove these waste products. You may experience symptoms of detoxification, which are similar to those of a viral infection: a runny nose, flulike symptoms, unexplained fatigue, skin eruptions, diarrhea, fever, bad breath, muscle aches, or headaches. This is your body telling you that you are eliminating waste products or cellular debris faster than your system can tolerate it. Side effects of excessive enzyme use include gas, bloating, and loose bowel movements. If these symptoms occur, reduce the dosage and/or frequency of supplementation until you reach a level that does not cause any symptoms. Or, you can begin using procedures from chapter 6, on detoxification, like coffee enemas, which increase the body's ability to eliminate waste products before they reach levels that cause detoxification symptoms.

PLANT-BASED DIGESTIVE-ENZYME SUPPLEMENTS

Susan often recommends that her patients who have digestive complaints use supplemental plant-based digestive enzymes as part of their treatment program. These enzymes supplement those normally made by the stomach and pancreas. Like the digestive enzymes produced within our bodies, they help in the digestion of starches, protein, and fats. They are a convenient digestive aid for people who eat primarily cooked foods and for those eating their meals on the road, with limited access to fresh food.

The most readily available plant-based supplemental enzymes are bromelain and papain, which are sold in natural-food stores and pharmacies. Besides assisting in the process of digestion, these enzymes are useful in the treatment of a variety of conditions, including pancreatic insufficiency, trauma due to sports injuries, surgery, respiratory-tract infections, angina, arthritis, prostatitis, painful menstruation, scleroderma, and phlebitis.

Bromelain

Bromelain refers to a family of enzymes extracted from the stem of the pineapple. It has been used over the centuries as a medicinal plant in tropical native cultures around the world and was isolated chemically over 100 years ago. In 1957, bromelain was introduced as a powerful therapeutic compound, used to aid protein digestion and reduce inflammation. Since then, over 200 scientific papers on its therapeutic applications have been published in the medical literature, ranging from treatment of the common cold to treatment of cancer. Following is a list of conditions that bromelain benefits, along with suggested dosages.

Digestion. As a digestive aid, bromelain can help to break down protein-rich foods such as red meat, poultry, dairy products, and wheat. Bromelain is most effective in improving digestion when it is taken with meals. Bromelain can also be used in the treatment of more severe digestive disorders such as gastric ulcers (an open sore or lesion of the mucous membrane of the stomach). An ulcer can produce symptoms of chronic pain, and if the erosion of the tissue is sufficient to cause bleeding, an ulcer can eventually be life threatening. It is thought that the uptake of two compounds, glucosamine (a substance present in mucus) and radioactive sulfur, by the gastric mucosa may speed the healing of ulcers. In an animal study published in 1976 in the *Hawaii Medical Journal*, researchers observed that bromelain increased the gastric uptake of glucosamine by 30 to 90 percent, and of radioactive sulfur by 50 percent.

Bromelain supplementation is helpful when there is diminished pancreatic function and a reduced ability to produce pancreatic enzymes (pancreatic insufficiency). Unlike most digestive aids, bromelain remains active both in the stomach and in the small intestine, and has been shown in studies to be an adequate replacement for our own protein-digesting enzymes, pepsin and trypsin. A 1981 research study appearing in the *Journal of the Association of Physicians of India* evaluated the effectiveness of an enzyme preparation containing bromelain, pancreatin, and ox bile for the treatment of malabsorption syndrome, a condition in which soluble nutrients are poorly absorbed from the digestive tract, leading to digestive symptoms and weight loss. With the bromelain preparation, patients experienced needed weight gain and a greater sense of well-being. They also reported less pain, gas, and frequency of bowel movements.

SUGGESTED DOSAGE: 500 to 1000 mg with or immediately following meals.

Inflammation. Nonsteroidal anti-inflammatory drugs (NSAIDs) such as Motrin, Naprosyn, and Ponstil are the most prescribed pharmaceutical agents in the United States, accounting for approximately 100 million prescriptions per year. Tens of millions of individuals also purchase anti-inflammatory medications over the counter, without a doctor's prescription. While these medications are useful in reducing the symptoms of inflammation of many common conditions, from menstrual cramps to arthritis, by suppressing the production of all prostaglandins, they also suppress the beneficial anti-inflammatory ones. In addition, they have no effect on dissolving fibrin clots. Furthermore, long-term use of NSAIDs can lead to liver, kidney, and gastrointestinal side effects.

Unlike NSAIDs, bromelain acts as a natural aspirin without any of the undesirable side effects. Bromelain reduces inflammation in several ways. While aspirin inhibits the synthesis of all prostaglandins (hormonelike chemicals produced within the intestinal tract, uterus, and other sites of the body), bromelain inhibits only the inflammatory ones, without affecting the anti-inflammatory ones.

Bromelain also interacts with fibrin, a tough, clotlike material made of protein that the body manufactures to seal off an injured area. When there is injury, caused by anything from a sports accident to bumping into the sharp corner of a desk, the blood vessels and capillaries in the injured area begin to dilate (expand) so the body's own healing substances can reach the area quickly. At the same time, fluids force their way into the surrounding tissue, causing congestion and resulting in pressure, swelling, heat, and pain. Helper cells then begin to seal off the damaged area, creating fibrin clots made of protein. In an effort to prevent the spread of bacteria and toxins generated by the injury, the fibrin also blocks blood and lymph vessels, which causes more swelling, a blockage of blood flow, and inflammation. The enzymes contained within bromelain help to reduce inflammation by digesting the fibrin clots.

In addition, supplemental bromelain helps to increase the oxygen level in injured tissue and stimulates the body's own natural enzymatic activity without suppressing the immune system, further accelerating the healing process.

SUGGESTED DOSAGE: Bromelain supplements, in standard dosages of 500 mg taken two to four times per day, should be combined with bioflavonoids and vitamin C, as these enhance the action of bromelain. Recommended dosages are 500 to 1000 mg of bioflavonoids taken three times a day, and 1 g of vitamin C taken two or three times a day apart from meals.

Sports injuries. Besides its usefulness in reducing inflammation due to illness, bromelain is also an effective treatment for a wide range of physical trauma. It is most typically used in the treatment of sports-related injuries. For example, if you strain your back playing golf on your day off, bromelain can speed your recovery and enable you to play again much sooner than you would otherwise expect.

In a 1995 research study reported in *Fortschritte Der Medizin*, fifty-nine patients (thirty-nine men and twenty women) with muscle strains, ligament tears, or contusions (a bruise or injury in which the skin is not broken) were given 500 mg of bromelain three times daily, thirty minutes before meals, for a period of one to three weeks. Patients were evaluated for pain at rest and during motion, for swelling, and for tenderness. Patients also rated their own symptom levels. In every case, patients reported a reduction in all symptoms, with pain during motion and tenderness when touched showing the most improvement.

Various professions have a high risk of injury: law enforcement agents, firefighters, emergency workers, Red Cross volunteers, tree trimmers, employees in heavy industry, and members of the active military. The use of bromelain can be quite helpful in limiting the extent of any injury. For example, bromelain has been used successfully in treating firefighters and police who have suffered injury in the line of duty. In Germany, prize fighters are directed to take enzymes before a fight to prevent the consequences of severe injuries. In many cases, the usual forced inactivity during a two-month rest period after major injury can be reduced to several weeks.

SUGGESTED DOSAGE: 500 to 1000 mg three to four times per day. Take between meals so that the bromelain is not used up in digesting food.

▲▲ Most public institutions and private businesses keep aspirin and other NSAIDs available to employees to reduce the pain of minor injuries on the job. Having bromelain available for these same purposes would be much more beneficial, since it is of greater assistance in resolving minor injuries.

Surgical wounds. Bromelain also speeds the healing of surgical wounds. An actress expressed her concern about how much time she would have to take off from work if she decided to undergo cosmetic surgery. Susan suggested a program of supplementation that included bromelain. The actress elected to have the surgery and immediately began Susan's program. To her delight, she found that she healed much more rapidly than expected.

According to a study published in the *Journal of Oral Medicine*, a group of sixteen patients received bromelain therapy four times a day, beginning seventy-two hours prior to undergoing oral surgery. Twenty-four hours after surgery, 38 percent of the patients receiving bromelain had only mild pain or none at all, as compared with 13 percent of the untreated patients. Furthermore, one day after surgery, 75 percent of the treated patients had only mild inflammation or none at all, while only 19 percent of the untreated patients experienced a comparable reduction.

Bromelain is also effective in reducing the inflammation resulting from dental procedures such as root canals, tooth extractions, and dental surgery. It can also speed the healing of gum tissue, which can become irritated during dental procedures. For maximum effectiveness, it should be taken shortly before the procedure and immediately after it and continued until healing is complete.

SUGGESTED DOSAGE: Begin the use of enzymes one to two days prior to the dental or surgical procedure and continue until the healing is complete—500 to 1000 mg four times per day apart from meals.

Respiratory-tract infections. Nasal congestion due to respiratory-tract infections is a nuisance, hampering almost any activity. There is scientific evidence that bromelain can be very useful in the treatment of upper-respiratory problems that generate mucus. Bromelain decreases the volume and viscosity of mucus so that it can be more easily cleared from the respiratory tract. This was demonstrated in a study appearing in 1978 in *Drugs Under Experimental and Clinical Research.* Volunteers included seventy men and fifty-four women, aged thirty-five to seventy-five, hospitalized with lung diseases such as chronic bronchitis, pneumonia, and pulmonary abscess. Patients were randomly given one of three therapies: amoxycillin plus 80 mg of bromelain, amoxycillin plus indomethacin, or amoxycillin alone, every eight hours, for at least eight days or as needed. The sputum (substance expelled by coughing or clearing the throat) of the patients was then analyzed for viscosity. The results of this study showed that bromelain significantly increased the fluidity of mucus. There was also evidence that bromelain combined with drug therapy enhanced the absorption of the amoxycillin.

SUGGESTED DOSAGE: 500 to 1000 mg four to six times per day. Take both with and apart from meals.

Using bromelain with antibiotics. Several studies in the scientific literature document the effectiveness of bromelain in enhancing the action of antibiotics. In one research study, published in 1961 in *Experimental Medicine & Surgery,* fifty-three hospitalized patients were given combined antibiotic and bromelain therapy to treat such potentially life-threatening diseases as pneumonia, bronchitis, thrombophlebitis, pyelonephritis, and rectal abscesses. Twenty-three of these patients had been unsuccessfully treated with antibiotic therapy alone. Of these, twenty-two responded favorably to the combined therapy. Researchers also compared the length of stay for patients taking antibiotics alone or the combined therapy. Patients with pneumonia or bronchitis who were treated with antibiotics alone remained in the hospital for an average of ten days, as compared with those who also received enzyme therapy, who were able to leave the hospital after only six days.

Another study, published in 1967 in the journal *Headache*, looked at the use of bromelain in combination with antibiotics for the treatment of acute sinusitis. Forty-eight patients were placed on standard therapy, which included antihistamines and analgesic agents, along with antibiotics, if indicated. Twenty-three patients received bromelain four times daily, while the remaining twenty-five received a placebo. Of the patients receiving bromelain, 87 percent had complete resolution of nasal mucosal inflammation, compared with only 52 percent in the placebo group.

▲▲▲ The next time you come down with an acute infection and your doctor writes you a prescription for antibiotics, be sure to supplement that medication with bromelain. Along with rest, supplementing with bromelain will help you return to your usual activities much more quickly.

Heart disease. Patients with cardiovascular disease may benefit from taking digestive enzymes since bromelain can help to reduce platelet aggregation or clumping. Platelets are a component of the blood that, when they clump, can increase the risk of heart attack and stroke. Use of digestive enzymes can reduce this tendency of platelets to be sticky. The first conclusive evidence that bromelain prevents clumping of blood platelets (aggregation) was reported in 1972 in the journal *Experientia*. Twenty volunteers with a history of heart attack or stroke, or with high platelet aggregation values, were given bromelain. In seventeen of the subjects, bromelain decreased aggregation of blood platelets. Oral pancreatic digestive-enzyme preparations are also regularly used in Europe to help dissolve clots in the veins. Numerous studies confirm their usefulness in dissolving small clots (microthrombi), which helps to prevent the development of large clots that may eventually trigger a vascular accident.

SUGGESTED DOSAGE: 500 to 1000 mg three to four times a day apart from meals.

Factors that can Inactivate Bromelain

Certain metallic compounds are known to render bromelain inactive, including copper and iron, which are found naturally in many foods, and the heavy metals lead, mercury, and cadmium, which are sometimes present as toxic pollutants in fish and other foods. Heavy-metal contamination can also be found in poor-quality, commercial-grade foods. Buying the highest quality organically grown foods will help you to avoid these enzyme inhibitors.

When shopping for a bromelain supplement, avoid those that combine the bromelain with copper or iron in the same tablet or capsule. Look for bromelain combined with magnesium or cysteine, bromelain activators that enhance its therapeutic effect. The quality of bromelain is expressed in gelatin-digesting units (g.d.u.). The higher the g.d.u., the higher the grade of bromelain and its activity. Keep in mind that bromelain is not heat stable, so supplements need to be stored in a cool place.

Papain

Papain is the enzyme derived from papayas. Best known as a meat tenderizer, it can also be used as a powerful digestant of protein either by itself or combined with bromelain and other digestive enzymes. Research has found that papain has many other clinical applications such as aiding in recovery from injuries and surgery and treating a number of inflammatory conditions such as gluten intolerance.

Digestive problems. Papain has been found to be helpful for digestive problems such as gluten intolerance. Gluten is the protein found in wheat; gluten intolerance can cause intestinal inflammation, bloating, cramping, and gas. An interesting case study, published in 1976 in *The Lancet*, documented the use of papain in the treatment of gluten intolerance. The authors reported that the patient studied was first put on a gluten-free diet, which produced symptom relief and some weight gain. However, the patient's steatorrhea (fatty stools) continued. He was then treated with papain. After four weeks of therapy, his intestinal absorption returned to normal. Subsequently, when the patient reintroduced gluten-containing foods in his diet, he experienced no further symptoms of gluten intolerance.

SUGGESTED DOSAGE: 200 to 300 mg with or immediately following meals, upon rising, and before bedtime.

Traumatic injuries. A variety of traumatic injuries, such as those resulting from playing sports, can be aided by the use of papain. A two-year study, published in 1969 in *Current Therapeutic Research*, followed the recovery time of 125 members of athletic teams, predominantly football, who received mild to moderate injuries during games or practice. The players were monitored for swelling, pain, and skin discoloration due to bleeding within tissues (ecchymosis). Of the sixty-five patients treated with papain (*Carica papaya*), nearly 70 percent showed a better than expected response to the therapy. Only 20 percent of the sixty untreated patients in the study had comparable recovery. The anti-inflammatory benefits of the papain allowed the players to return to their athletic activities sooner than anticipated.

SUGGESTED DOSAGE: 200 mg four times per day apart from meals.

Inflammatory conditions. Along with bromelain, papain is also useful in the treatment of inflammatory conditions that affect our cells and tissues, such as respiratory infections like colds, flus, bronchitis, arthritis, and thyroiditis.

SUGGESTED DOSAGE: 200 to 300 mg with or immediately following meals, upon rising, and before bedtime.

Minor surgery and dental procedures. Millions of individuals annually undergo minor surgery and dental procedures such as tooth extractions and root canals. While these procedures are usually not life threatening, they can cause significant pain and discomfort. The use of papain can reduce these uncomfortable symptoms and help speed up the healing process. Papain, like bromelain, is also an effective treatment for postoperative complications after oral surgery—specifically, after the removal of impacted molars, according to a study published in 1976 in the *Journal of the American Dental Association*. A group of 129 patients were given either papase or prednisolone (a synthetic form of the anti-inflammatory hormone cortisol) or were left untreated. Patients were given therapy postoperatively and evaluated for pain, edema (water retention in tissue), and trismus (the postsurgical spasm of the muscles of mastication). While no significant differences were found for edema between the treated and untreated groups, both papase and prednisolone were found to be effective at reducing trismus and pain. An added benefit of the natural-enzyme therapy is that there are virtually no side effects associated with its use.

SUGGESTED DOSAGE: 200 mg four times per day apart from meals.

Organic green papaya

Aside from papain, ground dried organic green papaya is also very high in its digestive-enzyme content. This can be found in natural-food stores or by mail order. Take to 1 to 3 tsp. with meals as a digestive aid and natural anti-inflammatory.

Side Effects of Plant Enzymes

While plant enzymes are not known to cause any serious side effects, they may cause increased intestinal gas. Gradually increasing your dosage can improve your tolerance and reduce the likelihood of gas. Plant enzymes should be avoided, as should most supplements, by pregnant women and people with any kind of bleeding disorder.

PANCREATIC ENZYMES DERIVED FROM ANIMAL SOURCES

Although commercial preparations of supplemental pancreatic enzymes are actually derived from the pancreas of animals, particularly cows and pigs, these enzymes are similar to those found in the human body. Pancreatic-enzyme products are unique because they are able to break down all three basic food substances found in our diets: carbohydrates, proteins, and fats. In other words, they contain protein-digesting (proteolytic), fat-digesting (lipolytic), and starch- and sugar-digesting (glycolytic) capability.

Pancreatic enzymes, whether produced within the body or taken as supplements, are necessary for normal digestive function. They are also powerful anti-inflammatory and anticlotting agents. Their action occurs at the tissue level in various parts of the body, including muscle and epidermal (skin) tissue. Supplemental pancreatic enzymes can also improve digestion, reducing the workload on the body's own pancreatic enzymes, and facilitate healing from sports injuries or other traumas or after surgery. Following is a list of health conditions benefited by pancreatic enzymes and the suggested dosages for the enzymes. While these can be taken alone, they are frequently combined in nutritional-supplement products with plant-based digestive enzymes.

Digestive problems

Pancreatic enzymes are helpful in supporting pancreatic insufficiency and digestive symptoms such as gas and bloating.

SUGGESTED DOSAGE: One to two 300 to 500 mg tablets with meals or directly following meals. Commercial products may vary between 100 and 500 mg, with many products in the 300 to 500 mg range.

Traumatic injuries

Numerous studies attest to the remarkable ability of these enzymes to speed recovery time and reduce the symptoms of sports injuries. According to a study published in *Practitioner*, enzymes were found to be of great benefit when used by English football (soccer) associations to treat soft tissue injury and damage to ligaments. In the 1964–65 season, the researchers gave enzymes for the first time to twenty-eight first-team players and kept track of their injuries. Up to that time, athletes were treated with the usual medical procedures as well as graded exercises, massage, and careful supervision. The researchers found that prior to enzyme therapy, athletes on the teams had lost an average of fifteen days of play during the preceding season. However, with enzyme therapy, the same players lost an average of only eleven days. In a further study, 131 soccer players who were not taking enzymes missed games because of injury, while only 90 athletes who were taking enzymes were unable to play.

As with soccer, karate injuries can occur in every area of the body. In a 1988 study, a variety of injuries responded quite rapidly to enzyme treatment. Ten karate fighters of both sexes were treated with enzyme tablets before competition, while a second group received no enzymes. During play, all the athletes had injuries comparable in severity. In the athletes treated with enzymes, hematomas (a swelling or mass of blood confined to a tissue and caused by a break in a blood vessel) disappeared within six and a half days, compared with nearly sixteen days in the untreated group. Swelling subsided after approximately four days in the treated group, compared with nearly ten days in the untreated group. Restriction of movement resolved after five days in the group treated with enzymes, compared with over twelve and a half days in the untreated group. In addition, inflammatory symptoms resolved rapidly, taking only four days to subside in the treated group, compared with ten and a half days in the players not taking enzymes.

Jim began to take advantage of the benefits of enzymes several years ago when he entered one of the numerous golf tournaments held at his country club. Usually, when a tournament lasted more than one day, he would notice stiffness or soreness on the second day. But when he began to use enzymes prophylactically, the second day of play felt as comfortable as the first. The remarkable ability of enzymes to heal or actually prevent the stiffness or soreness incurred by the occasional or weekend athlete have made participating in these events much more enjoyable.

SUGGESTED DOSAGE: One to two 300 to 500 mg tablets, four times a day, apart from meals.

▲▲ Many weekend warriors and people who like to take sports-oriented vacations can benefit from the use of supplemental pancreatic enzymes. If you plan to have several days of vigorous activity, skiing for the weekend or spending a week at a golf or tennis camp, be sure to supplement your diet with pancreatic enzymes during this period. Enzymes will minimize the stiffness and soreness you may feel after your first day's workout, and enzymes can provide prophylactic treatment of strains or injuries that may occur.

▲▲ Besides sports injuries, pancreatic enzymes can also be an important part of a healing regimen for injuries sustained on the job and accidents in general. Enzymes can be used to shorten employee time away from the office and may help to reduce disability. They should be a staple of on-site nursing facilities for companies whose employees have a higher risk of injury, such as construction workers and people working in assembly plants. Enzyme therapy can be a money-saving management strategy.

Repetitive-stress injuries

People who are required to use their hands for their work, such as computer programmers and casino dealers, may develop inflammation in the forearm, or tenosynovitis, caused by repetitive motion. In this ailment, the tissues that surround tendons (synovial sheaths) become inflamed. A person with this disease cannot use their hands in fine, delicate movements. A study appearing in 1973 in *Clinical Medicine* examined the effect of proteolytic-enzyme therapy in treating tenosynovitis. Sixty men who worked in South Africa as cane cutters (a type of work requiring repetitive movements over many hours and days) were divided into two groups. Twenty-eight of the volunteers were given enzyme therapy four times a day for five days, and their swelling, pain, and range of arm movement monitored. These disabling symptoms resolved far more rapidly in the treated group than for those workers not receiving enzymes.

SUGGESTED DOSAGE: One to two 300 to 500 mg tablets, four times a day, apart from meals.

Autoimmune disease

As discussed in chapter 3, pancreatic enzymes can reduce levels of circulating immune complexes (CICs). These are formed when large protein molecules, only partially digested in the small intestine, are absorbed into the bloodstream. The immune system treats these molecules as invaders. Antibodies couple with them and CICs are formed. CICs are found in such autoimmune diseases as thyroiditis, Crohn's disease, and rheumatoid arthritis.

German researchers found that a reduction in levels of CICs in patients with rheumatoid arthritis was associated with an improvement in health. In a study published in 1985 in *Zeitschrift für Rheumatologie*, forty-two patients with rheumatoid arthritis were given the pancreatic-enzyme preparation Wobenzym for a period of six weeks. During this time, researchers monitored the patients both for changes in their symptoms and for levels of CICs. At the end of the test period, over 60 percent of the patients had a reduction in their symptoms, and these improvements were positively correlated with a decrease in levels of CICs.

SUGGESTED DOSAGE: One to two 300 to 500 mg tablets, four times a day, apart from meals.

Surgery

Pancreatic enzymes can benefit surgical patients and patients experiencing delayed healing. One of the biggest concerns that Susan's patients facing surgery voice is their fear of getting behind in their work if they do not recover rapidly. This is a particular concern for people who are self-employed and cannot afford much time away from work since they have no corporate disability insurance to fall back on. The use of pancreatic enzymes can accelerate the surgical healing process and help people return to work and productive activity much more rapidly.

A powerful pancreatic-enzyme product produced in Germany has been tested in several clinical trials in the treatment of surgery patients. One such study, presented in 1990 at the FIMS World Congress of Sports Medicine, was conducted by researchers at a surgical clinic in Wiesbaden. They assessed the effect of enzyme treatment on recovery time after knee surgery. Using eighty volunteers, the researchers treated half of the patients with enzymes. Those receiving enzymes regained mobility more rapidly than the untreated patients, and had less postoperative edema (retention of fluid in the tissues). In a second study, the same researchers tested the effects of enzyme treatment given preoperatively on 120 patients awaiting surgical treatment of fractures. On the day of surgery, those patients receiving enzymes had far less edema and less pain than the untreated patients.

In a further study, published in 1967 in *Clinical Medicine*, digestive enzymes were shown to be effective for treatment of traumatic swelling due to oral and maxillofacial surgery. The enzyme chymotrypsin was given, four times daily, to twenty-two patients having maxillofacial (involving the jawbone) and routine oral surgery. Treatment was started at the time of surgery or immediately afterward. The actual swelling experienced by the patients after twenty-four hours was about one-third of that normally anticipated. In addition, the thirteen patients with maxillofacial injuries evidenced rapid, and in some cases, dramatic recovery.

SUGGESTED DOSAGE: Begin taking one 300 to 500 mg tablet one to two days before the surgery and continue until healing is complete. Take apart from meals.

Childbirth

Pancreatic enzymes can be very useful in obstetric care for women giving birth. Obstetricians will often perform an episiotomy, a small incision in the perineum made to avoid tearing of the tissues as the baby leaves the birth canal. The use of supplemental pancreatic enzymes can reduce the pain and edema associated with the procedure. In a 1966 double-blind study published in the *American Journal of Obstetrics and Gynecology*, of 204 episiotomy patients, 111 received proteolytic-enzyme treatment. The volunteers were evaluated for pain when moving, sitting, and at rest, plus edema and ecchymosis (skin discoloration due to bleeding within tissues). Enzymes were given as patients were admitted to the labor room and were continued for five days postpartum. The researchers noted that the enzyme treatment reduced edema during the three days after childbirth, when it is usually greatest, and that pain and ecchymosis were also reduced.

SUGGESTED DOSAGE: One to two 300 to 500 mg tablets, four times a day, apart from meals.

Pancreatitis

Pancreatic enzymes are used as replacement therapy in the treatment of chronic pancreatitis, a severe inflammatory condition, often caused by excessive alcohol use, that results in destruction of the structure as well as the enzyme-producing capability of the pancreas. In a 1977 study appearing in the *New England Journal of Medicine*, researchers monitored six patients with advanced pancreatic insufficiency (a condition in which the pancreas is no longer able to produce the requisite amount of enzymes needed for healthy digestive function). The patients were assessed for their response to treatment with pancreatin taken with cimetidine (a drug that decreases secretion of gastric acid during both the day and night), pancreatin taken alone, cimetidine taken alone, and no medication at all. With the combination of pancreatin and cimetidine, the digestive enzymes trypsin and lipase were restored after meals to significantly higher levels than with the medication alone. Further, this was the only treatment that fully prevented four of the six patients from having bowel movements that contained abnormally high levels of fat, which would normally be absorbed into the body. Pancreatin also allowed for better fat absorption when taken alone, as compared with neutralizing antacids.

Pancreatic enzymes have also been used in the treatment of a wide range of other inflammatory health problems, including sinusitis, hay fever, rheumatoid arthritis, and cystic fibrosis.

SUGGESTED DOSAGE: One to two 300 to 500 mg tablets four times a day, apart from meals to promote healing. Also consider using with meals to support better digestive function.

Cancer

Pancreatic enzymes have also been used in the treatment of cancer. The Scottish embryologist John Beard initiated the research on this, and certain modern alternative cancer treatment specialists have applied his theories, incorporating the aggressive use of pancreatic enzymes in their own cancer treatment programs. The most prominent of these specialists is Nicholas Gonzalez, who was trained as an immunologist. Gonzalez uses a protocol based on the work of William Donald Kelley. A dentist by training, Kelley was diagnosed with probable pancreatic cancer and cured himself by taking high doses of pancreatic enzymes. He also underwent an extensive liver detoxification program through the use of coffee enemas, as well as tailoring his diet to his metabolic type. Kelley subsequently treated many patients for a variety of cancers using these basic principles. While in medical school, Gonzalez had begun an informal study of the effectiveness of taking a nutritional approach to treating cancer. A friend told him about Kelley's work. Gonzalez met with Kelley and was so impressed that he eventually began a five-year research project under the direction of Robert Good, former president of the Memorial Sloan Kettering Institute. Gonzalez found Kelley's patient records to be meticulous, and he subjected Kelley's results to rigorous analysis. Gonzalez also searched out many of the patients Kelley had treated and was able to meet and/or talk with them firsthand. Gonzalez was able to confirm that Kelley's patients with pancreatic cancer, a cancer with negligible survival rates, had a remarkable survival rate using Kelley's protocols. Consequently, Gonzalez developed a protocol based on the Kelley program, and in 1989, began using this protocol with patients. In 1997, he completed a study in cooperation with the National Cancer Institute, in which he used enzymes to treat twelve patients with pancreatic cancer. The study began in December 1993, with a patient who had cancer that was inoperable. By 1997, of the twelve patients, seven were still alive and doing well, two who had not been fully compliant had died, and three who had been compliant also died. Current medical treatments for pancreatic cancer offer a survival time of six months. All of the patients in the study lived longer than had been predicted. Further, one reason that some of the patients did not survive is that they entered the program near death, or with cancers in a very advanced stage.

Dr. Gonzalez's program includes a specific diet and aggressive use of nutritional supplements, as well as both digestive-enzyme and pancreatic-enzyme therapy. Detoxification is also a critical part of the treatment to aid the body in eliminating the waste products and toxins that result from the breakdown of tumors. Gonzalez speculates that some of the poor survival rates of current treatment modalities result from the inability of the patient to eliminate the breakdown products from the tumors. To avoid any toxic buildup in the body, Gonzalez recommends coffee enemas. (This technique is fully explained in chapter 6.)

The German enzyme product Wobenzym, which is available in the United States, is used in complementary cancer therapy. It is recommended that the pancreatic enzymes be taken at other than mealtimes in order to maintain their tumor-destroying effects. The enzymes are often administered on a set schedule at intervals throughout the day and night. Obviously, making sure to wake up in the middle of the night to take these can be a nuisance. However, practitioners who prescribe enzymes have found them to be quite helpful in the treatment of a variety of tumors. Thus, disrupting one's sleep may be worthwhile, given the potential benefits.

If cancer is of specific concern, please contact an appropriate physician in your area. See the appendix for names, addresses, and phone numbers for associations of physicians practicing complementary medicine.

How to use pancreatic enzymes

Pancreatic-enzyme products are available in natural-food stores and are sold as tablets or capsules that can vary greatly in size of dose and potency.

The potency is indicated by a notation on the label, which is usually a number followed by an X, for instance, 4X or 10X. These have been strictly defined by the United States Pharmacopoeia (USP). In a 1X pancreatic-enzyme product (pancreatin), each milligram must contain at least 25 USP units of amylase activity, at least 25 USP units of protease activity, and at least 2.0 USP units of lipase activity. Any pancreatic enzyme of higher potency is noted with a whole number greater than 1 to indicate the degree of its greater strength. For example, a pancreatic extract, full-strength and undiluted, that is eight times stronger than the USP standard would be labeled 8X USP. Full-strength products are generally preferred, as lower-potency pancreatic products may be diluted with substances such as lactose, galactose, and salt.

Pancreatic enzymes are dispensed as powders, capsules, granules, and tablets, the last two available in enteric-coated forms (this means that they don't break down in the stomach). Pancreatic-enzyme supplements with enteric coating may have an advantage because the protective coating allows the pH-sensitive enzymes to pass through the hostile acidic environment of the stomach without being destroyed. Enteric-coated tablets are more likely to reach the small intestine intact, where they are normally used by the body to assist in the breakdown and digestion of foods.

SUGGESTED DOSAGE: A standard dosage of pancreatic enzymes is one to two tablets, taken with meals if they are meant to be used as a digestive aid. Follow the instructions on the bottle. If a stronger treatment is needed, buy a more potent enzyme product. If pancreatic enzymes are used to treat an anti-inflammatory disease such as rheumatoid arthritis, an accepted dosage is 300 to 1000 mg of high-potency pancreatic enzymes, taken three to four times a day, apart from meals. When pancreatic enzymes are used in this manner, the supplements need to be taken at least four times a day, because the enzymes are only active in the body for a maximum of five hours. It is essential that pancreatic enzymes be taken when the stomach is empty, preferably one-half to one hour before meals, because a considerable amount of the enzymes' ability to digest protein is lost in the acid environment of the stomach. Some enzyme products are enteric-coated, that is, buffered by chemicals like sodium bicarbonate so they will not be attacked by gastric acid or pepsin in the stomach. (See chapters 1 and 2 for a discussion of the dynamics of buffering and pH control.) However, numerous studies have found these to be no more effective, and in some cases, less effective, than uncoated enzymes.

Side effects of pancreatic enzymes

It is well documented in scientific studies that pancreatic enzymes are remarkably free of side effects. However, an excess dosage of these enzymes may cause diarrhea, especially in older patients, and bowel tolerance needs to be monitored. The need for these enzymes diminishes as health returns, and dosages can then be slowly decreased.

PART 3:
USE OTHER NATURAL ANTI-INFLAMMATORY AGENTS

FOR THE TREATMENT of acute and chronic inflammatory conditions, there are a number of natural anti-inflammatory agents that can be used in combination with digestive enzymes for even better results. These agents are available in most natural-food stores as nutritional supplements. A number of research studies attest to their ability to speed recovery time for many ailments. Because they have minimal or no side effects, they offer a safe way to treat a wide variety of inflammatory conditions.

MSM

Methylsulfonylmethane (MSM) is one of the most powerful anti-inflammatories derived from natural foods. MSM is a nontoxic, physiologically active sulfur compound that is a breakdown product of DMSO (dimethyl oxide). DMSO was originally used in the United States only as an industrial solvent. However, it is now recognized as having significant medical applications and is an FDA-approved treatment for interstitial cystitis, an inflammatory bladder ailment. DMSO is also used extensively by veterinarians for the treatment of a wide variety of inflammatory conditions in animals. A person taking DMSO may experience side effects such as dry skin and a fishy body odor. MSM is preferable as a therapeutic agent as it is odorless and virtually tasteless and causes no aftertaste when taken by mouth.

MSM functions as the flexible bond between proteins. When a cell dies, a new cell takes its place. Without the needed amount of MSM, cells and tissues lose their flexibility, and problems develop within the lungs and other parts of the body. In its role as an anti-inflammatory agent, MSM may facilitate the production of certain enzymes needed to counteract inflammation. As an antiparasitic, MSM is thought to block binding sites for parasites in the intestinal and urogenital tracts.

MSM is a component of all normal diets in vertebrates, but seems to be required in higher amounts than a typical diet provides. Cow's milk is a primary source of MSM for humans. However, since many people are allergic to or intolerant of cow's milk, they are unable to obtain MSM from this source. Since the body's levels of MSM tend to diminish with age, it is necessary to use supplemental sources after midlife to maintain essential tissue support.

Stanley W. Jacobs, a professor of surgery at the medical school of the University of Oregon, has conducted the primary research on MSM. According to an article by Jacobs and Herschler published in 1983 in the *Annals of the New York Academy of Sciences*, MSM has been shown to reduce the tendency toward food allergies and allowed food-sensitive individuals to eat foods that they would normally not have been able to tolerate. It also decreases the sensitivity to certain drugs such as anti-arthritic agents and antibiotics. Finally, MSM can function as an antacid and can be used for the treatment of constipation as well as parasitic and fungal infections. Dr. Jacobs has also found MSM to have analgesic (pain-relieving) and anti-inflammatory benefits when used to treat health problems such as interstitial cystitis, scleroderma, and systemic lupus erythematosus.

Supplemental MSM can also be used prophylactically before any strenuous physical activity. According to an article published in the winter 1997 newsletter of the *American Holistic Medical Association*, runners have found MSM to be of benefit when taken before a race to prevent joint pain, muscle soreness, and fatigue. The article also mentions that in veterinary medicine, MSM has been given to racehorses for many years to prevent them from having symptoms of physical stress after running a race.

SUGGESTED DOSAGE: 250 to 750 mg of MSM granules taken three times per day in divided doses with meals or before undertaking a strenuous activity.

COLLOIDAL SILVER

Reducing or eliminating infection, either bacterial or viral, will eliminate one of the major causes of inflammation. Inflammation results from the body's immune response as it tries to destroy the bacteria or virus. Further inflammation results from the highly acidic waste products eliminated by the bacteria or viruses.

For centuries, silver has been known to be an effective antibacterial substance. In ancient civilizations, water was stored in silver vessels to keep bacteria from growing in it, and people in the nineteenth century often put a silver dollar in milk to retard spoilage. In the early twentieth century, colloidal silver was shown to be a very effective antibiotic and antiviral substance for eliminating or preventing many minor internal and external infections. Today it is recognized that colloidal silver is effective against over 650 disease-causing organisms.

A colloid is a substance that consists of extremely fine particles suspended in another medium such as water. Colloidal silver is, therefore, submicroscopic clusters of pure metallic silver suspended in distilled water. It is created by electrolysis: An electrical current is passed between two poles, one of which is pure silver. The electric current breaks off microscopic pieces of the silver (a particle size of 0.0001 micron), and these particles stay suspended in the water due to their electrical charge. The particles are measured in parts per million (ppm); most commercially available products range from 5 to 500 ppm. Studies show that many viruses, bacteria, and fungi are rendered ineffective (in vitro) in three to four minutes after exposure to colloidal silver. Although the exact mechanism of action is not known, it appears that the silver affects enzymes in the cells of the bacteria, inhibiting their replication.

Colloidal silver is nontoxic at prescribed doses. It is tasteless and odorless and can be taken orally or applied to the skin by either spraying it on or using it in a salve form. It does not irritate the eyes, and when applied to wounds or scrapes, it does not sting. Even though it is a powerful antibiotic, when taken in prescribed doses, it does not destroy the "friendly" bacteria in the intestinal tract. Unlike pharmaceutical antibiotics, colloidal silver never permits strain-resistant pathogens to develop. Colloidal silver can be used wherever and whenever an antibacterial or antiviral agent is indicated. It can be used both to treat existing conditions and as a preventive agent.

Recent research indicates that many more health conditions may be caused by bacteria than had been previously thought. For example, peptic ulcers and rheumatoid arthritis are now thought to be caused, in part, by bacteria. In a study published in the February 1999 issue of the *Journal of the American Medical Association*, researchers found support that bacterial infections could be a cause of heart disease, the nation's number one killer. They found that people who have taken certain antibiotics may reduce their risk of heart disease—in effect, by containing or eliminating the causative strain of bacteria.

Colloidal silver can be purchased at health food stores or made at home using inexpensive battery-powered electrolysis units. It is available in dropper bottles in strengths varying from 5 to 500 ppm. (Lower strengths of 5 to 10 ppm are probably optimal.) When taking it orally, you should allow it to remain in the mouth for thirty to sixty seconds so that the microscopic particles of pure silver can be absorbed through the mucosal lining, bypassing the digestive tract. When using it on the skin, transfer the colloidal silver solution to a spray bottle and spray it on the affected area.

SUGGESTED DOSAGE: Take two dropperfuls every two to four hours for an acute infection, decreasing to every six to eight hours as symptoms begin to resolve.

COLOSTRUM

Colostrum is the first milk produced by all mammals after delivery of the newborn. While maternal milk provides important nutrients that are needed for growth and development, colostrum is crucial to the newborn's health since it enhances immunity. Studies have shown that breast-fed human infants have better resistance to a variety of diseases than bottle-fed ones. This is because colostrum contains cytokines and other low-molecular-weight protein compounds that act as biologic response modulators. These substances have profound anti-inflammatory and immunity-enhancing effects.

A number of research studies have found colostrum to be helpful in the treatment of diseases such as rheumatoid arthritis, endometriosis, prostatitis, gluten intolerance, allergies, colds, and herpes simplex infection. While human colostrum is not readily available and is very expensive, concentrated derivatives of bovine colostrum are now available in health food stores. Bovine colostrum supplements are available in either a spray or a chewable enzyme.

SUGGESTED DOSAGE: Use as a spray or lozenge twice a day. The product is usually held in the mouth for a minute or two to promote absorption through the mucosal lining. Treatment times vary between two weeks and six months.

ALKALINIZING AGENTS

Maintaining the cells and tissues of the body in their healthy, slightly alkaline state helps to prevent inflammation. In contrast, overacidity promotes the onset of painful and disabling inflammatory conditions as diverse as colds, sinusitis, rheumatoid arthritis, and interstitial cystitis. (This topic is covered in detail in chapters 1 and 2.) The use of alkalinizing agents like sodium and potassium bicarbonate in combination with digestive enzymes and other natural anti-inflammatory supplements can be extremely helpful in healing many different types of inflammatory conditions.

QUERCETIN

Quercetin, a natural substance, is a member of the flavonoid family. Flavonoids are substances found in nature in many plants that have anti-inflammatory, antiallergenic, antiviral, anticarcinogenic, and antimicrobial effects. Flavonoids are also potent antioxidants, free-radical scavengers, and metal chelators, which bind to iron and copper and help eliminate them from the body. Quercetin belongs to a subgroup of flavonoids called flavones and flavonols (commonly called bioflavonoids in products available in natural-food stores). Quercetin is naturally available in high amounts in plants such as onions. In experimental studies, quercetin displays the highest degree of activity of any flavonoid compound and is known to be highly effective in lowering inflammation.

Quercetin helps to maintain the strength of small blood vessels and to reduce vascular fragility. This counteracts the tendency toward bleeding problems and bruising, as well as lowering the trauma that occurs with tissue injury. It also inhibits the release of histamine and other inflammatory substances from mast cells. (Mast cells, which are widely distributed throughout the body and are found in highest concentrations in the lining of the respiratory and gastrointestinal tract, the skin, the lining of the joints, and the conjunctiva of the eye, are the usual sites of the allergic and inflammatory responses.) Because of its antioxidant activity, quercetin also inhibits the formation of leukotrienes, inflammatory compounds that are 1000 times more potent in stimulating inflammatory processes than histamine.

Susan has found quercetin to be particularly helpful in reducing sensitivity to allergens among her patients. One of her patients, Janet, suffered from environmental allergies since her teenage years. Her symptoms were particularly bad in the spring, when she would wake up in the morning feeling exhausted and suffering from severe symptoms of nasal congestion, which would continue throughout the day, not clearing until well into the evening. An artist by profession, she began to paint at night and sleep during the day as a survival strategy. She found all medications to be relatively ineffective in providing adequate symptom relief. However, after beginning a program of natural anti-inflammatory supplements, including quercetin, her symptoms resolved rapidly, and she was able to return to her former work schedule.

Besides environmental allergies, quercetin is also used in the treatment of food allergies, which occur with such common foods as milk, wheat, eggs, soy, strawberries, and peanuts in susceptible people. Quercetin is effective in the treatment of other inflammatory and allergic conditions including allergy, hay fever, asthma, eczema, arthritis and rheumatoid arthritis, gout, lupus, ulcerative colitis, and Crohn's disease, as well as diabetes and cancer. It has been successfully used to prevent injury and bruising in athletes and to speed recovery of acutely injured athletes and other performers. Quercetin is also beneficial for the heart, preventing platelet aggregation and promoting relaxation of cardiovascular smooth muscle. It also helps to regulate blood pressure and heart rate. Furthermore, quercetin has been shown to be effective in fighting viral disease and cancer.

SUGGESTED DOSAGE: Quercetin is not absorbed well by the body unless taken in combination with bromelain, which has been shown to increase its absorption and tissue concentration. Quercetin is available in various strengths; 300 to 600 mg, once or twice a day, is usually effective. Quercetin is well tolerated even in very large quantities. However, it can interfere with estrogen production and reduce menstrual flow. It should be used cautiously by menstruating women.

CURCUMIN (TURMERIC)

Traditional ethnic foods are often flavored with spices that have medicinal properties, which is good reason for regularly including more exotic dishes in your diet. Turmeric, an essential ingredient in curry powder, is a perennial herb of the ginger family and is extensively cultivated in India, China, Indonesia, and other tropical countries. Curcumin is the active medicinal ingredient contained in the thick rhizome of turmeric and gives turmeric its characteristic orange-yellow color.

For thousands of years, curcumin has been used in both Chinese and Indian systems of medicine as an anti-inflammatory agent and for the treatment of numerous health conditions. Modern research corroborates its use as an anti-inflammatory. A review article on curcumin, published in 1994 in the *American Journal of Natural Medicine*, summarized several studies done in India that document curcumin's usefulness as an anti-inflammatory agent. In one clinical trial, patients with rheumatoid arthritis were given either curcumin (1200 mg per day) or phenylbutazone (300 mg per day), an anti-inflammatory drug known to have serious side effects. The patients were then assessed for the length of time they were able to walk, persistence of morning stiffness, and degree of swelling in the joints. When the results were tabulated, the researchers found curcumin to be as beneficial as the drug therapy in reducing symptoms. In another study, curcumin was also found to be as effective as cortisone, a potent medical anti-inflammatory. This article noted that an added benefit of curcumin is that it does not normally cause side effects, providing a safe alternative to these powerful anti-inflammatory drugs, which can cause gastric irritation and even peptic ulcers in susceptible people.

Curcumin's therapeutic benefits occur through several mechanisms. Curcumin reduces inflammation by inhibiting leukotriene formation and platelet aggregation. It also promotes the breakup of blood clots and inhibits the inflammatory response to various stimuli. There is some indication that curcumin has an indirect effect on reducing inflammation through the adrenal gland or its hormones. The most likely explanation is that it increases the effectiveness of the body's own cortisone, one of the body's major anti-inflammatory hormones. Curcumin may do this by sensitizing or priming cortisone receptor sites, thereby potentiating cortisone's action. It may also act by increasing the half-life of cortisone through reducing its breakdown by the liver. While the long-term use of prescription cortisone has been associated with serious side effects, including adrenal atrophy, osteoporosis, and diabetes mellitus, curcumin has been found to be as effective as cortisone with no toxicity.

SUGGESTED DOSAGE: The recommended dosage for curcumin as an anti-inflammatory agent is 400 to 600 mg three times a day. It is often formulated with an equal amount of bromelain to enhance absorption. This combination is best taken on an empty stomach, twenty minutes before meals or between meals. Toxicity reactions have not been reported at standard dosage levels.

GINGER

Ginger is a pungent, spicy herb native to southern Asia. For thousands of years, ginger has been an important herb used in traditional Asian medicine. It is now cultivated throughout the tropics in countries as diverse as Jamaica, India, and China. It is used as a spice in many cuisines and as a flavoring agent for beverages such as ginger ale and in many baked goods.

Ginger is a powerful anti-inflammatory agent. It works through modulating or balancing the prostaglandin pathway. Chemicals in ginger have been found to inhibit inflammatory chemicals like thromboxanes and leukotrienes, which have been linked to conditions like asthma and coronary-artery spasm. On the other hand, these chemicals do not interfere with the production of beneficial anti-inflammatory prostaglandins. As a result, ginger has been found to reduce inflammation, pain, and fever in a variety of conditions. As such, its effects are similar to medications like aspirin, without the toxic side effects.

SUGGESTED DOSAGE: Dry, powdered ginger root can be used in dosages of 500 to 1000 mg per day. Tripling or quadrupling this dosage may provide more rapid relief. However, dosages should not be used beyond this level.

ESSENTIAL FATTY ACIDS

Essential fatty acids are fats that our body does not produce and that we must therefore obtain through our diet. They consist of two types of special fats called linoleic acid (omega-6 family) and linolenic acid (omega-3 family). While these essential fatty acids supply stored energy in the form of calories, they also perform many other important functions in the body.

They are components of the membrane structure of all cells in the body. They are required for normal development and function of the brain, eyes, inner ear, adrenal glands, and reproductive tract. These essential oils are also necessary for the synthesis of prostaglandins series I and III—hormonelike chemicals that, among other functions, reduce inflammation.

Linoleic acid (omega-6 family) is found in seeds and seed oils. Good sources include flaxseed oil, safflower oil, sunflower oil, and sesame seed oil. Linoleic acid is converted within the body to the anti-inflammatory series I prostaglandins. However, some individuals are unable to synthesize this conversion since their bodies cannot efficiently convert linolenic acid (omega-3 family) to gamma linolenic acid (GLA), an intermediary in the conversion process. Once GLA has been produced, the body can easily continue with the chemical processes needed for series I prostaglandin production. To bypass this potential block, individuals can take medicinal seed oils such as evening primrose oil, borage seed oil, and black-currant seed oil. These oils contain preformed GLA. The other common essential fatty acid, linolenic acid, is found in abundance in fish oil. The best sources are cold-water, high-fat fish such as salmon, tuna, rainbow trout, mackerel, and eel. The only good plant sources of this fatty acid are flax seeds, soybeans, pumpkin seeds, and walnuts.

In contrast, fats in red meat and poultry skin contain arachidonic acid. Arachidonic acid is converted within the body to the series II prostaglandins, which promote inflammation. To manage conditions that involve inflammation, the diet must predominate in linoleic and linolenic acids, rather than the fats found in animal foods.

SUGGESTED DOSAGE: Flaxseed oil can be used in a maximum dosage of 1 to 2 tbsp. of raw oil per day (do not cook with this oil since it is heat sensitive). Fish oil can be taken in dosages of one to two capsules once or twice per day. The therapeutic dosage for borage seed oil is two to four capsules per day, while evening primrose oil requires as many as thirteen capsules a day for maximum therapeutic benefit.

MAGNESIUM

Magnesium and calcium are essential minerals that make up the structure of the bones and also regulate the tone of the nerves and muscles. Calcium is present in beans, turnip greens, tofu, figs, hazelnuts, and blackstrap molasses. It is also present in dairy products, but because of the high incidence of lactose intolerance, may not be as well absorbed as the calcium contained within other foods. Foods that contain magnesium include soybeans, spinach, cashews, pumpkin seeds, and egg yolks.

Since calcium and magnesium have complementary and opposing effects, the objective of treatment is to raise cellular levels of magnesium while lowering levels of calcium. Magnesium helps relax muscles and stabilize mast cells, preventing them from bursting and releasing a flood of histamine, thereby triggering an allergic reaction. In contrast, calcium stimulates mast cells to release histamines. Magnesium is also particularly useful in the treatment of asthma by reducing inflammation and relaxing the smooth muscle in the lungs. Intravenous magnesium sulfate relaxes the smooth muscle and rapidly opens the bronchial tubes. Calcium also participates in inflammatory reactions as part of calcium-dependent carrier proteins, which transport proteins to seal off an area and increase inflammation. In individuals with inflammatory conditions, the normal calcium to magnesium ratio of 2:1 can be modified to 1:1 or even 1:2.

SUGGESTED DOSAGE: At many hospitals, intravenous magnesium sulfate is used, along with prescription drugs, to treat asthmatic attacks. While only a medical professional can administer intravenous magnesium, magnesium supplements taken orally can easily be found in most pharmacies and health food stores and are safe over the long term. A suggested dosage is 500 to 1000 mg per day. Magnesium does have a laxative effect when used in too high a dosage. If you begin to have loose bowel movements, cut back on the dosage.

VITAMIN C

Unlike most animals, who produce their own vitamin C, we humans must include it in our diet because our bodies are unable to synthesize it. Because vitamin C is water soluble, it does not accumulate in the body and is rapidly eliminated in urine and through perspiration. Most ingested vitamin C is excreted from the body within three or four hours. If high blood levels of vitamin C are needed, it must be taken at regular intervals throughout the day. In addition, its potency can be lost through exposure to light, heat, and air.

Vitamin C reduces inflammation by decreasing histamine levels in the blood. In an allergic response, histamine levels tend to rise. In a study published in 1975 in the *Journal of Nutrition*, oral supplementation of vitamin C at 1 g per day for three days in eleven volunteers reduced blood histamine levels in every case. This same paper noted that in evaluating 437 human blood samples, when plasma vitamin C levels fell below 1 mg/100 ml, whole blood histamine levels increased exponentially as the ascorbic-acid level decreased. Besides reducing histamines, vitamin C is also needed for the synthesis of adrenal corticosteroids, our body's own anti-inflammatory agents.

Vitamin C can have a laxative effect, enabling the patient to pass food through the intestinal tract more efficiently and completely. This too can be helpful in treating allergies. When a person is constipated, fecal material remains in the intestine long enough for toxins to be reabsorbed from the bowel back into the bloodstream. These reabsorbed toxins can exacerbate allergies. When vitamin C is combined with digestive enzymes and hesperidin (a bioflavonoid commonly found in citrus peel), it can also be used successfully to speed recovery time in sports injuries.

SUGGESTED DOSAGE: Since vitamin C has a laxative effect, initial doses should be low, such as 500 to 1000 mg, one to three times a day. Higher doses of vitamin C can be used safely, and people with inflammatory conditions may use as much as 5,000 to 10,000 mg of vitamin C as a total dosage. While high doses of vitamin C can be very helpful, not everyone can tolerate this because of bowel sensitivity and its laxative effect. If you want to experiment with dosages, start with 1 to 3 g per day, increasing your intake to bowel tolerance. If your stools become loose, drop to a level that permits a normal bowel movement. To accelerate recovery from injuries, 750 mg of citrus bioflavonoids, one to two capsules per day, can be used along with vitamin C.

Many people who are overly acidic tend to experience stomach or intestinal-tract discomfort when using vitamin C in the form of ascorbic acid. In such cases, be sure to use a buffered form of vitamin C. It can be buffered by the addition of alkaline minerals such as sodium, calcium, potassium, or magnesium and still maintain its active properties. Buffered vitamin C also reduces the laxative and gastric-irritant effects of ascorbic acid, which is helpful for people with poor bowel tolerance of this very important nutrient.

PART 4:
TAKE OTHER NUTRIENTS AND DEVELOP GOOD HABITS TO PROMOTE HEALTHY DIGESTIVE FUNCTION

IF YOU HAVE chronic digestive complaints such as gas, bloating, abdominal discomfort, or poor bowel function, usually more than simply weak pancreatic function is involved. Millions of people also suffer from such common conditions as irritable-bowel syndrome, colitis, intestinal food allergies, and gastritis. These conditions become particularly common after midlife and reflect the weakening and diminished functional capability of the digestive organs in general. In such cases, a nutritional program to support the function of the digestive tract may be helpful. We have included a number of substances in this section that can be helpful in supporting, and even restoring, better digestive function, as well as two good habits that you should try to develop to help your body's digestive process.

HYDROCHLORIC ACID

Hydrochloric acid (HCl) is produced by the parietal cells of the stomach, primarily to begin the task of breaking down proteins so that they can be properly digested. HCl is needed to lower the pH of the stomach. In fact, stomach acid is so strong that it is as much as 100,000 to nearly 1,000,000 times more acidic than water. HCl also activates the proteolytic enzyme pepsin, also found in the stomach. A lack of either or both will interfere with normal digestion. HCl also makes nutrients like calcium, iron, and vitamin B_{12} more absorbable and helps to suppress the growth of disease-causing bacteria in the stomach.

As we age, some individuals may produce less HCl. Several research studies have found reduced HCl production in more than half of volunteers examined over the age of sixty. Although other studies contradict these findings, you should be aware that a normal physiological decline in stomach acid can occur in certain individuals. This condition should be properly diagnosed and treated with HCl supplementation. Emotional stress, poor diet, and exposure to toxins can also impair our ability to produce HCl.

Low gastric acidity is associated with many diseases, including asthma, rheumatoid arthritis, and gallbladder disease. In addition, low gastric acidity may also contribute to the overgrowth of bacteria in the small bowel. Common symptoms of low gastric acidity are bloating, belching, flatulence immediately after eating, diarrhea, constipation, food allergies, and nausea after taking supplements.

▲▲ Individuals who are overly acidic may find that the use of hydrochloric acid worsens digestive symptoms such as heartburn and abdominal discomfort. If this applies to you, be sure to read the label of any digestive aid before buying it to make sure that it does not contain hydrochloric acid. If you have sufficient or even too much acid production, HCl may aggravate your symptoms, giving you heartburn, and should be discontinued immediately.

SUGGESTED DOSAGE: Begin by taking one tablet or capsule containing 10 grains (600 mg) of hydrochloric acid at your next meal. If well tolerated, take one tablet or capsule at the next meal and increase the dosage by one tablet or capsule at every subsequent meal. (That is, one at the next meal, two at the meal after that, then three at the next meal.) Continue to increase the dose until you reach seven tablets or until you feel a warmth in your stomach, whichever occurs first. After you have found the largest dose that you can take at mealtime without feeling any warmth, maintain that dose at all meals of similar size. You will need to take less at smaller meals, however. When taking a number of tablets or capsules, you should take them throughout the meal. It is very important not to take HCl on an empty stomach, and HCl is contraindicated in persons with peptic-ulcer disease. Because HCl can irritate sensitive tissue and can be corrosive to teeth, capsules should not be emptied into food or dissolved in beverages.

CIDER VINEGAR

Many people have found that taking 1 to 2 tbsp. per day of cider vinegar will have the same effect as supplementing with hydrochloric acid, with fewer negative side effects. Be sure to use raw, unpasteurized, unfiltered cider vinegar made from organic apples. For those whose stomach acid production is compromised, the cider vinegar seems to be less harsh to the stomach lining. The primary acid in cider vinegar is malic acid, and malate is a component of the Kreb's cycle, a series of chemical reactions involved in the conversion of food to energy.

▲▲ Overly acidic individuals should be conservative in their use of HCl or cider vinegar because it will add to their acid load and they will feel discomfort after taking it. Use these supplements with great caution, or not at all, if you have conditions related to overacidity. However, if you feel you may be deficient in stomach acid, you can try cider vinegar instead of beginning with commercial preparations of HCl.

LACTOBACILLI AND BIFIDOBACTERIA

Friendly bacteria like lactobacilli and bifidobacteria normally colonize the intestinal tract. These bacteria have many beneficial effects on digestion. Because they aid in the production of essential B vitamins as well as acetic and lactic acids, they prevent colonization of the colon by harmful bacteria and yeast.

However, overconsumption of alcohol or sugar, a high-fat diet, and the use of antibiotics can reduce the population of lactobacilli and predispose the body to an overgrowth of harmful bacteria and fungi. Pathogenic organisms like candida may flourish in this environment. Susan has worked with numerous patients who have been given antibiotics to treat such common health conditions as bronchitis and the flu and have consequently developed candida. The vaginal itching, burning, and discharge due to overgrowth of candida in the vagina and intestines then has to be treated as a separate infection.

To insure healthy intestinal flora, Susan recommends taking lactobacilli supplements on a regular basis. For maximum effectiveness, take these on an empty stomach, in the morning and one hour before meals. Various cultures are available as powders, capsules, tablets, and liquids, measured by the amount of viable bacteria per dosage. For those people who can tolerate dairy products, soured milk products such as buttermilk, yogurt, acidophilus milk, and kefir can also be used to help restore the levels of friendly bacteria. There are also nondairy acidophilus products, such as soy yogurt, for people who are allergic to dairy foods.

FIBER

Dietary fiber can improve the function and absorptive capacity of the intestinal tract. Insoluble fibers such as cellulose and hemicellulose are found in fruits, vegetables, nuts, and beans. Soluble fibers like pectins, gums, and mucilages are found in oatmeal, oat bran, sesame seeds, and dried beans. Because the refining process has removed most of the natural fiber from our foods, the average American's diet is grossly lacking in fiber.

Fiber helps prevent constipation, colon cancer, and many other intestinal disorders. (More than 85,000 cases of colon cancer are diagnosed each year.) Once ingested, fiber undergoes bacterial fermentation in the colon. This process produces butyrate, the main energy source for colonic epithelial cells, which are needed for a healthy, cancer-free colon. This effect was verified in a study published in 1996 in the *Scandinavian Journal of Gastroenterology*. Researchers followed the health of twenty patients who had undergone surgical treatment for colon cancer. The volunteers were given fiber in the form of psyllium seeds. After one month of supplementation, fecal concentration of butyrate increased by 47 percent.

Fiber may also help to decrease the tendency toward overacidity in the intestinal tract by reducing inflammation. This occurs because fiber improves the transit time of food as it moves through the intestinal tract; it also promotes the growth of beneficial intestinal flora. These flora are less acidifying and irritating to the intestines than are the less healthy flora that thrive when people eat low-fiber, high-fat, high-sugar diets.

High-energy activities and peak performance require proper bowel function, so that food moves quickly through the intestines and toxic waste products are eliminated. To increase your fiber intake, include in your meals whole-grain cereals and flours, brown rice, all kinds of bran, fruits such as apricots, dried prunes, and apples (unless you tend to be overly acidic), nuts, seeds, beans, lentils, peas, and vegetables. Several of these foods should be included in every meal. Moreover, when you eat apples and potatoes, enjoy them with their skins.

SUGGESTED DOSAGE: If you supplement your diet with fiber, start with small amounts and gradually increase your intake. Fiber like oat bran and psyllium should be used to a maximum dosage of 1 to 2 tbsp. per day. This should be taken mixed with 8 to 12 oz. of water and swallowed immediately after stirring, since psyllium can become gel-like in texture. Those suffering from Crohn's disease (an inflammatory condition of the small intestine that can cause abdominal pain, cramping, and change in bowel habits) should avoid supplemental fiber and only consume fiber in foods. Soluble fiber like guar gum and pectin (derived from apples and grapefruit) can be taken in the same manner. Combine $1/2$ tsp. guar gum and 500 mg of pectin and add this mixture to 8 to 12 oz. of water. Stir and drink immediately. Use one to three times a day.

HERBS

Herbs and spices are time-honored digestive aids. Many of Susan's patients use herbal teas as a healthy and satisfying alternative to acidic coffee. Susan also has many patients who drink coffee in the morning for a quick energy boost. However, this boost is only temporary; after an hour or two, most individuals have difficulty staying alert enough to focus on work and meet deadlines without drinking additional coffee. Ginger and peppermint teas are made from mildly stimulating herbs and can produce more subtle but sustained increases in energy. Many herbs can be used as a delicious morning beverage and have beneficial effects on both mental alertness and digestive function without causing the side effects and addiction of caffeine. Peppermint tea also helps alleviate gas by acting as a stomach sedative and powerful antispasmodic. Chamomile tea soothes the digestive tract and also acts as a natural antispasmodic, reducing pain and discomfort. Fennel disperses gas and dispels bloating. (For this purpose, a traditional Indian curry dinner ends with a bowl of fennel.) Finally, licorice, the sweet-tasting herb used to flavor candy, has been found to be quite effective in the treatment of peptic ulcers. Research studies have shown that licorice strengthens the protective lining of the intestinal tract and helps to prevent ulcer formation.

WATER

For optimal digestive health and hydration of body tissues, drink eight to ten glasses of water a day. This should be done apart from liquid taken with meals. Fluids stimulate the production of saliva, bile, and gastric, pancreatic, and intestinal juices. The water should be drunk at room temperature. Nonchlorinated spring or filtered water is best. There is ongoing controversy over whether taking fluids with meals dilutes digestive enzymes or stimulates their production. Susan recommends reducing fluid intake with meals and drinking most of your water between meals.

TWO GOOD HABITS

You can also improve your digestive function by developing two simple habits that will make an important difference in your health: (1) chew your food thoroughly, and (2) eat your last meal of the day in the early evening.

Chew your food thoroughly

This maternal advice still holds true. The longer you chew your food, the longer the enzymes in your mouth have to begin the work of digestion. The starch-digesting enzyme ptyalin helps to break up starches even before they are swallowed.

Chewing is critical for digestion of all foods, because enzymes only act on the surface area of food particles. The more time you spend chewing, the more surface area of food will be exposed to enzymes, leading to better digestion. Raw fruits and vegetables, although good sources of living enzymes, need to be chewed thoroughly because they contain indigestible cellulose membranes that must be broken before nutrients can be released and the food digested.

Chewing also triggers the body's production of digestive-tract enzymes and stimulates the secretion of pancreatic fluids, intestinal juices, and bile (an emulsifying agent produced by the liver that is essential for the digestion of fats). Gulping down a sandwich in ten minutes so that you can use the rest of your lunch hour for catching up on work does not serve your health in the long run.

Eat your last meal of the day in the early evening

Eating late at night puts stress on the digestive organs. It is preferable to complete your final meal of the day by 7:00 P.M. It is also important to eat in a relaxed state and not to try to negotiate a major deal over dinner. To maintain the health and stamina you need to be successful in business or any creative endeavor, you need to make mealtime a peaceful and relaxing experience.

SUMMARY OF TREATMENT OPTIONS
FOR RESTORING YOUR DIGESTIVE ENZYMES

Diet
Choose enzyme-rich foods
Avoid foods that stress the pancreas
Drink blenderized drinks, if indicated
Eat pureed foods, if indicated

Supplemental digestive enzymes
Plant-based digestive enzymes
    Bromelain
    Papain
Pancreatic enzymes derived from animal sources

Other natural anti-inflammatory agents
MSM (methylsulfonylmethane)
Colloidal silver
Colostrum
Alkalinizing agents
Quercetin
Curcumin (turmeric)
Ginger
Essential fatty acids
Magnesium and calcium
Vitamin C

Digestive aids
Hydrochloric acid
Cider vinegar
Lactobacilli and bifidobacteria
Fiber
Culinary herbs
Water

5

How Detoxification Benefits Peak Performance and Health

WESTERN CULTURE IS firmly rooted in the pleasure principle. Many people enjoy eating rich foods, drinking alcoholic beverages, and even smoking cigars to increase their enjoyment of life or as a reward for working hard and accomplishing their goals. Many people use cigarettes, drugs, and alcohol to reduce their level of stress and buffer them from the fears and anxieties that would otherwise dampen their mood. When things go wrong, many of us tend to look for a quick fix. We value convenience in many areas of our lives above all else, regardless of its cost or possible deleterious effects on our health. Examples of modern conveniences that have potential health hazards include spraying the lawn with herbicides instead of digging out weeds, eliminating insects with pesticides, and using toxic solvents for cleaning. Similarly, Western medicine treats most health problems by using drugs to suppress symptoms rapidly but may cause potentially toxic side effects.

All of these pleasures and conveniences of modern life generate enormous amounts of toxic residues that we ingest or are exposed to on a daily basis through the air we breathe or even take into our bodies through our skin and mucous membranes. In order to remain in good health, the body must break down and eliminate all of these toxins on a continual basis. In addition, the body must similarly process the by-products of its own metabolism, which, if allowed to accumulate in the body, could cause serious illness or even death.

Detoxification, therefore, is one of our body's most crucial physiological functions. Detoxification refers to the process of neutralizing or transforming substances that would normally be poisonous or harmful, and eliminating them from the body. Without proper detoxification, toxic substances would accumulate within the body and impair our health by interfering with the function of all our vital organ systems.

The many benefits of good detoxification, for both peak performance and health, are listed in the following chart.

Benefits of Detoxification

Peak-Performance Benefits

1. Increased physical vitality and stamina (helps improve work productivity)

2. Enhanced mental clarity and acuity

4. Increased ability to get along with other people (permits enjoyment of extensive social and business entertaining)

5. Increased ability to remain calm under pressure

8. Increased resistance to illness

Health Benefits

- Eliminates toxins from the body
- Protects the nervous system and brain from unmetabolized toxins
- Reduces the risk of heart disease
- Decreases the risk of PMS, fibroid tumors, endometriosis, and breast cancer
- Promotes sexual performance and maintains libido
- Is used as a complementary therapy for the treatment of cancer

---

The liver is our primary organ of detoxification. It is the main interface between both ingested and internally created toxins and all the cells of our bodies. If the liver can handle the toxic load we put on our bodies, we can perform at our best and remain healthy. If liver function is impaired, however, performance is negatively affected in many different ways. Poor detoxification function is linked to chronic low-grade fatigue, brain fog upon arising in the morning, muddled thinking, or reacting with inappropriate behavior (usually anger) to many of life's inconsequential annoyances.

In this chapter we will describe how critical healthy detoxification is to peak performance and ultimately success. In fact, most peak performers have the Chemistry of Success, in part, because of their excellent detoxification capabilities. You will also gain an understanding and appreciation of how valuable the liver is to optimal health. In addition, you will learn how our modern lifestyle has tended to overload this crucial function in millions of Americans and why many so-called behavioral abnormalities may even be traced to poor liver function. In the following chapter, you will learn invaluable techniques for restoring liver function and, thereby, regaining your ability to perform to your maximum potential.

To help you assess whether or not your body has the kind of detoxification ability that you need for good general health as well as peak performance, work through the following checklist (photocopy it if you don't want to write in the book), and refer to it as you read through the chapter. Detoxification can also be tested medically; see page 300.

CHECKLIST: DO YOU HAVE ADEQUATE DETOXIFICATION?

Although the following checklist does not provide a definitive diagnosis of detoxification ability, seeing which items apply to you, in conjunction with your reading of this chapter, can help you to determine whether your own system is working adequately. If the results of this exercise suggest that your liver function is weak, you can learn ways to improve your ability to detoxify in the next chapter.

Lifestyle/environmental factors

Put a check mark beside those statements that are true for you.

❑ My diet is high in sugar.

❑ My diet is high in fat.

❑ I tend to eat a lot of fast food.

❑ I regularly consume caffeinated beverages, including coffee, tea, and colas.

❑ I regularly consume alcohol.

❑ I regularly consume food additives and artificial sweeteners such as aspartame.

❑ I use excessive amounts of prescription drugs, over-the-counter medications, and recreational drugs.

❑ I have been exposed to synthetic pesticides and herbicides.

❑ I have been exposed to industrial chemicals and cleaning agents.

Performance indicators

❑ I experience brain fog upon waking in the morning.

❑ I am frequently unable to think clearly and use good judgment.

❑ I am often unable to remain calm under stress.

❑ I have difficulty socializing and mixing easily with people because of food and alcohol intolerances.

❑ I am often unable to perform tasks effectively.

❑ I suffer from chronic fatigue.

❑ I am often irritable.

❑ I have a tendency to be impatient, arrogant, and resentful.

❑ I often get angry when driving.

❑ I have an explosive or impulsive personality.

Physical indicators

❑ I have vitamin and mineral deficiencies, especially the fat-soluble vitamins and vitamin B complex.

❑ I have high cholesterol.

❑ I have high levels of circulating estrogen.

❑ I am over seventy years old.

❑ I have frequent episodes of tiredness, dizziness, nausea, and a racing pulse.

❏ I have a marked distaste for oily foods.

❏ I experience soreness in the liver area under moderate fingertip pressure.

❏ I often have poor digestion, gas pains, constipation, and a feeling of fullness in the stomach and intestines.

❏ I have low levels of stomach acid and digestive enzymes.

Medical history

❏ I have a history of hepatitis or other liver disease.

❏ I have had a diagnosis of heart disease, such as congestive heart failure, cardiac arrhythmia, enlarged heart, or coronary heart disease.

❏ I have a history of nervous-system diseases, such as polyneuritis.

❏ I generally lack resistance to infectious disease.

❏ I have a history of disease of the gastrointestinal tract, such as gastritis, esophagitis, pancreatitis, or ulcers.

❏ I have a history of gallstones.

Now that you have a preliminary understanding of the importance of detoxification to peak performance and optimal health, as well as some idea from the checklist of your own functioning in this area, you are ready to decide what to read next. To learn more about the chemistry of detoxification, read the following section. To learn how diet and lifestyle affect detoxification, read section 2, on page 268. For a detailed discussion of how detoxification affects peak performance, read section 3, on page 276. For a detailed discussion of how detoxification affects general health, including specific conditions caused or exacerbated by inadequate detoxification, read section 4, on page 295. (Ideally, these latter two sections should be read consecutively, as the effects of detoxification on peak performance and health are intricately intertwined.) Finally, for information on how to restore and strengthen your ability to detoxify, read chapter 6.

SECTION 1:
THE CHEMISTRY OF DETOXIFICATION

TWO KINDS OF toxins must be processed by the body in order to maintain health: those that are generated in the environment and those that are generated within the body.

ENVIRONMENTAL TOXINS

Beginning early in this century and accelerating in the last four or five decades, there has been an enormous increase in the number and amount of environmental pollutants that we are exposed to on a daily basis. Our ability to process and excrete these toxins is crucial for survival. Our bodies are being assaulted on a daily basis by chemicals such as pesticides, herbicides, and contaminants from industrial manufacturing that are in the air, water, and food supply. The amount of toxic chemicals we are exposed to in our environment is staggering. Each year, the average American is exposed to fourteen pounds of food preservatives, additives, waxes (used to preserve produce), colorings, flavorings, antimicrobial agents, and pesticide and herbicide residues. U.S. production of synthetic pesticides exceeds 1.4 billion pounds a year, and the Environmental Protection Agency (EPA) estimates that there are approximately 70,000 various chemicals in foods, drugs, and pesticides that we may be exposed to, any of which the human body must be prepared to deactivate and remove.

In addition, most of us consume highly processed foods that are laden with artificial chemicals and food additives like MSG (monosodium glutamate), a widely used flavor enhancer; aspartame, an artificial sweetener used in many calorie-reduced foods; and trans fatty acids. These trans fatty acids, which are not found in nature, are polyunsaturated vegetable oils that have been chemically altered by hydrogenation, which converts a fat that is liquid at room temperature into one that is solid, like margarine. All of these artificial chemicals must be detoxified and eliminated by the body.

Toxins also accumulate in the body through the ingestion of addictive substances such as alcohol, caffeine, sugar, and nicotine. Manufacturers promote these addictive substances with billions of dollars of advertising, and many of our social customs support their usage. We have every opportunity to indulge in these substances thanks to daily coffee and cigarette breaks at work and the universal availability of these products in every imaginable channel of distribution.

The body must also detoxify prescription and over-the-counter drugs as well as recreational ones. Drugs are commonly broken down by the liver and eliminated through excretory organs like the kidneys. Many Americans routinely take as many as two to three drugs per day in an attempt to quickly fix a health complaint that is often the result of a poor lifestyle choice. Older Americans have been known to be on ten to twenty or more different drugs for various ailments. Over time, this puts enormous strain on the liver.

SELF-GENERATED TOXINS

Beside the toxins we take into our bodies from the outside, our bodies also create endogenous toxins (originating from inside the body), which must also be broken down and eliminated. These are chemicals that we produce internally as by-products of metabolism. When the detoxification process is working efficiently, these toxins are usually neutralized or excreted without unduly stressing the body. However, if allowed to circulate unaltered through the body, these chemical substances can be highly toxic. For example, when you have a protein-rich meal like a steak dinner, the by-product of the chemical breakdown of the protein is ammonia, which is highly toxic if allowed to accumulate in the body. Normally, ammonia is immediately converted by the liver into a harmless substance called urea that can then be excreted from the body through the kidneys. In patients with severe liver disease, however, this ability to convert ammonia is compromised and ammonia can become elevated to dangerously high levels.

When toxic substances are not properly neutralized and excreted from the body, they are stored in the cells, particularly in fatty tissue. Our cells and tissues can store toxins for months, even years, releasing them during times of low food intake, exercise, or stress. When they are finally released into the bloodstream, the toxins can trigger unwanted symptoms as the body reacts to these poisons, including tiredness, dizziness, nausea, and a racing pulse. Many chronic and even deadly diseases such as coronary heart disease and diseases of the nervous system, liver, pancreas, and other vital organs have been linked to impaired detoxification. Both the health and performance consequences of poor detoxification have been corroborated by many research studies.

THE BODY'S MAIN ORGAN OF DETOXIFICATION: THE LIVER

When the liver is working efficiently, it buffers the body internally from the harmful effects of both ingested toxins and environmental pollutants as well as the by-products of our own metabolism. Most people are unaware of the vital role the liver plays in maintaining health, equating it only with a food that tastes good when cooked with onions. However, an understanding of how this vital organ functions is crucial for maintaining high performance levels and overall good health.

The liver is one of the most complex and metabolically active organs in the body. It is also the largest organ in your body, normally weighing about four pounds. The liver lies in the upper right portion of the abdominal cavity beneath the diaphragm. Its large size reflects the multiple functions it performs. It carries out hundreds, if not thousands, of enzymatic reactions along numerous metabolic pathways, playing a pivotal role in maintaining health. The liver is so crucial to health that it is the only organ that can completely regenerate itself when part of it is removed or damaged. Up to 25 percent of the liver can be removed, and it can still perform its tasks. Moreover, its powers of regeneration are awesome: Within a short period of time, the liver will grow back to its original shape and size.

As harmful chemicals and bacteria circulate through the liver, they pass through a network of blood vessels called the portal system. Unlike other organs of the body, the portal system does not receive blood from the heart. Instead, the liver receives much of its blood directly from the intestinal tract. This allows the liver to process the nutrients and any ingested pollutants before they reach the general circulation. The liver processes about three pints of blood, or an average of 29 percent of a person's total cardiac output, per minute.

The liver deactivates and removes the toxic chemicals that circulate throughout the body by two methods. The first method consists of filtering channels called sinusoids. Cells that line the sinusoids surround and break down foreign debris, bacteria, and toxic chemicals via phagocytosis, the process in which one molecule digests another. The second method consists of an extensive two-step system of enzymes that facilitate the deactivation and elimination of toxins.

There are two phases to this process. Phase I involves a group of enzymes called the cytochrome P-450 system. This system contains between fifty and a hundred enzymes, each of which detoxifies specific types of chemicals. In this phase, toxins undergo oxidation and reduction, in which electrons are transferred between molecules. They are also rendered more water soluble.

Most harmful chemicals—such as pesticides, herbicides, alcohol, and drugs—are fat soluble when they first enter the body, which allows them to be stored in our fatty tissue and therefore makes them more difficult to eliminate from the body. But when toxins are rendered water soluble, they can be more easily excreted through the kidneys and intestinal tract. Phase I of the detoxification process reduces the toxicity of chemicals that would be harmful to the body if they were allowed to remain in their original state. After this phase, toxins are either neutralized, excreted from the body through the intestines or urinary tract, or converted into an intermediate form suitable for further processing by the phase II detoxification system. As these intermediate products are formed, free radicals are generated, and antioxidants are necessary to keep these free radicals from damaging the liver. Because these intermediate products are potentially dangerous, it is important that phase II of detoxification be functioning properly to be able to complete the metabolism of these toxins. Foods such as broccoli, brussels sprouts, cabbage, oranges, tangerines, dill, and caraway seeds can support this function. Broccoli, brussels sprouts, and cabbage contain indole-3-carbinol and oranges, tangerines, dill, and caraway seeds contain limonine, both of which stimulate the phase I detoxification enzymes.

In phase II of the detoxification process, the intermediate compounds generated in phase I are transformed into harmless metabolites (breakdown products) that can then be excreted by the body. Phase II enzymes act directly on some toxic substances through a process called conjugation, in which these substances are bound with a protective compound. This process either inactivates or neutralizes the toxins or enables them to be more readily eliminated from the body. Phase II detoxification occurs through the production of glutathione, a substance composed of three amino acids, cysteine, glutamic acid, and glycine, and other sulfer-containing compounds such as sulfuric and glucorunic acid. Several amino acids—including glycine, glutamine, arginine, ornithine, and taurine—along with acetyl CoA and methyl groups (which originate from the amino acid methionine), also combine with and neutralize toxins in phase II. Conjugation removes toxins from their free state, in which they could ordinarily cause cellular stress or damage. Conjugated toxins are then excreted through the urinary tract or the intestines.

An example of substances that must be detoxified by the liver are the many hormones produced within the body. Hormones like estrogen, testosterone, adrenaline, and insulin must be efficiently metabolized and excreted from the body. Otherwise, they would accumulate to toxic levels, producing a variety of adverse effects. Hormones circulate throughout the body, being transported in the blood to various tissues and organ systems. As hormones pass through the liver, they are inactivated by being bound to sulfuric and glucuronic acid and converted to less potent forms. This process of binding hormones with other chemicals makes them unable to attach to the specific hormone receptor sites within the cells. Once hormones have been detoxified by the liver, they are then secreted with the bile into the small intestine and eliminated through the bowels.

The detoxification of alcohol also occurs in the liver. Detoxification lessens the toxic effects of alcohol on the liver by helping to convert the alcohol into less harmful end products. When this process does not function properly, alcohol residues can cause serious inflammatory changes within the liver. Many medications, insecticides, heavy metals, and nicotine from cigarette smoke are examples of other toxic substances treated by phase II detoxification.

OTHER LIVER FUNCTIONS THAT AID DETOXIFICATION

The liver performs many other important functions that assist in and support the process of detoxification. These include the liver's production of bile as well as its functions as a storage reservoir for blood and as a filter of bacteria and viruses. The liver also aids in the digestion, absorption, storage, and utilization of many vitamins, minerals, protein, sugar, and fat. While not specifically needed for detoxification, these other functions are all crucial for the maintenance of good health and peak performance.

Bile production

The liver produces bile, a yellowish-green fluid that is stored in the gallbladder and secreted into the intestine to emulsify (disperse into smaller droplets) and facilitate the digestion of fats. Toxins are also secreted into the bile and then eliminated from the body through the intestinal tract. Thus, adequate bile production helps to reduce the workload of the liver. Within the liver, bile is transported through small ducts into larger canals and, finally, into the gallbladder where it is stored and concentrated. The emulsifying agent in the bile, lecithin, transforms large fat globules into tiny ones, which are more water soluble and more readily assimilated. Bile helps the body excrete breakdown products from the blood, neutralizes stomach acid, promotes intestinal peristalsis, and increases the absorption of the fat-soluble vitamins, A, D, E, and K.

Blood storage

Since the liver is an organ that can expand and contract, it is capable of serving as a reservoir for blood when there is excess volume in circulation. It is also capable of supplying extra blood to the rest of the body when blood volume is low. The normal blood volume of the liver is about 10 percent of the body's total blood volume. Only one-quarter of the blood that circulates through the liver is derived from general circulation; the remaining three-quarters comes from the portal blood flow, which is derived from the intestines, stomach, spleen, and pancreas. This portal blood carries bacteria picked up from the intestines. The liver is said to cleanse this blood through the action of cells within the liver that digest and destroy these bacteria.

The proper release of blood from the liver is critical for good health. The liver is also involved in the formation of blood, creating serum proteins such as albumin, which maintain fluid balance through osmosis and act as transport molecules. Traditional Asian medicine has long recognized the importance of the liver's blood storage function, using terms such as "blood deficiency" and "blood stagnancy" to explain the origins of various health problems. For example, visual problems, muscle spasms, and menstrual-bleeding abnormalities are all diagnosed in terms of liver blood flow.

Virus and bacteria filtration

Blood flowing through the intestinal capillaries picks up many bacteria from the intestines. Within the liver, the Kupffer cells line the hepatic sinuses. These cells engulf and digest about 99 percent of the bacteria present. Only the remaining 1 percent of the bacteria escapes destruction within the liver and is able to pass through the liver into the general circulation. Bacteria and yeast can also form toxins that are absorbed into the bloodstream and carried throughout the body. These microbes are implicated in various diseases, including ulcerative colitis, thyroid disease, allergies, and immune disorders. The healthy liver filters out these pathogens, further reducing stress on the immune system.

OTHER IMPORTANT FUNCTIONS OF THE LIVER

Besides its detoxification functions, the liver also plays an important role in the metabolism of protein, fat, and carbohydrates. In addition, numerous compounds essential to the growth, repair, and maintenance of body tissues are either stored or manufactured in the liver, including glucose, cholesterol, and lipoproteins. Many important nutrients are also stored in the liver, including the vitamins A, D, E, and B_{12}; and the minerals iron and copper. Healthy liver function is also necessary to regulate the blood sugar level.

SUMMARY

The liver plays a pivotal role in maintaining health. It performs so many functions and is so crucial to the body that it is the only organ that can completely regenerate itself. The liver is the main organ of detoxification, cleansing the blood of harmful chemicals, viruses, and bacteria; it produces bile, which is essential in the digestion of fat; it stores extra blood; it helps to metabolize protein, fat, and carbohydrates; and it stores important nutrients.

SECTION 2:
HOW DIET AND LIFESTYLE AFFECT DETOXIFICATION

GIVEN THE LIVER'S crucial role as our primary organ of detoxification, any physical or chemical stress that lessens its ability to carry out this function will strongly compromise many aspects of performance and health. Fortunately, many of these stressors are due to lifestyle habits that are under our control. By supporting liver function through healthy lifestyle practices, one can maintain the ability to detoxify at effective and peak levels well into old age.

THE AGING LIVER

The decrease in the liver's detoxification capability is not readily apparent in standard medical testing. While the liver does go through some structural changes as the body ages, these changes consist of only minor alterations, a slight shrinking in the size of the liver and some changes in cell structure. This decrease in size parallels a similar decrease in overall body size, a process that continues from age fifty to seventy. However, research studies show no significant alterations with age in the most common laboratory indicators of liver function—serum bilirubin, serum glutamic oxaloacetic transaminase (SGOT), and serum glutamic pyruvic transaminase (SGPT)—which are all low in people with normal liver function. Hepatic blood flow does decline somewhat with age, but only with the normal decrease in cardiac output.

However, declines in the liver's detoxification capability do occur in some individuals and are often accelerated by external factors related to exposure to environmental toxins and lifestyle habits. These include lack of B vitamins, infectious disease, overconsumption of alcohol, overuse of drugs, and exposure to industrial chemicals. Over time, the cumulative effect of these toxins can cause chronic liver damage.

Alcohol

The most common cause of liver stress and damage in the United States today is the overconsumption of alcohol. It is estimated that more than 100 million Americans consume alcoholic beverages. When the liver's ability to detoxify alcohol is overwhelmed, peak-performance capability is significantly diminished. Moreover, chronic overconsumption can cause inflammatory changes within the liver, which can finally lead to fibrosis and permanent damage to the liver's cells. As many as a million liver cells can be destroyed by a single alcoholic drink.

Numerous studies document the specific ways in which alcohol impairs liver function. Habitual overconsumption of alcohol can increase the risk of developing a number of degenerative diseases, including hepatitis and cirrhosis, as well as gastritis and ulcers, pancreatitis, hypoglycemia, diabetes, gout, nerve and brain dysfunction, immune suppression, and some types of cancer. The overconsumption of alcohol also increases a person's susceptibility to other toxins such as carbon tetrachloride. It has been estimated that the overconsumption of alcohol can shorten a person's life span by ten to fifteen years.

People who regularly drink alcoholic beverages are particularly susceptible to multiple vitamin and mineral deficiencies. Because alcohol contains very few nutrients itself and also suppresses appetite, a person drinking alcohol eats less and takes in fewer vitamins and minerals. Finally, the alcohol molecule is small and easy to absorb, so it is preferentially assimilated before other, more nutrient-rich foods can be metabolized.

Alcohol consumption also leads to an increase in daily caloric intake. One ounce of hard liquor is 80 calories, five ounces of wine 100 calories, twelve ounces of beer 140 calories, and various mixed drinks made with juices, sodas, and sweeteners can be between 100 and 250 calories. The average social drinker obtains 5 to 10 percent of their calories from alcohol, while alcoholics may consume more than 50 percent of their calories as alcohol. The empty (meaning, nutrient-poor) calories in alcohol can also lead to weight gain, especially as the toxins in alcohol disrupt fat metabolism.

While alcohol adds significant calories to the diet, it simultaneously impairs digestion and absorption of many nutrients from the small intestine, including the fat-soluble vitamins, A, D, E, and K, plus thiamine, vitamin B_6, vitamin B_{12}, choline, folic acid, and some minerals. Alcohol has a diuretic effect as well, promoting the excretion of nutrients in the urine. Numerous research studies document the close correlation between alcohol intake and specific nutrient deficiencies. Alcoholics frequently show low levels of beta-carotene, thiamine, zinc, and vitamin B_6. Magnesium deficiency often occurs in chronic alcoholics due to increased loss of magnesium through the urinary tract, which is exacerbated by magnesium deficiency in the diet.

OVERCONSUMPTION OF PROTEIN, FATS, AND SUGAR

The standard American diet abounds with foods high in protein, fats, and sugar—everything from hamburgers and milk shakes to filet mignon and strawberry cheesecake. These foods place tremendous stress on the liver, which has to process them and convert their residue into waste products that can be eliminated from the body. One indication that the liver is not handling this task adequately is poor digestion. Common signs are gas pains, constipation (less than one bowel movement per day), a feeling of fullness in the stomach and intestines, loss of appetite, marked distaste for oily foods, and a soreness in the liver under moderate fingertip pressure.

Protein

Only a finite amount of protein can accumulate within the cells of the body. Once the cells have been filled to their limit, excess amino acids are degraded by the liver so that they can be either used as a source of energy or stored as fat. This degradation begins with a process called deamination. Ammonia, a toxic by-product similar to the ammonia in bottled cleaning solutions, is generated during this process. Ammonia is a strong-smelling and extremely potent poison. In order to avoid the accumulation of toxic levels of ammonia in the blood, the liver metabolizes it into urea, a harmless substance that can be eliminated via the kidneys. When a person's diet is very high in protein, though, more ammonia is generated and the liver must work harder to metabolize it. Ammonia will accumulate in the blood of individuals with severe liver disease; this accumulation is toxic to the brain and can lead to coma.

Fats

The high fat content of the American diet contributes approximately 40 percent of all calories consumed. This excessive amount of fat in the diet stresses the liver by adding to its workload. The liver must process the fat, converting it into fuel and various building blocks of the cells such as cholesterol and phospholipids. The liver must also produce bile to help break down the excess fat to prepare it for excretion.

Some of the saturated fats that we consume are converted into hormones such as estrogen, which the liver must eventually deactivate. Specifically, diets high in the saturated fats found in red meat and dairy products tend to promote high levels of estrogen in the body and increase the detoxification load on the liver. Research studies have shown that vegetarian women eating a low-fat, high-fiber diet excrete two to three times more estrogen in their bowel movements and have 50 percent lower blood levels of estrogen than women eating a diet high in dairy and animal fats.

In addition, large amounts of dietary fat can also stress the liver indirectly by causing excessive amounts of estrogen to be reabsorbed from the intestinal tract into the general circulation, thereby increasing the amount of estrogen that the liver must detoxify. Research studies done at Tufts University Medical School in the 1980s found that the composition of the diet strongly affected the type of bacteria present in the intestinal tract. A high-fat diet promoted the growth of intestinal bacteria that secrete an enzyme called beta-glucuronidase. The estrogen that has been bound and deactivated by the liver can be cleaved by this enzyme and thus reconverted back into free estrogen. Estrogen can then be reabsorbed back into the general circulation, thereby increasing the estrogen load presented to the liver. In contrast, a diet low in fat and high in fiber promotes the excretion of estrogen from the body, decreasing the amount circulating through the body—and, in particular, the liver.

Sugar

Sugar stored in the liver can also impair its function. Yet Americans eat an extraordinary amount of refined sugar, and the quantity continues to rise. According to the Economic Research Service of the USDA, U.S. consumption of total caloric sweeteners was 128.6 pounds per capita in 1986, and rose to 154.5 pounds per capita in 1997. When the liver stores too much glucose as well as toxins, the canals through which bile flows can become compressed, which decreases bile flow and impairs digestion. Excess stored glucose therefore makes the liver work harder to produce bile and essential digestive enzymes.

A study published in 1983 in the *American Journal of Medicine* noted signs of possible liver injury associated with the typical high-sugar American diet. Twenty-one normal adult males consumed a typical diet containing 25 to 30 percent sucrose for eighteen days and a "calorically diluted" diet containing less than 10 percent sucrose for twelve days. Levels of SGOT and SGPT, two enzymes that are released from liver cells into the bloodstream when these cells are acutely damaged, rose significantly when the men were on the high-sucrose diet and returned to baseline levels when they were on the low-sucrose diet.

Prescription, Over-the-Counter, and Recreational Drugs

Frequent use of medications causes the liver to work overtime in order to metabolize them. When drugs are used in moderation and the liver is healthy, it can normally detoxify them quite efficiently. However, when large amounts of medication or recreational drugs are ingested, especially when combined with other toxic substances such as alcohol, these substances can easily overwhelm the liver's detoxification ability.

Although over-the-counter (OTC) products such as anti-inflammatory medications are usually less toxic than prescription drugs, they are also more frequently abused, since they can be readily obtained without visiting a doctor and are less expensive. In America, there are over 50 million regular users of aspirin, with 20 to 25 billion tablets taken each year. Though most consumers usually consider OTC drugs harmless, the excessive use of them can cause dangerous side effects and even be life threatening—in part because the liver's ability to detoxify them is overwhelmed.

An interesting case study, published in the *Journal of Family Practice*, documents the history of a thirty-seven-year-old closet drinker who was taking multiple prescription and OTC medications. After taking a cough medication for an upper-respiratory infection, she arrived in the emergency room with markedly elevated liver enzymes. The patient was given intensive support but died ten hours later. In this tragic case, the chemically overloaded liver was unable to clear the cough medication rapidly enough from her body. As a result, her body went into a state of toxic overload.

Recreational or street drugs, including cocaine, speed, crack, opium, methadone, and heroin, are particularly toxic to the liver. Substances such as THC (the active ingredient in marijuana) and nicotine remain in the body for several weeks or even months.

Certain prescription drugs have well-documented side effects involving the liver. For example, the use of cimetidine (sold as Tagamet), an antiulcer medication, may result in liver damage in susceptible individuals. Older people are particularly susceptible to the toxic effects that medications may have on liver function: Not only have they cumulatively taken more medications in their lifetime, in general, but they also typically consume more prescription and over-the-counter medications than younger people.

INDUSTRIAL CHEMICALS

In the normal course of the day, we may be exposed to extremely toxic chemicals on the job and in the products we buy. For instance, chlorinated solvents such as carbon tetrachloride and chlorobenzene are used for degreasing and cleaning many types of machinery. Furniture strippers that contain chlorinated solvents may have been used on woodwork in your home. Chlorinated solvents can also strip the naturally protective oils from the skin, lung tissue, and eyes, causing damage on the cellular level. These solvents in drinking water have also been associated with chronic liver problems, as well as weakness of the kidney and heart. They are also suspected of causing certain types of cancer. Such chronic exposure to this myriad of chemical substances will, over time, weaken the liver's detoxification capability.

MEDICAL CONDITIONS

Some medical conditions affect the liver's ability to detoxify, including a vitamin B deficiency and hepatitis. Cirrhosis of the liver is the most serious, and usually fatal, liver disease.

Vitamin B deficiency

Vitamin B complex plays a special role in maintaining liver health. When there is a deficiency of the B vitamins, a person's ability to detoxify is greatly hindered. A deficiency of vitamin B complex and its link to liver disease was first researched in the 1940s by Morton S. Biskind, in both animal and human studies. In an animal study published in 1942 in *Endocrinology*, Biskind demonstrated that a B-complex deficiency could impair the liver's ability to deactivate a form of estrogen. Furthermore, Dr. Biskind noted that female patients with signs and symptoms of vitamin B deficiency also suffered from symptoms of excessive estrogen such as menorrhagia (heavy menstrual bleeding), premenstrual tension, and chronic cystic mastitis (painful breasts). He found that supplementation with B vitamins such as thiamine, riboflavin, and niacin helped to resolve the symptoms of excessive estrogen.

Hepatitis and cirrhosis

Hepatitis is an inflammatory disease of the liver that can be caused by exposure to a virus, chemical toxins such as alcohol or drugs, tainted food, or a blockage of the duct leading from the liver to the gallbladder. Symptoms of hepatitis include nausea, vomiting, jaundice, loss of appetite, tenderness in the upper-right abdomen, aching muscles, and joint pain.

While many individuals do recover from hepatitis and, over time, even regain normal liver function, not everyone does. In certain individuals, hepatitis does not resolve, and chronic liver disease develops. This often occurs with long-term exposure to pathogens like viruses. With end-stage liver disease, a condition called cirrhosis develops in which the inflammation of liver cells gradually leads to damage of cell structure. The gradual loss of liver function results, as living cells become surrounded by pockets of scar tissue, thereby shutting off the flow of portal blood to the remaining healthy tissue. As mentioned earlier, liver cells have the capacity to regenerate following many forms of illness, but cirrhosis is not one of them. Cirrhosis is usually fatal, as toxins accumulate in the body. It can be caused by anything from ingestion of toxic chemicals such as carbon tetrachloride, to viral diseases such as infectious hepatitis, to infectious processes in the bile ducts. However, alcoholism is the most common cause.

SUMMARY

A variety of dietary and lifestyle factors can harm the liver, including the overconsumption of alcohol, protein, fats, sugar, and drugs. Toxic chemicals in the environment are also harmful. Changes in lifestyle can eliminate or greatly limit these stressors, as the liver responds well to a healthy lifestyle, and aging does not greatly affect its detoxification capacity.

Section 3:
Detoxification and Peak Performance

A properly functioning liver can greatly assist you in performing at a peak level and attaining many of your goals and aspirations. This is because healthy detoxification helps us to maintain our level of physical energy, our cognitive function, the ability to make sound decisions, and the ability to remain calm during times of stress. It also helps us to maintain healthy social and business relationships by allowing us to enjoy social situations without any limitation on the types of food and drink we can ingest. Individuals who need to restrict their alcohol or food intake can undoubtedly survive at social occasions, dinner, and banquets where choice is minimal, but their options may be few.

1 Physical Vitality and Stamina

Success in most areas of life requires a tremendous amount of physical energy and stamina—which cannot be maintained without healthy detoxification capability. Most people are unaware of the crucial role that detoxification plays in maintaining one's level of energy. However, all of us have witnessed individuals who maintain their level of energy, even under adverse circumstances, because their detoxification capability is functioning effectively. These are the people who can work all day in hermetically sealed office buildings, with pollutant-laden recirculated air, and still feel energetic and fresh at the end of the workday. Unlike millions of chemically sensitive people, these individuals seem to be impervious to the chemical pollutants commonly found in such environments, such as benzene, formaldehyde, and toluene. Many of our modern sealed buildings with their synthetic carpeting and furnishings expose their occupants to high levels of such toxic chemicals. Only individuals with superfunctioning detoxification capability can thrive and maintain their physical energy and stamina after years of exposure to such toxic environments. In addition, these same individuals are often able to eat rich food accompanied by fine wines, drink at social and business affairs, smoke cigars, and generally expose themselves to a wide variety of pollutants that the body must detoxify. Yet, because they have inherently strong liver function, they are able to detoxify all of these pollutants and continue to have a tremendously high level of energy.

One of Jim's business associates, Michael, typifies this link between the ability to detoxify and physical energy. Michael is able to enjoy rich food and to drink large amounts of alcoholic beverages. Yet, he still maintains a tremendous level of vitality and energy even though he is now in his mid-sixties. Michael's business requires that he travels internationally for several months each year. He uses time on the plane to relax and catch up on his reading. While Michael takes full advantage of the hospitality in first class, and requests many refills of the wines and aperitifs he is served, he never experiences a drop in his energy level after drinking. He arrives at his destination, be it Singapore or Mexico City, without a hangover and ready to go to work. While he is totally committed to his work, he also engages regularly in strenuous physical activity. Wherever in the world he is traveling, he gets up early and does his daily jog. Slowing down his pace is unimaginable to him: While he will retire from his firm in a few years, he is already making plans for a second career.

The millions of Americans who do not have superfunctioning detoxification systems, however, take daily hits to their energy and stamina because they are unable to efficiently metabolize the vast ocean of toxic chemicals in which we are all immersed. Morning grogginess and brain fog are a daily concern for many of us, because toxins accumulate during the night and are not broken down by the liver and eliminated from the body. When the liver is unable to detoxify efficiently, the toxic substances generated within the body while a person is asleep are not fully metabolized until later in the day, after the liver has become more active. This can lead to a slow start in the morning. The tendency to feel tired and groggy is even greater if a person has eaten a heavy meal or consumed alcoholic beverages late the night before. Many people need that first cup of morning coffee to clear their head and restore their physical energy. They will drink coffee throughout the morning, until their liver has finally cleared the accumulated toxic load. Some of Susan's patients report that they drink as many as four to six cups of coffee or other caffeinated beverages in the morning; this consumption then tapers off in the afternoon, once their energy level picks up.

Susan has found that poor liver detoxification is often an important causal factor in patients who complain of chronic fatigue. Some of these patients also have symptoms of poor liver function or even a history of prior liver disease such as hepatitis. Symptoms of digestive distress due to poor liver function—such as bloating, discomfort in the upper-right abdominal area, and the inability to tolerate rich or fatty foods—can be seen in these patients. They also tend to be intolerant of alcohol. If they are women, they may also suffer from many common female problems such as PMS, heavy and/or irregular menstrual flow, and fibroid tumors of the uterus due, in part, to their liver's inability to detoxify estrogen.

Many of those with poor detoxification capability complain about underperforming in important areas of their lives because they simply lack the physical energy and vitality to do so. These people are genuinely upset by their inability to participate in many of the joys of living. Susan has found that many of these individuals benefit greatly from a liver detoxification program of the type described in the next chapter. Once the liver's detoxification ability is restored, they are often able to reduce their dependence on stimulants while regaining their physical energy and stamina.

A good example is Christine, a local real-estate agent who was in her late forties when she first consulted Susan about her chronic fatigue. During her twenty-year career, Christine always had sufficient energy to perform the many functions required of realtors. Success in the real-estate business requires an enormous amount of physical energy: Realtors are expected to be available to show houses at any time of the day or night, including weekends. There are constant tours, open houses, and staff meetings. Negotiations between the buyer and seller are often highly stressful, with deals sometimes falling through after weeks of effort. As part of her work, Christine enjoyed socializing frequently with her clients and coworkers. She would often enjoy a glass or two of wine after work and continued to drink into the evening at the social events she attended three to four nights a week.

However, in the year before her consultation with Susan, Christine began to find the physical demands of her job difficult to meet. To sustain her flagging energy, she began to increase her coffee intake significantly, starting with a mug of black coffee as soon as she got out of bed. She even kept a thermos in her car so she could get a caffeine hit while driving. Upon evaluation, Susan found that Christine's liver function tests were mildly elevated, probably due to her overconsumption of alcohol. She also had many symptoms typical of compromised liver function, such as bloating after eating fatty food and mild abdominal discomfort. Given these facts, Susan recommended that Christine begin a liver-cleansing program as well as reduce her intake of alcohol and fatty foods. Over a period of several months, Christine noted an improvement in her level of energy and was able to decrease her dependence on caffeine down to one cup of coffee per day, which she used for enjoyment rather than as a necessity.

▲▲ Blood tests to assess the health of the liver are often normal or only mildly elevated until the liver is severely damaged from alcohol abuse, illness, or toxic chemical exposure. The ability of the liver to detoxify may be greatly reduced, yet standard medical tests may still be within the normal range. If you suspect that you have compromised liver function based on symptoms of fatigue, inability to process moderate amounts of alcohol, abdominal bloating, intolerance to fatty foods, and needing to drink significant amounts of coffee to get started in the morning, it may be helpful to try the liver-strengthening suggestions described in the next chapter. Try them for a month or two to see if your symptoms begin to diminish. If so, you may want to maintain a liver restoration program until your symptoms improve further. If you do not notice any benefit, however, your problem may not be liver related. In any case, consult with your own physician for a proper diagnostic evaluation.

◀2 MENTAL CLARITY AND ACUITY

The excessive ingestion of alcohol has deleterious effects on cognitive thinking. Millions of Americans are either alcohol abusers or consume alcohol beyond their ability to metabolize it effectively. This can cause significant impairment of their mental sharpness and ability to think clearly. Most people have experienced, at least to some degree, the negative effect that alcohol has on cognitive function. Anyone who has had a drink and become mildly inebriated has experienced the mild signs of toxicity—blurred thinking and a slight lack of coordination. Because alcohol is rapidly absorbed and can cross the blood-brain barrier, the effect is felt rapidly.

Most teenagers and young adults can more easily metabolize all the alcohol they consume. Jim remembers friends in college with prodigious detoxification capability who could drink large quantities of beer at night and still show up for early classes clear-headed and do well on exams. However, most people, by the time they reach their thirties and forties, can no longer drink with abandon and still perform high-level cognitive functions. Beyond the fifth decade, it is only individuals with superfunctioning detoxification systems who can continue to consume large amounts of alcohol and still function as peak performers intellectually.

Numerous studies have shown that elevated levels of alcohol have a direct toxic effect on the brain and nervous system. For example, studies have found significant degenerative changes in the brains of chronic alcohol abusers compared to nonalcoholics. One such study, published in 1993 in the *Lancet*, compared the brains of fifty-five chronic alcoholics with those of eleven nonalcoholics at autopsy. The study confirmed that the brains of alcoholics suffer much more degenerative damage, losing white matter, the part of the brain consisting mainly of nerve fibers.

Frequent alcohol consumption that continues into midlife and beyond may begin to cause an impairment of cognitive abilities, because alcohol becomes more difficult to metabolize with age. Many studies confirm that chronic alcoholics, who have lost their detoxification abilities over the years, score poorly in cognitive testing. One such study, published in 1994 in *ACTA Neurologica Scandinavica*, stated that 50 to 70 percent of chronic alcoholics exhibit mild to moderate cognitive impairment. This study compared cognitive deterioration in fifty-four chronic alcoholics as compared to thirty nonalcoholics. Researchers found that alcoholics had significantly lower intellectual and visual-spatial scores than the nonalcoholics.

When a person drinks beyond their ability to process alcohol over a long period of time, the intellectual skills required in business can be impaired and careers eventually ruined. A good example of this is Frank, a business acquaintance of ours, who used to be a much sought after consulting engineer. He was known for his ability to accurately assess a construction project, prioritize activities, and finish the job on time. But his drinking destroyed his formerly crisp, linear thinking. As he continued to drink and his health deteriorated, Frank began to make basic technical mistakes in his work. Equipment installations that should have been easy began to go awry. Frank submitted disorganized, incoherent written reports, used exceptionally poor judgment in business situations, and finished projects late. However, he failed to make the connection between his excessive drinking and his diminished mental capabilities. Frank continued his excessive overconsumption of alcohol; over time, he lost his consulting business and his life's savings, and his health continued to deteriorate.

The brain and nervous system are sensitive to the negative effects of other toxins besides alcohol. Petrochemical-based pollutants such as pesticides, herbicides, and the thousands of industrial and household chemicals to which we are all exposed can also affect cognitive function. These chemicals are fat soluble and tend to accumulate in the brain and nervous system, which are predominantly made up of fats or lipids. Exposure to these pollutants can slow our thought processes and hamper both logical thinking and creative abilities. In addition, many chemicals form metabolites that, if not properly detoxified, will also impair one's ability to concentrate, causing symptoms like brain fog and dizziness.

One example is a toxic chemical called trichloroethylene, which forms a metabolite in the body called chlorhydrate. Chlorhydrate can cause significant brain fog and fatigue in susceptible individuals. Common chemicals found in new homes or office furnishings and building materials—such as styrene, toluene, xylene, and formaldehyde—can release a significant amount of gas into the indoor environment, causing an inability to concentrate, spaciness, and fatigue. In addition, individuals working in research laboratories, dry-cleaning establishments, and beauty salons are exposed to these types of toxic chemicals daily. Susan remembers having had significant exposure to chemicals such as toluene and formaldehyde both as a teenager and as a college student working in a medical laboratory, as well as during her years of medical training. At that time, she had no idea how destructive to the liver these chemicals were and did not take precautions. She suspects that the accumulated residues of these chemicals strongly contributed to the bout of chronic fatigue she suffered in her late thirties. Fortunately, a liver detoxification program helped restore her mental energy.

Susan has had many patients who have complained about impairment of their cognitive function, both from exposure to chemical pollutants in the workplace and from exposure to toxins released by building materials and furnishings in the home. One of her patients, Elizabeth, moved into an apartment that had just been refurbished with new carpeting, drapes, and furniture, all of which were made from synthetic materials. After moving in, she immediately began to suffer from brain fog, fatigue, and dizziness as well as a constant runny nose. Recognizing that the chemicals emanating from the new furnishings were probably causing her symptoms, she began to stay with friends and found new housing as quickly as possible. Her symptoms resolved as soon as she was no longer living in a toxic environment. Another patient, Stan, reported feeling weak, nauseated, and unable to think clearly whenever he walked near lawns that had recently been sprayed with herbicides. And another patient, Maria, had to quit her job as an administrative assistant because she could not handle the toxic load of chemicals that she was exposed to in the hermetically sealed office building in which she worked.

All of these individuals noted impaired cognitive function from exposure to environmental chemicals that their livers were unable to effectively detoxify. They all had to either change location or avoid contact with these offending chemicals. In addition, they began to follow nutritional and cleansing programs to restore their liver's detoxification ability and build up their resistance to those environmental chemicals that we are all inevitably exposed to.

 Avoid, if at all possible, living or working in an environment where you are constantly breathing airborne pollutants. If you are buying or renting a new home or apartment and suffer from chemical sensitivities, find out if new carpets or furnishings have recently been installed. Often, these are made of synthetic materials that can release toxic gases into the indoor environment.

One of the most effective ways to eliminate airborne petrochemical-based pollutants, viruses, bacteria, mold, fungi, or just plain unpleasant odors is through the use of an ozone generator (ozone is an activated form of oxygen). Portable ozone generators are available for home or office, and corporations should investigate the use of large-scale ones to protect office workers in sealed buildings or in factories where they are working with toxic chemicals. See chapters 7 and 8, on oxygenation, for more information.

4 THE ABILITY TO GET ALONG WITH OTHER PEOPLE

The social consequences of poor detoxification touch our lives in many ways. The newspapers are full of stories about accidents caused by road rage, violent crimes, and acrimonious litigation. There appears to be an increase in aggressive behavior throughout society. Inconsequential and minor behavioral actions, such as the minor driving errors that sometimes trigger road rage, are being met with increasingly hostile reactions.

An article published in 1997 in the *San Francisco Chronicle* provided statistics assembled by the National Highway Traffic Safety Administration on road rage and the frequency of motor-vehicle fatalities. According to this federal agency, aggressive behaviors were factors in nearly 28,000 of the 42,000 highway deaths in 1996, and the problem is getting worse. Antisocial behaviors included tailgating, weaving through busy lanes, honking or screaming at other drivers, exchanging insults, using angry hand signs, speeding, changing lanes illegally, running red lights, and even gunfire. While several factors are involved in every car crash, rage is involved in two-thirds of the deaths and one-third of the nonfatal crashes, resulting in 3 million injuries. And, according to the *Chronicle* article, the AAA Foundation for Traffic Safety's study of 10,000 aggressive-driving accidents estimated that in 35 percent of cases, a vehicle was used directly as a weapon.

The explosive emotions and violence associated with poor liver function are even expressed through art, books, movies, and TV shows. One of the most noted writers of the 1950s and 1960s, Allen Ginsberg, had a lifetime history of liver disease. Ginsberg made a successful career writing poems full of anger and defiance; in 1956, he published a book of free verse, *Howl and Other Poems*, which is considered the preeminent poetic work of the Beat movement of the 1950s. Ginsberg suffered for many years from hepatitis C, which eventually led to cirrhosis of the liver. He was later diagnosed with cancer of the liver, and he died in 1997 from cardiopulmonary arrest with secondary liver disease.

At the level of interpersonal interaction, poor detoxification capability also affects business and personal relationships. While some employees clearly have emotional or character disorders that make them difficult to work with, the inability to detoxify efficiently can also wreck havoc on one's ability to maintain productive relationships in the workplace. For example, a liver that is grossly malfunctioning due to substance abuse such as alcohol or drug addiction can cause an individual to behave in an abusive or aggressive manner toward their coworkers.

This issue is typified by the predicament of a patient Susan saw a number of years ago. Craig was a young scientist who had recently begun to work in a large research facility. He initially consulted with Susan because of headaches and chest pain, which turned out to be stress related. Craig's work situation was particularly difficult, in that his supervisor disliked him and made his work life miserable with constant criticism. She also gave him so much extra paperwork that he had to spend outside time to complete it. The fact that Craig heard from other employees that this supervisor was "difficult" for everyone to deal with was of no consolation to him.

Luckily for Craig, the vice president, who had been protecting and even encouraging his supervisor's behavior, left the company. The new vice president was tipped off by other employees about the supervisor's inappropriate and demoralizing behavior. Upon looking into the situation, he found that her behavior toward Craig and others was unacceptable; he also discovered that she was a closet alcoholic. Having determined that she was a real liability for the company, harming both morale and productivity, he fired her.

▲▲ Traditionally, organizations have dealt with difficult and disruptive personality traits in their employees or members by either firing them or requiring them to undergo psychological counseling. There has rarely been any recognition that an individual's aberrant behavior may have biochemical origins. The importance of making this distinction between a biochemical and a psychiatric disorder is particularly crucial for employees who have previously performed well. If an individual's behavior, which had previously been acceptable, suddenly begins to deviate from their past performance, and there are no obvious stress factors to explain it (such as divorce, illness, death in the family, or financial reversal), the individual should be advised that their problem could be biochemically based and should be promptly evaluated by a physician.

Susan often sees the negative effects of poor detoxification on relationships within her patients' families. Alcohol abuse can be a major cause of upset between family members, resulting in toxic relationships that often end in divorce. Further, the children of alcoholics may suffer abuse, both mental and physical, from their alcoholic parents and may need to spend years in support groups trying to recover from the damage.

One example of how impaired liver detoxification can adversely affect family relationships is in women who suffer from premenstrual syndrome

(PMS). The single most common problem that these women complain of is the emotional changes that they experience premenstrually—and the deterioration of social relationships that these changes can cause.

Research studies have suggested that there is a close relationship between PMS and the liver's ability to detoxify hormones efficiently. This link was first noted over fifty years ago by Morton S. Biskind, who discovered that the liver is responsible for detoxifying estrogen. Elevated estrogen levels during the second half of the menstrual cycle are thought to predispose women to PMS symptoms, since it is known that estrogen affects brain function and is a strong determinant of mood. Elevated estrogen levels have been linked to such common PMS symptoms as anxiety, panic, irritability, and mood swings. Biskind's initial studies, on both laboratory animals and human beings, found that the liver is responsible for detoxifying and inactivating estrogen as it circulates through the body in the bloodstream. Poor liver function can lead to elevated levels of estrogen, thereby increasing the tendency toward PMS.

Susan's PMS patients often describe themselves as short-tempered, grouchy, and highly critical. Research studies that discuss the behavioral changes that occur in women with PMS have found that the aberrant behavior varies from milder symptoms of poor social function to antisocial and highly destructive behavior. In women with severe PMS, marital conflict is common. Some women even complain about their tendency to abuse their children, both emotionally and physically, during the premenstrual period. Women may develop phobias and sleep disturbances for one or two weeks out of the month, and they may experience depression and lethargy. At the far end of the spectrum, various studies demonstrate that women tend to have high rates of aberrant behavior, psychiatric episodes, and even crimes of passion during their premenstrual phase.

Because alcohol is a known liver toxin, women with PMS may be particularly susceptible to its deleterious effects. This link was evaluated in a study published in 1986 in *Obstetrics and Gynecology*. Researchers evaluated two separate groups of women, 95 who received treatment for PMS and 147 who did not. The women were screened for alcoholism and were assessed using a questionnaire followed by an interview. The researchers found that 72 percent of the PMS patients had a history of alcohol abuse, as compared with only 45 percent of the non-PMS sufferers. Women with PMS may be equally intolerant of other foods that compromise liver function, such as saturated fats and refined sugar.

One of the first steps that Susan often takes in treating her PMS patients is to recommend a liver-cleansing program. This helps to restore the liver's detoxification capability and allows the liver to metabolize hormones, such as estrogen, more efficiently. The benefits of a liver restoration program begin to be evident within a few weeks. Often, within several menstrual cycles, PMS sufferers report that their moods are substantially improved. Women with families state that they have more patience in dealing with their children and are able to stop themselves before they begin to bicker with their husbands or significant others during the premenstrual period. They also report more socially appropriate behavior and are more even tempered at work or with friends.

Healthy liver function and social entertaining

Another benefit of having healthy detoxification function is being able to fully participate in many different types of social events, such as receptions and dinner parties, where food and drink are part of the hospitality. Invariably, alcohol is served as well as foods high in fat, such as canapés, cheeses, heavy sauces on entrées, and rich desserts. A person with optimal detoxification capability can enjoy this food and drink with no ill effects. However, someone with marginal liver detoxification capability may instinctively avoid much of what is being served, or will indulge and then pay the penalty the next day, with fatigue, brain fog, or even inappropriate behavior.

For many politicians, corporate executives, public relations personnel, brokers, agents, and sales reps, the ability to entertain clients often and to eat and drink without fear of a severe hangover or energy drop can be a prerequisite for career success. Of course, there are also many people who work nine-to-five jobs, whether schoolteachers, hospital personnel, or government workers, whose careers do not depend on entertaining, but who love to eat rich meals with good wines just for the pleasure of it. These people, like those who must entertain for business, can only keep this pattern up if their livers can efficiently detoxify. Once this ability is compromised, a person will likely suffer indigestion, have severe hangovers, and suffer disturbed sleep, making entertaining more of a chore than a pleasure. Being unable to detoxify effectively can therefore limit how much a person can eat and/or drink and how often they are able to enjoy the pleasures of entertaining.

Alcohol is served at virtually all work-related events here in the United States as well as in Europe and Asia. The person who can share a convivial drink with coworkers, clients, and potential customers is perceived as mixing well with others and being more socially accessible. Again, we are referring to someone who can manage their alcohol intake, uses it as a social facilitator, and, of course, knows when to quit, not someone who becomes habitually drunk.

Ted is the head of a major corporation who is legendary for his ability to drink with the troops. His ability to tolerate and to recover from alcohol allows him to drink with his salespeople late into the night and then be up early the next day for a power breakfast with his investment bankers. He attends all the company events and socializes with everyone in the organization, and has earned a reputation for being very likable and extremely accessible. Because the people who work for him feel relaxed and comfortable with him, they feel free to speak their minds. This gives him invaluable information about his company and its customers. In short, because of his ability to socialize, Ted can gather information and generate goodwill at the same time. Ted also uses this capability to maximum effect with customers, suppliers, bankers, and lawyers to the benefit of the corporation.

For some people, who are working in careers in which socializing with one's coworkers and clients is an important part of being successful, the benefits of being able to tolerate moderate amounts of alcohol can be quite useful in the early stages of their careers. When people are in their twenties and thirties, alcohol can, if used appropriately, facilitate one's advancement in their chosen field of endeavor. Camaraderie, social bonding, storytelling, and other pleasures of social interaction can be enhanced and facilitated by alcohol. These social interactions often build the networks that will be used for future business or professional careers. (Of course, this is not to say that people who do not tolerate or don't enjoy alcohol can't be equally successful.) However, as people age, their ability to tolerate alcohol diminishes. The overconsumption of alcohol can then actually become a liability in business. The downsides of alcohol consumption in middle age are memory loss, weight gain, and, perhaps worst of all, the inability to act appropriately at all times.

One very public example of this career-ending problem is former New York Yankees manager Billy Martin. Throughout his tumultuous career, Martin was known for his drinking habits and his fiery temperament. He had a reputation for irrational behavior, and his bar-room brawls elevated him to celebrity status. The Yankees hired him and fired him as their manager five different times. In 1989, on Christmas Day, he died in a car accident, the result of drunk driving.

▲▲ Many individuals place exceptional stress on their liver's ability to detoxify. If your job requires frequent socializing or entertaining, or if one of your great pleasures in life is enjoying rich food and drink, a preventive liver maintenance program will serve you well. Prevent the wear and tear on your liver that rich food and alcohol consumption will inevitability create. Follow the liver restoration treatments discussed in the following chapter.

How social and business entertaining affects women

Research studies have shown that, in general, women are markedly less able to tolerate alcohol than men. Women metabolize alcohol more slowly than men and take longer to recover from alcohol's toxic effects. Furthermore, because of women's smaller body size and higher body-fat content, alcohol tends to become more concentrated in their bodily fluids. Many of Susan's women patients complain that after one or two drinks, they feel sleepy and often have hangovers the next day. Susan herself notices that she is more susceptible to the effects of alcohol than Jim is.

A review article published in 1998 in the *Female Patient Supplement* examined women's relative intolerance of alcohol and the effects that this has on their careers. The article noted that, while women do tend to drink less than men, those women who are alcohol abusers suffer greater career and social consequences. Male alcohol abusers are treated with more sympathy than female abusers in a job setting. Women are more likely to be fired for alcohol abuse. They are also less likely to use workplace-based rehabilitation programs. Because alcohol has a sedative and depressant effect, a significant percentage of female alcohol abusers are likely to suffer from depression, which can further hamper job performance.

The deleterious effects of alcohol are not limited simply to women's relative intolerance to this substance. An article on alcohol and the liver, published in 1994 in *Gastroenterology*, stated that for women compared to men, only half as much alcohol intake resulted in a statistically significant increase in cirrhosis of the liver. The review article also presented evidence that women are more likely than men to have liver disease progress to severe liver damage.

In today's fast-paced business climate, women are finding themselves having the same entertaining and socializing responsibilities as men. Throughout most of this country's history, women have not been employed in positions where entertaining and socializing were a requirement of the job. Women were primarily in back-office or staff positions with little direct customer or client responsibilities. However, this has changed completely, with many women in positions such as account executives, brokers, and sales as well as senior and middle management, with the responsibility of developing and maintaining business relationships. In addition, many women now own or run their own businesses and must perform all of these jobs themselves. As with men, women now engage in business as well as social entertaining as representatives of their organizations. This often means eating rich meals, consuming alcoholic beverages, getting to bed late, and then having to be up early the next day to do it all again. During our numerous consulting engagements, we have seen a dramatic increase in women being the focal points for entertaining. Women, because they are more sensitive to the effects of alcohol than men, have to exercise more care in business situations where alcoholic beverages are served.

▲▲ Women whose work includes socializing on a business and professional basis need to know how to gracefully decline alcoholic drinks if they lack the ability to handle them and order a socially acceptable nonalcoholic beverage instead. Luckily, the prevalence of women professionals in virtually every career, from business to the arts and sciences, has coincided with the growing acceptance of nonalcoholic beverages such as mineral water or nonalcoholic beers. Many men are also forgoing or reducing their consumption of alcoholic beverages at professional lunches and dinners, often for health reasons but also for performance reasons.

▲▲ If you do plan to indulge in alcoholic beverages and want to avoid the energy drop that can follow, the old saw about not drinking on an empty stomach applies. To slow down the rapid absorption of alcohol, it is important to precede its ingestion with fatty or oily foods. Starting courses such as smoked salmon,

a salad served with an oil-based dressing, or even bread and butter can prevent the liver's detoxification capability from being
overwhelmed by alcohol consumed on an empty stomach. Some
women may prefer to use flaxseed oil capsules, thereby gaining a
health advantage as well as moderating the amount of alcohol
their liver must process.

5 THE ABILITY TO REMAIN CALM UNDER PRESSURE

Peak performers in every major area of life tend to be those individuals
who are able to think and strategize calmly under pressure. For example,
in sports, the ability to remain calm under stress is often more important
than having the physical skills to win. Every weekend, millions of people
watching sports on television see poise, emotional control, and positive
focus winning over raw talent that has lost its composure. A figure skater
almost stumbles on a triple axel but rights herself and finishes the program with a flourish. A champion golfer hits the ball into a difficult lie in
the deep rough but plays it out onto the green, positioned for a par-saving
putt. A college basketball player sinks two free throws with almost no
time left to seal a come-from-behind victory in the noisy arena of a rival.

Tennis champion Chris Evert dominated the world of women's tennis for many years even though she did not have the greatest athletic ability or foot speed. However, she was always able to play her best under the
stress of competition. When she hit a bad shot or a call went against her,
she was able to remain calm and in control of her thoughts and actions.
She never showed anger or fear, saving all her energies and skills for winning the next point.

Another classic example of an athlete who performs well under pressure is Michael Jordan. Countless times in his career, he has hit the winning shot or made the steal that sealed a victory in the waning seconds of
a game. He so frequently dominated in the decisive fourth quarter that
sportswriters and fans began to refer to that period as "Jordan time."
Indeed, one of the traits that defined Jordan's greatness as a basketball
player was his unique ability to perceive the less obvious determining
moments within the flow of a game—and to insert the dagger at precisely
that point. After the game had ended, observers could say that that was
the key basket or steal, the play that deflated his opponents' morale or
inspired his own teammates. But at the time, only Jordan understood the

potential of the moment. He was so calm under pressure that he could perceive and seize potential turning points that others could see only in retrospect.

Although few people need to perform at the level of intensity and composure of professional athletes, many people are engaged in careers where remaining internally calm and centered during periods of stress is a prerequisite for success. Professional securities traders or emergency-room doctors and nurses are constantly making critical decisions with incomplete information under chaotic conditions. For the trader, split-second decisions to buy, hold, or sell a security can mean millions of dollars in gains or losses for a client or their firm. For the emergency room doctor or nurse, the need to make rapid decisions in a crisis situation often has life-or-death consequences.

Healthy liver functioning is a physiological prerequisite for being able to remain calm and perform well under stress. Individuals with healthy detoxification function tend to be more even tempered, are more likely to demonstrate good judgment, and are better able to solve problems in a logical and impartial manner. The deleterious effects that impaired detoxification capability has on temperament and judgment have been confirmed in a number of research studies. When liver function is impaired, toxic chemicals such as alcohol, recreational drugs, and even industrial pollutants are not properly metabolized and their toxic by-products will accumulate within the tissues of the body. These toxic by-products can cloud judgment, affect emotional stability, and reduce the ability to perform well under stressful conditions. Individuals whose liver function is compromised are more likely to have emotional outbursts and lose their focus under duress. These people, under pressure, will tend to make poor decisions, reacting to a situation rather than calmly dealing with the issues at hand and creating effective solutions.

Many people in various walks of life limit their chances of succeeding because they have poor detoxification function and are unable to remain calm under stress or maintain appropriate behavior. Years ago, Jim found himself working briefly with such a person. Bill, the manager of the project, had spent most of his career raising capital for start-up ventures in which he often took on some form of operational responsibility; however, a number of these projects had been mismanaged, so his performance history was inconsistent. As Jim began to work with him, he began to understand why Bill's record was so poor. Although Bill had an excellent education and was extremely bright and physically very strong, he had also been a heavy drinker. He had an aggressive personality, which his drinking had only worsened. When inevitable differences of opinion and communication snags arose while working on a project, Bill's response was to become overly aggressive, threaten everyone involved, and often institute legal action. Because he was unable to stay calm and find constructive solutions to problems, he routinely alienated people and developed serious interpersonal animosities.

By the time Jim started to work with him, Bill had actually quit drinking and was attending AA meetings. Susan, who met Bill on a number of social occasions, noted that despite his discontinuance of alcohol, his diet was not supportive of healthy detoxification function. Instead of alcohol, he was continually drinking highly sugared cola drinks and coffee, snacking on chocolate chip cookies, and eating a high-fat, red meat–based diet, always finishing with rich desserts. All of these foods continued to put stress on his liver, which exacerbated his belligerent and aggressive behavior. Within a year, his overly aggressive personality, abrasive behavior, and poor decisions caused him to be removed from the project.

▲▲ Individuals with a history of alcohol abuse who have ceased their consumption of alcoholic beverages should also avoid using substitutes that continue to damage liver function. Soft drinks, fruit juice, tonic water, coffee or black tea, and even carbonated water should be rigorously avoided because of their high content of sugar, caffeine, and carbon dioxide (an acidic waste product of our own body's cells). All of these substances are detrimental to healthy liver function. Instead, drink plenty of spring or filtered water or herbal teas such as peppermint and chamomile, which are traditionally used in herbal medicine to support and restore healthy liver function. In addition, highly sugared or fat-laden meals should be avoided during the period of recovery from alcohol abuse. These dietary guidelines are equally helpful for individuals recovering from other chemical addictions, such as the use of recreational drugs, or from toxic environmental exposure, since all toxic chemicals tend to compromise liver function.

Susan has had many patients over the years who have complained about their inability to remain calm and centered during times of stress.

Often, impaired detoxification capability has played a role in causing their problem. Many of these individuals have had a history of alcohol or drug abuse. They would often describe a tendency toward overreacting to seemingly small issues with panic, upset, and even rage. For some of these individuals, years of counseling and stress management training had not produced the desired behavioral changes. It was only when they began to treat the chemical basis of their overreactivity to stressful situations that they finally achieved mastery over their own responses. Improving the liver's ability to detoxify has been an important facet of these therapeutic programs.

▲▲ If you, like the individuals described above, have always been capable of operating in a calm and centered manner under stressful or adverse conditions, but have found in recent years that you are beginning to respond with less equanimity and more upset or anger, your liver's detoxification capability may be part of the problem. These changes are often early-warning signs that your crucial detoxification function is beginning to break down, which could be due to the effects of aging or accumulated wear and tear from unhealthy lifestyle habits. In such a case, it is helpful to eliminate obvious dietary and environmental toxins and to have your detoxification capability evaluated by a health-care professional.

8 RESISTANCE TO ILLNESS

Good detoxification is a major factor in preventing illnesses. It prevents toxic chemicals from accumulating in the body, which can cause a wide variety of distressing symptoms such as brain fog, aching joints and muscles, digestive symptoms, and even cold and flulike symptoms. Over the years, Susan has seen a number of patients develop cold and flulike symptoms when exposed to toxic chemicals like formaldehyde, toluene, or benzene. She has also seen these symptoms in patients whose livers could not handle prescription drugs that were prescribed by their physicians for specific medical purposes. She has seen patients develop a runny nose, sneezing, and even chills when administered a local anesthetic for minor surgery. She has even seen these types of symptoms after patients ingested synthetic hormones like Synthroid, a replacement therapy for low thyroid

function, or Provera, a synthetic form of progesterone, as well as prednisone, an adrenal hormone used to treat many inflammatory conditions.

The cold and flulike symptoms did not abate in these individuals
until they were able to avoid exposure to the environmental toxins that
they could not tolerate or until they discontinued the use of the offending
drug. Symptoms often continued after minor surgery until the anesthetic
was finally detoxified by the body. Prescription drugs are not the only cul-
prits. Susan has also found that some patients develop nausea, bloating,
and other symptoms of poor liver function after taking oil-based nutritional supplements such as vitamin E, evening primrose oil, and certain
herbs.

The individuals who suffer from such extreme susceptibility to environmental chemicals, medications, and nutrients are unable to detoxify
them efficiently due to poor liver function. All of these substances must
be broken down by the enzyme systems of the liver and then excreted
from the body so as not to accumulate to toxic levels. Healthy people,
whose detoxification systems are intact, tend to metabolize and excrete
specific drugs at the same rate. This rate is measured as the half-life of the
drug, or the amount of time required for 50 percent of it to be eliminated
from the body. Drugs with long half-lives remain in the body a longer
period of time in their active form and only need to be used once a day. A
drug with a shorter half-life, like aspirin, may need to be taken every four
to six hours to maintain therapeutic activity. However, when an individual patient has impaired liver function, the half-life of the drug may be
considerably longer, due to their inability to metabolize or excrete it. In
this case, either the drug dosage may need to be revised or its use discontinued entirely.

▲▲ The symptoms of colds and flus are performance and success
saboteurs—making you feel miserable and often resulting in lost
work time. If you frequently suffer from these symptoms, it is
important to differentiate between the symptoms caused by
infectious disease and reactions that are due to exposure to a
toxic substance you cannot tolerate. While colds and flus need to
be treated by suppressing the pathogens and restoring your
body's buffering, enzyme, and oxygenation functions, similar
types of symptoms due to toxic chemical exposure need to be
treated differently. Toxic chemicals need to be detoxified and

eliminated from the body through healthy liver function. Remember that cells within the liver also help to destroy disease-causing bacteria. If you are susceptible to specific drugs or nutrients, their use should be discontinued and further use avoided. However, be sure to consult with your physician before discontinuing any prescription drugs. If your symptoms seem to be due to the use of nutritional supplements, use non-oil-based substitutes. In addition, your should follow a liver restoration program such as the one described in the next chapter to help restore your detoxification capability.

SUMMARY

Good detoxification is important for anyone who wants to be at their best in the work world. It promotes a number of peak-performance traits, including physical vitality and stamina, mental clarity and acuity, the ability to get along with people, the ability to remain calm under pressure, and resistance to illness. A healthy liver allows us to participate fully in social and business events that involve alcohol and rich foods, and helps us to resist illnesses caused by toxins in the environment.

SECTION 4:
DETOXIFICATION AND HEALTH

WHEN THE LIVER'S ability to detoxify is weakened, blood levels of improperly metabolized chemicals begin to rise. Normally, toxins such as alcohol, drugs, environmental pollutants, and even hormones produced within the body are inactivated and broken down into harmless residues by a healthy liver. When allowed to accumulate, however, such chemicals can be an important contributing factor to a number of diseases such as chronic fatigue, environmental allergies, alcoholic heart disease, gastrointestinal illnesses, inflammatory conditions of the nervous system, and even cancer. The overconsumption of alcohol, fats, and refined sugar can cause hormone imbalances in both males and females, leading to elevated estrogen levels. This can increase the risk of PMS, fibroid tumors of the uterus, endometriosis, and even uterine cancer in women and abnormal breast development and alterations in sexual function in men. Finally, the overconsumption of alcohol can lead to alcoholic hepatitis and cirrhosis of the liver, resulting in severe and permanent liver damage. The major health conditions caused by poor detoxification are discussed below.

CHRONIC FATIGUE AND ENVIRONMENTAL ALLERGIES

As mentioned in section 3 of this chapter, the exposure to a wide variety of environmental toxins can be causal factors in both chronic fatigue states and environmental allergies. When improperly detoxified, such common substances as lawn and garden pesticides and herbicides, cleaning solutions, perfumes and hair care products, and building materials can trigger allergic symptoms. These include fatigue, poor cognitive function, runny noses, eye irritation, skin rashes, headaches, nausea, joint pains, and mood changes. If these cases of chronic fatigue and environmental sensitivity due to poor detoxification capability remain undiagnosed, the individuals affected may languish for months or years, unable to function properly at work or participate fully in their personal lives. Proper diagnosis of these conditions is mandatory. Individuals with these symptoms should seek out the help of physicians who deal with environmental illness and are knowledgeable about detoxification therapies.

NERVOUS-SYSTEM DISEASE

The inability of the liver to detoxify alcohol is a main cause of nervous-system disease and impairment. A liver that is able to clear alcohol from the system as it is consumed acts as a protective barrier, preventing the toxic by-products of its breakdown from reaching the brain and nervous system, which are particularly vulnerable. In chronic alcohol abuse, the liver's ability to detoxify alcohol slowly erodes over time, and there is an increase in circulating levels of alcohol in the blood. As liver disease advances, brain cells are destroyed, resulting in serious nervous-system disorders, including polyneuritis (nerve inflammation), premature senility, and encephalopathy (chronic degenerative brain syndrome).

Research suggests that one possible cause of the destruction of brain cells may be an accumulation of manganese in the brain due to poor clearance by the liver. The intake of normal amounts of manganese is required for good health, but in higher amounts it can be toxic. In a small study appearing in 1994 in the *Annals of Neurology*, researchers investigated this association. The patients, aged forty-nine to sixty-five, had cirrhosis of the liver coupled with neurologic dysfunction. The researchers noted that these patients had elevated blood levels of manganese and also an accumulation of this mineral in the brain, suggesting that with impaired liver function, even normal amounts of dietary manganese can accumulate to toxic levels within the tissues.

ALCOHOL-RELATED HEART DISEASE

An efficiently functioning liver protects not only the brain but also the heart from being damaged by alcohol. Circulating alcohol is toxic to the heart. Alcohol decreases heart muscle action and electrical conductivity and can, over time, lead to congestive heart failure, cardiac arrhythmias, and cardiac enlargement. There is some evidence that low to moderate alcohol consumption may reduce the risk of deep venous thrombosis and pulmonary embolism in older individuals, according to a study published in the *Journal of the American Geriatric Society*. But many studies also document the association of excess alcohol intake and potentially dangerous cardiac disease. One study, published in 1995 in the *Journal of the American Medical Association*, examined the heart health of 100 asymptomatic, alcoholic men and fifty asymptomatic, alcoholic women, compared with fifty nonalcoholic women as a control group. Of the men, 39 percent showed evidence of alcohol-related heart damage. This was found to be the case for an even higher percentage of the alcoholic women studied. In almost a third of the men, their alcohol intake was found to be a causal factor. Furthermore, women showed an even greater susceptibility to the toxic effects of alcohol as a risk factor for their disease.

ELEVATED ESTROGEN LEVELS

As mentioned earlier, efficient metabolism of estrogen by the liver helps to regulate hormone levels in women. Through its detoxification function, the liver helps to modulate the amount and control the type of estrogen circulating through a woman's body. Estrogen is secreted by the ovaries in a highly potent form called estradiol. The liver metabolizes this form of estrogen so that it can be eliminated from the body, first by converting estradiol to an intermediary form called estrone and finally to a weaker form called estriol. The liver's ability to efficiently convert estradiol to estriol is important because estriol is the safest and least chemically active form of estrogen. In contrast, estrone and estradiol are very active stimulants in breast and uterine tissue.

Excessive intake of alcohol, fat, and refined sugar in females has been associated with both lack of ovulation and elevated estrogen levels. Excess estrogen can worsen the congestive symptoms of menstrual pain and cramps and cause fluid and salt retention in the body, particularly during the premenstrual and menstrual phases. Excess estrogen can also trigger the growth and spread of endometriosis implants, thereby worsening menstrual cramps and pain. Overconsumption of alcohol has also been linked to heavy bleeding and spotting in women with fibroid tumors of the uterus and endometriosis. Finally, excess estrogen is a risk factor for the development of breast cancer.

Alcohol abuse also elevates estrogen levels in men. Like women, men produce estrogen, but in much smaller amounts. Normally, a healthy male secretes as much estrogen as a woman does after menopause, about 10 to 25 percent of the amount she produces during her reproductive years. In male alcoholics, their liver may be unable to detoxify the small amount of estrogen that they produce, leading to an elevation of their blood estrogen levels. This can lead to breast enlargement and other mild symptoms of feminization. Research scientists have also observed estrogen-induced cellular changes in the prostate glands of patients with liver disease.

SEXUAL PROBLEMS

Many people think of alcohol as a stimulant because it reduces inhibitions and, when consumed in moderation, increases social interactions. But it is actually a sedative, suppressing emotions and potentially causing impotence. Research studies have confirmed the negative effect that alcohol has on sexual desire and performance. This is due, in part, to hormonal imbalances caused by impaired liver detoxification. Besides elevating the estrogen levels in male alcoholics, overconsumption of alcohol can also lead to a reduction in testosterone levels. This can cause both a decrease in libido and the aggressive impulse that many men direct into their careers and hobbies. These men may experience extreme mood swings, which can have further negative effects on their social and business relationships. It has also been found that heavy alcohol use by teenage boys may delay sexual maturity.

CANCER

The development of cancer may be related to liver function, as evidenced by the link between alcohol intake and the incidence of esophageal, liver, and breast cancer. A number of recent studies suggest that drinking alcoholic beverages, even in moderate amounts, increases the risk of breast cancer. A study conducted at the Harvard School of Public Health followed the dietary habits of 89,538 women nurses between the ages of thirty-four and fifty-nine for four years. Women who ingested between three and nine drinks per week had a 30 percent increase in their risk of breast cancer. Those who had more than nine drinks per week had a 60 percent increase. In another study published in the *New England Journal of Medicine*, 188 women between twenty-five and seventy-seven were followed over a ten-year period. Researchers observed that the women who consumed alcohol regularly, as compared with those who did not, had a 50 percent greater risk of developing breast cancer.

When a person is undergoing chemotherapy or any cancer treatment that results in the killing of tumor cells at an accelerated rate, it is imperative that both the toxic by-products of this tumor cell destruction and the drugs themselves be quickly eliminated from the body. If these toxic chemical residues remain in the system, they can overburden the liver's detoxification capabilities and greatly increase the risk of death. Complementary physicians usually recommend that cancer patients do everything possible to support their liver's ability to detoxify these harmful substances. (See the following chapter for more information on liver detoxification techniques.)

LABORATORY TESTS TO EVALUATE LIVER FUNCTION

Traditionally, physicians have assessed liver health by ordering blood tests to measure the levels of enzymes produced by the liver, such as SGOT and SGPT. These enzymes become elevated when there is significant damage to the liver. However, newer tests are available that allow health care professionals to measure not only liver pathology but also the health of the liver's detoxification function.

Blood tests

When there is liver damage or inflammation, an elevation in the blood levels of liver enzymes can occur. Elevated levels can indicate liver damage due to excessive alcohol intake, exposure to toxic chemicals, or infectious diseases such as hepatitis. The two enzymes most commonly monitored are serum glutamic oxaloacetic transaminase (SGOT) and serum glutamic pyruvic transaminase (SGPT), which are released by liver cells when there is acute cellular destruction. Of the two enzymes, SGOT is more sensitive to cellular damage and is released even when there is only mild injury. However, SGOT is found in several types of tissue, including significant amounts in the heart, making it a less specific indicator of liver disease. SGPT requires somewhat more extensive or severe cell damage to rise above normal levels, but it is a reliable indicator of liver damage because virtually all of SGPT originates in the liver, making it a more specific test.

Detoxification profile

A detoxification profile is a relatively new procedure that tests the ability of the liver to detoxify various substances. Their metabolites are then measured in the urine, blood, or saliva. The profile measures substances that are active either in phase I or phase II of the detoxification process. To measure the function of the phase I detoxification system, a premeasured amount of caffeine is ingested. If salivary testing is done, saliva samples are taken during the eight hours after ingestion. The caffeine's rate of clearance can be used to assess phase I detoxification activity. To test the phase II detoxification system, individuals are given aspirin, acetaminophen, or sodium benzoate (which is used for individuals with salicylate sensitivity). The metabolites are then measured. Individuals show great variation in their ability to detoxify, depending on the health of their liver.

SUMMARY

Healthy liver function is essential to many aspects of peak performance as well as good general health. As we will see in the next chapter, we can support our liver's ability to detoxify our bodies in a number of ways, including dietary choices, nutritional supplementation, and several very effective liver-cleansing techniques.

6

Restoring Your Ability to Detoxify

In order to maintain good health and maximum performance, the liver must be able to detoxify pollutants that the body ingests or absorbs from the environment as well as those that the body generates itself in the process of metabolism. Fortunately, there are many effective techniques that a person can use to restore their health by reestablishing the liver's ability to detoxify. In this chapter, we have included a powerful three-part program to enable you to restore your detoxification ability. This program is very effective and will begin to work rapidly to help support and rebuild your liver so that your detoxification capability can return to optimal functioning. The program consists of specific dietary regimens (described in part 1) as well as the use of special liver restorative nutrients (part 2), which will help the liver metabolize and rid the body of toxic pollutants, chemicals, and the waste products generated by our own metabolism. We also provide you with a number of very effective liver-cleansing techniques (part 3), which will accelerate the healing of the liver as well as help it detoxify and eliminate many potentially toxic substances from the body.

Over the years, Susan has found that when her patients have followed a program to support liver function and enhance detoxification, they usually begin to notice a rapid reduction in their symptoms. The liver responds quickly, especially if the intake of toxic substances that burden it is significantly reduced.

A Caution on Starting Your Detoxification Program

When you are customizing your own liver detoxification program, it is important to both cleanse the liver and strengthen and restore its functional capacity at the same time. Since powerful reactions such as headaches, fatigue, and even a runny nose can occur with any detoxification program, you must start slowly and gradually work up to suggested levels. As with all health programs, you must experiment within known safe ranges to find the levels that work for your individual biochemistry.*

Pick the colon-cleansing techniques that you are most comfortable with, and use it as frequently as your occupation and lifestyle permit. As you reduce your intake of toxins like alcohol or recreational drugs, your body will begin to try to eliminate these and other toxins that have been stored at the cellular level. The colon-cleansing techniques, in particular, will allow for the accelerated excretion of these toxins without the body having a healing crisis as the liver unloads toxins into the bloodstream and the small intestine. Colon cleanses are one of the most important things you can do while rebuilding your liver function.

PART 1:

THE DETOXIFICATION DIET

THE FOLLOWING SECTION provides guidelines on what foods to eat and avoid as well as a modified approach to fasting.

DIETARY GUIDELINES

To restore the liver's detoxification capability, it is important to eat a predominantly vegetarian diet, with an emphasis on raw foods. Daily meals should incorporate a variety of salads, fresh vegetables, whole grains, and legumes. These foods, which are made up of simple molecules of starch, cellulose, fruit sugars, antioxidants, and other easy-to-metabolize substances, place minimum stress on the liver. If animal protein is desired,

---

* Anyone beginning a nutritional supplement program should begin at one-quarter to one-half the recommended dosages given in this book. They can then increase their dosages slowly over the course of several weeks until they have reached either the full recommended dosage or a dosage that is therapeutic for them—whichever level comes first. Some individuals will experience therapeutic benefits at doses that are well below the doses recommended in this book. Also, while the dosages provided in this chapter are appropriate for most people, there are certain groups who should continue to use less than the recommended dosages. Children, the elderly, and individuals with a frail constitution or who are extremely sensitive to drugs and nutritional supplements usually do best at therapeutic dosages of no more than half the recommended levels. Consult your physician or nutritional consultant if you have any questions about the advisability of using a particular nutritional supplement or to determine the dosage most appropriate for you.

small amounts of easy-to-assimilate fish and eggs can be added. Oils should be high-quality cold-pressed monounsaturated and polyunsaturated vegetable oils—used only in small amounts in the early stages of recovery.

Traditional Chinese medicine recommends the use of certain plant-based foods as part of a dietary regimen for restoring liver function. Susan has found in her clinical practice that the following foods are well tolerated and seem to accelerate the healing of liver-related problems: beets, broccoli, cabbage, Brussels sprouts, turnips, kale, parsley, lettuce, cucumber, green foods such as spirulina, chlorella, and barley grass, beans and peas, sprouts, tofu, rice, millet, rice bran syrup, barley malt syrup, maple syrup (all sweeteners should be used in small amounts), and fruits in small quantities, preferably consumed during the summer months. However, Susan recommends avoiding vinegar and citrus fruits since many individuals with liver conditions are also overly acidic.

In contrast, a diet that includes large amounts of red meat, dairy products, and fatty foods burdens the liver, which must break down the large and more complex structures of these proteins and fats into triglycerides, prostaglandins, and an array of waste products that can be excreted by the body. When the liver cannot process fats, they accumulate inside liver cells, creating fatty degeneration of the liver. In time, these fats will be deposited in the arteries, leading to eventual heart problems and stroke.

To decrease stress on the liver, it is also critical to avoid certain substances, such as refined white sugar and flour, alcohol, caffeine, and drugs (other than needed prescribed medicines), because the breakdown of these products leaves toxic residues that the liver must neutralize. Following a lighter, fresher diet allows the liver to go through a gradual self-cleansing process, without causing further stress.

▲▲ Eat only those foods that do not add to the stress load on the liver. Constantly experiment with the suggested food groups and find those you like and tolerate best. Incorporate these foods into recipes you enjoy or find recipes that use these food groups. Remember, it is virtually impossible to rebuild and restore liver function without eliminating foods that are high in fat and sugar content.

▲▲ Individuals who are following a program to restore their detoxi-fication capability may still want to enjoy an occasional meal of animal protein. The following suggestions will put the least strain on your liver. Eat eggs prepared simply, either soft- or hard-boiled. Avoid eggs prepared with fats and oils such as dev-iled, fried, or scrambled eggs or eggs prepared as omelettes. Choose soft-textured, easy-to-digest fish such as salmon over red meat such as pork, lamb, or beef, which are high in saturated fat and more fibrous in texture.

▲▲ While you are restoring your liver function, eliminate all alco-holic beverages. Switch to mineral water and herbal teas such as chamomile and peppermint, which are therapeutic for the liver. Once liver function is restored, alcohol intake should be limited to an occasional, single beverage.

▲▲ Individuals with impaired detoxification function should make an effort to avoid eating after 6:00 P.M. or 7:00 P.M. at the very lat-est. In addition, eat your heaviest meals early in the day, with your last meal being the lightest. This will help to prevent undue stress on the liver during the night when it should be repairing and restoring itself rather than trying to metabolize the residues of a heavy meal. Eating late at night can significantly retard a liver restoration program. Susan's patients have found that avoiding heavy meals eaten late at night significantly reduces morning grogginess and brain fog.

▲▲ All dietary changes that are made to improve liver function should be done gradually, over several weeks to several months. Too extreme and rapid a change in one's diet can induce waste products to be eliminated more rapidly than the liver can handle, triggering symptoms like nasal congestion, flulike symptoms, diarrhea, bad breath, and aches and pains.

MODIFIED FASTING

Many books on detoxification recommend fasting as the quickest and most efficient way to rid the body of accumulated toxins, but true fasting is very difficult for the average American. A true fast means consuming only water or diluted liquids such as juices, broths, or herbal teas for a prescribed period of time. Fasting has been practiced for thousands of years by the people of nearly all cultures all over the world. Used for purification, penance, during periods of mourning, and to strengthen mental, physical, and spiritual powers, fasting is an ancient practice with modern applications.

However, most of us in the United States live busy, stressful lives, with myriad responsibilities at home, school, and work. We don't often have the luxury of a large block of time without responsibilities to undertake the intensity of a true fast. Fasting can accelerate the elimination of toxins from the body. Such rapid detoxification can trigger any of several troublesome symptoms, including a displeasing taste in the mouth, a thick coating on the tongue, skin odor and/or eruptions, headaches, and digestive upset. A person may develop flulike symptoms or a nasal discharge for a day or two. Most people who go on a rigorous, traditional fast experience a drop in their energy level and have constant thoughts of food. Some people experience even more serious symptoms, such as faintness or an irregular heartbeat, which should be reported to a physician immediately.

If you are working and active, a true fast can be very disruptive. However, it is possible to follow a modified fasting program of two or three light meals a day consisting of vegetable juices; low-sodium and low-fat broths; herbal teas; light, easy-to-digest solid foods, such as uncooked or lightly steamed organic vegetables and sprouts; and thoroughly cooked starches, grains, and legumes. Such a program will gradually begin to clear toxins from the liver.

You should consume only organic vegetables during a modified fast, because if you are trying to eliminate toxins from the body, consuming foods covered with chemical pesticides and fertilizers is counterproductive. Vegetable juices should be prepared fresh, used within a day or two, and always kept refrigerated. Some bottled vegetable juices may be used when fresh ones are unavailable. Preferred vegetable juices are carrot, beet and beet green, parsley, celery, cucumber, and spinach. To enhance the cleansing action of these juices, add a little garlic or wheatgrass juice. However, don't drink fruit juices because they are highly acidic and high in concentrated sugars. If you can't live without some fresh fruit juice, the best ones are papaya and melon, preferably diluted by 50 percent with water. But if you are hypoglycemic or suffer from fatigue, you should avoid them completely. The simple sugars found in fruit juices will cause an overproduction of insulin by the pancreas. This, in turn, will trigger the roller-coaster effect of quick highs and sudden lows in blood sugar levels.

PART 2:

TAKING NUTRIENTS TO RESTORE LIVER DETOXIFICATION

THERE ARE MANY nutrients that help to repair the liver and maintain optimal liver function. These include antioxidants such as vitamins C and E, the B-complex vitamins, lecithin, amino acids, and essential fatty acids. Poor nutritional status is common in liver disease. The following section discusses in detail those nutrients especially important to the various chemical reactions that make up the detoxification process.

ANTIOXIDANTS

The health of the liver depends on having sufficient levels of antioxidants in the liver tissue to scavenge free radicals that interfere with liver functioning. A free radical is a type of oxygen molecule that freely moves inside cells, reacting with proteins, fats, and DNA, changing their structure and disrupting their functions. Free radicals are generated by the metabolism of oxygen and other chemicals, including cigarette smoke, unsaturated fats, food additives, and environmental chemicals—and even by aerobic exercise. It is estimated that about 17 percent of our total oxygen consumption turns into free radicals. The process of detoxification itself also generates a certain amount of free radicals as by-products of the chemical reactions involved, and an accelerated detoxification process, such as that which occurs during a modified fast or cleansing program, will generate even higher levels of free radicals than normal.

Antioxidants unite with free radicals and deactivate them, preventing them from doing damage. A variety of substances have an antioxidant function, including vitamin C, vitamin A, beta-carotene, vitamin E, selenium, and glutathione. It is important to either include all of the antioxidants in the diet or take them as supplements. Selenium, for example, increases the effectiveness of vitamin E. A 1992 study in the *Journal of Hepatology* found low levels of selenium in both alcoholic and nonalcoholic liver disease. The liver itself produces two important antioxidant enzymes, superoxide dismutase (SOD) and glutathione peroxidase (GP). Because these antioxidant enzymes are unstable and cannot be supplemented, it is especially important to maintain their production and function.

Both human and animal studies document a variety of ways in which antioxidants support liver health. In a paper published in 1990 in the *Journal of the American College of Nutrition*, thirteen healthy males were given supplemental ascorbic acid (vitamin C) along with alcohol. The vitamin C allowed the liver to clear the alcohol more easily by accelerating its breakdown. In addition, vitamin E has been shown to have a protective effect on the liver after exposure to carbon tetrachloride, a known liver toxin.

SUGGESTED DOSAGE FOR VITAMIN E: 400 to 1200 IU (International Units) per day, preferably taken in the d-alpha-tocopherol form. While vitamin E rarely causes side effects, occasional cases have been reported of an elevation in blood pressure in individuals with preexisting hypertension. Vitamin E might also affect insulin requirements in diabetics. In both of these cases, it is best to err on the side of caution and begin taking vitamin E at lower dosages, preferably 100 IU, and increase gradually, monitoring either blood pressure or blood sugar levels as needed. Susan has rarely seen any problems arising from vitamin E use; probably fewer than ten patients out of the many thousands she has worked with in the past twenty-four years have had problems. These few patients reported minor side effects like digestive upsets and skin rashes using vitamin E. Given the millions of people who take vitamin E in this country and rarely report any unpleasant side effects, it is a remarkably safe nutrient for the vast majority of people.

Note: Use natural vitamin E instead of the synthetic form. Research studies have primarily used natural vitamin E derived from wheat germ oil. To tell the difference, read the label on the bottle. Natural vitamin E is listed as d-alpha while the synthetic is listed as d'l-alpha. Although the synthetic form is less expensive, there is some concern that it is also less effective.

SUGGESTED DOSAGE FOR VITAMIN C: 1 to 5 g per day, in divided doses. If taking 2 g, take these in the morning and evening; 3 g, one at each meal; 5 g, divided as two in the morning and evening and one with lunch. Because vitamin C is water soluble and is quickly excreted, for maximum benefit, you must take this vitamin several times during the day. Individuals who are overly acidic should use buffered vitamin C (see chapter 2 for more information). Vitamin C is not toxic in large doses, but taking more than the body needs will cause diarrhea, a reliable sign of overdose.

SUGGESTED DOSAGE FOR BETA-CAROTENE: 25,000 to 75,000 IU per day. Beta-carotene in standard dosages is not toxic. Symptoms of toxicity include nausea, enlargement of the liver and spleen, blurred vision, and skin rashes. In extremely rare cases, high doses color the skin orange. Symptoms disappear in a few days if the vitamin is withdrawn.

B-COMPLEX VITAMINS

The vitamin B complex includes thiamine (B_1), riboflavin (B_2), niacin (B_3), pantothenic acid (B_5), vitamin B_6, vitamin B_{12}, folic acid, biotin, choline, and inositol. They are water soluble and are not stored well in the body, requiring that some be consumed each day, in food or supplements. People who eat a diet of mostly processed foods high in white sugar and flour, as well as those who consume a lot of alcohol, need greater amounts of B-complex vitamins. The richest source of B vitamins is brewer's yeast, but other good sources include the germ and bran of cereal grains and animal liver. Some B vitamins are also made in the intestines. Antibiotics such as sulfa drugs and tetracycline can interfere with this production, so when taking medications such as these, it is important to supplement your diet. B vitamins are critical for the production of energy within the cells and are also vital for the metabolism of fats.

The B vitamins play many roles in maintaining the health of the liver. They are necessary for the deactivation of excess estrogen, which was initially documented in studies by Morton S. Biskind in the early 1940s. Thiamine is needed for the metabolism of alcohol to degrade it to nontoxic carbon dioxide and water. Animal studies indicate that niacin protects against carbon tetrachloride poisoning and lowers cholesterol and triglyceride levels in the blood. And folic acid and vitamin B_{12} have been shown to counteract fatty liver (accumulation of fat within the liver).

Vitamin B deficiencies are common factors in most liver diseases. The treatment of alcoholic liver disease, for example, requires supplementation with thiamine, vitamin B_6, and folic acid. Macrocytic anemia, which is associated with liver disease, requires folic acid and vitamin B_{12}.

SUGGESTED DOSAGE: A standard dose for most B-complex nutritional supplements is between 25 and 100 mg per day. (However, some of the nutrients contained within these products, like folic acid, biotin, and B_{12}, are included in smaller amounts, measured in micrograms.)

LECITHIN

Lecithin is made up of two B-complex vitamins: choline and inositol. It is a main building block of cell membranes, making up 65 percent of the membranes of liver cells. Consequently, it is one of the most important nutrients for the liver. Metabolism of various pollutants, alcohol, viruses, drugs, and other toxins occurs on the surface of cell membranes, and in this process, the detoxification enzymes produce reactive metabolites that attack liver tissue. According to an article published in 1996 in the *Alternative Medicine Review*, two decades of clinical trials provide evidence that supplemental lecithin speeds the regeneration of damaged tissue. Lecithin is used in the treatment of hepatitis, fatty liver, and alcoholic liver disease. Lecithin also helps to prevent atherosclerosis by inhibiting low-density lipoproteins from interacting with arterial receptors, according to a study published in 1976 in *Atherosclerosis*. Good sources of lecithin are egg yolks, brewer's yeast, wheat germ, fish, peanuts, leafy green vegetables, and animal liver.

The components of lecithin, choline and inositol, are classified as lipotropic factors (substances that help prevent the accumulation of fat in the liver), and as components of bile, which accelerates fat excretion. Choline is a very sensitive compound, easily destroyed by alcohol, estrogen, sulfa drugs, and cooking. In a double-blind study published in 1982 in *Liver*, choline was given for three days to fifteen patients with chronic active hepatitis. A significant reduction in disease activity was noted in patients receiving the choline. The body has large stores of inositol, which is found in whole grains, citrus, and unrefined molasses, and is depleted by drinking coffee.

SUGGESTED DOSAGE: To supplement your diet with lecithin, take 2 tbsp. stirred into 4 oz. of water, once a day. The range of dosage for both choline and inositol is 50 to 500 mg.

AMINO ACIDS

While many people take vitamins and minerals, supplementing with amino acids, the building blocks of protein, is less common. Nonetheless, certain amino acids, such as methionine, glutathione, and cysteine can aid in the process of detoxification and can be taken as nutritional supplements. They are generally available in natural-food stores as well as certain pharmacies.

Methionine

Methionine is an essential amino acid, which means that it cannot be made within the body and must be supplemented or supplied by the diet. Good dietary sources of methionine include beef, chicken, beans, eggs, yogurt, onions, and garlic. It is one of the sulfur-containing amino acids and is a powerful detoxifier with a long list of functions. For example, methionine can rid the body of heavy metals such as lead and mercury. It functions as an antioxidant, scavenging free radicals generated by the breakdown of toxins such as alcohol. Methionine promotes the production of lecithin, which is required in the breakdown of fats, preventing their accumulation in the liver. If unchecked, fatty accumulation can lead to cirrhosis of the liver. Several human and animal studies show abnormalities in methionine pathways as one cause of this disease. Methionine also maintains the body's reserves of glutathione peroxidase, the powerful antioxidant enzyme.

SUGGESTED DOSAGE: Dosages for methionine used for detoxification range from 200 to 1000 mg per day. The supplement has a meaty, sulfurous odor. It tends to be packaged in 100 to 500 mg capsules. Methionine is normally converted within the body to a substance called homocysteine, which is toxic to the heart. To prevent the buildup of homocysteine, 25 to 50 mg of vitamin B_6 should be taken with methionine.

Glutathione

Glutathione is an extremely important amino acid in the detoxification process. It is a compound amino acid composed of cysteine, glutamic acid, and glycine. It is used by complementary medical practitioners for the prevention and treatment of a variety of degenerative conditions associated with the aging process.

Like vitamins A, C, and E, glutathione is a deactivator of free radicals in the body and assists in slowing the cross-linking of collagen fibers. Cross-linking of protein fibers is a characteristic sign of aging in which the tissues become constricted and tight. It is most noticeable in older persons whose skin has taken on a leathery characteristic. However, that is just the external deterioration; cross-linking is going on throughout the entire body. Studies have shown that glutathione also acts as an immune system enhancer and assists the body in removing heavy metals such as mercury, lead, and aluminum. Glutathione is especially important for the liver in that it helps prevent damage from alcohol by assisting in the detoxification of liver peroxidation. Through the action of glutathione-S-transferase, the liver can break down toxins into substrates for excretion via bile into the small intestine. Glutathione is available from the diet through eating fresh fruits and vegetables, fish, and meat. Supplementary oral glutathione can be purchased in health food stores; however, it is not particularly well absorbed when taken orally. In addition, 500 to 2000 mg of vitamin C per day can elevate glutathione levels within the body by helping the body to manufacture it.

SUGGESTED DOSAGE: 1000 to 2000 mg per day.

Cysteine

Methionine gives rise to the amino acid cysteine, the precursor to glutathione, which the body uses to synthesize the detoxification enzymes glutathione peroxidase and reductase. These antioxidant enzymes prevent the oxidation of fats and help break down toxins from car exhaust, smoke, drugs, radiation, and other carcinogens. In a study conducted in Ghana, published in 1994 in the *Journal of International Medical Research*, researchers concluded that low levels of cysteine and glutathione may increase the risk of liver toxicity from oxidants.

SUGGESTED DOSAGE: The dosage of cysteine is 200 mg twice a day, taken with meals. Cysteine should be taken in conjunction with 50 mg of vitamin B_6 three times per day and with supplemental vitamin C (ascorbic acid) to prevent kidney stones.

N-acetyl cysteine (NAC)

Body levels of glutathione can also be increased by supplementing with N-acetyl cysteine (NAC), which converts to glutathione once inside the cells. NAC is more beneficial as a supplement than glutathione itself, which is not well absorbed. Not only does NAC boost our detoxification capability, but it also improves immune function. Research studies have found that it can reduce flu symptoms when 600 mg are taken twice a day.

SUGGESTED DOSAGE: A standard dosage is 300 to 600 mg once or twice per day.

Glycine and taurine

Glycine is an essential part of glutathione, along with cysteine and glutamic acid. Thus, it plays an important role in healthy detoxification. Along with taurine, glycine conjugates or binds with bile acids to maintain the solubility of fats and cholesterol in bile, thereby helping to prevent the formation of gallstones. (Bile is a substance secreted by the liver which is stored in the gallbladder and then secreted into the small intestine.) Bile has an emulsifying effect on the fat contained in food.

SUGGESTED DOSAGE: Take glycine and taurine together on an empty stomach. A standard dosage is 500 mg of glycine and 100–500 mg taurine once or twice a day.

ESSENTIAL FATTY ACIDS

Because the liver is prone to inflammatory disease and all toxins cause an inflammatory reaction, it is important to consume certain oils that counteract the inflammatory response. These are the omega-3 fatty acid oils, like flaxseed oil, which have a high percentage of linolenic acid and are beneficial to liver health. In contrast, excessive consumption of saturated fats such as those found in red meat, dairy products, and palm kernel oil promotes inflammation.

The omega-3 and the omega-6 fatty acids found in plant oils such as sesame and sunflower make up the cell walls of the mast cells, which are distributed throughout the body. These cells protect us against viruses, bacteria, and allergens by releasing material that is toxic to these invaders. When there are sufficient omega-3s in the diet, the structure of the mast cell walls is stable, but when there is a predominance of omega-6s, the cell walls can break down more readily, releasing the fatty acids. These fatty acids enter the general circulation and are eventually metabolized by the liver. Within the liver, their chemical structure is altered, both desaturating and elongating the fatty acids.

As the omega-6 fatty acids are metabolized, they may enter the arachidonic cascade, which is a series of chemical reactions that generate primarily arachidonic acid and secondarily series II prostaglandins and leukotrienes. These are hormonelike substances that can trigger an inflammatory response and impair liver function. Studies have shown that the production of leukotrienes increases the risk of inflammatory liver diseases. Red meat and dairy foods also contain arachidonic acid, and these foods as well can lead to inflammation. In contrast, the breakdown of omega-3 fatty acids does not enter the arachidonic pathway and therefore does not trigger the same inflammatory reactions.

To promote healthy liver function and prevent inflammation, there should be a balance of these fats and oils in the diet. While omega-6 fatty acids and the saturated fats found in red meat and dairy products need to be consumed judiciously, they should not be avoided completely. In fact, the omega-6 fatty acids contribute to the health of the liver in ways unrelated to their participation in the inflammatory pathways. A 1991 study in *Alcohol and Alcoholism* found evening primrose oil, which contains high amounts of omega-6 fatty acids, to be effective in preventing liver damage caused by alcohol and in reducing alcohol withdrawal symptoms. However, as many as eight to thirteen capsules of evening primrose oil must be taken on a daily basis to attain therapeutic levels. A more practical option is to use borage seed oil, which contains a more concentrated form of beneficial fatty acids. Two to four capsules per day of borage seed oil is sufficient to reach therapeutic levels.

It is important to buy oils that are unrefined and cold-pressed to avoid the toxic by-products that occur in processed oils during the extraction process. Flaxseed oil is delicate and requires special handling. As it breaks down quickly when exposed to light, oxygen, and heat, it should never be used for cooking but only added to foods just before eating them. Flaxseed oil is usually sold in small quantities in an opaque container, found in the refrigerator section of natural-food stores. The date at which the oil was processed is found on the container, and the oil should be used only during the time specified.

SUGGESTED DOSAGE: To supplement your intake of essential fatty acid, take 1 to 2 tbsp. of flaxseed oil a day. Good supplemental sources of omega-6 fatty acids are evening primrose oil, eight to thirteen capsules per day, or two to four capsules of borage oil per day.

▲▲ Individuals with poor liver function should begin fatty-acid therapy in very small amounts. Use one-quarter to one-third the recommended dose and increase gradually to therapeutic levels. People with poor liver function may find that fatty-acid use may initially cause nausea, abdominal bloating, and even diarrhea. In such cases, an accelerated liver-cleansing program (discussed later in this chapter) and more readily tolerated liver restorative nutrients such as lecithin and antioxidants should be instituted for several months before starting fatty-acid therapy.

▲▲ Whole flaxseeds, ground up in a blender or food processor and used as a cereal or in shakes, provide an excellent alternative to the use of flaxseed oil. Besides their high oil content, flaxseeds are extremely rich in a wide variety of nutrients that are beneficial for the entire body, as well as the liver. Ground flaxseeds contain the entire range of essential amino acids in an easy-to-assimilate form as well as large amounts of valuable alkaline minerals such as calcium, potassium, magnesium, and zinc. They are also an excellent source of fiber, mucilage, and lubricants, which promote the excretion of fats and other waste products from the body, thereby reducing the load on the liver. Organically grown flaxseeds are inexpensive and available in bulk at most health food stores. We developed the following flaxseed recipes many years ago.

FLAX SHAKE No. 1

4 tablespoons raw flaxseeds

1 ripe papaya

2 cups spring or filtered water

flavoring agents such as rice bran syrup, cinnamon, or nutmeg, if desired

Combine all the ingredients in a blender or food processor and run it on high speed for 60 to 90 seconds or until the drink is totally liquefied. Add more water if a thinner drink is desired. Drink immediately.

Provides a complete meal for 1 person.

FLAX SHAKE No. 2

4 tablespoons raw flaxseeds

1 ripe banana

2 cups soy or other nondairy milk

flavoring agents such as rice bran syrup, cinnamon, or nutmeg, if desired

Combine all the ingredients in a blender or food processor and run it on high speed for 60 to 90 seconds or until the drink is totally liquefied. Add more nondairy milk if a thinner drink is desired. Drink immediately.

Provides a complete meal for 1 person.

INSTANT FLAX CEREAL

4 tablespoons raw flaxseeds

$^2/_3$ cup soy or other nondairy milk

$^1/_2$ ripe banana, sliced

flavoring agents such as rice bran syrup, cinnamon, or nutmeg, if desired

Grind the flaxseeds into a powder using a seed or coffee grinder. Place the powder in a cereal bowl and slowly add the nondairy milk, stirring until the mixture thickens to a texture similar to that of cream of rice or oatmeal. Top the cereal with the sliced banana. Add sweetener and eat right away.

Serves 1.

HERBS

The following herbs are proven tonics for the liver. They have a wide range of therapeutic benefits. Many herbs increase the flow of bile from the liver. They also stimulate increased blood flow through the liver, removing debris, old cells, and toxins. These herbs also protect the liver from a wide variety of everyday environmental toxins, such as cleaning agents and cigarette smoke, and encourage the production of enzymes that facilitate detoxification. Some of these herbs stimulate the growth of new liver cells when there is damage to the liver.

▲▲ We recommend that the herbs discussed in this section be taken primarily as capsules or as teas (if palatable). Susan does not advise the use of tinctures and extracts for her patients with liver conditions or for those who are attempting to restore liver function, if the tinctures and extracts are processed with and preserved in alcohol. Alcohol, of course, adds to the toxic load of the liver and should be avoided when using herbs for liver restoration.

Silymarin

Milk thistle plant has been used for centuries as an herbal medicine. A group of the most potent and medicinally active flavonoids found in the seed of the milk thistle plant are known collectively as silymarin. In Europe, silymarin has long been prescribed for both acute and chronic liver disease. Its effectiveness has been confirmed by more than 300 studies conducted since the late 1960s.

Silymarin is used to treat jaundice, hepatitis, cirrhosis, fatty liver, and congestion of the bile ducts, as well as disorders of the spleen, gallbladder, and digestive tract. In a double-blind study published in 1982 in the *Scandinavian Journal of Gastroenterology*, forty-seven patients, primarily with alcohol-induced liver disease, showed significant improvement with silymarin treatment. This was evidenced by a reduction in the enzymes SGPT and SGOT, which become elevated when the liver is damaged.

Silymarin protects the liver from environmental pollutants, including smoke from tobacco, coal, oil, and incense; X-rays and the side effects of radiation therapy; and industrial toxins including carbon tetrachloride. Animal studies demonstrate silymarin's action to be comparable to that of penicillin in counteracting poisons. There is also some documentation of silymarin's ability to protect against nonmelanoma skin cancer and leukemia. Studies indicate that silymarin functions as a powerful antioxidant, scavenging free radicals that can damage liver cells. It also inhibits depletion of glutathione, one of the liver's most important antioxidant enzymes.

When liver cells are damaged by poisons, silymarin accelerates the rate of protein synthesis and regeneration of liver cells. It also prevents the reabsorption of poisons once they leave the liver and pass through the gastrointestinal tract. This reduces the toxic load on the liver and spares the cells not yet poisoned so that they can act as centers for the generation of new liver cells. With time, complete restoration of the liver is possible.

SUGGESTED DOSAGE: Milk thistle extract is considered completely safe to take in normally prescribed amounts. However, some people may experience loose stools during the first few days of taking this herb. Products containing milk thistle extract in combination with other liver restorative herbs are also available. Milk thistle extract is combined in these products with herbs such as turmeric, artichoke leaf, dandelion, or licorice. Milk thistle extract standardized to 80 percent silymarin is available in 150 to 175 mg capsules. Take one to three capsules per day.

Dandelion

Dandelion, which can grow rampant in your lawn, is a low-growing perennial plant used medicinally for over a thousand years. Arab physicians in the tenth century prescribed dandelion as a diuretic, and by the seventeenth century the English herbalist Nicholas Culpepper incorporated dandelion as the foundation of many medicinal remedies. The early English colonists introduced dandelion to North America, where it grows in many regions of the continent.

Dandelion is often prescribed to help detoxify the liver and also to prevent gallstones. Dandelion increases the flow of bile from the liver, facilitating the detoxification process. This is supported by German research, and German physicians routinely prescribe dandelion to prevent gallstones. Herbalists also often use dandelion, because of its diuretic properties, in the treatment of conditions involving fluid retention, such as PMS, obesity, high blood pressure, and congestive heart failure. As a diuretic, dandelion helps eliminate toxins from the body via the urine. It is also high in easily assimilated minerals, adding to its benefits.

SUGGESTED DOSAGE: Dandelion is included in the FDA's list of herbs generally regarded as safe. In sensitive individuals, dandelion may cause a skin rash. It should not be used by women who are pregnant or nursing. When used as a food, dandelion leaves can be enjoyed in a salad. Mixed with other greens, they lend a slightly bitter sharpness. The leaves can also be taken as an infusion. Make a tea using $1/2$ oz. of dried leaves per one cup of boiling water and steep ten minutes, drinking a maximum of three cups a day. Dandelion is also available in 150 mg capsules. Take one to three capsules per day.

Artichoke

The artichoke is a thistlelike plant that actually belongs to the daisy family. It is prescribed extensively in Europe to protect against toxins and to encourage the regeneration of liver cells. The principal active compound in artichokes is cynarin.

Artichoke helps prevent the accumulation of fats in the liver and arteries and is used in the treatment of atherosclerosis and arteriosclerosis. In a controlled trial published in 1975 in *Drug Research*, two groups of thirty patients with hyperlipidemia (elevated blood fat levels) were treated for fifty days with cynarin (500 mg) or a placebo. Cynarin produced a significant reduction in blood cholesterol levels, lipoprotein levels, and body weight. Artichoke is also effective in preventing elevated cholesterol when toxins such as alcohol are present. As a bile stimulant, artichoke can also help prevent gallstones and liver damage from environmental toxins.

Cynarin decreases the rate of cholesterol synthesis in the liver and increases its conversion into bile acids. It also facilitates the flow of bile from the gallbladder and increases the contractive power of the bile ducts. In studies, artichoke has been shown to increase the production and volume of bile flow by as much as four times in a twelve-hour period. Artichokes also interrupt the enterohepatic circuit that would otherwise recirculate toxins between the gastrointestinal tract and the liver. Finally, artichokes stimulate the regeneration of liver cells.

SUGGESTED DOSAGE: Artichoke is generally recognized as safe by the FDA. Persons who are experiencing an acute episode of pain and spasm due to inflammation of the gallbladder should not take artichoke as it may aggravate the symptoms. Artichoke is available in 160 mg capsules; take one to two capsules three times per day.

Turmeric

Turmeric is an indispensable part of the mixture of spices known as curry powder. The medicinally active compound in turmeric is curcumin, the rich orange-yellow pigment that gives turmeric its characteristic color. Turmeric has been used for thousands of years in Indian cooking and in India's traditional Ayurvedic medicine. The turmeric plant, grown from India to Indonesia, is related to ginger and has pulpy, orange, tuberous roots that grow to about two feet in length.

Turmeric is widely used in indigenous medicine in the treatment of jaundice and liver disease. Herbalists prescribe it to prevent liver damage from alcohol and other toxins. Turmeric is also known to promote circulation, dissolve blood clots, and treat irregular menstruation of all kinds.

Animal studies have shown curcumin to be an effective treatment for acute and chronic inflammation, and curcumin is used in the treatment of gallstones, acute and chronic inflammation of the gallbladder, and inflammation of the bile duct. In India it is applied topically to treat fresh wounds, bruises, and insect bites.

In a 1970 study in the *Journal of Nutrition*, curcumin lowered serum and liver cholesterol by one-half to one-third. Turmeric is also used as a digestive aid, facilitating the digestion of fats—hence its medicinal usefulness in curry.

Curcumin increases bile secretion and the contraction of the gallbladder, thereby facilitating detoxification and potentially lowering cholesterol. Curcumin also functions as an anti-inflammatory and anticoagulant agent. It has been shown to increase levels of glutathione-S-transferase and UDP glucuronyl transferase, two liver enzymes important for the promotion of phase II detoxification reactions. In addition, curcumin has been shown to have an antibacterial action and to block tumor growth.

SUGGESTED DOSAGE: Turmeric is on the FDA's list of herbs generally regarded as safe. However, because turmeric has a potential anti-clotting effect, anyone with a blood-clotting problem or who is currently taking anticoagulant medications should consult with their physician before taking this herb. Turmeric should not be taken by pregnant or nursing women. Turmeric is available in 400 or 500 mg capsules; take one capsule two to three times per day.

Licorice root

The use of licorice has a long history, appearing prominently in the first great Chinese herbal *The Pen Tsao Ching (Classic of Herbs)*, written more than 5000 years ago. Licorice today is one of the most prescribed herbs in the Chinese pharmacopoeia, second only to ginseng. Licorice has also long been used in the West for medicinal purposes. Bundles of licorice sticks were found amid the treasures of King Tut's tomb, and licorice appears in European herbals (an herbal is a book about plants) from the Renaissance to modern times, usually prescribed and referenced as a diuretic.

The primary active component in licorice is glycyrrhizin, which has a broad range of benefits. The licorice root is fifty times sweeter than sugar. In studies, licorice has been used effectively to control hepatitis and improve liver function in people with cirrhosis.

Contemporary herbalists recommend licorice for its soothing effects on the respiratory and gastrointestinal tracts. In a 1962 study published in the *Lancet*, fifty patients with gastric ulcers were successfully treated with licorice, which was as effective as treatment with a drug such as cimetidine. Licorice also has important anti-inflammatory properties. It stimulates cell production of interferon, the body's own antiviral compound. Licorice can also be used in nutritional programs to treat bacterial and fungal infections.

SUGGESTED DOSAGE: Licorice is included in the FDA's list of herbs generally regarded as safe. Overdose reports have involved highly concentrated licorice extracts used in some candies, laxatives, and tobacco products. There have been no reports of problems caused by licorice sticks or the powdered herb. However, licorice should not be used by pregnant and nursing women or by anyone with a history of diabetes, glaucoma, high blood pressure, stroke, or heart disease, as licorice can cause water retention and a rise in blood pressure. To take licorice as a decoction, gently boil $1/2$ tsp. of the powdered herb in one cup of water for ten minutes. Drink up to two cups a day. Licorice root is also available in 300 mg capsules; take one capsule between meals two times per day.

A Caution on the Use of Herbs

The use of herbs in individuals with impaired detoxification capabilities can be a double-edged sword: Certain herbs have very powerful liver-cleansing and restorative effects. However, very sensitive individuals may not be able to process these herbs, which then overwhelm the very detoxification system that needs to be strengthened. These individuals may have immediate unpleasant side effects such as nausea, abdominal bloating, and congestion, and discomfort in the region of the liver. Such individuals should avoid the use of liver-cleansing herbs entirely until their detoxification capability is greatly strengthened. If you want to try an herbal program and are unsure of your tolerance for herbs, start with one-quarter of the suggested dosages. If this is well tolerated, you can gradually increase your intake over several weeks to therapeutic levels.

GREEN FOODS

Green foods are important ingredients in herbal cleansing programs because chlorophyll, which imparts the green color to these foods, helps to neutralize and remove toxins. The greener the plant, the greater the amount of chlorophyll. Foods high in chlorophyll also help heal digestive disorders, provide energy, boost immunity, and prevent deficiency diseases such as anemia. Certain grasses and algae, which are described below, are especially high in chlorophyll.

As cited in an article published in 1986 in *Mutation Research*, the National Institute for Occupational Safety and Health estimated that millions of workers in the manufacturing sector have been exposed to potentially hazardous chemicals, many of which cause genetic mutation and promote cancer. This same article reports on a study that shows the effectiveness of chlorophyll in counteracting the mutagenic effect of pollutants such as cigarette smoke, coal dust, and diesel-emission particles. Chlorophyll was extremely effective at inhibiting the mutations of the various nitrogen compounds, aromatic amines, and hydrocarbons found in these substances. Chlorophyll also protected against harmful compounds in fried beef and pork, red grape juice, and red wine. Chlorophyll has also been used successfully to treat iron deficiency anemia and peptic ulcers.

Pure extracted liquid chlorophyll is available in health food stores. Always use chlorophyll that has been extracted from alfalfa or other plants; avoid the chemically manufactured variety. There is a benefit to consuming the plant itself as a source of chlorophyll, since grasses and algae offer their own additional properties.

SUGGESTED DOSAGE: 100 mg two or three times a day.

Wheat grass and barley grass

Cereal grasses, such as wheat grass and barley grass, are high-chlorophyll foods. Commercially, they are available fresh and as supplements, in both powder and tablet form. It is also possible to grow wheat grass at home. Both have nearly identical therapeutic properties, although barley grass may be digested a little more easily by some. People with allergies to wheat and other cereals can usually tolerate these grasses since grain in its grass stage rarely triggers an allergic reaction.

These grasses contain about the same quotient of protein as meat, about 20 percent, as well as vitamin B_{12}, chlorophyll, vitamin A, and many other nutrients. Wheat grass is capable of incorporating more than 90 out of the estimated possible 102 minerals found in rich soil.

Wheat and barley grasses have been used to treat hepatitis and high cholesterol, as well as arthritis, peptic ulcers, and hypoglycemia. They are both effective in reducing inflammation and contain the antioxidant superoxide dismutase (SOD), which slows cellular deterioration, plus various digestive enzymes that aid in detoxification.

SUGGESTED DOSAGE: Combine 1 to 2 tbsp. of the powder or 1 to 2 oz. of the fresh juice in 8 oz. of water.

Microalgae

Spirulina, chlorella, and wild blue-green algae contain more chlorophyll than any other foods. These algae are aquatic plants, spiral-shaped and emerald to blue-green in color, and have been used medicinally for thousands of years in South America and Africa. Today they can be purchased, dried, in health food stores. They are also the highest sources of protein, beta-carotene, and nucleic acids of any animal or plant food, as well as containing the essential fatty acids omega-3 and gamma linolenic acid. The protein in spirulina and chlorella is so easily digested and absorbed that two or three teaspoons of these microalgae are equivalent to two to three ounces of meat. Further, unlike animal protein, the protein in algae generates a minimum of waste products when it is metabolized, thereby lessening stress on the liver.

Spirulina. Spirulina detoxifies the kidneys and liver, inhibiting the growth of fungi, bacteria, and yeasts. Because spirulina is so easily digested, it yields quick energy. It is also strongly anti-inflammatory and therefore useful in the treatment of hepatitis, gastritis, and other inflammatory diseases. Spirulina strengthens body tissues and protects the vascular system by lowering blood fat. Athletes use spirulina for energy and for its cleansing action after strenuous physical exertion, which can stimulate the body to rid itself of poisons.

SUGGESTED DOSAGE: A standard dosage of spirulina is 1 to 2 tbsp. stirred into 8 oz. of water per day. Green foods are very concentrated, so start with a half dose and increase gradually to make sure it's well tolerated.

Chlorella. This well-known algae is an especially effective detoxifier and anti-inflammatory agent because it is high in chlorophyll, which stimulates these processes. Chlorella is notable for its tough outer cell walls, which bind with heavy metals, pesticides, and carcinogens such as PCBs (polychlorinated biphenyls) and then carry these toxins out of the body. Because of chlorella growth factor, this algae also promotes growth and repair of all kinds of tissue. Animal studies show that it reduces cholesterol and atherosclerosis.

SUGGESTED DOSAGE: 1 tbsp. taken in 8 to 12 oz. of water. Green foods are very concentrated. Be sure to begin with a partial dose and increase gradually.

Wild blue-green algae. Wild blue-green algae grows in Klamath Lake in Oregon and is processed by freeze-drying. It is sold under various trade names, frequently as a mail-order product. Wild blue-green algae is very energizing and can improve an individual's mental concentration. However, a sign of overuse is weakness and a lack of mental focus, and certain forms are known to be highly toxic.

Many of Susan's female patients who are in their late thirties and forties report that taking blue-green algae helps lessen the fatigue and mood swings associated with PMS and perimenopausal hormone imbalances. While Susan has not found it to be helpful in reducing physical symptoms such as bloating, breast tenderness, and menstrual irregularity, it does seem to promote more efficient liver function. Since the liver has a crucial role in detoxifying and deactivating estrogen, healthy liver function helps to bring estrogen levels into balance, thereby relieving the fatigue, depression, and moodiness often found in perimenopausal women.

SUGGESTED DOSAGE: 1 tbsp. daily in 8 to 12 oz. of water. It is important to buy wild blue-green algae from a reputable company that processes the algae in an FDA-approved laboratory. To avoid certain wild blue-green algae that is highly toxic, never collect it yourself or consume any that you have gathered.

Various green foods can be combined in an easy-to-digest, highly nutritious drink. As with all concentrated foods, begin with small amounts and work up to your final level. In our personal recipe, we use 1 tbsp. of a wheat and barley grass combination and 2 tbsp. of spirulina. Add water to a consistency you enjoy, and combine using either a whisk or a blender. If you use a blender, be sure to empty the container and then add back some additional water to remove all the green foods, as they are expensive and you do not want to waste them.

PART 3:
LIVER-CLEANSING TECHNIQUES

BOTH COFFEE ENEMAS and liver flushes are very effective detoxification techniques that directly stimulate the liver and gallbladder to release accumulated poisons. They are best used as part of an overall detoxification program that incorporates a modified diet, nutritional supplements, adequate water, exercise, and rest.

Because a rigorous detoxification program can be extremely disruptive to a person's life, Susan recommends a slower, gentler, more gradual process of detoxification accomplished with a lighter diet (as outlined on pages 302–304), which will cause fewer side effects. When it comes to detoxification, intense is not necessarily better. A rigorous cleanse is more appropriate for times of relaxation and retreat when a person has nothing to do but take a sauna, lounge in the sun, and read books. However, if you want to take a more aggressive approach, you may want to experiment with the following cleanses, which accelerate detoxification. These include a coffee enema, liver flush, colon cleansing, sauna, and dry-brush massage.

USING COFFEE FOR A POWERFUL DETOXIFICATION TECHNIQUE

Although the procedure may sound unusual, coffee enemas have been used as a detoxification technique for at least 100 years. As cited in the April 1996 *Townsend Letter for Doctors & Patients*, animal studies conducted in Germany in the 1920s found that a caffeine solution administered rectally tends to stimulate the production of bile. Max Gerson, a pioneer in liver detoxification techniques, incorporated coffee enemas into his now well-known cancer protocol. He recommended that a regimen of coffee enemas be strictly followed, both in the clinic and at home, for at least eighteen months. The noted New York immunologist Nicholas Gonzalez also includes coffee enemas as part of an overall program to treat cancer. According to Gonzalez, the enemas facilitate elimination of the waste products and toxins that can accumulate as tumors break down.

Coffee enemas flood only the sigmoid, or lower, portion of the bowel. When coffee is taken into the lower bowel, nearly all of the caffeine in it is absorbed, first into the hemorrhoidal veins, then into the portal veins, and eventually into the liver. The caffeine causes these blood vessels and the liver's bile ducts to dilate (expand), thereby increasing the release of bile. The fluid in the bowel dilutes the bile, triggering a further increase in bile flow. Furthermore, a coffee enema significantly increases levels of glutathione-S-transferase, an enzyme that catalyzes the release of bile.

A coffee enema that lasts ten to twelve minutes can facilitate significant purging of toxins from the liver and colon. In addition, caffeine causes smooth muscle in the liver and gallbladder to relax, which can be therapeutic for individuals with spastic colon and irritable-bowel syndrome.

Ingredients and equipment

It is important to use coffee that is both caffeinated and organic. Using nonorganic coffee beans, most of which are sprayed with pesticides, would undermine the purpose of the technique, which is to purge the body of toxins. When making the coffee, use water that is free of chlorine and fluorides. The water can be distilled, filtered, or spring water from a glass container (water stored in a plastic container may contain toxic chemicals that leached into it from the plastic).

Procedure

The actual procedure for a coffee enema is relatively simple and can become routine.

First, make the coffee. Use three rounded tablespoons of organic drip ground caffeinated coffee to one quart of pure water. Boil the coffee for five minutes, then lower the heat and simmer it for fifteen to twenty minutes. Strain the coffee and cool it to body temperature.

Next, lay a towel on the floor. Put the enema bag in the sink with the catheter closed, and pour 8 to 16 ounces of the prepared coffee into the bag. Loosen the catheter clamp to allow the coffee to flow to the tip of the catheter, and reclamp it when all the air is removed from the tubing. Then hang the filled bag from a door handle or towel rack near where you are going to lie down to generate a gentle flow of liquid.

Lie down on the towel on the floor and insert the catheter into the rectum a few inches, using a lubricant if needed. Lie on your right side in a fetal position, with both thighs drawn close to the abdomen. Release the clamp and slowly let the coffee flow into the colon. Breathe deeply. If you experience any discomfort or fullness, immediately close the clamp.

Retain the fluid for ten minutes to insure that caffeine reaches the bile ducts of the liver. Feel free to change position to insure the greatest degree of comfort. When the time limit is reached, be sure to expel the enema completely as with normal elimination. If you have an immediate urge to release the coffee, do so to empty the colon of stool, then repeat the procedure. When you are done, rinse the enema bag thoroughly with soap and water and hang it to dry. You can also clean it using boiling water or peroxide to prevent mold growth.

Cautions for coffee enemas

Complementary physicians who recommend this technique report that coffee enemas can be taken once or even several times a day during the early stages of a detoxification program without toxic effects. There is no indication that enemas disrupt normal voiding; in fact, people often report less constipation. There is also little risk of flushing out vitamins and minerals because these are absorbed from the stool before it reaches the sigmoid portion of the bowel. If symptoms of toxicity occur—such as headache, fever, nausea, intestinal spasms, and fatigue—take the enemas less frequently or stop their use entirely. Individuals with chronic diarrhea or inflammatory bowel disease should use this technique cautiously or not at all.

LIVER FLUSHES

A liver flush is a drink of fruit juice and olive oil, which increases the flow of bile from the liver, helps to eliminate toxins, and thereby assists in the restoration of liver function. For a gradual cleanse, liver flushes may be done on several consecutive days. It is beneficial to consult an experienced complementary health care professional if you wish to do a series of these, since different practitioners may suggest various programs. However, if you want to do a liver flush on an unsupervised basis, they may be done for a period of up to ten days. Since the flush is made up, in part, of low-pH citrus fruit juices, it should be used cautiously or avoided entirely by overly acidic individuals. This type of flush is best tolerated by individuals with healthy, balanced buffer systems and high alkaline producers. (See chapters 1 and 2 for more information.) The following liver flush has a pleasing taste and can be made as follows:

1. Combine 6 oz. of an orange/grapefruit juice mixture with 2 oz. of either lime or lemon juice. This mixture will taste relatively acidic and astringent (it may make your mouth pucker). Such mixtures are traditionally used to neutralize the deleterious effects of a high-fat, high-protein diet on the liver and help to promote liver cleansing.

2. Pour the juice mixture into a glass jar with a tight-fitting lid (or in a blender), and add one or two cloves of fresh-squeezed garlic and $1/2$ tsp. grated fresh ginger.

3. To this juice and herb mixture, add 1 tbsp. extra-virgin olive oil. Finally, dilute this mixture with up to 6 oz. of spring or filtered water. Close the lid securely and thoroughly shake the mixture to combine the ingredients, or blend in the blender.

4. Drink the liver flush slowly. It is best to take the flush early in the morning, apart from meals, and to follow it with an herbal tea such as peppermint or chamomile, both of which have a mildly cleansing effect on the liver.

COLON CLEANSES

Colon cleanses are an important component of detoxification. A colon cleanse removes toxins from the walls of the intestines, where they may have accumulated over time; it can also lessen the stress of toxins on the liver. Waste products are excreted either via the kidneys, intestines, or skin, but the majority of waste products leaving the liver pass from the body through the bowels. How efficiently and quickly the body can rid itself of these toxins directly depends on how well the colon is cleansed, which can speed transit time of conjugated chemicals and prevent their reabsorption into the body.

Fiber, dietary or supplemental, is a very effective colon cleanser. A diet that lacks fiber is usually high in fat, and this combination promotes the reabsorption of cholesterol and hormones. In contrast, a high fiber diet binds both cholesterol and estrogen effectively, and enhances their elimination from the body from the intestinal tract. There are two main types of fiber, insoluble and soluble. In addition, clay products can have similar effects to those of fiber.

Insoluble fiber

Insoluble fiber is mostly indigestible cellulose, which makes up the skin of fruits and vegetables and the cover of cereal grains such as wheat germ. Eating an apple along with its skin or brown rice rather than white provides insoluble fiber. Other fibers include the hemicelluloses. A good example is psyllium seed husks, which are an essential part of colon cleanses, binding the toxins released from the liver during detoxification. Psyllium is able to hold water, thereby softening and moisturizing the intestinal tract as it passes through the bowel. And because psyllium is similar to the mucosa of the intestines, it is able to keep debris from sticking to the walls of the intestines. Sometimes psyllium treatment is accompanied by the use of an herbal laxative such as senna, which speeds the elimination of bound toxins. Susan usually recommends 1 to 2 tbsp. of psyllium stirred into 12 to 16 oz. of water. This should be drunk immediately, as psyllium will tend to form a gel.

Soluble fiber

Guar gum is a soluble fiber that is extracted from the guar plant, grown in the Middle East. It is included in detoxification protocols as an intestinal binder and laxative. It easily absorbs cold water, forming a thick, pastelike substance (the reason it is often an ingredient in commercial ice cream and cheese spreads). As a dietary fiber, it also assists the liver in managing cholesterol levels, lowering LDL cholesterol (which is associated with a higher risk of heart disease), increasing bile secretion, and reducing the absorption of cholesterol. Stir $^1/_2$ tsp. of guar gum into 8 to 12 oz. of water and drink immediately.

Pectin is another soluble fiber, found in most plants and particularly in fruits and vegetables such as apples and citrus. Pectin has a neutral, nonassertive flavor and is used as a food stabilizer and thickener. It is also a binding agent, prescribed extensively in Russia for the removal of environmental toxins from the body. As a supplement for detoxification, use 1 tsp. in 8 to 12 oz. of water, mix well, and drink immediately, before it jells. This drink can be taken twice a day. Guar gum and pectin can be combined. Pectin is also available in 500 mg capsules; take three capsules, one to three times per day.

Clays

Some holistic health care practitioners use clay products in a detoxification regimen. Bentonite is a powdered clay composed of minute particles that give the clay a very large surface area in proportion to its volume, allowing it to collect as much as forty times its weight in toxins. Liquid or hydrated bentonite is most frequently used for internal detoxification, but any powdered clay can be added to water and soaked overnight for use the next day. Bentonite is available in premeasured regimens in natural-food stores.

A fiber success story

One of Susan's patients, Alan, a forty-five-year-old health care practitioner, had great success using fiber to improve his health. He had a busy and demanding practice, with little time to eat lunch. He often sent his assistant to one of the surrounding fast-food restaurants to bring back a quick meal consisting of a burger or tacos. He came to Susan complaining of constipation, with bowel movements only every three or four days, bloating, morning brain fog—symptoms typical of toxicity and poor elimination. He was twenty-five pounds overweight, and his cholesterol was quite elevated, a particular concern since he had a strong family history of heart disease: His father had died of a heart attack while only in his fifties.

With Susan's counsel, Alan slowly improved his overall diet, and he began to take bag lunches with him to work, which included raw vegetables like carrots and celery, and whole grain breads for fiber. If he ate a burrito or taco, it was homemade with brown rice, beans, and with no added fat. Alan also began to take a daily fiber-rich drink made with 1 tsp. guar gum and 1 tsp. pectin dissolved in 12 oz. of water. In addition, he took 2 tbsp. of psyllium mixed with water every day. When he came back to Susan's office for a three-month checkup, Alan reported having bowel movements once or twice a day; he had lost fifteen pounds and his cholesterol had dropped significantly. He was very pleased with the results and totally committed to continuing the program.

Maintaining intestinal flora

Colon cleanses can remove healthy flora from the intestines, so it is important to reintroduce live, friendly bacteria into the intestines after a program of detoxification is completed to maintain proper digestion. Yogurt and other fermented foods such as kefir contain the beneficial bacteria *Lactobacillus acidophilus*.

Prebiotics, a therapy developed in Japan, is designed to feed the beneficial bacteria. Fructo-oligosaccharides (FOSs) are naturally occurring carbohydrates that promote the growth of the healthful bacteria Bifidobacteria and lactobacilli. As a supplement, FOS comes in dry powder form and as a syrup. FOS is readily available in natural-food stores. Follow the directions listed on the packaging of the product you buy. These carbohydrates are also found in honey, garlic, asparagus, tomato, onions, banana, rye, barley, and triticale.

THERAPEUTIC BATHS, SWEATS, AND SAUNAS

The skin is the largest organ of elimination in the body. Besides excreting essential minerals when we perspire, the skin is also a route for the excretion of waste products. Any detoxification program must include regular bathing and, during times of leisure, can be enhanced by activities that accelerate sweating, such as saunas and exercise.

Many people are aware that spending some time in a hot tub or sauna hydrates and relaxes the body, but few think of the health benefits in terms of detoxification. Relaxing in this way also benefits the internal organs of elimination, the liver and kidneys, by lessening the amount of toxins they must process. When taking sweats and saunas, be sure to drink ample water, and supplement your diet with potassium, calcium, and magnesium to replace the minerals lost in perspiration. Combinations of these nutrients are available in natural-food stores. Also, avoid becoming overheated. Some people take niacin, which causes flushing and additional perspiring. To avoid an exaggerated niacin flush, which can be stressful, begin by supplementing with only 10 to 50 mg daily, gradually increasing to a maximum dose of 100 mg per day.

A Home-Spa Cleansing Treatment

When you have some leisure time to yourself, plan a few days of juice fasting (see page 305) and thirty minutes to an hour of regular aerobic exercise, plus a niacin flush and a sauna or hot tub each day. Such days of renewal are best spent quietly in contemplation or meditation. Most people find that they feel greatly refreshed after spending even a few days doing such a program.

Dry-brush massages

You can easily incorporate dry-brush massage into a program of cleansing, adding it to your normal daily routine of washing. Dry brushing removes dead surface skin and increases superficial circulation throughout the body. Many alternative healers use dry-brush massage to facilitate detoxification, on the theory that it stimulates the lymphatic system. The lymphatic system is the network of ducts or channels that transport lymph, the clear fluid that accumulates in the spaces between cells and in the capillaries. Like the circulatory system, the lymphatic system helps to move fluid through the body and carries toxins to the liver for breakdown and excretion.

To give yourself a dry-brush massage, use a moderately soft, natural vegetable-fiber bristle brush, and rub the skin vigorously to stimulate it and remove dead cells. Then brush your body, front, back, and limbs, using light but brisk short strokes. Start at the extremities and stroke in the direction of your navel, moving from the wrists to the armpits, the chin to the navel, and the feet up to the groin. Brush gently at first, as some parts of the body may be especially sensitive. The massage should take no more than ten minutes daily. As your body becomes accustomed to the massage, this routine can be done daily for three months, and then twice a week as part of a preventive-maintenance program. Putting sea salt on the brush will cause the pores of the skin to open further for an even more cleansing effect.

Sea salt and soda baths

Taking a bath in water that contains dissolved salts will draw toxins out of the body. Sea salt and soda baths are pleasant, gentle ways to detoxify the body and can be enjoyed several times a week. Fill a tub with warm water and add one cup of baking soda (sodium bicarbonate) plus one cup of sea salt or one pound of Epsom salts. To fully mobilize the toxins out of the skin, stay in the bath for twenty to thirty minutes.

Regular Exercise

Aerobic exercise such as walking helps the body to detoxify since circulation is enhanced and toxins are more efficiently excreted through the urinary tract, bowels, and skin. Exercise also increases metabolic rate and tones the liver so that it can metabolize fats better, as well as burning calories. If you are consuming potentially toxic substances such as alcohol and sugar, regular aerobic exercise is essential and should be done, most beneficially, nearly every day or at least every other day for thirty minutes to one hour. During an aerobic workout, the heartbeat should remain elevated for at least thirty minutes. After exercising, be sure to shower to wash away the toxins excreted in perspiration, which may be reabsorbed if they remain on the skin.

OXYGEN THERAPIES

Oxygen therapies can increase oxygenation and circulation through the liver, thereby enhancing the detoxification process. They can be tremendously useful in restoring liver function and are used in treating liver diseases such as hepatitis. Oxygen therapies are discussed in detail in chapters 7 and 8.

SUMMARY OF TREATMENT OPTIONS FOR RESTORING YOUR ABILITY TO DETOXIFY

Diet
    The detoxification diet
    Modified fasting

Nutrients to restore liver function
    Lecithin
    Amino acids
        Methionine
        Glutathione
        Cysteine
        N-acetyl cysteine (NAC)
    Essential fatty acids
    Herbs
        Milk thistle plant (silymarin)
        Dandelion
        Artichoke

Nutrients to restore liver function, (cont.)
> Curcumin (turmeric)
>> Licorice root
> Green foods
>> Wheat grass and barley grass
>> Microalgae

Liver-cleansing techniques
> Coffee enema
> Fiber intake
> Maintaining intestinal flora
> Dry-brush massage
> Sea salt and soda baths
> Regular aerobic exercise
> Oxygen therapies

7

How Oxygen Benefits Peak Performance and Health

Success and peak performance are virtually impossible without superior oxygenation. This should be no surprise, since the body contains more oxygen than any other element. Because oxygen is fundamental to our very existence, having sufficient levels within the body is a prerequisite for every aspect of peak performance. Sufficient oxygen is necessary for the energy and vitality, drive and determination, mental clarity, good social skills, and ability to recover from illness, injury, and exertion that are mandatory for a high level of success in every area of life. For a detailed list of the benefits of oxygen on peak performance and optimal health, see the chart on page 336.

Oxygen is an essential nutrient and a major component of our structure; it is fundamental to our very existence. Along with food, oxygen is the primary nutrient that cells use to generate energy for all their functions. Even a slight deficiency of oxygen in the cells can have a profound effect on our physical and mental performance as well as set the stage for the development of many diseases. For laboratory tests of oxygen levels, see the appendix.

Checklist: Do You Have the Oxygen Levels Needed for Peak Performance and Health?

To begin to learn whether your ability to oxygenate your body is at a level consistent with peak performance and optimal health, work through the following checklist (photocopy it if you don't want to write in the book), and refer to it as you read through the chapter. Doing so will help you to assess how well your body is oxygenated. Putting a check mark beside any of the items listed could mean that your body is not receiving sufficient oxygen. If you find that a number of the statements in the checklist apply

Benefits of Healthy Oxygenation

Peak-Performance Benefits

 Increased physical vitality and stamina (helps improve work productivity)

 Enhanced mental clarity and acuity

 Strengthened determination and perseverance in pursuing goals

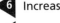 Increased ability to get along with other people (permits enjoyment of extensive social and business entertaining)

 Increased ability to remain calm under pressure

6 Increased optimism and vision

7 Hastened recovery from illness, injury, and exertion (includes inflammation from colds, flus, sinusitis, bronchitis, and allergies; athletic and repetitive-stress injuries; minor surgery; and dental procedures)

8 Increased resistance to illness

Health Benefits

- Promotes healing and prevention of infectious diseases due to bacteria, viruses, and parasites
- Lowers the risk of cardiovascular disease
- Is used as a complementary therapy for the treatment of cancer
- Helps in the treatment of gastrointestinal disorders
- Promotes healing of joint and bone diseases
- Helps in the treatment of neurological diseases such as multiple sclerosis
- Relieves cluster headaches
- Reverses age-related degeneration of vision
- Improves symptoms of skin conditions
- Promotes health of the teeth and gums

to you, you should implement a program to restore your oxygen levels. Your responses to this checklist can also help you decide whether you need to exercise more, change your diet, or make a more conscious effort to breathe deeply. You may also realize that your environment needs upgrading to provide you with better-quality air to breathe or water to drink. As always, consult a health care professional if you think that you may have a serious health condition.

Lifestyle/environmental factors

Put a check mark beside those statements that are true for you.

- ❏ I rarely eat fresh fruits and vegetables.
- ❏ I eat mostly overcooked foods and foods that are processed.
- ❏ I smoke cigarettes.
- ❏ I walk or exercise along streets filled with traffic.
- ❏ I lead a sedentary lifestyle.
- ❏ I tend to stand and move with a stiff, military posture.
- ❏ I habitually feel stressed and uptight.
- ❏ I regularly spend long hours engaged in desk work.
- ❏ I spend much of every day working at a computer.
- ❏ I live in a major metropolitan area.
- ❏ My home is in a city with a smog problem.
- ❏ I recently moved into a new house or apartment.
- ❏ My floors are covered with carpets made of synthetic fibers.
- ❏ I regularly burn wood in the fireplace.
- ❏ I cook on an unvented stove.
- ❏ I work in a building that has sealed windows.
- ❏ My profession involves exposure to chemical toxins (for example, I am a painter, firefighter, hairstylist, or health care worker or I work in a dry-cleaning establishment).
- ❏ I work in a factory where there is dust from cotton, synthetic fibers, sugarcane, aluminum, or talc.
- ❏ I work in an oil refinery or in a plant that produces or utilizes toxic chemicals.

Performance indicators

- ❏ I have little energy for recreational activities or spending time with family and friends.
- ❏ I often have difficulty concentrating.
- ❏ I rarely participate in meetings and have difficulty coming up with new ideas.
- ❏ I am often unable to remember names.
- ❏ I am frequently unable to see a project through to completion.
- ❏ I lack goals and inspiration.
- ❏ I am slow to recover from injury, illness, and physical exertion.
- ❏ I have limited stamina and endurance while exercising.
- ❏ I am easily fatigued and usually tired at the end of the day.
- ❏ I find myself out of breath after running for the phone.
- ❏ I am out of breath after climbing a flight of stairs.
- ❏ I lack close social and personal relationships.
- ❏ I am introverted and don't enjoy social gatherings.
- ❏ I am generally pessimistic.

Medical history

- ❏ I have frequent episodes of colds, flus, bronchitis, pneumonia, allergies, or sinusitis.
- ❏ I tend to be anemic.
- ❏ I have a history of emphysema, chronic bronchitis, lung infections, or asthma.
- ❏ I suffer from cardiovascular or vascular disease.
- ❏ I suffer from chronic-fatigue syndrome.

C Now that you have a preliminary understanding of the importance of oxygenation to peak performance and optimal health, as well as some idea from the checklist of your own functioning in this area, you are ready to decide what to read next. To learn more about the chemistry of oxygenation, read the following section. To learn how aging, lifestyle, and general health affect oxygenation, read section 2, on page 343. For a detailed discussion of how oxygenation affects peak performance, including how the various oxygen therapies work, read section 3, on page 352. For a detailed discussion of how oxygenation affects general health, including specific conditions that oxygen therapies are used to treat, read section 4, on page 376. (Ideally, these latter two sections should be read consecutively, as the effects of oxygenation on peak performance and health are intricately intertwined.) Finally, for information on how to restore your oxygen levels, read chapter 8.

SECTION 1:
THE CHEMISTRY OF OXYGENATION

OXYGEN IS A clear, odorless gas that easily dissolves in water. Because it combines readily with other elements, it is the most abundant element on Earth, constituting about 50 percent of the weight of the Earth's crust, seawater, and atmosphere. Oxygen makes up approximately 20 percent of the composition of air by volume. The body itself consists of four primary elements—oxygen, carbon, hydrogen, and nitrogen—which make up approximately 95 percent of the total mass of the body. Over two-thirds of this amount is oxygen. Each molecule of oxygen consists of two oxygen atoms and is described chemically as O_2.

Oxygen is the most important element needed to sustain life. Humans can survive without food for many weeks and can go without water for several days but can only survive without oxygen for a matter of minutes. We inhale between twelve to twenty times a minute while at rest, and much more frequently when we are engaged in strenuous physical activity. On average, we breathe in 2500 gallons of air every day. Although oxygen is needed by all the cells and tissues of the body, much of the oxygen in the air we breathe is used by the heart, the liver, and especially the brain, which requires a disproportionate amount of oxygen. Even though the brain represents only about 2 percent of the weight of an average adult, it uses over 20 percent of the body's oxygen supply.

HOW OXYGEN IS TAKEN INTO THE BODY

Oxygen is primarily taken into the body by the lungs during respiration. The lungs are two cone-shaped spongy organs. The wider part of the cone rests on the diaphragm just above the stomach. The left lung has an indentation to accommodate the heart, which sits slightly to the left between the two lungs. When we breathe, the lungs expand and contract like a bellows. This continuously repeating movement also depends on the flexibility and movement of the various structures around the lungs. When we inhale, the diaphragm moves downward and the ribs elevate, increasing lung volume and capacity. When we exhale, the diaphragm automatically relaxes, the ribs lower, and the abdominal muscles contract. The lungs are then compressed, sending air out of the body.

When air is taken in through the mouth and nose, it moves toward the lungs. From the windpipe, air passes into two large bronchial tubes, which branch out into the bronchi and then into tiny bronchioles. Air finally enters the alveoli; these microscopic air sacs are the smallest compartments of the lung. There are 300 million alveoli in each lung. Because of this branching into smaller and smaller components, the lungs contain the equivalent of about 600 square feet of surface area. This enormous surface area allows for the efficient exchange of one of the body's primary waste products, carbon dioxide, for life-sustaining fresh oxygen.

Because of the structure of the alveoli, oxygen is able to diffuse into the blood. Although the walls of the alveoli are very thin, they contain a dense network of interconnecting capillaries, the smallest pathways through which blood circulates. Within the alveoli, oxygen from the air is now in close proximity to the capillaries and can enter the circulatory system. At this point, it is now considered to be inside the body, but the oxygen still has a long way to go before it reaches its final destination.

The circulatory system is made up of miles of capillaries and blood vessels that bring blood and oxygen to the tissues and cells throughout the body. Oxygen first travels to the heart and then through these blood vessels. In turn, the veins collect waste products that accumulate in the cells, primarily carbon dioxide, which is generated in the production of energy. The veins bring the carbon dioxide back to the lungs. The carbon dioxide diffuses into the alveoli and then passes through ever-widening air passageways until it is exhaled. Well-oxygenated blood in the arteries tends to be bright red, while the venous blood carrying all the waste products, especially carbon dioxide, tends to be darker. About 97 percent of the oxygen in the blood is carried in combination with hemoglobin, an iron-containing protein within the red blood cell. This allows oxygen to be delivered efficiently to all the cells of the body.

HOW OXYGEN IS USED WITHIN THE BODY

Oxygen is the primary fuel that supports all of the biochemical processes that occur in our tissues and cells. It supplies the energy for the maintenance, growth, and repair of all our cells and tissues, and is crucial for maintaining our level of health and well-being. The oxygen we breathe reacts with glucose (sugar), which is derived from the foods that we eat and from the breakdown of starches and fats in the body. This reaction produces carbon dioxide, water, and energy. The energy that is created from this reaction, which is a form of combustion, is stored in the body as adenosine triphosphate (ATP), which is often referred to as the basic energy currency of the body.

Because of its role in energy production, oxygen is essential for all of the tasks the cells must perform to maintain the health and integrity of the body, such as the transport of molecules, the synthesis of chemical compounds, and mechanical work like muscle contraction. Hundreds of thousands of these reactions are going on at all times. Because of these reactions, the heart is able to pump blood, the immune system to fight infections, the gastrointestinal tract to digest foods, and the nervous system and brain to process information. Oxygen-generated energy is also fundamental to our ability to perform all physical movements. Oxygen is also an important structural component of the organic compounds used by the body as essential nutrients, such as vitamins, carbohydrates, and fatty acids. In addition, oxygen also has an important role in removing waste products from the body. When food is broken down and converted into energy, carbon residues can accumulate and must be removed from the body. This carbon combines with oxygen to form carbon dioxide, a waste product of metabolism that is excreted from the body through the lungs.

Oxygen is also alkaline and thereby helps the cells to maintain the slightly alkaline pH necessary for peak performance and optimal health. When a cell is highly oxygenated, it is able to create energy (ATP) through oxidative combustion, maintain its alkalinity, and sustain an environment that is incompatible with most disease-causing microorganisms. However, when the amount of oxygen in the body is reduced below optimal levels, this creates an environment in the cells that is conducive to the growth of infectious microorganisms. Most pathogens are anaerobic— that is, they thrive in an environment that is low in oxygen and has an acidic pH. In fact, infectious microorganisms such as bacteria, viruses, fungi, and parasites as well as cancer cells produce their energy (ATP) through the fermentation of glucose instead of through oxygen. These pathogens are unable to survive in a cellular environment that is oxygen rich and slightly alkaline, which is why it is so critically important for peak performance and optimal health that we remain highly oxygenated and maintain our pH in a slightly alkaline state.

When a person becomes unable to fully oxygenate, an environment is created in which our energy begins to decline. We become fatigued, and disease and illness begin to occur with greater frequency. Over time, chronic conditions like heart disease and even cancer can develop. Finally, continued low levels of oxygenation increase the degenerative processes associated with aging and infirmity.

SUMMARY

Oxygen, the most abundant element on Earth, is also the most important element needed to sustain life. Breathed in by the lungs, it is carried through the body, largely by hemoglobin, and is used by our tissues and cells to help create the energy needed for normal metabolic function. When the body is not properly oxygenated, energy begins to decline, which can lead to fatigue, chronic illnesses, and degenerative processes. The following section explains how aging, the way we live, and our health all affect our ability to oxygenate our bodies.

Section 2:
How Aging, Lifestyle,
and Health Affect Oxygenation

A WIDE VARIETY of environmental and lifestyle factors, as well as certain diseases and the aging process itself, can cause oxygen levels in the body to decline. Outside of serious lung disease, atherosclerosis , or anemia, no single factor alone can significantly reduce oxygen intake, but often a combination of factors can have a significant impact on a person's ability to maintain optimal oxygenation. For example, if a person does not exercise, is a moderate to heavy smoker, and develops a respiratory infection, then the ability to oxygenate can be seriously diminished, and the effects on performance and health can be significant. Very serious health conditions often develop from circumstances like these.

Aging

The cells of the body become damaged with age and cannot carry out their normal metabolic function, including the cell's ability to use oxygen. Damage to the cellular machinery occurs spontaneously during normal metabolism and also by contact with the large number of environmental pollutants and toxins to which people are exposed on a daily basis. These include heavy metals, pesticides, air pollution, outgassed toxins from indoor carpets and furniture, and a variety of other toxic agents with which people come in contact.

As people age, their lungs and cardiovascular systems become much less efficient in extracting oxygen from the air and delivering it to the cells. It also becomes more difficult for the cells to create energy through the metabolism of food and oxygen. There are many reasons for this decline in function. Chronic muscle tension can become more of a problem as people age. This tension causes the muscles to lose their suppleness and flexibility, which restricts the action of the diaphragm and lungs. The aging process also brings about a loss of elasticity to all tissues, including the lungs. Much of the deterioration in breathing rate, lung capacity, and the ability to exchange gases is due to this loss. The rib cage, which expands and contracts with each breath, also becomes less elastic and pliable, and eventually the muscles in the lungs will weaken.

The very structure of the lungs changes over time, as airways narrow, the alveoli become flattened, and the alveolar ducts enlarge. All these factors contribute to a decrease in the ability of the body to take in oxygen. In addition, with age, cells throughout the body can become damaged simply from normal functioning and become less able to use the oxygen they receive.

LIFESTYLE

The air we breathe, the amount of stress we experience, and the food we eat all affect our oxygen levels. Our patterns of living, from our environment to our daily habits, are important indicators of the amount of oxygen we take in. Even the quality of the air we breathe can affect our oxygen levels.

Air pollution

It is estimated that over half the population of the United States regularly breathes unsafe, polluted air. Poor air quality is now commonplace in many of our leading cities, and many types of work expose people to air that is dangerous to breathe.

For example, smog is a photochemical haze caused by the action of ultraviolet radiation on atmospheric pollution. It contains various toxins, including hydrocarbons and oxides of nitrogen from automobile exhaust. Nitrogen oxide is a primary industrial pollutant that reacts with sunlight and forms nitrogen dioxide, a brownish toxic gas. A person may also be exposed to toxic airborne substances in the workplace, which can also limit the ability of the lungs to provide the body with sufficient oxygen. Factory workers may be exposed to dust generated in the manufacture of certain products. Breathing dust composed of cotton, synthetic fibers, sugarcane, aluminum, or talc may be unavoidable. Workers in oil refineries may breathe sulfur dioxide, and people handling commercial refrigeration may be exposed to ammonia fumes. Servicing swimming pools exposes a person to chlorine-containing products, while health care professionals, roofers, woodworkers, welders, custodians, and firefighters often touch and handle toxic substances on a daily basis. Printers, lab workers, and painters breath vapors from solvents and other toxic chemicals.

Our homes often contribute to the number and amount of airborne pollutants that we breathe in. Certain synthetic materials used in home furnishings such as carpets and upholstery can outgas—that is, they can emit volatile organic compounds such as toluene and xylene, known carcinogens such as formaldehyde and benzene, and pesticides that are toxic to our bodies. We also breathe fumes given off by cleaning agents, waxes, and polishes. Offices, schools, stores, churches, and car interiors—any place that is furnished with products that outgas—can be a source of toxic substances. Another home pollutant is nitrogen oxide, which can originate from space heaters, unvented cooking stoves, and wood smoke.

When we inhale these toxic fumes and airborne pollutants, we breathe in less oxygen. In addition, these toxic substances can damage lung tissue and impair lung function, further limiting oxygen uptake. Normally, pollutants are blocked from entering the body as they pass through the upper airways of the respiratory system, the nose, sinuses, and throat. The upper airway cleans the air, clears it of particles, and inactivates microbes. However, after heavy and/or prolonged exposure to air pollution, the system can become overwhelmed by toxins. At first, this may cause annoying symptoms such as sneezing, coughing, congestion, and inflammation similar to an allergic reaction. But if exposure persists, pollution can lead to lung damage. The lungs may become less flexible, and their ability to exchange carbon dioxide for oxygen may become impaired, causing the lungs and heart to work harder. Bronchitis and other chronic lung conditions may also develop.

Studies done in the past few years have examined the effects of pollution on the health of people living in cities with heavy levels of air pollution. For example, several studies have examined air quality and its impact on the health of people in Mexico City, where air pollution can far surpass acceptable levels. Residents of Mexico City showed significantly more signs of lung damage than people living in unpolluted cities in Mexico. In addition, even visitors suffered from respiratory irritation when exposed to high levels of smog-ridden air. These changes persisted even after the visitors had returned home, abating only several weeks later.

Many people living in cities make a special effort to exercise outdoors to bolster their health and well-being. However, if exercise is performed on smoggy days or near highways, this well-intentioned physical activity may often do more harm than good. When a person does vigorous exercise, they breathe through the mouth, and air does not pass through the nose to be cleaned. A person jogging in smog will inhale dirty air deep into their lungs, where it can affect the health of the lungs and oxygen intake.

Smoking

One particularly lethal form of air pollution is cigarette smoke, whether a person smokes and inhales the toxins directly or inhales it secondhand from someone else's cigarette. Smoking limits the amount of oxygen that reaches our cells and tissues in several ways. Cigarette smoke irritates lung tissue, particularly the cilia. Cilia are threadlike projections that line the respiratory passages and normally sweep back and forth, moving debris out of the lungs. Cigarette smoke paralyzes the cilia, especially the smoke from menthol cigarettes. In response, the lungs produce mucus, which covers the cilia and further prevents them from doing their job of cleaning. As debris accumulates, the alveoli become damaged, impairing the uptake of oxygen into the circulation. Cigarette smoke also decreases the amount of hemoglobin in the blood. As a result, the blood cannot carry as much oxygen to the cells. Smoking can also lead to health problems that are associated with low levels of oxygen such as respiratory infections, pneumonia, chronic bronchitis, and lung cancer. These diseases, in turn, often damage the lungs, which further impairs oxygen uptake.

Carbon monoxide

Carbon monoxide is formed by the combustion of carbon in oxygen when there is an excess of carbon. It is generated in coal stoves, furnaces, and gas appliances that do not get enough air. It is also present in the exhaust of automobiles. Early symptoms of carbon monoxide poisoning include headaches and drowsiness, followed by unconsciousness, respiratory failure, and death. Carbon monoxide can be a particularly lethal component of air in that it has no odor, so a person isn't aware of inhaling it. According to an article published in 1998 in the *Journal of the American Medical Association*, there are approximately 2100 deaths from carbon monoxide poisoning in the United States each year. Hemoglobin (the oxygen-carrying protein in red blood cells) has a much greater affinity for carbon monoxide than oxygen. As carbon monoxide in the air we breathe is only a very recent phenomenon, the body is not designed to block it from entering the system. In the alveoli of the lungs, where gases from the outside are exchanged with gases from within the body, hemoglobin, which usually carries molecules of oxygen through the body, is over two hundred times as likely to grab onto a molecule of carbon monoxide instead. Therefore, any exposure to carbon monoxide limits the amount of oxygen uptake as well as the quantity reaching the cells.

Stress

Being caught in a seemingly unending traffic jam or spending the day hunched over a computer trying to finish a late report causes physical and emotional stress that can affect breathing by causing our muscles to tighten. Stress also causes breathing to become rapid and shallow. A person may even stop breathing altogether and hold their breath for brief periods without realizing it. All of these changes in breathing patterns cause less oxygen to be taken in through respiration, which decreases the oxygen available to the muscles and internal organs. Under stress, a person will also tense muscles in certain parts of the body, commonly the shoulders and neck, involuntarily preparing for a fight as the automatic stress response sets in. Blood vessels also constrict, reducing circulation to the tense muscles and preventing oxygen from reaching these areas and carbon dioxide from being eliminated. If a person leads a life in which nearly every day is stressful, such muscle tension can become chronic. Over time, this constant tension reduces the amount of oxygen that reaches the cells, and performance and health begin to suffer as a result.

Techniques for retaining physical flexibility, such as stretching and yoga, can serve several purposes. By promoting muscular flexibility, these techniques significantly enhance the the mechanics of breathing, thereby assisting the flow of oxygen to the cells and the removal of carbon dioxide. These slow, methodical exercises also reduce muscle tension. As you relax, the other effects of stress are gradually reduced. Also, stretching exercises and yoga can be practiced almost anywhere, which is a great benefit to travelers.

Lack of aerobic exercise

A sedentary lifestyle can weaken the lungs, heart, and blood vessels, reducing the amount of oxygen taken into the body and transported to the tissues. Lack of exercise reduces the efficiency of lung function. The lungs are not able to fully expand and fill with air. The heart will not pump as forcefully to circulate blood and oxygen throughout the body. One benefit of physical activity is to dilate (expand) the network of blood vessels so blood reaches the muscles and vital organs as well as the small capillaries. When a person does not exercise, this expansion of the circulatory system is diminished.

Diet

Foods that are highest in water content, such as raw vegetables and fruit, are also highest in their oxygen content. A diet that contains plenty of fresh, raw vegetables and fruit can significantly contribute to our supply of oxygen. Unfortunately, processed and refined foods usually have a much lower water content than the original fresh ingredients. This can even be true of frozen foods, such as strawberries: Once defrosted, they lose most of their water content. Also, the foods that make up the standard American diet are highly processed and refined. These foods tend to be highly acidic, further reducing the stores of oxygen within the body.

HEALTH CONDITIONS

A number of diseases limit how much oxygen is taken into the body. These include a wide variety of conditions, including some lung diseases such as asthma, bronchitis, and pneumonia. Whatever the cause of the damage to the lung, the end result is the same: The lungs are less able to breathe in oxygen and transfer it to the blood for circulation throughout the body. Atherosclerosis, anemia, and chronic-fatigue syndrome also affect the amount of oxygen in the body.

Sinusitis

The term *sinusitis* refers to an infection lodged in any of the four sacs of air cells that surround both sides of the nose. Sinuses have openings into the nose that are quite small and easily blocked by thick secretions and swelling. When blockage occurs, the warm, moist environment within the sinuses is a ready breeding ground for bacteria. As a result, breathing becomes more difficult.

Chronic bronchitis

Shallow breathing can also occur with chronic bronchitis. This ailment involves persistent inflammation of the air passageways within the lungs. It is often characterized by the excessive secretion of mucus and a chronic cough. Smokers are at higher risk of developing this condition.

Emphysema

In this disease, the alveoli are destroyed, impairing the exchange of oxygen and carbon dioxide, and oxygen does not as readily diffuse into the blood. The lungs enlarge, but they work less efficiently, often painfully and with great effort.

Asthma

Asthma is usually due to an allergic reaction to a substance such as pollen. It can also be triggered, in some individuals, by strong emotions. When a person has an asthmatic attack, tissues in the passageways of the lungs swell and become narrower. The muscles involved in breathing may contract. Exhaling can become very difficult, and the proper exchange of oxygen and carbon dioxide is prevented.

Pneumonia

Pneumonia is an infectious disease in which the alveoli become infected with bacteria. The membranes within the alveoli become inflamed and porous. The alveoli become filled with fluids and blood cells. Symptoms of pneumonia can include coughing, sputum production, and a high fever.

Tuberculosis

In recent years, there has been an increase in the incidence of tuberculosis, a potentially dangerous bacterial disease, especially in inner cities. In tuberculosis, fibrous tissue usually forms to wall off the infected area. This is the body's way of limiting the spread of the disease. However, in about 3 percent of cases, this process fails, and the disease spreads throughout the lungs. This reduces the total amount of functional lung tissue, limiting the amount of oxygen the lungs can hold and the amount of oxygen that diffuses into the blood.

Atherosclerosis

The circulatory system consists of miles of arteries and capillaries that bring oxygen to the tissues. Anything that causes a narrowing or occlusion of these blood vessels can affect oxygenation. Plaque, an accumulation of cholesterol and fibrous tissue on the arterial walls, is one of the most common causes of such narrowing. The buildup of plaque is often referred to as "hardening of the arteries," or atherosclerosis. The plaque may accumulate sufficiently in certain places to decrease blood flow and obstruct circulation. In these areas, oxygenation and the flow of nutrients to the tissue can be drastically reduced. Hypertension (high blood pressure) can also limit oxygenation since it causes the blood vessels to contract. This forces the heart to work harder to move the same amount of blood to the tissues.

Anemia

It is estimated that as many as 20 percent of all American women suffer from anemia, which is a deficiency of red blood cells or a reduction in hemoglobin (the oxygen-carrying protein in red blood cells). Anemia may be due to blood loss, diminished blood production, a failure of the red blood cells to mature because of a lack of vitamin B_{12} or folic acid, or hemolysis, in which the red blood cells break apart.

Anemia reduces the amount of oxygen available to all cells of the body. As a result, less oxygen is available for energy production by the cells. Important processes such as muscular activity and cell building and repair slow down and become less efficient. As a result, anemia can be debilitating and result in profound physical fatigue.

Because of this reduction in blood cells, individuals who are anemic tend to be pale with poor skin color and tone. They often appear washed-out and seem listless. Individuals with anemia usually feel extremely fatigued. Because muscular activity is inhibited, those suffering from anemia lack endurance and physical stamina. Susan has had many physically active patients who had to stop pursuing vigorous aerobic exercise programs when they developed anemia. These people simply lacked the physical energy to continue their active exercise regimens once the anemia became too severe. Many people who are chronically tired are suffering from a low-grade anemia that needs to be treated.

Chronic-fatigue syndrome

Chronic-fatigue syndrome (CFS), a condition in which fatigue is debilitating if not incapacitating, has been diagnosed in 3 million Americans. The onset of fatigue is often sudden; many individuals can pinpoint exactly when it started. The fatigue is so severe that even minor exertion, such as a short walk or light housework, can be difficult to accomplish. Many people with CFS curtail their activities and take naps during the day, or sleep more hours at night. However, increased bed rest does not improve the energy level of those with this problem.

The most widely accepted hypothesis is that CFS is due to a viral infection, although this has not been definitely proven. Most of the attention has focused on the herpes family of viruses, such as Epstein-Barr virus. In addition, though, people who have CFS tend to be poorly oxygenated. Patients may indeed be infected by a virus, but viruses thrive in oxygen-depleted environments. A wide variety of environmental and lifestyle factors may also contribute to CFS by stressing the immune system. Many of Susan's CFS patients report extreme and prolonged emotional stress, anxiety, and depression, and a history of poor nutritional habits predating the onset of CFS. Environmental pollutants and contaminants may also play a role in weakening the body and allowing CFS to develop. All these related conditions further reduce oxygen within the body.

SUMMARY

Often a combination of factors negatively affects a person's ability to take in oxygen. These include air pollution, exposure to cigarette smoke, stress, lack of exercise, and aging. Several diseases also affect oxygen levels, including lung diseases such as emphysema and tuberculosis and such common conditions as atherosclerosis and anemia.

SECTION 3:
OXYGENATION AND PEAK PERFORMANCE

THE LEVEL OF oxygen in the body affects every-peak performance trait discussed in this book. When individuals are well oxygenated, they are more likely to be energetic, mentally sharp, optimistic, and able to focus on accomplishing goals and aspirations. Abundant levels of oxygen within the body also tend to make us more outgoing and sociable, and enhance our ability to perform at peak levels by increasing our resistance to disease and allowing for rapid recovery from colds, flus, and allergies as well as injury, physical exertion, and even surgical procedures. The therapies discussed below help to increase oxygen levels within the body, thereby supporting peak performance.

OXYGEN THERAPIES

There are many ways of increasing the amount of oxygen in the body besides taking it in through the air we breathe. Many of these therapies are used as disinfectants or for the treatment of a variety of medical conditions. They can also be used to enhance many peak-performance traits. These therapies include the use of pure oxygen as well as ozone therapy, hydrogen peroxide therapy, and hyperbaric-oxygen therapy.

Oxygen therapies can act on the body in two ways. One is by supplementing the oxygen in the body, thereby increasing the amount of oxygen in the blood and tissues. This process is referred to as oxygenation. Another is through the chemical reaction known as oxidation. In the process of oxidation, an electron (a subatomic particle with a negative electrical charge) transfers from one molecule to another. (The molecule that loses the electron is said to be oxidized.) The electron that splits off is free to interact with other substances. For example, when it reacts with pathogens such as bacteria and viruses, it will inactivate or destroy them. Some of the oxygen therapies that we discuss oxygenate the body, whereas others primarily work through oxidation. Some therapies, such as ozone, do both.

Pure oxygen

Pure oxygen is an oxygen therapy that makes use of elemental oxygen, which is the same as the oxygen in the air we breathe. The only difference is that while air contains about 20 percent oxygen, along with nitrogen and other gases, pure-oxygen therapy supplies 100 percent pure oxygen.

The chemical symbol for oxygen is O_2. In this form, it is a stable gas. Pure oxygen is usually stored in a tank, and a patient will inhale the gas through a tube inserted in the nose or by using a mask. A doctor will prescribe pure-oxygen therapy for use in the hospital or for home care. It is used to treat patients with chronic lung disease such as emphysema and chronic bronchitis. In these conditions, the lungs have lost their elasticity and lung tissue is damaged, making breathing very difficult. The patient is no longer able to inhale enough oxygen or exhale enough carbon dioxide, which then accumulates as a waste product in the body. When a person with chronic lung disease breathes pure oxygen, the oxygen stores of the body are increased.

Ozone

Ozone, also known as activated oxygen, is a naturally occurring, pale-blue gas. (It turns deep blue when it is condensed to a liquid at very low temperatures.) While an oxygen molecule is made up of two atoms of oxygen, ozone (O_3) is composed of three. Ozone is very unstable. Within twenty to forty-five minutes, half of it will revert back to stable oxygen and a singlet oxygen. This singlet oxygen is itself unstable and will search for another electron, which converts it back into stable O_2. Ozone surrounds the earth and is formed in the atmosphere when oxygen and ultraviolet radiation from the sun interact. It can also form during electrical storms when lightning acts on oxygen. The stimulating, fresh scent in the air that we sometimes notice after a thunderstorm is due to ozone. Turbulent air also causes a small amount of the ozone in the upper atmosphere to descend to lower altitudes.

Ozone is often labeled "smog" in the popular media, but this is an incorrect notion. Ozone is simply pure, activated oxygen. However, when it combines in the lower atmosphere with toxic chemicals produced by industry or vehicular exhaust such as hydrocarbons or oxides of nitrogen, a petrochemical haze is formed consisting of new and highly toxic pollutants. While ozone itself has many health benefits, both as a disinfectant and as a medical treatment, smog is toxic to the human body.

Whether used as a disinfectant to purify air or water, or to treat medical conditions, ozone is formed in the same way. Pure oxygen (O_2) passed over an electrical arc or an ultraviolet light will be converted into ozone (O_3). In these reactions, only a small percentage of the oxygen (ranging from less than 1 percent to 6 percent) is converted to ozone. As mentioned above, while oxygen is very stable, ozone is very unstable. It rapidly begins to break down into a stable oxygen molecule and an intermediate unstable product called a singlet oxygen. When ozone/oxygen mixtures are administered to the body for the treatment of various health conditions, the stable oxygen effectively supplements the oxygen levels in the tissues and cells. However, the singlet oxygen has an oxidative effect, as it searches for an electron to allow it to regain stability. Many of the therapeutic benefits of ozone are due to the singlet oxygen attaching to bacteria, viruses, fungi, parasites, and tumors for its needed electron and, in the process, destroying them. It also combines with the membranes of the red blood cells, making those cells more flexible and fluid, which promotes better blood flow and enhances circulation throughout the body. Ozone also has a powerful alkalinizing effect, since it has a pH of between 7 and 9. In addition, it dissolves remarkably well in water, being absorbed twelve times faster than oxygen itself.

When used properly, for either household or medical purposes, ozone is remarkably safe and effective. In fact, its safety record is much better than that of medication or virtually any other type of medical therapy. A German study done in the 1980s evaluated the incidence of side effects in over 5.5 million ozone treatments given by health care providers. The study found an astonishingly low level of only forty incidences of side effects, or less than 1 in 100,000 adverse effects noted. After reviewing hundreds of research studies on ozone therapies for many different types of medical conditions, we have also been impressed by its remarkable record of safety over many decades of clinical use throughout the world.

Hydrogen peroxide

Hydrogen peroxide is a liquid made up of molecules composed of two atoms of hydrogen and two atoms of oxygen (H_2O_2). This compound is much less stable than water and ultimately breaks down into water and oxygen. When you are drenched in a rainstorm, a small amount of the rainwater that falls on you is actually hydrogen peroxide. Water interacts with ozone in the atmosphere, and hydrogen peroxide is produced. There are even small amounts of hydrogen peroxide in the foods we eat, such as asparagus, watercress, apples, watermelons, wild herbs, and liver. Hydrogen peroxide is also found in significant amounts in the waters of legendary healing springs such as those at Lourdes in France and Fátima in Portugal. Hydrogen peroxide is also produced by the cells of the body. When hydrogen peroxide is mixed with other compounds, it can potentially generate tremendous energy. It is a component of the fuel that sends rockets roaring into space, when combined with such substances as kerosene or hydrazine. The energy is generated because hydrogen peroxide oxidizes the other substance. In the oxidation process, hydrogen peroxide collects electrons, which are small units of negatively charged energy. Because of this ability to transfer energy, hydrogen peroxide affects every biochemical reaction, including every enzyme reaction that occurs within the body.

Although hydrogen peroxide was discovered in 1818, it was not until 1984 that Charles H. Farr, a distinguished American physician who was nominated for the Nobel Prize in Medicine in 1993, clarified its function within the body. Dr. Farr described hydrogen peroxide's role within the body as being primarily oxidative rather than oxygenating. Through Farr's research, it became clear that hydrogen peroxide had therapeutic value because of its ability to oxidize other substances. This has greatly expanded our understanding of hydrogen peroxide therapy. Hydrogen peroxide is used to treat a wide variety of diseases. It can destroy and inactivate bacteria, viruses, parasites, and other pathogens. It also enhances the immune response and is an effective adjunct therapy for cancer.

Hyperbaric-oxygen therapy

Divers who come to the surface too quickly can suffer from decompression sickness (commonly called the bends) and air embolism (a condition in which a blood vessel is blocked by air). In the 1930s, the military needed to find a solution for these problems and developed hyperbaric-oxygen therapy (HBOT). When people today receive hyperbaric-oxygen therapy, they are placed in a snugly fitting tube about seven feet long and twenty-five inches in diameter. The tube is sealed and the air pressure slowly increased until it reaches the equivalent of the pressure found fifty feet under water. Pure oxygen is then flowed into the chamber, and the person inhales this for thirty to sixty minutes. Because of this higher pressure, oxygen is forced into the body and travels to tissues where circulation is poor or the cells have become devitalized. Cells starved for oxygen begin to revive. Many health conditions can be treated and prevented using HBOT. An even newer method of delivery involves a hyperbaric chamber that accommodates several people at once, with oxygen delivered individually through a mask. The advantage of using this multiperson chamber is that patients can receive personal care and be removed quickly if they react adversely.

There are about 300 hyperbaric chambers in the United States today, most associated with hospitals and other health care facilities. Hyperbaric-oxygen therapy has been used in American hospitals to treat wounds and burns as well as smoke inhalation and carbon monoxide poisoning. However, physicians in Europe treat a far wider range of health problems with this therapy, and alternative physicians have also broadened its uses. Patients with problems related to poor circulation—such as stroke, tinnitus (a ringing in the ears), migraines, and traumatic injuries—have all benefited from breathing pressurized oxygen. Hyperbaric oxygen has even been used successfully to treat complications arising from AIDS.

PHYSICAL VITALITY AND STAMINA

Most people think that the food they eat provides the fuel needed by their body to produce physical energy. However, this is only partly true. While we do depend on the health of our digestive tract to absorb and assimilate the food we eat and the water we drink, converting this food into usable energy can only proceed efficiently when there is enough oxygen available. Food must undergo a series of chemical transformations within the cells before energy can be released. The oxygen that we breathe in through our lungs is an essential factor in this conversion. As a result, being able to breathe deeply and maximally fill the lungs with oxygen is a prerequisite for physical energy, stamina, and endurance.

The edge that healthy oxygenation confers is apparent in many careers, sports, and hobbies. For example, competitive swimmers, runners, opera singers, and musicians who play horn instruments are successful, in part, to the extent that they can take in and absorb oxygen through their lungs. Maximal oxygenation allows these people to swim harder, run faster and longer, project their voice more effectively, and play their instruments with more versatility than those with lesser respiratory capability.

In comparison, people who tend to be poor oxygenators are often deficient in their level of physical energy. These individuals tend to be either shallow breathers or to have suffered damage to their lung tissue that limits the amount of oxygen they can take in from the environment. Damage to the lungs often occurs from chronic exposure to chemical pollutants or tobacco smoke or from infections. In addition, people who are depressed or fearful tend to unconsciously restrict their movements, including breathing. Depressed and fearful individuals are often more immobile and less animated in their gestures. They are much more likely to be shallow breathers than people who are more exuberant, outgoing, and extroverted. People who spend many hours each day at a desk or in front of a computer also tend to be shallow breathers because of their relative immobility and their focus on mental rather than physical tasks. These individuals spend a great deal of their time reading reports or research material, evaluating data, and solving problems through logical or abstract thinking. When people are deeply engaged in complex mental work, they often lose awareness of their physical body. They may be totally unaware that they are breathing shallowly or sitting in a cramped position.

Unlike these individuals, who still have the capability to take a deep breath and reexpand their lungs, people with chronic lung diseases such as emphysema and chronic bronchitis are not physically capable of oxygenating efficiently. In these circumstances, the disease process itself causes damage to the lungs such as the destruction of the alveoli or the overproduction of mucus in the airways. Over time, this damage impairs both the act of respiration and the ability to absorb oxygen into the circulation.

The aging process also causes changes to the structure and capacity of the lungs. One measurement of the relative vitality of the lungs, called forced vital capacity (FVC), diminishes with age. This is a measurement of the amount of air that can be expelled with effort after taking a deep breath. Forced vital capacity is an important indicator of a person's level of energy and vitality. Researchers have found that the greater the decline in a person's FVC, the closer they are to dying. With age, the chest muscles and lung tissue also lose their elasticity, so the bellowslike movement of the lungs becomes restricted. This limits the amount of air one can take in through breathing. In addition, fibrous material accumulates in the lungs and thickens the walls of the air passages and the alveoli. With all of these changes, as oxygenation diminishes, the levels of physical energy, stamina, and endurance also decline. Fortunately, the level of oxygen within the body can be increased through aerobic exercise and a variety of oxygen therapies.

Aerobic exercise

The very act of engaging in physically demanding activities tends to make people better oxygenators. Frequent aerobic exercise, in particular, will help to increase the level of oxygen within the body. This exercise includes such popular activities as walking, jogging, dancing, bicycling, tennis, and swimming. Aerobic exercise requires that the activity be done in a moderate, relaxed fashion so that oxygen levels are restored rather that depleted, which occurs in activities that require hard physical exertion (anaerobic exercise).

Aerobic exercise conditions the heart and lungs to work more efficiently. A healthy heart is a well-functioning pump. It beats slowly and forcefully, circulating blood and oxygen throughout the body with each stroke. The lungs function more efficiently with exercise, too. They expand more fully and are able to take in more oxygen from the surrounding air. Exercise also helps to maintain the elasticity of the chest muscles and lung tissue; it will also help to promote better circulation through the lungs and better exchange of oxygen for carbon dioxide, our main waste product, at the junction between the lungs and the blood vessels.

Research studies have shown that aerobic exercise can actually slow down and possibly even reverse the aging of the lungs. For example, regular aerobic exercise helps to maintain our maximal oxygen uptake (VO_2max). This refers to the largest amount of oxygen that the body can take in during vigorous exercise. VO_2max declines with age at the rate of about 1 percent per year after age twenty-five. Thus, a sixty-year-old person will have approximately 33 percent less VO_2max than a twenty-year-old. However, researchers have found that individuals who engage in frequent aerobic activity do not show the expected decline in VO_2max for their age. Other studies have shown that when elderly individuals engage in aerobic-fitness programs, their VO_2max can actually be increased.

Ozone

Ozone is both an oxygenating and an oxidative therapy. This means that it both supplements the total level of oxygen in the body and creates a whole host of beneficial metabolic effects. Individuals who use ozone therapy on a regular basis (to purify the air in their home or office, drinking water, hot tub, or pool), either for the treatment of a medical condition or to enhance the quality of their life, frequently find that their level of physical energy improves greatly.

One reason for this might be that ozone therapy greatly improves circulation, bringing more oxygen to tissues and cells throughout the body. In fact, many research studies have found ozone to be beneficial in the treatment of a variety of circulatory conditions, including heart attacks, strokes, and peripheral vascular disease. Ozone combines with the fatty acids in the membranes of red blood cells, creating microscopic gaps in the membrane. As a result, the red blood cells become less rigid and much more flexible and pliable, which allows them to migrate into areas of the microcirculation that they might not normally be able to enter. Since oxygen is transported throughout the body by binding to the hemoglobin of the red blood cell, ozone therapy can promote better oxygenation and improved energy production in tissues that have been relatively oxygen deprived. Ozone in low concentrations also causes blood vessels to dilate as well as relaxation of tense, constricted muscles. These changes can further improve one's level of physical energy.

Using ozone in its various forms—for purification of your air and drinking water, for bathing and hot tub—should be strongly considered by individuals who would like to boost their level of physical energy by increasing their levels of oxygen. Specific information on these methods is provided in the next chapter.

We personally know a health care professional nearly eighty years old who experienced an increase in physical energy after using ozone therapy. Martha had a busy clinical practice for nearly fifty years, retiring in her mid-seventies after the death of her husband. She became quite despondent after his death. She also had two severe episodes of pneumonia, which left her with residual lung damage as well as chronically fatigued. Then she began to use ozone therapy on a regular basis to prevent further lung infections. She found that ozone therapy increased her level of physical energy significantly, and she was able to begin a program of walking and yoga. After four years of retirement, her energy level was so dramatically improved and her boredom with her forced inactivity so high that she decided to start seeing patients again at an age when many of her peers were either retired, disabled, or deceased.

Hydrogen peroxide

Hydrogen peroxide has been found to improve energy by facilitating the flow of blood through the circulatory system. This helps to promote the exchange of gases, thereby helping to rid the body of energy-depleting carbon dioxide and improving oxygenation. Ozone and hydrogen peroxide can also increase physical energy and vitality because of their immunity-enhancing effect. They both have antibacterial, antiviral, and antifungal effects, thereby helping to rid the body of energy-depleting microorganisms. However, while ozone can be used effectively on a self-care basis, hydrogen peroxide is best administered by a physician.

◢2 MENTAL CLARITY AND ACUITY

The brain requires a large share of the body's oxygen supply. Even though the brain makes up only 2 percent of the body by weight, it uses 20 percent of the oxygen that we inhale. Individuals who are engaged in complex mental tasks tend to deplete their brain's supply of oxygen much more rapidly than individuals who are not engaged in intellectual pursuits. As we have discussed, this problem is compounded by the shallow breathing, relative immobility, and muscle constriction that can accompany long hours of mental effort. In addition, the aging process also takes its toll on the brain's supply of oxygen. The age-related decline in memory and cognitive function that is commonly seen in elderly individuals is due, in part, to a reduction in the brain's oxygen levels. The loss of elasticity and fibrosis of the aging lungs and atherosclerosis of the blood vessels that feed the brain all contribute to this problem. Both exercise and ozone therapy can help to increase oxygen levels.

Aerobic exercise

Anyone who is engaged in strenuous mental activity should participate in frequent aerobic exercise. Without continually replenishing the supply of oxygen to the brain and nervous system, individuals who are engaged in intellectual work will, at some point, experience mental exhaustion and burnout. Regular aerobic exercise is crucial if one is to maintain one's mental edge. Similarly, elderly individuals who are engaged in regular physical activity will maintain better cognitive function than their housebound or sedentary peers.

Walking, swimming, bicycling, and dancing all improve mental alertness and cognitive function when practiced on a regular basis. Aerobic exercise does this by improving oxygenation and circulation to the brain and nerves and by opening up and dilating blood vessels of the head and brain. Thus, more nutrients can flow into and more waste products can be removed from this vital system. Research studies done on adults who exercise on a regular basis compared with similar groups who are sedentary show striking differences in a variety of mental functions. Adults engaged in an active exercise program have better concentration and clearer and quicker thinking and problem-solving abilities. In addition, reaction time and short-term memory improve with exercise. Not only does regular physical activity induce functional improvements in the brain, it also dramatically alters brain chemistry in a positive way through the increased production of neurochemicals like dopamine and beta-endorphins, which greatly increase alertness and produce a sense of elation and well-being.

The importance of physical activity in maintaining cognitive function is illustrated by one of Susan's patients who had been a remarkable peak performer during his younger years. This individual accumulated great wealth and prestige quite easily in his chosen field. Besides being well read in a number of areas, he was also quick and witty, often the life of the party. However, by the time he reached his seventies, generalized circulatory disease had reduced the supply of oxygen to his brain significantly.

He found that he was beginning to forget facts that had previously been easy for him to recall. He told Susan that he only felt like his old energetic, mentally alert self after playing tennis or swimming.

Ozone therapy

Supplementing with ozone can help to support and maintain mental alertness and mental clarity during long bouts of exhausting mental work. Ozone/oxygen mixtures go directly into the brain, where they increase its supply of oxygen and blood flow. While ozone can help healthy people to perform at peak levels in the intellectual arena, it may even be of benefit to individuals with severely compromised cognitive function. Several promising studies indicate that ozone therapy may be helpful in the treatment of senile dementia or Alzheimer's disease. Two studies conducted in the early 1990s in Havana, Cuba, and presented at the Eleventh World Ozone Conference found that a high percentage of patients treated with ozone showed an improvement in cognitive function and social behavior. In one study, sixty elderly patients with senile dementia were treated with either pure oxygen or an ozone/oxygen mixture for a period of twenty-one days. All of these patients were evaluated by neurological testing as well as standardized tests of intelligence, behavior, and emotional responses. In the ozone/oxygen-treated group, more than 80 percent showed an improvement in cognitive function, with a similar portion demonstrating an improved ability to manage their daily activities. They also showed improved ability to interact socially with other people. In contrast, no improvement was noted in the control group.

In another study, 120 male and female elderly patients who suffered from cerebrovascular disease (in which there is a lack of blood flow and oxygen to the brain) were treated with an ozone/oxygen mixture five days a week for three weeks. As part of the study they were given psychological testing and assessed for their level of social functioning. Ozone/oxygen therapy produced the best results in patients who had been the most recently diagnosed. Nearly half of the chronic patients improved, and 100 percent of the acute cases showed improvement. In addition, no side effects of ozone therapy were observed in either study. Intravenous hydrogen peroxide therapy has also been found to improve cognitive function in individuals with cerebrovascular disease. Hydrogen peroxide therapy lessened confusion, disorientation and slurred speech in affected individuals.

◀3 Determination and Perseverance in Pursuing Goals

A person with drive and determination will often outperform their more talented peers. Drive and determination are based on willpower and inspiration but also require physical energy and stamina. The continuity of action that we think of as perseverance requires a high level of physical and mental energy. As previously mentioned, these traits depend on having sufficient levels of oxygen within the body. Many of history's greatest leaders, such as Winston Churchill and Dwight D. Eisenhower, demonstrated the physical and mental vigor typical of strong oxygenators during their years in public office. These individuals had the drive and determination to enact ambitious social, political, and economic agendas and see them through to their successful conclusion despite strong opposition. The men and women who pioneered this country, encountering every possible physical adversity as they explored and eventually settled the western half of the United States, are other good examples of individuals whose drive and determination were supported by the physical vigor that comes from being well-oxygenated. Many entrepreneurs who have built successful companies demonstrate this same level of drive and dedication to achieving their goals, which is supported by a tremendous level of physical vigor and vitality.

In contrast, individuals who are poor oxygenators lack this degree of physical vitality. They are often forced to be more modest in their goals and aspirations. Susan has seen this often in patients who describe having had a much greater ability to set and achieve challenging goals for themselves when they previously had much higher levels of physical energy. These individuals tend to lose interest in pursuing their once cherished goals and aspirations as their level of physical energy diminishes. People lose their drive and perseverance as their ability to oxygenate declines.

▲▲ Regaining one's level of physical energy is well worth the effort if one has meaningful goals and aspirations. Giving them up because of a lack of physical energy, rather than a lack of will or desire, is unnecessary once you understand the important role that oxygenation plays in supporting one's goals. Improving one's level of oxygenation through the four-part program described in the following chapter can help you to achieve any goal you wish to attain.

◀4 THE ABILITY TO GET ALONG WITH OTHER PEOPLE

People who are well oxygenated are more likely to be outgoing and socially adept. These individuals often have a certain charisma that others are attracted to. If inclined towards social activities, these people, who tend to be genial and jovial, are in high demand at social events. Because of their high level of physical energy, they are able to put in the time and make the effort required to build and sustain friendships. They also tend to build strong career networks because they have the physical energy needed to meet and socialize with people in their chosen field. They also maintain their prior contacts from their years in school, military training, professional training, and prior jobs.

Aerobic exercise

When people are depressed, they tend to become introverted and to isolate themselves from contact with other human beings. They will often curtail their level of physical activity and become more housebound. They also tend to restrict their movements and inhibit the expansion of their lungs, which results in shallow breathing. While the standard treatment for depression is psychotherapy and antidepressant medication, a number of studies have shown that exercise significantly helps relieve moderate depression. One such study, done at the University of Virginia, observed depressed college students. Those who jogged regularly during the study period showed a significant reduction in symptoms of depression, while those who did not exercise showed virtually no change in their symptoms.

Oxygen therapies

Oxygen therapies help to relieve depression and enhance sociability because of their positive stimulatory effects on brain chemistry and mood. Ozone therapy is particularly beneficial in this regard. Not only does it help to uplift the mood and promote greater sociability in relatively normal individuals, but it also appears to enhance sociability even in severely compromised individuals with senile dementia. This was confirmed in a study that was conducted in a hospital in Havana, Cuba, in the early 1990s. In this study, which was presented at the Eleventh World Ozone Conference in 1993, elderly patients with senile dementia were administered either an ozone/oxygen mixture or pure oxygen alone for a period of twenty-one days. Not only did the majority of the patients receiving the ozone/oxygen mixture show an improvement in their neurological status, but they also showed an improved ability to interact socially with other people and manage their daily activities. In addition, many patients showed relief of symptoms of depression. In contrast, no improvement was noted in the control group.

5 THE ABILITY TO REMAIN CALM UNDER PRESSURE

An important trait of all peak performers is the ability to remain calm and centered during times of stress. Successful outcomes do not occur when one is frantic, upset, or angry. It is only by remaining calm and maintaining your ability to rationally think through a solution to a problem that you improve the odds of a successful outcome. Good oxygenators are more likely to have a balanced emotional response to stressful situations because their production of stress-coping chemicals is enhanced when sufficient oxygen is present. The positive chemical support that one draws from good oxygenation is more likely to leave one with a feeling of innate strength and confidence.

There is some evidence that oxygen therapies, such as ozone and hydrogen peroxide, can produce these types of benefits. Because of the analgesic properties and mood-elevating effects of these therapies, people using them will literally feel less emotional pain and tension surrounding difficult circumstances and decisions. Yet they are still able to maintain their alertness and ability to think clearly. Good decision making occurs best under these circumstances. In contrast, stress depletes the oxygen levels of the body dramatically in poorly oxygenated individuals. This depletion can exaggerate the feelings of fear and panic that one might feel when confronted with a stressful situation. Over time, it can also lead to exhaustion and burnout.

6 OPTIMISM AND VISION

Having a sufficient level of oxygen within the body is a prerequisite for vision and optimism. The brain depends on a steady supply of oxygen in order to produce the wide variety of neurochemicals, such as dopamine, serotonin, pregnenolone, and beta-endorphins, that are necessary to maintain a positive mental state and promote feelings of well-being. While having a positive outlook on life cannot be reduced to a series of chemical reactions, maintaining a positive frame of mind does require that the brain receive sufficient oxygen. In contrast, people who are oxygen deprived tend to feel mentally dull, listless, and even depressed. Oxygen deprivation does not create the fertile ground from which great visions and aspirations arise. Individuals who are well oxygenated are more likely to be able to see the possibilities and opportunities in everyday circumstances.

The link between oxygenation and vision is exemplified by the inspirational speaker and author Anthony Robbins. Robbins's highly energetic presentations have captivated more than a million people who have attended his seminars. In addition, he has sold 24 million personal-development audiotapes in the past five years, according to an April 1998 article in *Success Magazine*. Robbins motivates people with inspirational stories and tips on how to achieve their goals. His charisma, dynamic presentation, and high level of physical energy are typical of a person with a superoxygenated body. Even his large-chested physique is typical of an individual who is an excellent oxgenator. His work includes frequent travel as well as presenting workshops and seminars in diverse geographical locations. Much of this activity takes place in poorly oxygenzated environments like airplanes and hotels. Only individuals with superior oxygenating capabilities (as well as healthy acid/alkaline balance) have the physical energy and stamina to sustain this lifestyle for long periods of time. Interestingly enough, in his book *Giant Steps*, Robbins emphasizes the importance of oxygenation and aerobic exercise in creating the high level of physical energy needed for peak performance.

Aerobic exercise

Regular aerobic exercise greatly improves blood flow and oxygenation to the brain. This can dramatically alter brain chemistry in a positive way through the increased production of the neurochemicals, like dopamine and beta-endorphins, needed to produce a mood-elevating effect and a sense of elation. This state of mental well-being is necessary for optimism and vision.

For example, beta-endorphins, chemicals released from the pituitary gland, act as natural opiates. They are chemically similar to the pain reliever morphine but 200 times more potent. Endorphins have a dramatic effect on mood. When levels in the body are high, they improve an individual's general sense of well-being. Aerobic exercise significantly increases the production of beta-endorphins. Research studies demonstrate that brisk aerobic exercise like running can increase beta-endorphin levels as much as fivefold. Measurements of beta-endorphins taken a half hour after exercise showed that beta-endorphin levels were still higher than at starting. In fact, beta-endorphins are thought to be responsible for the runner's high that marathoners experience. Individuals who exercise regularly report related feelings of elation, euphoria, and even bliss. This supports the high level of vision and optimism that many of the greatest inspirational figures in various professions demonstrate.

Other individuals may effectively suppress their vision and optimism with negative self-talk. Often this self-talk includes fearful thoughts and worries about stressful life situations or even imagined concerns. Such individuals may even have difficulty relaxing or falling asleep when their negative self-talk is mixed with strong anger, hostility, and upset toward a person or difficult situation. Susan has had patients tell her that they have tried strong sleeping medications or alcoholic beverages to induce sleep; however, their upset feelings would override the sedative effects of the medication or alcohol.

Exercise can help to reduce negative self-talk, improve one's ability to relax, and even reduce insomnia by working off nervous energy and diffusing the fight-or-flight response. When you engage in regular aerobic exercise, the production of mood-elevating chemicals like beta-endorphins can help to create a shift in your habitual patterns of thinking: Pessimism and doubt can change to vision, optimism, and a sense of mastery over your environment.

Oxygen therapy

Research studies suggest that oxygen therapy can have a profound mood-elevating effect. For example, it has been noted that when these therapies are used to reduce pain and discomfort, patients are less likely to be depressed. In a study done by Charles H. Farr, which was published in 1987 in the *Townsend Letter for Doctors*, normal, healthy volunteers who received intravenous infusions of hydrogen peroxide reported various degrees of mood elevation and even elation. When a person's mood is elevated, they are likely to be more optimistic. Ozone has a definite and significant mood-elevating effect when used in low concentrations, which have a stimulatory effect on the body. Regular use of ozone not only improves cognitive function, but also promotes the production of brain chemicals related to a positive mental state, vision, and optimism.

7 SPEEDY RECOVERY FROM ILLNESS, INJURY, AND EXERTION

Peak performers have an amazing ability to bounce back quickly from all types of physical stress. Absenteeism is not an issue for them. Very successful individuals in any field strive to meet their deadlines and attend all of their scheduled meetings. To be successful, athletes must be ready to play on the day of a scheduled game or meet, and actors must attend all their rehearsals and be on stage when the curtain goes up for a performance.

The ability to recover quickly from all kinds of physical trauma is very important, given the large number of injuries, illnesses, and surgical procedures that occur each year. According to the Consumer Product Safety Review, an agency that collects injury data, nearly 2 million people are injured each year just by slipping on stairs, ramps, landings, and floors. In addition, millions of individuals undergo either major or minor surgery (including dental surgery) each year. There are also millions of athletic injuries each year.

When a traumatic injury occurs, the area of tissue damage will become deficient in oxygen. With swelling and leakage of blood into the affected area, circulation to the injured area is diminished. This reduces oxygen delivery to the area. Fortunately, various types of oxygen therapy can be used to help restore the level of oxygen to devitalized tissue and promote wound healing.

Ozone therapy

The ability of ozone therapy to accelerate the healing of traumatic injuries was dramatically documented in a Russian study presented in 1993 at the Eleventh World Ozone Conference. In this study, researchers monitored the progress of sixteen children, ranging in age from twenty days to eighteen years, who had been admitted to the emergency room of a Russian hospital. These children had experienced a variety of traumatic injuries caused by fires, explosions, bullet wounds, automobile accidents, and carbon monoxide poisoning. They were then treated with an ozone/oxygen mixture over a forty-eight-hour period. These treatments helped to accelerate the healing process and prevented further devitalization of tissue in the affected area. Pain at the site of injury was also reduced.

Susan has seen a number of patients who have consulted her following a surgical procedure. Some of them were disappointed in how slowly their surgical incision healed and in their inability to rapidly bounce back. They continued to feel more fatigued and depressed than they had felt prior to the procedure. However, these symptoms can be countered by the use of ozone therapy. Several studies have shown that ozone therapy, administered prior to and following a minor surgical procedure, such as cosmetic surgery or liposuction, may enable a person to return to work more rapidly as well as resume their normal level of activity sooner.

A French study examined the ability of ozone to promote patients' relaxation prior to surgery, prevent postoperative infections, and speed the healing process. This study, which involved 100 patients, was presented at the Ninth World Ozone Conference in 1989. Prior to surgery, patients received one to two ozone treatments per week for a total of five treatments, plus five treatments postoperatively. The ozone treatments promoted healing of the surgical incisions. Patients healed faster and without complications like infections. Other studies have found that ozone can help to reduce the amount of bleeding during surgery when administered at the site of the operation.

Not only does ozone help to heal surgical incisions, but it also helps to resolve poorly healing postoperative wounds and bedsores (decubitus ulcers), which patients sometimes develop after protracted periods of being confined to bed. The role of ozone in healing postoperative wounds and bedsores was discussed in a study presented in 1991 at the Tenth World Ozone Conference. In this study, fifty-one patients with postoperative lesions were healed by the administration of ozone therapy over two to four months. All of these patients had previously had poor responses to other types of therapy. Similar positive results were found in a three-year study conducted in England in which ozone therapy was given to 200 hospital patients with bedsores and wounds due to injury or surgery. This study, which was reported in 1979 in the journal *Physiology*, found that ozone both accelerated the healing process and caused a marked reduction in pain.

Finally, physicians have found ozone to be useful in the treatment of burns. A burned area can be given a gentle shower of ozonated water while being cleansed and the dead tissue removed. Topical ozone has also been found to facilitate the grafting of new skin and to help prevent infections that can occur as a result of the grafting procedure. Ozone is also used as an antiseptic when a burn area is incised in an effort to prevent fluid from accumulating in the tissue.

Hydrogen peroxide and hyperbaric-oxygen therapy

Hydrogen peroxide has also been shown to speed recovery from wounds and injuries. A study published in the *American Journal of Surgery* reported on the work of researchers at Baylor University Medical Center, in Dallas. In this study, researchers administered intra-arterial hydrogen peroxide to patients with tissue damage due to skin ulcers, varicose-vein ulcers, stasis ulcers of the foot, leg, and jaw, and radiation therapy. The researchers found that hydrogen peroxide helped to speed up the healing of these wounds and injured areas. They attributed the healing produced by hydrogen peroxide to its superoxygenating effects.

Similar results have been seen with the use of hyperbaric-oxygen therapy (HBOT). This has been confirmed in a number of studies. One such study, published in 1996 in *Diabetes Care*, followed the progress of approximately seventy diabetic patients suffering from diabetic foot ulcers. Thirty-five of these patients received hyperbaric-oxygen therapy, and an equivalent number did not. HBOT was found to significantly reduce the need for amputation in diabetic patients in the treated group. The Undersea and Hyperbaric Medical Society approves the use of HBOT for the treatment of poorly healing wounds, infections in devitalized tissue, and crush injuries.

◀8 RESISTANCE TO ILLNESS

In previous chapters, the roles of acid/alkaline balance, digestive enzymes, and healthy detoxification were discussed as important functions needed for resistance to illness. In this section, we will discuss the tremendous benefits that can occur with the use of oxygen therapies.

Ozone therapy and respiratory illnesses

A number of research studies have found ozone to be an effective therapy for many types of acute respiratory conditions. In bacterial infections of the respiratory tract, ozone works by disrupting the integrity of the bacterial cell membrane. It does this by combining with and chemically altering the phospholipids and lipoproteins found in the cell membrane. With viral infections, ozone damages the protein coat of the virus. It also interferes with the reproductive cycle of the virus by interrupting the virus-to-cell contact. Peroxides are formed through the interaction of ozone with the fatty acids of the cells. Cells that have previously been infected by viruses can be destroyed by the high levels of peroxides produced by this process. In addition, the production of mucus and the accumulation of fluid in the tissues is reduced by ozone therapy.

In a 1993 study presented at the Eleventh World Ozone Conference, ozone in combination with vitamin C and B vitamins was used instead of antibiotics to treat several cases of pneumonia. Ozone was administered daily for twelve days. Not only were symptoms reduced, but marked improvement was noted on X-ray examination of the lungs. Another study, also presented at the Eleventh World Ozone Conference, examined the therapeutic benefits of ozone in treating asthma. In this German study, eighty-four patients were treated with ozone therapy, and 69 percent of them either experienced a full remission or noted a significant improvement in their asthmatic symptoms. These are remarkable results given the tenacity of this disease. Similarly, a French study noted a significant improvement in symptoms in patients with asthma who received twice-weekly ozone treatments over a period of several months.

Judy exemplifies the beneficial effects of ozone for respiratory conditions. She is prone to recurrent episodes of colds and bronchitis. She has been using ozone successfully for several years to prevent recurrences of these respective conditions. Prevention of these conditions has helped her economic survival since she is a self-supporting woman whose previous episodes of respiratory infections left her incapacitated and unable to work for periods of up to four to six weeks. She could not afford the loss of income that these infections caused and incurred financial hardship as a result. The use of ozone has been tremendously beneficial in improving her resistance to and greatly reducing her episodes of respiratory infections.

Respiratory symptoms of allergy such as nasal and sinus congestion, middle-ear congestion, and itching and tearing of the eyes can also be treated with ozone therapy. These symptoms can be triggered by seasonal pollens, grasses, and indoor allergens like dust mites, feathers, and cat and dog dander. Ozone has proven an effective treatment when standard therapies have proven ineffective. The 1993 German study that used ozone for the treatment of asthma also reported on the results of thirty-nine patients with allergies who were treated with ozone/oxygen therapy. Fifty-five percent of these patients reported having either a full remission of or significant improvement in their allergic symptoms, while 22 percent reported some improvement in their symptoms.

We saw dramatic evidence of the benefit of ozone in a business associate with severe mold allergies to whom we loaned our ozone air-purification machine for three weeks. Linda lived in a fog belt area of San Francisco and was constantly suffering from the ill effects of the mold and mildew that she was unable to eradicate from her house. However, after only one day of using our air-purification machine, she noticed such a significant improvement in her symptoms that she kept our machine until she could obtain her own. The ozone air-purification machine began to powerfully eradicate the mold that had been stressing her immune system for several years, causing chronic nasal congestion and coughing.

Charles H. Farr of Oklahoma City, Oklahoma, was a world-renowned expert in the use of hydrogen peroxide therapy for the treatment of many medical conditions. In papers published by Dr. Farr in various journals, he discussed the successful application of intravenous hydrogen peroxide therapy for the treatment of infectious bronchitis, viral influenza, asthma, allergic reactions, and even chronic lung diseases like emphysema and chronic bronchitis. He has found that many patients with acute respiratory conditions responded to therapy in twenty-four to forty-eight hours. For example, many bronchitis patients had a reduction in their coughing and sputum production and were breathing more easily within twenty-four hours. These patients also reported increased levels of energy. Many allergy patients also responded rapidly to hydrogen peroxide therapy, within two to three treatments. Patients who had had allergic problems for longer periods of time responded more slowly. However, Dr. Farr found that most patients had improved within ten weeks when hydrogen peroxide treatments were given weekly.

In 1989, Dr. Farr used hydrogen peroxide therapy to treat individuals suffering from type A/Shanghai influenza. A seasonal epidemic of this influenza occurred in Oklahoma during the 1989–90 winter flu season. Many of the victims developed fever, chills, sore throat, cough, headache, aching in the joints, and intestinal symptoms. Full recovery from this influenza normally required twelve to eighteen days. Dr. Farr treated twenty flu patients, aged sixteen to seventy-eight, with intravenous hydrogen peroxide at their first visit. They were asked to return for a second treatment the next day, if symptoms persisted. Seven of the patients returned for a second infusion, and two required a third infusion. (The latter two patients were both over seventy years of age.) The patients who were treated with hydrogen peroxide fared significantly better than patients in the control group, who had been treated with conventional medical therapy consisting of antibiotics, decongestants, and pain-relieving medication. The control group showed a 50 percent improvement in flu symptoms after 4.1 days and a 75 percent improvement after 7.8 days. Ninety percent had recovered by eleven days. In contrast, patients treated with hydrogen peroxide experienced a 50 percent improvement in symptoms after only 1.9 days, a 75 percent improvement after 3.2 days, and 90 percent recovery after 5.5 days. Even more noteworthy, in terms of performance and productivity, is the comparative number of days of work missed by patients in each group. Flu patients treated with hydrogen peroxide, as a group, missed only 5 days of work, while those in the control group missed a total of 41.5 days.

One of Jim's friends, Phillip, an executive in the computer industry, developed a severe viral respiratory infection several years ago that he was unable to resolve. After several months of functioning well below his usual level of efficiency, he finally consulted a physician, who used intravenous hydrogen peroxide as part of his treatment program. After one intravenous hydrogen peroxide treatment, his symptoms resolved entirely. Phil was astonished by the effectiveness of the treatment.

There are many reasons why hydrogen peroxide is so effective. As an oxidizing agent, it is able to inactivate bacteria and viruses. In addition, it plays a crucial role in promoting a strong immune response within the body. White blood cells, or granulocytes, produce hydrogen peroxide as a defense against bacteria, viruses, fungi, and parasites. Supplemental hydrogen peroxide strengthens this function. Hydrogen peroxide therapy has also been found to stimulate the immune response by increasing the production of various types of white blood cells that fight infection. These include monocytes, which kill bacteria; T-helper cells, will help coordinate the immune response; and gamma interferon, a protein that acts as a cellular messenger and is present when cells are exposed to viruses. Hydrogen peroxide also functions as a vasodilator. It increases blood circulation through the lungs, improving the uptake of oxygen into the body.

▲▲ If you are prone to severe and recurrent respiratory conditions, you may want to consider consulting with a physician who specializes in oxygen therapies. Information about these physicians is available from complementary medical associations. A list of these organizations can be found in the appendix of this book.

Ozone therapy and environmental illnesses

Individuals who are well oxygenated tend to have good detoxification capability. Oxygen promotes healthy functioning of the liver, so those who are well oxygenated are often able to drink excessive amounts of alcohol or even work and live in chemically polluted environments without apparent ill effect. They have such excellent detoxification capability that they are able to metabolize and eliminate these toxins from their bodies.

Other individuals are not so fortunate. People who are poor oxygenators are more prone to sensitivity reactions to environmental pollutants, due to the reduced efficiency of their detoxification mechanisms. Symptoms of toxicity from pollutants can include sneezing, nasal congestion, coughing, fatigue, digestive symptoms, and brain fog. The brain and nervous system are particularly vulnerable to chemical pollutants. Inhaled toxins such as hydrocarbons and chemical solvents rapidly diffuse into the brain. In the brain, chemical pollutants readily combine with the fatty tissue, which is a large component of this organ. Severely affected individuals often find that they must take extreme measures to avoid a particular substance. They may have to move from their home or leave their job. Even worse, the offending material may never be identified. Fortunately, treatment with ozone has been found to eliminate adverse reactions to chemical pollutants as well as accelerate these pollutants' breakdown to less toxic substances.

While ozone therapy improves liver function and the ability to detoxify, ozone itself acts chemically upon environmental pollutants that have been absorbed into the body by converting them into carbon dioxide and water. These substances can then be excreted from the body through the lungs or urinary tract. Ozone destroys and eliminates herbicides, pesticides, and many of the synthetic chemicals present in modern furnishings and building materials, such as benzene, toluene, styrene, xylene, hexanes, trichloroethylene, and phthalates. A person may be exposed to these chemicals after moving into a new apartment building or in the workplace. In recent decades, many buildings have been designed to seal in heat and air-conditioning to reduce operating costs. These so-called "tight" buildings also tend to recirculate airborne chemical pollutants and do not allow fresh air to enter.

Carpeting made from synthetic materials can also release pollutants into the air. Until the invention of synthetic fibers in this century, all carpeting was made out of natural fibers such as cotton, wool, and silk. However, today's mass-produced carpeting may contain as many as 120 chemicals, some of which are toxic to the nervous system or are carcinogenic. According to a 1997 article in *Medical & Legal Briefs*, an independent laboratory tested new carpet samples on mice, who were exposed to air blown over the carpet. The researchers found that 25 percent of the carpet samples caused severe health problems in the animals involving respiration as well as the nervous system and muscles.

Another toxic substance that millions of people are exposed to is formaldehyde, which is a component of building insulation as well as particle board and plywood. Formaldehyde is also found in such everyday products as detergents, paper, adhesives, dyes, paint, clothing, leather goods, insecticides, and fertilizers. Workers who produce these goods are regularly exposed to this toxic chemical.

Hotel rooms can be another source of toxic-chemical exposure. Travelers may find themselves in rooms described as nonsmoking that still have a strong odor of cigarettes. Rooms may have also been sprayed with synthetic chemical deodorizers. In tropical climates with damp, humid air, mold and fungi, which thrive in such conditions, may also be present. The research assistant who worked with us on this book recalls spending a week in a motel in Florida during a business trip. She sneezed and coughed continually during her stay because of her sensitivity to mold. Upon looking closely at her room, she found evidence of mold on the bathroom tiles, window ledges, and carpeting.

Ozone air-purification machines should be used in any home, office building, or manufacturing plant in which airborne chemical pollutants are present. These machines will greatly improve the quality of your indoor air, eliminating pollutants as well as bacteria, viruses, mold, mildew, spores, pollen, and cigarette smoke. You will be amazed at how fresh and pure ozonated air smells. These machines are described in greater detail in the next chapter.

SUMMARY

Oxygen levels affect all eight of the peak-performance traits. Aerobic exercise and the various oxygen therapies—pure-oxygen, ozone, hydrogen peroxide, and hyperbaric-oxygen therapies—can improve oxygenation and thereby benefit physical vitality and stamina; mental clarity and acuity; determination and perseverance in pursuing goals; the ability to get along with other people; the ability to remain calm under pressure; optimism and vision; speedy recovery from illness, injury, and exertion; and resistance to illness.

SECTION 4:
OXYGENATION AND HEALTH

GOOD OXYGENATION HELPS the body maintain its healthy, slightly alkaline pH. This enables the activation of enzymes to occur and crucial physiological functions like digestion and the immune response to proceed most effectively.

When oxygen levels are deficient, people are at greater risk of developing a wide range of diseases, including infectious diseases, circulatory problems, cancer, and many other health conditions. Various types of oxygen therapy, including ozone, hydrogen peroxide, and hyperbaric-oxygen therapies, have been used successfully to treat these conditions. In some cases, oxygen therapy alone is sufficient to eliminate symptoms and reverse the course of the disease. In other instances, the oxygen therapy is a highly beneficial adjunct to more conventional therapies. This has been documented in thousands of research studies. For an in-depth discussion of the various oxygen therapies, see the next chapter.

INFECTIOUS DISEASES

Ozone therapies have proven useful in the treatment of a variety of bacterial, viral, and fungal infections as well as parasitic infections. As early as the mid–nineteenth century, various researchers in Europe demonstrated the ability of ozone to kill bacteria. Since then, hundreds of articles have been published documenting the disinfectant and antimicrobial properties of the various oxygen therapies, particularly ozone and hydrogen peroxide. Not only has ozone has been used for decades to eradicate microorganisms, but it has also been used as a disinfectant in the treatment of water and to sterilize equipment in hospitals. Hydrogen peroxide has been used to disinfect food and food containers as well as to treat infections in human beings. Furthermore, unlike antibiotic therapies, which are becoming less effective because of the increased resistance of microorganisms to the therapeutic agents, oxygen therapies are incredibly effective at eradicating a wide variety of pathogens.

Bacterial infections

Ozone is able to destroy many kinds of bacteria, including dangerous pathogens like *Escherichia coli*, a common food contaminant that can cause symptoms of food poisoning; *Staphylococcus aureus*, which can cause infections in hospitals; or *Mycobacterium tuberculosis*, which causes tuberculosis. Ozone destroys bacteria by attaching to the cell wall that encases the bacteria and reacting chemically with the phospholipids and lipoproteins in the cell membrane. This process produces peroxides, which destroy the bacterial cell membrane. In addition, ozone penetrates the cell membrane of diseased cells and alters the DNA within the cell. In a research paper presented in 1989 at the Ninth World Ozone Conference, researchers stated that while ozone can alter the DNA of unhealthy cells, it is unable to do this in healthy human cells, which are more capable of repair.

Ozone was used as a disinfectant to treat water as far back as 1899. It was first used for this purpose in Lille, France. Ozone is used today in many European countries to purify drinking water and swimming pools. It acts more rapidly and can be used in lower concentrations than chemical disinfectants like chlorine. Compared with chlorine, ozone is effective against a far wider range of infectious agents, including viruses, molds, and algae. While chlorine has an unpleasant taste, ozonated water tastes remarkably fresh and delicious. When chlorine reacts with organic compounds, it can produce carcinogens such as trihalomethane. In contrast, ozone breaks down rapidly in water and does not generate toxic by-products.

Research studies investigated the use of ozone in hospitals as a sterilizing agent for surgical instruments. Even the movie industry has considered the use of ozone as a sterilizing agent. During the 1950s, when 3-D movies were at the height of their popularity, there was concern about transmitting infections of the eye, scalp, and skin via the 3-D glasses, since these glasses were reused by different audiences. In a paper published in 1953 in the *American Journal of Public Health*, researchers recommended that movie theaters use ozone as a disinfectant to clean the 3-D glasses.

Not only can ozone be used to purify water, but it can also be taken internally as a powerful antibacterial agent. Early studies done in the 1940s and 1950s investigated the antibacterial effect of ozone for possible internal use. In a study presented at the 1956 International Ozone Conference held in Chicago, *E. coli* were exposed to an ozone solution and after one minute of contact, all of the bacteria were destroyed. This occurred in an all-or-nothing fashion: Once a certain concentration of ozone was reached, all the bacteria died. Another study, published in 1947 in the *Journal of the American Pharmaceutical Association*, found that ozone was able to kill other common types of bacteria including several forms of staphylococci as well as streptococci. Since there is growing concern that the overprescribing of antibiotics during the past decades has led to the evolution of strains of bacteria resistant to antibiotics, ozone therapy may well offer an effective treatment alternative.

Hydrogen peroxide is also used to treat bacterial infections. Hydrogen peroxide works primarily through oxidation, a process in which electrons are transferred from one molecule to another. Through this process, hydrogen peroxide destroys unhealthy, devitalized cells as well as pathogenic bacteria. In addition, hydrogen peroxide therapy supplements the hydrogen peroxide normally produced by our cells. As a protection against bacterial invasion, hydrogen peroxide selectively destroys disease-producing bacteria.

As part of the immune response, white blood cells, called granulocytes, produce hydrogen peroxide, which is injected directly into the part of the cell containing the microorganism. Initially, microorganisms multiply more quickly than they can be destroyed. However, the balance then shifts as microorganisms die off and the production of hydrogen peroxide increases. Hydrogen peroxide also stimulates the production of cytokines (hormonelike chemicals that act as chemical messengers to regulate immune function) as well as other cells needed for healthy immune function such as T-helper cells and monocytes.

Viral infections

Many common diseases such as poliomyelitis, mumps, measles, influenza, and hepatitis are caused by viruses. While antibiotics are ineffective as treatments for viral infections, oxygen therapies have been found to be quite useful as antiviral agents. The mechanism by which ozone and hydrogen peroxide inactivate viruses is similar. Both of these therapies interfere with the ability of a virus to bind with and infect other cells. A virus is contained within an envelope, called a capsid, made of fats or lipids. Examples of viruses with lipid envelopes are the HIV virus and the herpes family of viruses, which includes the herpes simplex and Epstein-Barr viruses. Growing from the virus envelope are spikes containing tiny bulbs that function as receptors. It is through these receptors that a virus connects with other cells to infect them. Both ozone and hydrogen peroxide can inactivate these spikes by structurally altering the receptors. As a result, the virus is no longer able to infect other cells. Ozone will also react with the fats within the envelope, forming lipid peroxides that can disrupt the viral envelope. Once inside the virus, ozone can also disrupt the DNA and RNA that make up its genetic machinery.

When a cell is infected with a virus, it normally produces hydrogen peroxide to defend itself. Supplemental hydrogen peroxide, together with the hydrogen peroxide produced by the cell, will kill the virus. Both ozone and hydrogen peroxide therapies also increase the oxygen levels within the cells, thereby improving their health. Following is a list of various viral infections and information on the oxygen therapies that are used to treat them.

Poliomyelitis. An early laboratory study, published in 1943, compared the effectiveness of both ozone and chlorine in inactivating the poliovirus. Under experimental conditions, ozone inactivated the poliovirus within two minutes, while chlorine required between one and one-half and three hours to achieve the same result. A subsequent study, published in 1974 in the *American Water Works Association Journal*, confirmed these results. Researchers investigating different methods of water treatment to eliminate the poliovirus from sewage found that using a relatively low level of ozone killed 99 percent of the poliovirus within ten seconds. By comparison, a relatively greater amount of chlorine achieved the same results in 100 seconds. Iodine, which can be used as a disinfectant, was even less effective, requiring 100 minutes to destroy the poliovirus.

Hepatitis. The use of ozone therapy for the treatment of hepatitis has been well documented in a number of studies. Ozone therapy shortens the healing time from viral hepatitis and helps to prevent the disease from becoming chronic. A study on the use of ozone for the treatment of hepatitis was conducted by Horst Kief, a German physician. In this study published in 1983, Kief discussed twelve cases of chronic hepatitis that were treated with ozone therapy. Ozone therapy was administered once a week for three to four weeks, at which point the interval was increased to fourteen days or longer to give the body time to develop an immune response. The average treatment time of this study was about three months, during which time most of the patients showed significant improvement. In addition, there were virtually no side effects or relapses with the ozone therapy.

Similar results were reported in a paper presented in 1991 at the Tenth World Ozone Conference. In this study, fifteen patients were treated with ozone given intravenously twice a week until laboratory values were no more than 50 percent above normal. Patients received a total of six to ten ozone treatments. Their progress was monitored by clinical assessment and laboratory testing. Of the fifteen patients, twelve showed evidence of improvement, a success rate of 80 percent.

Herpes. Herpes is a viral infection of the skin and mucous membranes. It commonly causes lesions on the lips, in the genital area, buttocks, or thighs. It is characterized by shallow-based ulcers caused by the breakdown of the skin. Lesions can cause itching or burning and usually take a week or two to clear. Research studies have found ozone therapy to be an effective treatment for this disease. One such study, conducted by Heinz Konrad of Brazil and presented at the Tenth World Ozone Conference in 1991, used ozone to treat herpes. A total of 243 patients with oral or genital herpes were given one or two ozone treatments per week for a total of ten to twelve sessions. With the ozone treatments, the infections were milder and of shorter duration.

AIDS. Ozone therapy benefits AIDS patients in a variety of ways. It inactivates HIV, which is considered to be the virus responsible for the development of AIDS. It can also cure the patient of the opportunistic diseases that AIDS patients are vulnerable to contracting. This was confirmed in several in vitro studies. One such study, published in 1991 in the journal *Blood*, found that, depending on the concentration, ozone was able to inactivate 97 to 100 percent of HIV. Another study, conducted by Michael Carpendale and Joel Freeburg at the University of California, San Francisco, found the HIV virus 99 percent inactivated when treated with a low concentration of ozone. These results were published in 1991 in *Antiviral Research*. Dr. Carpendale subsequently presented a clinical study in 1993 at the Eleventh World Ozone Conference, where he reported on two AIDS patients who had experienced good therapeutic results with ozone therapy. These patients followed a treatment regimen of an ozone/oxygen mixture taken as a rectal insufflation (or enema) daily for twenty-one days. They then took one treatment every three days for sixteen weeks, followed by weekly treatments for fifteen weeks. The patients then continued on a maintenance program of periodic ozone treatments. Both of the patients improved, reporting a decrease in their symptoms. In addition, their blood counts improved. Over a six-year period, one patient not only had a significant increase in his T4-helper cells, an important indicator of immune system health, but also became classified as HIV negative. The other patient survived for six years, dying of a pneumonia unrelated to AIDS. This patient had remained essentially infection free during the preceding period but did not lose his HIV-positive status. Dr. Carpendale also published a study in the *Journal of Clinical Gastroenterology* in which he treated AIDS patients who were suffering from severe diarrhea with ozone rectally. Daily treatments were taken for twenty-one to twenty-eight days. Three of the patients were completely cured of the diarrhea, while a fourth had no change in his symptoms.

Some clinics also use hyperbaric-oxygen therapy (HBOT) to treat AIDS. This form of treatment is available at a unique facility, called Lifeforce, Inc., in Baltimore, Maryland, which is headed by Michelle Reillo, BSN, RN. Lifeforce is one of the few independent facilities, apart from hospitals and university centers, that use HBOT. Treatments are provided in multiplace hyperbaric chambers, which can seat several patients at once. In an interview, Reillo related that patients who had come to her eight years ago with full-blown AIDS are still alive and continue to participate in her program. Reillo regards HBOT as a beneficial adjunct therapy in the treatment of AIDS, having seen clinical proof of its ability to promote weight gain, help fight opportunistic infections, and lessen symptoms of the over 500 health problems that can be associated with AIDS. She believes that HBOT should be part of the first line of treatment in newly infected patients since it lessens the fatigue and lack of physical energy that is almost always associated with this disease. In addition, HBOT also helps the body to detoxify the drugs used to treat AIDS, thereby reducing the severity of the side effects that these drugs can cause.

Fungal infections

Ozone can act as an effective antifungal therapy. In fact, one of the early medical applications of ozone in the early 1900s was for the treatment of yeast infections. While ozone therapy is not commonly used to treat such conditions today, some physicians do use it to treat these types of infections. This kind of therapy has also been found particularly effective in the treatment of candida.

Candida. The effectiveness of ozone in the treatment of *Candida albicans* infections is well documented. This disease is due to a parasitic fungus that is found most commonly in the intestinal tract. Candida is a normal inhabitant of the digestive tract and usually lives in balance with the friendly bacteria that help to maintain healthy digestive function. However, when the balance between the bacteria and the fungi is upset, candida may proliferate, infecting tissues of the digestive tract, vagina, and mouth. The toxins released by the fungi weaken the immune system, allowing candida to penetrate throughout the body and spread to other systems, such as the bladder and respiratory system. Candida infections are more common in diabetics and have been linked to the prolonged use of antibiotics, cortisone, or birth control pills. Diets that are high in refined sugar or yeast promote the growth of candida within the body. Intravenous hydrogen peroxide has also been used successfully to treat candida infections. One of the most experienced physicians in the use of this treatment is Charles Farr. He has used intravenous hydrogen peroxide successfully to treat hundreds of patients with candida infections.

Parasitic infections

Ozone is also used for the treatment of parasites. As early as 1944, an article published in the *American Journal of Tropical Medicine* described a study conducted at the University of Southern California and Los Angeles County Hospital. This study compared the effects of chlorine and ozone in the treatment of the parasitic cysts of *Entamoeba histolytica*. The results of this study showed that ozone killed the parasites much more rapidly than did chlorine.

Malaria is a disease commonly found in the tropics. It is estimated that malaria infects several hundred million people and is known to kill more than 2.5 million persons each year. Hydrogen peroxide may eventually prove to be a useful treatment for malaria. Laboratory and animal studies have shown that some species of malaria parasites are killed by even slight concentrations of hydrogen peroxide.

In the United States, many people are infected with *Giardia lamblia*. This parasite is found in contaminated municipal drinking water and in freshwater sites that campers use for their water supply. *Giardia lamblia* is a protozoal parasite that can infest the human intestinal tract, causing diarrhea, weight loss, nausea, vomiting, and intestinal cramps. It is often very resistant to medical treatment. A presentation in 1991 at the Tenth World Ozone Conference reported on a study of eighty patients with *G. lamblia*. Half of the patients were treated with ozonated water four times a day for twelve days, while the remaining forty patients were given an ozonated oil for five to ten days. Patients were assessed for continued presence of the parasites in their stools and intestinal tract. The treatments were highly successful, with a cure rate of 97.5 percent for each group.

CIRCULATORY PROBLEMS

Circulatory problems such as heart attacks, strokes, and peripheral vascular disease are among the leading causes of death and disability in the United States. Research studies have confirmed that oxygen therapies have a remarkable ability to restore blood flow to devitalized tissues, reduce the symptoms of vascular disease, and improve the health of the heart and blood vessels. In fact, the results of various oxygen therapies are so dramatic that individuals should consider adding the appropriate one (described below) to the treatment program for their specific condition.

Ozone therapy

Ozone increases the level of oxygen within the blood vessels by increasing the fluidity of the blood as well as the pliability of red blood cells. In circulatory diseases as well as many other chronic illnesses, clumping or aggregation of the red blood cells occurs. This aggregation hinders blood flow and promotes clotting. In addition, blood that aggregates has less surface area, reducing the amount of oxygen that can be transported by the hemoglobin of the red blood cells.

Ozone therapy works by altering the electrical charge on the surface of the red blood cells, thereby reducing the tendency of these cells to aggregate. Ozone also increases the elasticity and flexibility of the red blood cells. A Swiss study, presented in 1989 at the Ninth World Ozone Conference, suggested that this occurs because ozone breaks the double bonds of the fatty acids contained within the outer membrane of red blood cells. This breakage produces microscopic gaps in the membrane, making them more flexible and allowing them to flow more readily into constricted areas of the microcirculation, thereby improving blood flow to tissues throughout the body. Ozone therapy also increases the level of oxygen in devitalized tissue. The health conditions described below benefit from ozone therapy.

High cholesterol. Studies have confirmed that ozone can reduce cholesterol in patients who have already suffered from angina, heart attacks, or strokes, as well as patients who have previously undergone bypass surgery. Ozone can lower the total cholesterol level within the bloodstream, thereby helping to reduce an important risk factor for heart attacks and strokes. A Cuban study examined the usefulness of ozone therapy in reducing cholesterol levels. This study, presented in 1993 at the Eleventh World Ozone Conference, examined the effect of ozone therapy on blood lipids in twenty-two adult males, aged forty-six to seventy-six. All of these individuals had suffered a heart attack during the previous year. They were given ozone treatments, administered intravenously, five days a week for a total of fifteen sessions. In all cases, there was an average decline in the total cholesterol of approximately 10 percent. Concentrations of LDL (low density lipoprotein) cholesterol, which is associated with heart disease, declined by an average of nearly 20 percent. Other studies have shown similarly positive changes in cholesterol levels with ozone therapy.

Heart disease. The therapeutic value of ozone therapy in the treatment of heart disease was confirmed in a Russian study presented in 1993 at the Eleventh World Ozone Conference. In this study, thirty-nine patients who had experienced symptoms due to lack of blood flow to the heart and brain were given ozone intravenously. Each patient received a total of five ozone treatments. Following these treatments, patients had significantly fewer episodes of angina and required only a third of their normal dosage of nitroglycerine, a medication given to dilate blood vessels. In addition, 82 percent of the patients reported an increased ability to tolerate physical activity, being half as likely to experience dizziness.

Other studies have found oxygen therapy to be useful for the treatment of strokes. When a stroke occurs, especially in older people, there is likely to be a deterioration in mental function and motor control. In a study conducted in Cuba and presented in 1993 at the Eleventh World Ozone Conference, 120 elderly patients, sixty-four males and fifty-six females, were given ozone rectally five days a week for three weeks. Patients were then evaluated for their level of social functioning and psychological health. Those patients with the most recent diagnosis showed the greatest improvement in their medical and mental symptoms: All of them improved, while 47 percent of the patients with long-term disease also showed improvement.

Peripheral vascular disease. Vascular disease reduces blood flow to the affected parts of the body, usually the extremities. Symptoms can include rapid tiring of the muscles and a sensation of coldness in these areas. Symptoms can advance to intermittent lameness or limping, pain, and even gangrene. Ozone therapy has been shown to be a highly effective therapy for this condition. An Austrian study published in *Circulation* assessed 232 patients grouped according to the stage of their peripheral vascular disease. Ozone was given intravenously and, in some cases, also applied directly to the affected limbs. Before treatment, the stage II patients, who normally suffered from pain due to poor blood flow to the limbs, were able to walk without pain for only 100 meters. After ozone therapy, this increased to 1000 meters. In stage III patients, at-rest and nightly pains were relieved in 70 percent of the cases following ozone therapy. Stage IV patients had severe vascular disease, in which breakdown of the tissues and even gangrene can occur. In this group, ozone treatment healed over 50 percent of the ulcers and soft-tissue gangrene and reduced the length of the patients' stay in the hospital. In another study, published in 1985 in *Australian Family Physician*, ozone therapy was used in the treatment of leg ulcers. The results of this study were also positive. After seventy-three patients were treated for four to six weeks, the researchers evaluated the lesions and found that fifty-nine patients showed evidence of healing, with only fourteen showing no response.

Hydrogen peroxide

Hydrogen peroxide also has therapeutic benefits for a variety of cardio-vascular and vascular diseases. Hydrogen peroxide dilates blood vessels both in the heart and in the general circulation. It increases the efficiency with which the heart works, lowering the resistance of the blood vessels so that blood can circulate more easily throughout the body. In cases of heart attacks, the use of hydrogen peroxide therapy can improve the chance of a patient being resuscitated. Hydrogen peroxide can also be used to treat tachycardia, or rapid heartbeat. It helps to slow the heart rate and can normalize an irregular heartbeat. Hydrogen peroxide has been used to treat ventricular fibrillation, a dangerous condition that can lead to fatalities.

Research studies investigating the therapeutic benefits of hydrogen peroxide therapy were conducted at Baylor University Medical Center, in Dallas, in the 1960s. In an animal study published in the *Journal of the New York Academy of Medicine*, dilute solutions of hydrogen peroxide, coupled with DMSO (dimethyl sulfoxide), were used to maintain the functioning of the heart despite the laboratory animals undergoing an ischemic episode, in which the heart tissue is deprived of oxygen. In another animal study, published in *Circulation*, hydrogen peroxide was able to reverse ventricular fibrillation or cardiac arrest when infused into the affected area, enabling the regular rhythm of the heart to be restored. In contrast, animals who were treated by standard methods could not be revived. In human studies, hydrogen peroxide therapy was also found to reduce arterial plaque.

Hyperbaric-oxygen therapy

Researchers have found that hyperbaric-oxygen therapy (HBOT) is a valuable treatment for patients who have suffered heart attacks. When used as part of an emergency treatment program, HBOT minimizes cell damage and can even prevent cell death by preventing edema (or fluid accumulation) within the heart cells. It also enhances the therapeutic benefits of clot-dissolving drugs like tissue plasminogen activator (TPA). HBOT also helps to relieve chest pain more rapidly than TPA alone in heart attack sufferers. Research studies conducted in the Soviet Union have found that HBOT also has cholesterol-lowering benefits, helps to normalize the heart rate and rhythm, and can even improve the ability of the heart to perform physical work.

One complication of advanced diabetes is impaired circulation to the extremities. In such cases, breakdown of the tissues can occur and foot ulcers can develop. In severe cases, amputation of the extremity may be necessary. An Italian study, published in 1996 in *Diabetes Care*, examined whether HBOT was able to arrest the progress of the disease and prevent amputation. The researchers divided sixty-eight diabetic patients into two groups, giving one group daily HBOT. All of the patients were given antibiotics and had their dead tissue surgically removed. The initial results of this study demonstrated the therapeutic value of hyperbaric-oxygen therapy, with only 9 percent of patients treated with HBOT requiring amputation above or below the knee. In contrast, 33 percent of those in the control group required amputation.

CANCER

Oxygen therapies have great potential for the treatment of many different types of cancer. Not only are some of these therapies useful in destroying tumors, but they are also used to counter some of the side effects of chemotherapy and repair tissue damaged by radiation. Early research in elucidating the role of oxygen in the development of cancer was done by Otto Warburg, a distinguished scientist. In 1931, Dr. Warburg won the Nobel prize for discovering that a deficiency of oxygen is a predisposing factor for the development of cancer within the body. In healthy cells, glucose is converted to energy in the presence of oxygen. However, cancer cells tend to be oxygen deficient and must use a more primitive form of metabolism called fermentation to meet their energy needs. A probable reason for this is that the mitochondria, the energy-producing organelles of the cells, are damaged in cancer cells. In fermentation, glucose is inefficiently metabolized and releases much smaller amounts of energy, with lactic acid generated as a by-product. This primitive form of metabolism is also seen in simple organisms like bacteria and fungi. A cancer cell may contain as much as ten times the lactic acid as a normal cell. Tumors thrive under these conditions of high acidity and low oxygen. It was thought that increasing the level of oxygen within the body could help prevent tumor growth. Since Warburg's initial discoveries, his work has been greatly amended. What is very clear is that there are great differences in the biochemistry of normal cells versus those that are malignant.

Ozone therapy

As early as 1910, ozone began to be used in the treatment of cancer. It appears to disrupt cancer cell metabolism, selectively blocking the multiplication of cancer cells while leaving normal cells unaffected. Ozone also increases the body's production of tumor necrosis factor, a chemical produced by the body that helps destroy cancers. This effect was investigated in a study done at the Institute of General Physiology, in Sienna, Italy. The results of this study were published in 1991 in *Lymphokine and Cytokine Research*. Researchers exposed blood samples to different concentrations of ozone for thirty seconds. Midrange concentrations stimulated tumor necrosis factor activity, while doses much higher or lower did not.

Ozone also generates the production of peroxides and free radicals as it breaks down into stable oxygen and a singlet oxygen, and this can lead to the breakdown of the cancer cell. Research has shown that, unlike normal cells, tumor cells are unable to inactivate peroxide, since they lack the necessary enzymes. Ozone also detoxifies many carcinogenic compounds that can enter the body and damage healthy cells, such as tar from cigarette smoke, soot from contaminated air, as well as chlorinated and nonchlorinated hydrocarbons that are components of alcohol and certain drugs. Ozone converts these substances into harmless compounds that can be eliminated from the body.

When used with conventional cancer treatment, ozone can counteract the adverse effects caused by these therapies. For example, ozone helps to heal tissue damage caused by radiation. Because it has a direct antitumor effect, ozone also enhances the effect of conventional treatments, reducing the amount of chemotherapy needed to achieve a reduction of the tumor mass. Finally, as an antiseptic, ozone lowers the risk of infection that can occur with cancer surgery.

In animal studies, ozone has successfully reversed various cancers. An ozone/oxygen mixture injected directly into mammary cancer in mice caused immediate cell death and increased the life span of the animals, according to a study published in 1985 in the *Journal of Holistic Medicine*. Another study, presented in 1989 at the Ninth World Ozone Conference, found that ozone treatment greatly reduced the number of lung cancers in mice. The antitumor effects of ozone have also been tested in the laboratory on cancer cells taken from breast, lung, and uterine cancers in human beings. In a study by Frederick Sweet, appearing in 1980 in *Science*, ozone was shown to selectively inhibit the growth of these cells while normal cells were unaffected. Low dosages of ozone, given over eight days, inhibited the growth of cancer by more than 90 percent. A German study, presented in 1989 at the Ninth World Ozone Conference, found that ozone improved the therapeutic effectiveness of chemotherapy after cancer cells had become resistant to this treatment. The researchers found that ozone in combination with 5-fluorouracil was able to kill a line of cells resistant to 5-fluorouracil alone.

In clinical practice, ozone is used as part of a comprehensive treatment program by complementary physicians in the United States. It is used for the treatment of a variety of tumors such as cancers of the lung, breast, stomach, liver, pancreas, kidney, bladder, adrenals, brain, prostate, colon, uterus, cervix, and ovary. It is also used to treat lymphomas, melanomas, sarcomas, and leukemias. The German surgeon Joachim Varro has had excellent results using ozone therapy with hundreds of cancer patients to reduce and even eliminate the side effects commonly seen with surgery and radiation therapy. He has found that when ozone therapy is used in combination with standard therapies, the spread of cancer is arrested for longer periods of time and the survival time of patients is lengthened. He found this to be true even in cases of inoperable cancer and cancers not responding to radiation therapy. In addition, Varro reported that patients had more energy, better appetite, and experienced less pain when they were treated with ozone therapy. Many of his patients who received ozone therapy soon after having surgery were able to return to work full-time. Another German physician, Horst Kief, treated thirty-one patients with intravenous ozone therapy. These patients had been diagnosed with a variety of tumors, including carcinomas, lymphomas, and sarcomas. Ninety percent of these patients reported an improvement in vitality and quality of life, and 70 percent had less pain as a result of the treatment. Ozone has also been used as an adjunct therapy in the treatment for cancers of the female reproductive tract, such as endometrial cancer, ovarian cancer, and cervical cancer. Intravenous ozone is especially valuable, but vaginal and rectal ozone has been used as well. The French physician Jean-Claude Delafons has used ozone therapy in his practice to treat cervical cancer. In one case study, intravenous injection of ozone over a six-week period reduced the size of the tumor.

Hydrogen peroxide

Hydrogen peroxide's antitumor effect is thought to be due, in part, to its ability to promote the release of tumor necrosis factor, a chemical produced by the body that helps destroy cancer cells. Tumor necrosis factor is a cytokine (cytokines are biochemical messengers that play an active role in the healing process, helping to regulate immune functions and inflammation). Other cytokines, such as interleukin-2 and interferon, also help to destroy cancer cells. Hydrogen peroxide also stimulates the production of natural killer cells, which prevent cancer cells from spreading. There is even evidence that hydrogen peroxide directly kills tumor cells.

In animal studies, hydrogen peroxide has been found to be a very powerful cancer-fighting agent. In a study conducted at the Rockefeller University, in New York, published in 1981 in the *Journal of Experimental Medicine*, cancerous mice were injected with a solution of hydrogen peroxide. Tumor cells were then collected and assessed. These researchers observed that hydrogen peroxide contributed to the breaking apart of the tumor cells, with no harm done to the animal itself.

Physicians who use hydrogen peroxide for the treatment of cancer have found that hydrogen peroxide can cause a significant reduction in tumor size and even lead to complete recovery in some cases. Research involving hydrogen peroxide and its applications to the treatment of cancer were conducted at Baylor University Medical Center in Dallas. One of these studies was published in 1962 in the *Southern Medical Journal*. In this study, researchers reported that hydrogen peroxide was found to be a useful adjunct to radiation therapy for the treatment of cancer in both laboratory animals and humans. As oxygen levels increased through hydrogen peroxide therapy, the cancer cells became more sensitive to destruction by radiation. Another study done by Baylor University researchers also found that hydrogen peroxide could cause large abdominal tumors to shrink in size, making them easier to treat surgically.

Hyperbaric-oxygen therapy

Hyperbaric-oxygen therapy (HBOT) can greatly increase the level of oxygen in the body by delivering it under pressure. HBOT is used to heal tissue that has been damaged by radiation therapy: It is administered only after chemotherapy or radiation therapy has been completed and the patient is free of active cancer, since certain cancers can proliferate in the presence of oxygen. Trish Planck is the founder of the Hyperbaric Clinic of Santa Monica, in California, and the Hyperbaric Clinic of Nevada, in Reno. In a conversation with Planck, she explained that hyperbaric-oxygen therapy can be used to revive tissue virtually anywhere in the body, including bone tissue and tissues of the throat and face. Cancers of the head and neck can be terribly disfiguring, requiring reconstructive surgery. Patients who have been treated for cancer will come to Planck's clinic for HBOT before having reconstructive surgery done in order to improve the health of their tissues. HBOT is then also administered after surgery to promote healing of the surgical wounds. Hyperbaric-oxygen therapy can also be used to counteract the debilitating effects of chemotherapy and help restore a patient's level of general health so that healing can proceed more efficiently.

BONE AND JOINT DISEASES

Oxygen therapies have been used to help heal a wide variety of bone and joint diseases including osteoporosis, arthritis, and arthrosis (a degenerative disease involving the breakdown of the joints).

Osteoporosis

Osteoporosis is a common degenerative disease, affecting as many as one-third of all American women. It is a condition in which mineral loss from the bones results in a reduction in bone mass. Osteoporosis significantly increases the risk of bone fractures in the elderly. While this condition was relatively rare at the turn of the century, the incidence of osteoporosis, particularly in postmenopausal women, has grown to near epidemic proportions. Hormone replacement therapy, weight-bearing exercise, diet, and calcium supplementation are usually prescribed to slow the progress of the disease. However, recent research suggests that ozone therapy may also help to increase bone density.

One such study was done by E. Rive Sanseverino, of the University of Bologna, Italy. His findings were published in 1988 in the journal *Europa Medicophysica*. In this study, a total of 225 women with the disease were divided into three treatment groups. Group A received only prescription drugs like hormones. Group B received the same treatments as group A plus ozone treatments administered intravenously. Group C received both of the above treatments and were also given an exercise program. Ozone treatments were administered twice a week for six weeks, with this regimen repeated three times a year. Patient progress was assessed by successive measurements of bone density. The researchers found that bone density increased with the more therapies a patient received. Drug therapy combined with ozone treatments and exercise was found to be the most beneficial. A combination of hormone therapy and ozone also produced a reduction in bone pain after only three to four weeks of treatment.

Rheumatoid arthritis

Rheumatoid arthritis is an inflammatory disease of the joints that typically affects small joints like those in the fingers and wrists. The disease tends to be chronic and progressive and can result in crippling deformities. Common symptoms include pain, swelling, stiffness, and decreased mobility of the joints. When used for the treatment of rheumatoid arthritis, ozone has been found to be more effective than anti-inflammatory drugs, resulting in less pain, stiffness, and swelling and greater strength, according to a report presented at the Eleventh World Ozone Conference in 1993. In research conducted in Germany, ozone therapy was compared with the drugs traditionally used to treat this disease, such as immuno-suppressive agents and anti-inflammatory steroids. Ozone was found to be more effective than conventional antiarthritic therapy. Patients treated with ozone initially reported symptom relief, with more than a 50 percent decrease in pain. Several weeks later, there was also a reduction in laboratory indicators of inflammation.

Symptoms of gouty arthritis can also be reduced with ozone therapy, according to a study presented in 1989 at the Ninth World Ozone Conference. There was a significant improvement in patients who were treated with intravenous ozone for eight to ten sessions over four to six weeks, plus ozone injections once or twice a week. These patients had reduced morning stiffness and less inflammation of the joint.

Osteoarthritis

Osteoarthritis is characterized by a progressive deterioration of the cartilage that cushions the joint. With age and excessive wear and tear, the cartilage can literally wear away. This condition occurs mostly in older people and in obese individuals. Osteoarthritis can also develop due to repeated injury or overuse of a joint. This can occur in individuals engaged in heavy physical labor and also in those people who participate in sports such as football where traumatic injuries are common. In studies of osteoarthritis involving the knee, injections of ozone into the joint resulted in symptom relief in nearly all patients. Symptom relief is rapid, often occurring after the first few sessions. Ozone treatment produces a reduction in inflammation, greater mobility of the affected joint, and a disappearance of pain.

Arthrosis

Arthrosis is a degenerative disease that occurs in joints. The use of ozone as a treatment for this condition has been researched in Cuba. One Cuban study was presented in 1991 at the Tenth World Ozone Conference. This study involved 234 arthrosis patients, many of whom had tried conventional treatments with poor results. They were given intramuscular injections of a low concentration of ozone daily for ten days, followed by treatment three times a week up to a total of twenty sessions. Pain relief was dramatic with ozone therapy. Eighty-nine percent of volunteers reported having almost total relief of their pain symptoms, while 10 percent experienced a reduction in pain. Ozone therapy was ineffective in only 1 percent of the patients. The analgesic benefits of ozone were noticeable after the third treatment session. If symptoms or pain recurred, an additional four to six injections, given twice a week, were often sufficient to eliminate the pain. Signs of inflammation were also reduced.

Hydrogen peroxide

Hydrogen peroxide has also been used successfully to treat diseases of the bones and joints. A leading exponent of hydrogen peroxide therapy, Charles H. Farr, has treated several thousand patients with hydrogen peroxide and has found it to be highly beneficial, especially when injected into trigger points in soft tissues and joints. He has also injected nerves, ligaments, tendons, and muscles, when indicated, with hydrogen peroxide. Hydrogen peroxide works quickly to relieve the pain associated with rheumatoid arthritis, providing symptom relief in twelve hours to seven days. Inflammation responds more slowly and requires one or two weeks to resolve. Most patients require only one injection or, at most, two. Furthermore, Dr. Farr has found that in 98 percent of cases, there have been no side effects or complications. Many physicians specializing in sports medicine also report rapid healing of injured tissues with injections of hydrogen peroxide.

GASTROINTESTINAL DISORDERS

Ozone therapy has been used to treat a variety of intestinal complaints, including diarrhea caused by food poisoning, microorganisms, and parasitic infections. It is an important complementary treatment for food poisoning due to *Staphylococcus aureus*. This is the organism that can develop in picnic foods such as potato salad and cold fried chicken that are left in a warm place for a period of time. Ozone also counteracts food poisoning from *E. coli*, a common toxin in restaurant and processed food due to human fecal contamination. Ozone is also used for the treatment of irritable-bowel syndrome, ulcerative colitis, Crohn's disease, and duodenal ulcers. Celiac disease, a condition due to sensitivity to gluten (the protein found in wheat), can also be treated with ozone therapy, along with eliminating gluten from the diet.

A large study was conducted on the medical use of ozone to alleviate the symptoms of a nonbacterial form of gastroenteritis (a condition in which the intestinal tract and stomach are inflamed) in children. Diarrhea is a common symptom of this condition. In this study, 2757 children, with ages ranging from one month to 18 years, were divided into four groups. The largest group, 1932 children, were treated with an ozone/oxygen mixture administered rectally. The remaining children were divided into three control groups, receiving either a restricted diet, rectal insufflation with room air, or rectal insufflation with oxygen. The results of this study clearly demonstrated the effectiveness of ozone. Diarrhea persisted in those children treated with diet alone, room air, or oxygen, and continued for three to six days after the treatment ended. In contrast, all of the children treated with ozone had no further diarrhea after undergoing ozone therapy. Diarrhea caused by bacteria also responds well to ozone therapy. Ozone is given either as ozonated drinking water, by rectal insufflation (or enema), or, if infection is systemic, administered intravenously. Fluids and electrolytes are also provided, to reestablish acid/alkaline balance, since diarrhea can cause the loss of electrolytes such as sodium and chloride through the bowel.

DISEASES OF THE LIVER AND PANCREAS

Certain diseases of the liver and pancreas respond to ozone therapy, including hepatitis and acute pancreatitis due to alcohol abuse. Habitual overconsumption of alcohol can impair liver function in susceptible individuals. Symptoms include loss of appetite, nausea, vomiting, and tenderness in the upper-right abdomen, as well as achiness of the muscles and joints. In some cases, hepatitis does not resolve, and chronic liver disease can develop. If this continues, a condition called cirrhosis can occur. In cirrhosis, chronic inflammation of liver cells gradually leads to permanent damage. This disease is usually fatal. Ozone can be administered rectally, in small amounts, to treat these various types of liver disease. With rectal insufflations, ozone is absorbed through the mucosa of the colon and is carried through the portal circulation to the liver. Ozone also improves the liver's detoxification capability. In addition, rectal ozone can be used to treat hemorrhoids related to poor liver function. About 80 percent of the cases of acute pancreatitis are also triggered by excessive alcohol intake. With this condition, the pancreas becomes inflamed, and the pancreatic enzymes, normally carried to the small intestine, begin to digest cells of the pancreas instead. Ozone helps to reduce and limit pancreatic inflammation.

MULTIPLE SCLEROSIS

Multiple sclerosis (MS) is an autoimmune disorder in which the protective covering of the nerves, the myelin sheath, is destroyed. Damage occurs in a patchy fashion throughout the brain and spinal cord. Richard A. Neubauer, director of the Ocean Hyperbaric Center in Lauderdale-by-the-Sea, Florida, has successfully treated MS with hyperbaric-oxygen therapy (HBOT). There are plentiful case histories attesting to the effectiveness of HBOT. By Dr. Neubauer's count, 12,000 MS patients in fourteen countries have been treated with HBOT, plus 1,500 of his own patients, whom he has treated over a period of twelve years. While not a cure for MS, HBOT does help to stabilize the disease. Dr. Neubauer has documented relief of pain as well as improvement in bladder control, mobility, coordination, vision, and speech. He has witnessed rapid improvement, including a patient who arrived for her first appointment in a battery-powered cart, and after three hours of oxygen treatment, was able to walk out using crutches. An average course of therapy, usually consisting of twenty sessions, is administered at a frequency of one or two treatments per month.

HEADACHES

Oxygen therapy has been shown to be of benefit in treating cluster headaches. Cluster headaches are seen in one out of every 250 men and with less frequency in women. They tend to be more prevalent in hard-driving men with type A personalities. Typically, a cluster headache is one-sided and occurs in a series of episodes usually lasting a half hour. Symptoms include severe pain, tearing, congestion, and redness of the face. Breathing pure oxygen can help to arrest these headaches when they first occur. Breathing pure oxygen for fifteen to twenty minutes, at seven to ten liters per minute, is usually sufficient to relieve symptoms. However, this treatment should not be continued for longer than an hour. Researchers studying the use of oxygen therapy report that breathing pure oxygen can prevent a cluster headache from developing in 80 percent of the cases.

Eye Diseases

As a person ages, eyesight often deteriorates. While this may require nothing more than wearing reading glasses, some people are faced with eye problems that are far more serious. One such condition is age-related macular degeneration (AMD), which refers to the loss of vision that occurs in old age when the macula (the central part of the retina) is damaged. The macula is composed of a layer of cells located at the back of the eye that functions like film in a camera. Light passes through the front parts of the eye, such as the lens and iris, which focus this light. Cells in the retina register both light and color. The macula makes possible sharp, detailed vision and enhances color perception.

In most cases, this damage is due to the breakdown of cells in the macula that are sensitive to light, but in a small percentage of cases, AMD can be caused by blood vessels that leak within the eye. A person with AMD will have difficulty reading, driving, and even recognizing the faces of people they know well. Such loss can impinge on every area of performance. AMD can be treated by laser surgery, but only if it is caught in the first few weeks after its onset. Some cases of AMD have also been successfully treated with ozone, according to a study published in 1990 in *Panminerva Medica*. This study involved twenty patients with AMD. Ozone was administered intravenously during two treatment periods, one lasting a month and the other lasting six weeks, with a month in between when no treatment was given. Patients were assessed by testing for visual acuity as well as the circulation of the eye. Nine of the patients experienced an improvement in visual acuity of about 40 percent, while the other patients showed no improvement. However, all of the patients, including those without an improvement in their vision, reported an increase in their well-being, with indicators such as appetite, sleep, mood, muscle tone, mental concentration, and work capacity improving with the ozone treatments.

Other studies have indicated that ozone can be useful in the treatment of retinitis pigmentosa, a chronic progressive disease that begins in early childhood. In this condition, cells in the retina degenerate, and the optic nerve atrophies. Loss of vision can result. Ozone therapy has been found to either improve this condition or arrest the deterioration in many of the individuals treated.

SKIN CONDITIONS

Ozone therapy has been used to treat a wide variety of skin problems, including such common problems as eczema and psoriasis. Ozone is usually applied topically by wrapping the affected portion of the body in an ozone-resistant plastic bag. An ozone/oxygen mixture is then pumped into this bag to treat conditions such as skin rashes and gangrene. Another way of administering ozone is by pumping the gas into water in which the patient then bathes. Some practitioners also ozonate sunflower or olive oil, which is then rubbed on the skin.

At the Eleventh World Ozone Conference, held in 1993, a German physician, Horst Kief, reported on his successful use of ozone therapy on three patients with neurodermatitis. This condition is characterized by skin rashes and intense itching. These patients were treated for four weeks, with 90 percent of the patients going into full remission. Ozone is also used for the treatment of viral conditions of the skin or mucous membranes such as herpes infections and warts, bacterial skin infections such as impetigo, and fungal infections in areas such as toenails.

DENTAL HEALTH AND DENTISTRY

As a disinfectant and sterilizing agent, ozone has many applications in treating dental problems. Ozonated water was first used in 1920 to reduce inflammation in the mouth. It can be applied directly to diseased areas of the mouth as well as used to cleanse dental equipment. Fritz Kramer, a pioneer in the use of ozone therapy in dental practice, gives ozonated water as a mouth rinse to cleanse and disinfect the tissues between the teeth in cases of gingivitis (an inflammation of the gums characterized by swelling, redness, and a tendency to bleed). He also uses it to treat individuals with yeast infections of the mouth, and when the mouth in general is inflamed (stomatitis).

During dental procedures, Dr. Kramer works with ozone to disinfect and cleanse cavities when treating tooth decay. He also uses it when capping teeth, as well as when performing root canals and during dental surgery. Healing of tissues in the mouth is also accelerated, since oxygen levels are increased within the oral cavity. Several studies have been published in which ozone has been used to sterilize dental equipment, as well as to disinfect the water and air used to rinse and dry the patient's mouth.

Another report, presented in 1993 at the Eleventh World Ozone Conference, described the usefulness of ozone as a disinfectant for dental impressions. The material used to make dental impressions is alginate, which is derived from kelp, a type of seaweed. Alginate absorbs water from conventional antiseptic solutions. Researchers exposed alginate impressions to bacteria, and then treated a portion of these with ozonated water for twenty-five minutes. The ozone-treated alginate was free of bacteria, while the untreated alginate showed a wide spectrum of bacterial growth.

The use of hydrogen peroxide, in a 3 percent solution, has been a popular home remedy to retard plaque and gingivitis. Studies show that hydrogen peroxide, taken as a mouthwash, prevents the colonization and multiplication of many kinds of bacteria and retards plaque formation. People using hydrogen peroxide mouthwash and toothpastes report that their mouths feel fresher and cleaner after doing so.

SUMMARY

Oxygen therapies have been shown to be effective in helping to alleviate a wide range of health conditions, including a number of infectious diseases, circulatory problems, cancer, bone and joint diseases, gastrointestinal disorders, diseases of the liver and pancreas, multiple sclerosis, cluster headaches, eye diseases, and some skin conditions, and have also been found useful in dentistry.

LABORATORY TESTS FOR OXYGEN LEVELS

Direct testing of oxygen levels in the blood is not done routinely on normal healthy people. Such tests are given only in a hospital for patients with serious diseases such as chronic lung disease. However, several tests that can be done in an office setting on an outpatient basis assess lung capacity and the relative health of the lungs. One test is the forced vital capacity (FVC). This is the measurement of the amount of air that can be exhaled after taking a deep breath. The lower a person's FVC, the less functional capability the lungs possess. This test also appears to be a good indicator of the general level of health and vigor of a person's body, as well as a biomarker of aging. Another test is the maximal oxygen uptake, or VO_2max. This refers to the greatest amount of oxygen that one can take in during vigorous exercise. For a man, on average, this declines by approximately 1 percent a year beginning in his thirties. At age thirty, a man is likely to be able to inhale 6 quarts of air with each breath, 5.4 quarts at age forty, 4.5 quarts at age fifty, 3.6 quarts at age sixty, and 3 quarts at age seventy. Thus, between the ages of thirty and seventy, VO_2max can decline by as much as half. However, if they stay physically fit throughout their lives, athletes can maintain their VO_2max without showing the normal age-related declines. Both of these tests can provide a good assessment of one's ability to take oxygen into the body.

8

RESTORING YOUR OXYGEN LEVELS

HAVING SUFFICIENT OXYGEN is necessary for every peak performance trait discussed in this book. In addition, sustaining optimal health is virtually impossible without adequate oxygenation. This chapter outlines a four-part plan to help you boost the oxygen in your tissues and cells to peak-performance levels: (1) Use oxygen therapies to supplement your body's own level of oxygen; (2) take antioxidants such as vitamin E, vitamin C, and beta-carotene so that oxygen therapies can be used safely and without side effects; (3) use other nutritional supplements to reinforce the benefits of oxygen therapies;* and (4) develop oxygen-healthy habits, such as eating an oxygen-rich diet, doing regular aerobic exercise, practicing deep breathing, and practicing stress reduction techniques. These good habits will help to increase your intake of oxygen and optimize its transport and delivery to your cells and tissues.

PART 1:
OXYGEN THERAPIES

THIS SECTION PROVIDES specific, detailed information on how to use and administer various types of oxygen therapy on a self-care basis. It also describes the conditions for which oxygen therapy can be used most

---

* Anyone beginning a nutritional supplement program should begin at one-quarter to one-half the recommended dosages given in this book. They can then increase their dosages slowly over the course of several weeks until they have reached either the full recommended dosage or a dosage that is therapeutic for them—whichever level comes first. Some individuals will experience therapeutic benefits at doses that are well below the doses recommended in this book. Also, while the dosages provided in this chapter are appropriate for most people, there are certain groups who should continue to use less than the recommended dosages. Children, the elderly, and individuals with a frail constitution or who are extremely sensitive to drugs and nutritional supplements usually do best at therapeutic dosages of no more than half the recommended levels. Consult your physician or nutritional consultant if you have any questions about the advisability of using a particular nutritional supplement or to determine the dosage most appropriate for you.

effectively and safely in a home or office setting, as well as when these therapies should be administered in a clinical setting by a qualified health care professional.

PURE OXYGEN

Pure oxygen is usually administered, on the recommendation of a physician, to patients with chronic lung diseases such as emphysema and chronic bronchitis. In these conditions, there is structural damage to the lungs and destruction of the lung tissue, which reduce the ability to breathe in oxygen from the surrounding air. In addition, individuals with chronic lung disease are unable to exhale carbon dioxide efficiently, which further reduces the oxygen levels within the body and causes acidosis. Pure-oxygen therapy is also prescribed by some physicians for the treatment of painful cluster headaches.

Oxygen is usually supplied by a tank that can be rented from a medical supply store or hospital. The oxygen is inhaled either through a tube inserted into the nose or by using a mask. Unlike the air we breathe, which contains only about 20 percent oxygen along with other gases, medical-grade oxygen is supplied to patients in its pure form as 100 percent oxygen. When used to treat headaches, pure oxygen is breathed at seven to ten liters per minute for up to twenty minutes, not to exceed more than one hour per day.

Some healthy individuals with access to pure oxygen, such as airplane pilots, have discovered its performance-enhancing benefits and may use it occasionally to relieve fatigue, boost energy, and even help recover from a hangover after a night of excessive drinking. (Oxygen helps the liver metabolize alcohol more quickly and efficiently.)

OZONE THERAPY

Ozone therapy is one of the most powerful oxygenating techniques available, providing the body with large amounts of supplemental oxygen. Individuals whose careers, avocations, or participation in sports require that their bodies be extremely well-oxygenated should consider using ozone for its superoxygenating benefits. This can easily be done on a self-care basis through the use of various types of ozone-generating equipment. Ozone air-purification machines can be used to purify and clean the air you breathe, and ozone water-purification devices can remove chlo-rine from tap water and increase the oxygen content of your drinking water. You can also increase the level of oxygen in your body through bathing in water that has been enriched with ozone/oxygen mixtures. You can do this while soaking in bathtubs, spas, and hot tubs.

Complementary physicians who use ozone in their treatment regi-mens can administer it in a variety of ways. As a medical treatment, ozone has several benefits. Not only does ozone increase the level of oxygen within the body but, because the ozone molecule is unstable, consisting of three oxygen atoms bonded together, it rapidly reverts back to stable oxy-gen, or O_2. In the process, it releases a singlet oxygen. And this singlet oxy-gen has powerful antibacterial, antiviral, antitumor, antiarthritic, and circulation-promoting benefits.

Ozone air-purification machines

Traditionally, people have used air filters as well as spray and wick prod-ucts to clean indoor air. However, none of these methods have proved to be particularly useful. Spray and wick products consist of perfumed chemicals, which can cause sensitivity reactions in allergic individuals. Air filters have proven to be only partially effective in cleansing and purifying the air. In contrast, ozone air-purification devices are extremely effective in destroying and eliminating airborne pollutants, fumes, tobacco smoke, mold, fungi, bacteria, and viruses from homes, offices, and industrial plants. These devices can also be very effective in eliminating airborne chemicals and fumes from beauty salons, animal shelters, and smoke-filled conference centers and hotel rooms. Many individuals are extremely sen-sitive to chemicals such as formaldehyde that outgas from new carpeting, drapes, and furniture in apartments, homes, and office buildings. Outgassing can cause flulike symptoms (achiness, chills, nasal congestion, and sneezing) as well as indigestion, brain fog, and fatigue in susceptible individuals. The use of an ozone air-purification machine can be enor-mously helpful if you are forced to work or live in such a setting. For example, ozone is one of the few substances we know of that can be used to treat petrochemical-based pollutants, which are converted by ozone into the less harmful substances carbon dioxide and water.

Ozone is generated through relatively inexpensive and portable equipment that can clean as much as 1500 square feet of space for home use. More powerful generators can be used for even larger areas, up to 2500 square feet. Ozone machines should not be placed on the floor. Since ozone is heavier than air, it will circulate better if the air-purification machine is placed on an elevated surface. When an ozone molecule encounters a pollutant or pathogenic organism such as bacteria, one of the oxygen atoms will break away from the ozone molecule and attach itself to the pollutant or pathogen, thereby destroying it through the process of oxidation.

Air that has been ozonated smells incredibly pure and fresh; individuals who use these generators often comment on the improved air quality of their home or office. We have been using an ozone air-purification machine at home for nearly a decade. We frequently lend it to friends who suffer from recurrent respiratory infections due to mold and mildew in their homes or who have moved to new homes furnished with outgassing materials. Every one of these individuals has commented on how much better they felt after using the machine for two or three weeks, and they have all bought their own units. Our friends have commented to us that the quality of their home or office air is improved and that they are sleeping better. They have also found that nasal congestion is reduced or eliminated, brain fog has cleared, and their resistance to allergies or respiratory infections is strengthened.

▲▲ Ozone is extremely effective in quickly eliminating fumes from cars when chemicals used as cleaning agents have been applied to interior surfaces and upholstery. Simply place the ozone generator on the seat of your car and run an extension cord from your house or office to the ozone machine. Close all of the car windows, and run the ozone generator for several hours. You will be amazed at how effectively ozone eliminates noxious chemicals from the interior of your car.

▲▲ Companies whose offices are located in hermetically sealed buildings or have production plants that generate chemical pollutants and fumes should consider using ozone equipment to improve the air quality and, therefore, the energy level and productivity of their personnel. Everyone, including management, office employees, and plant workers, can benefit from the use of ozone air purifiers.

▲▲ Businesspeople who are required to travel frequently as well as individuals who travel often for pleasure should consider taking a portable ozone machine with them for use in hotel rooms. Many hotel rooms contain residual cigarette smoke from previous guests as well as fumes from the strong chemicals used to clean these rooms. In addition, the windows of many hotel rooms are sealed and cannot be opened to let fresh air circulate.

▲▲ Occasionally, individuals with severe allergies to molds, pollen, dust, or airborne pollutants may find that breathing the ozone generated by an air-purification machine can be somewhat irritating. In such cases, it is preferable to run the machine when you are away from your home or office. The machine can run safely for many hours, clearing the air of pollutants or fumes, while you are off-site. It can then be turned off when you return.

Ozone water-purification devices

Many people are concerned about the health of their drinking water. Municipal water is treated with chemicals such as chlorine, a common water disinfectant, to reduce the level of dangerous pathogens. Unfortunately, exposure to these chemicals may be equally dangerous to your health. For example, chlorine combines with organic matter to form substances like trihalomethanes, which are carcinogenic. In addition, trace amounts of toxic metals like aluminum can also be found in our water supplies.

Ozone water-purification units can be used as sinktop devices to clean the water coming out of your kitchen or bathroom faucet. Larger units can also be installed to clean the entire water supply of your house. Not only is ozonated water as effective (if not more so) than chlorine in killing pathogenic organisms, but it will eliminate the chlorine itself as well as undesirable heavy metals. Ozone causes heavy metals to clump or flocculate, which allows them to be filtered out of your drinking water more readily. Ozonated water also removes unpleasant odors and has a clean, pure taste. In addition, ozone rapidly converts back into pure oxygen, thereby increasing the oxygen level of the water itself. (Ozone has a half-life of only twenty to forty minutes.) Over 3000 cities worldwide, including Moscow and Los Angeles, now use ozone to disinfect their water supplies.

Many people find that the chlorine and bromine used to disinfect and clean their swimming pools, spas, and hot tubs are irritating to their skin and eyes. These chemicals also tend to dry the skin and hair, causing hair to split and break more easily. Ozone can be used instead to keep the water in pools and spas clean and fresh. The ozone is usually generated by passing air into a sealed chamber across an ultraviolet light source. The ultraviolet light will convert some of the oxygen in the air to ozone. This ozone-enriched air is then discharged into the pool or spa water. Using ozone can reduce the need to use pool chemicals like chlorine or bromine by 50 to 90 percent, depending on the size of the ozone generator. In addition, since ozone tends to cause particulate matter to clump or flocculate, it can be readily cleaned out by the pool or spa filter, thus allowing the water to remain clear and clean.

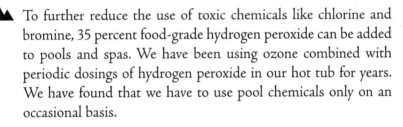 To further reduce the use of toxic chemicals like chlorine and bromine, 35 percent food-grade hydrogen peroxide can be added to pools and spas. We have been using ozone combined with periodic dosings of hydrogen peroxide in our hot tub for years. We have found that we have to use pool chemicals only on an occasional basis.

Small portable ozone generators that can be attached to your bathtub are now available. These generators can be used to neutralize the chlorine and allow you to bathe in superoxygenated water. Since ozone/oxygen mixtures can be absorbed through the skin, bathing in highly oxygenated water is tremendously healthful, particularly when done on a regular basis. See also pages 411 and 412 for other techniques, such as the use of ozonating spas, saunas, or ozone body bags and body suits. These methods also permit absorption of ozone/oxygen mixtures through the skin and can help to increase one's physical and mental energy.

Ozone generators for medical treatment

Medical ozone generators have been used to treat various diseases since the turn of the century. Much of the pioneering work on the use of medical ozone was done by physicians in Germany. During World War I, ozone was used by the German army to treat battle wounds and severe infections. It was in Germany that the first medical ozone generators were developed that could accurately produce ozone within specific therapeutic dosage ranges. Currently, ozone therapy is used medically in countries throughout the world for the treatment of infectious diseases, circulatory diseases, cancer, arthritis, and AIDS, to name but a few conditions. Clinics using ozone are found in such diverse locales as certain states within the United States, Europe, Russia, and Cuba.

While medical-grade ozone generators have not yet been approved by the FDA for specific health care conditions, these devices are sold by a number of companies and are generally available. Ozone generators can be sold to clinics, physicians, and even consumers within the United States as long as the companies that sell the machines do not make medical claims for their use. However, physicians and clinics in states such as New York, Alaska, and South Carolina, among others, are permitted to administer ozone to patients. These states have passed freedom-of-practice laws that allow consumers access to any potentially effective treatment. As a result, some physicians in these states now offer ozone therapy as part of their treatment regimens.

Medical-grade ozone is generated by a device that passes pure oxygen through a closed chamber. The oxygen is then converted into ozone by passing 100 percent pure oxygen across either an ultraviolet light source or an electrical arc. This will convert a small amount of the oxygen into ozone. Normally, 1 to 5 percent is converted for medical use. Lower concentrations, between 1 and 3 percent, enhance circulation and help to heal wounds. Higher concentrations, between 4 and 5 percent, act as a disinfectant, cleanse wounds, and inhibit cell division. The amount of ozone generated depends on how much oxygen flows past the electrical arc or ultraviolet light, the voltage, and the distance between the arcs. The oxygen is provided either by a tank containing 100 percent pure, medical-grade oxygen or by an oxygen concentrator, a device that can extract oxygen from the environmental air at about 92 to 95 percent efficiency. The oxygen is then passed through a plastic tube to the ozone generator. As the ozone/oxygen mixture is created, it flows from the ozone machine through a second, outflow tube to the user.

Buying and Using an Ozone Generator

If you are considering buying an ozone generator for your personal use, be sure to buy a machine that is made of stainless steel, Teflon, or glass parts. No medical-grade ozone generator should be manufactured with any other metal besides stainless steel (which is ozone-resistant). This is particularly true of the chamber in which ozone is formed. All other metals, like aluminum and copper, will react chemically with ozone and can cause toxic accumulation of these metals within the body.

Ozone-resistant tubing should be used for the outflow tube that transports the ozone/oxygen to the user. Do not use the tubing commonly found in hardware stores. Much of this tubing is made of polyvinyl chloride, or PVC. Ozone will cause PVC to leach out of the tubing, which is definitely not desirable. Reputable dealers will usually provide consumers with ozone-resistant tubing.

Ozone is normally administered in an ozone/oxygen mixture containing between 1 to 5 percent ozone. When administered in this concentration, ozone is exceptionally safe to use. A 1993 study presented at the Eleventh World Ozone Conference evaluated the dosage at which damage to blood cells becomes visible after treatment by various concentrations of ozone. In this study, samples of blood were exposed to different concentrations of ozone for 45 seconds and then examined under an electron microscope, which provides detailed visualization of the blood cell membrane and its internal structure. Structural damage to the blood cells was clearly visible at concentrations of 9 percent ozone and higher. However, this is much greater than the percentage of ozone normally used in medical therapies, thus providing a wide margin of safety in its use. Moreover, the concentration of ozone produced by an ozone generator can be carefully controlled through proper use of the machine.

How ozone is administered to the body

Ozone can be administered to the body through various methods. While many of these methods are appropriate only when applied in a medical setting, several can be done safely on a self-care basis.

Major and minor autohemotherapy. In a clinical setting or medical office, ozone is often administered via an intravenous drip. When this technique was first developed in Germany, it was called major or minor autohemotherapy. A small amount of blood is removed from the patient's body. An ozone/oxygen mixture is then added to the blood, which is then returned to the patient's body via an intravenous drip. The difference between major and minor autohemotherapy depends on the amount of blood withdrawn from the body. Fifty to 100 ml is often withdrawn for major autohemotherapy, and 10 ml for minor autohemotherapy. This technique has been one of the most widely used historically. The indication for its use are manifold and include the treatment of viral infections, hepatitis, asthma, allergies, diabetes, arteriosclerotic vascular disease, hyperlipidemia, carcinomas, postmenopausal osteoporosis, and arthritis. Its drawbacks are that it is cumbersome and requires that the patient be injected several times by needles, which many people dislike.

Direct intravenous injections. Direct intravenous injections of ozone/oxygen mixtures are as effective as autohemotherapy and bypass the need to remove blood from the body and reinject it back after it has been ozonated. This method of treatment dates back to 1935 and was initially used in Germany to treat both venous and arterial circulatory problems such as intermittent claudication and cerebrovascular insufficiency. This method can also be used to treat a wide variety of health conditions. By injecting the gas mixture directly into the general blood circulation, ozone can be used to treat cancer, arthritis, infectious diseases, inflammatory conditions, pain syndromes, and deficiency states of the glands and organs. The ozone/oxygen mixture must be injected very slowly into the circulation to avoid side effects. Although the incidence of side effects is extremely low with any type of ozone application, studies suggest that intravenous application presents the greatest possibility of risk (although even this is very small).

Intramuscular injections. Ozone/oxygen mixtures can be administered by intramuscular injection. With this method, a small amount, up to 10 ml, is injected, usually into the buttocks. These injections are normally administered to patients suffering from inflammatory diseases or cancer.

To avoid causing pain, it is important that the injections be administered very slowly.

Intra-articular applications. Ozone administered in this fashion is usually done for orthopedic conditions such as joint problems as well as arthritis and arthrosis (a degenerative disease involving a progressive breakdown of cartilage in the joints and spine). Ozone can be injected directly into joints such as the hip, wrist, and knee. Orthopedic physicians in Europe use intra-articular ozone with beneficial therapeutic results.

Rectal insufflations. With this method, an ozone/oxygen mixture is infused slowly and gently into the large bowel through a flexible plastic intravenous bag. Ozone gas is diffused into the colon through a sterile tip inserted into the rectum. The intravenous bag is then slowly compressed, which empties the ozone/oxygen mixture into the colon. Research studies have shown that the ozone/oxygen mixture diffuses through the colon wall and is distributed into the general circulation, thereby increasing the level of oxygen within the body. Elevated levels of oxygen as high as 250 percent above normal have been recorded in the intestinal wall, venous blood, and portal vein, as well as the liver. Other research studies have documented that the oxygen content of the general blood circulation increases after rectal applications. Ozone insufflations have therapeutic benefits for people suffering from a variety of gastrointestinal problems, including cancer of the colon, irritable-bowel syndrome, ulcerative colitis, hemorrhoids, constipation, and diarrhea. It is also a very effective treatment for cancer of the prostate, other prostate conditions, and male impotence since it enhances blood flow and oxygenation to the penis.

Because rectal insufflations increase the level of oxygen within the general circulation, individuals who use this technique may report an increase in their level of physical and mental energy, due to an increase in the oxygen levels throughout the entire body.

Vaginal douches. With this technique, an ozone/oxygen mixture is introduced into the vagina using the same techniques as for rectal insufflation. Because of ozone's virucidal, fungicidal, and bactericidal efficacy, some physicians have found it to be an extremely effective treatment for vaginal yeast infections as well as other vaginal and pelvic infections. By promoting improved circulation and oxygenation to the pelvic region, ozone has also been found to help promote reproductive health and menstrual regularity. While vaginal douches are usually done under a physician's care, some women do use vaginal douches at home on a self-care basis.

Application into the ear canal. With this therapy, the outflow tube of the ozone generator is placed next to the opening of the outer ear canal. Ozone is allowed to gently flow into the outer ear canal for one to two minutes per treatment. This is useful for the treatment of infections of the outer ear canal, middle ear infections, and fluid in the ear. When doing this treatment, you should be careful not to breathe in the ozone, and your eyes should be closed to avoid any possible irritation.

Topical applications. Historically, topical applications have involved "bagging" the skin surfaces and extremities, with a subsequent application of an ozone/oxygen mixture to the enclosed area. The bag used must be made of an ozone-resistant material. This treatment has traditionally been used by physicians for the healing of skin ulcers, wounds, and osteomyelitis. Since ozone is readily absorbed from the skin, large amounts of the ozone/oxygen mixture can be taken into the body without ill effects.

Some individuals use a variant of the ozone-bagging technique to increase their total body oxygen levels. This technique involves running ozone into a steam cabinet or hot tub, thereby taking ozone and oxygen in through the skin. Large ozone-resistant plastic bags or body suits made out of rip-stop nylon used in parachutes are also available and can be used for the same purpose. Ozone-resistant bags or body suits enclose the body up to the chest or neck. The ozone outflow tube is placed into the bag or body suit, which is then tightly sealed around the body to avoid breathing ozone. The concentration of ozone used is generally 2 to 4 percent. Sessions can last between thirty minutes and one hour. This is an extremely powerful technique for healthy individuals wanting to increase their oxygen levels for peak performance. This technique increases one's level of physical and mental energy, so it is useful for individuals with strenuous work schedules and activity demands. It improves energy, stamina, and endurance as well as shortening the recovery time after exertion. Increasing the level of oxygen within the body also improves one's resistance to disease of all types.

Bathing in ozone-enriched water. With this therapy, which is done in a clinic or spa, warm water is ozonated and the patient reclines in a full-body bath. Clinics use bathing in ozonated water for the treatment of skin problems such as eczema, localized skin ulcers, circulatory problems, and arthritis. Ozone can also be bubbled through water in a hot tub. The outflow tube can be run through the water-recirculating and filtering system of the hot tub. With this system, ozonated water will come through your hot tub jets. This treatment also helps to reduce muscle tension and joint aches and pains. Ozone can also be used in steam baths. Some spas use ozonated steam baths and saunas to both beautify the skin and promote relaxation.

Ozone Bathing at Home

If you wish to use ozone to improve and maintain your peak-performance capability, you may want to consider ozonating your spa or tub. Most spa maintenance services will know how to install either a pool- or spa-ozonating device or can install the outflow tube in your water-recirculating and filtering system. A diffuser can also be used to reduce the size of the ozone bubbles.

Soaking daily in a hot tub or bath treated with ozone will make your skin softer, smoother, and healthier in appearance. Unlike chlorine, which actually has a drying effect on the skin, ozone helps to remove the outer layers of the skin, which are often drier and rougher in texture.

Ozone-enhanced drinking water. High concentrations of ozone can be diffused through drinking water just prior to consumption by use of a simple, inexpensive plastic diffuser that allows the ozone to be dispersed in small bubbles throughout the water. As a result, the water is able to absorb the ozone/oxygen mixture. Besides improving the quality of the water, some physicians recommend the use of superoxygenated drinking water for patients with upper-gastrointestinal-tract problems such as gastritis, indigestion, dyspepsia, and peptic-ulcer disease. Ozonated drinking water is also an effective treatment for problems of the mouth and throat such as sore throats, thrush, and periodontal (gum) disease. Like bathing in ozonated water, drinking superoxygenated water can easily be done at home.

▲▲ If you are making your own drinking water, use a diffuser to break the ozone gas into a stream of small bubbles so that it can dissolve more readily in water. Plastic diffusers, which are ozone resistant, can be bought through companies selling ozone machines or even at some pet stores, where they are sold for use in aquariums. Diffusers can also be used in hot tubs and baths that are treated with ozone.

Safety and Side Effects of Ozone

Ozone has been found to be a completely safe therapy when applied properly. Direct inhalation of ozone should therefore be avoided, since it can be irritating to the lungs. Ozone is also irritating to the eyes and should be kept away from the face. It can also cause local irritation when intravenous injections are improperly administered. The safety of ozone was thoroughly evaluated in a study done in the 1980s by the German Medical Society for Ozone Therapy. This study evaluated the experience of 644 health care professionals who used ozone with 384,775 patients. Approximately 14.5 ozone treatments, on average, were administered to each patient, for a total of 5,579,238 treatments. There were only forty cases of side effects due to ozone therapy reported out of the more than 5 million treatments. This represents a rate of adverse side effects of less than 1 treatment in 100,000, an incredibly low rate compared to the number of side effects normally incurred with the use of standard medical treatments. After reviewing hundreds of medical studies on ozone therapy, we have been impressed with both the efficacy and the safety of this treatment.

HYDROGEN PEROXIDE

Hydrogen peroxide has a long history of commercial use, being used since the 1800s as a bleaching agent, disinfectant, and purifying agent. It is currently available in different grades, depending on the purpose for which it is used:

- 3 percent hydrogen peroxide: This very dilute form can be bought in drugstores and supermarkets. It is commonly used as a disinfectant for superficial wounds and abrasions, to clean household surfaces, and to wash fruits and vegetables. It should not, however, be ingested since it contains a variety of stabilizers like phenol.

- 6 percent hydrogen peroxide: This form is used as a bleaching agent, primarily by hairstylists to lighten the color of hair, or by individuals who wish to bleach their hair at home.

- 30 percent reagent-grade hydrogen peroxide: This form can be purchased from chemical-supply stores. It is used by laboratories and, when properly diluted, by clinics in intravenous injections for the treatment of a variety of medical conditions. Individuals who handle reagent-grade hydrogen peroxide should avoid skin contact since it can cause burning and whitening of the skin. Breathing its vapors or ingesting it should also be avoided since it can be corrosive to tissues. It should only be used as a medical therapy when properly diluted to safe levels.

- 35 percent food-grade hydrogen peroxide: This form has been used for its disinfectant and antibacterial properties to treat foods such as fruits, vegetables, and eggs and food containers. When diluted, it can also be used to superoxygenate bath water. Food-grade hydrogen peroxide does contain stabilizers such as tin and phosphate, so it should not be used internally as a medical therapy.

- 90 percent hydrogen peroxide: This extremely concentrated form of hydrogen peroxide is used in space exploration and by the military as a propellant in rocket fuel.

Hydrogen peroxide can be safely and effectively used for a variety of health and household purposes. However, it is much less versatile than ozone in its ability to be used on a self-care basis to improve either performance or health. As a medical therapy, hydrogen peroxide is most effectively administered by a physician as an intravenous injection. Given intravenously, it is an amazingly effective and fast-acting therapy.

Topical disinfectant

Three percent hydrogen peroxide is commonly found in medicine cabinets as a safe and handy first-aid treatment. It can be applied to cuts and minor wounds as a disinfectant. It will bubble up and foam as it kills bacteria and cleans superficial wounds. It is also used in toiletries such as toothpastes and mouthwashes for its cleansing and purifying benefits. (However, these products should never be swallowed.)

▲▲ Foods such as fresh fruits and vegetables can be washed in 3 percent hydrogen peroxide before eating them to eliminate surface bacteria and dirt. However, do not use the form commonly available in drug stores and supermarkets for this purpose because stabilizers are used in its manufacture. Instead, get reagent-grade hydrogen peroxide from a chemical-supply store. This type of peroxide is much more concentrated but does not contain stabilizers like phenol. You will need to dilute 30 percent reagent-grade hydrogen peroxide with distilled water in a 10:1 ratio, thereby creating a 3 percent solution.

Peroxide baths

Six ounces of 30 percent reagent-grade or 35 percent food-grade hydrogen peroxide can be mixed into a tub of warm water to create a superoxygenated bath. A hydrogen peroxide–enriched bath is useful for individuals who suffer from joint stiffness and muscle tension. A soak can be done for twenty to thirty minutes and will leave you feeling relaxed and refreshed. However, 30 or 35 percent hydrogen peroxide needs to be handled with extreme care due to the corrosive effects of hydrogen peroxide on the skin. Peroxide in these concentrations should never be ingested since it will erode the tissues of the digestive tract.

A Caution on the Oral Ingestion of Hydrogen Peroxide

The oral use of hydrogen peroxide is controversial. Practitioners who recommend using it often advise taking ten drops of 35 percent food-grade hydrogen peroxide in an 8 oz. glass of distilled water several times a day on an empty stomach. Unfortunately, there are several drawbacks to using hydrogen peroxide in this manner. First of all, it is extremely harsh and unpalatable. Hydrogen peroxide cannot be combined with juice, milk, or other beverages since this will cause the destruction of the hydrogen peroxide itself, thereby neutralizing its effectiveness. In addition, hydrogen peroxide is harmful to the entire intestinal tract, which is lined with a very delicate mucous membrane. Its use may lead to erosive changes within the stomach or intestines. Therefore, Susan recommends against the oral ingestion of hydrogen peroxide.

Intravenous injections

Intravenous hydrogen peroxide should only be administered by trained health care professionals in a medical office or clinical setting. Physicians who use it find it to be an extremely effective treatment for a variety of conditions including bacterial, viral, fungal, and parasitic infections such as influenza, herpes simplex, herpes zoster, *E. coli*, *Candida albicans*, and *Trichomonas vaginalis*. Intravenous hydrogen peroxide is also used for the treatment of many other diseases, including cardiovascular, cerebrovascular, and peripheral vascular disease, emphysema, asthma, multiple sclerosis, migraine headaches, rheumatoid arthritis, metastatic cancer, and chronic pain syndromes.

Hydrogen peroxide therapy is administered intravenously one to three times a week with the duration of each treatment lasting between one and three hours. The dosage of hydrogen peroxide given intravenously is very dilute—in fact, it is about 100 times more dilute than the 3 percent hydrogen peroxide sold in pharmacies and supermarkets. While side effects are uncommon, intravenous use can cause a stinging and burning sensation and, rarely, inflammation at the site of the injection.

Thirty percent reagent-grade hydrogen peroxide is normally used in the preparation of intravenous solutions. Food- or cosmetic-grade hydrogen peroxides are avoided for medical use because they may contain tin and phosphate compounds to stabilize the peroxide molecule. Health care workers who are required to handle hydrogen peroxide need to avoid skin contact since peroxide may cause skin to turn white from the oxidation of the superficial layers. If allowed to remain on the skin, hydrogen peroxide can cause pain and discomfort. If hydrogen peroxide is accidentally spilled and comes in contact with the skin, it should be washed off immediately.

HYPERBARIC-OXYGEN THERAPY

With hyperbaric-oxygen therapy (HBOT), pure oxygen is administered under pressurized conditions. Hyperbaric-oxygen therapy cannot be done on a self-care basis and is normally administered in a clinic or hospital setting. There are currently 300 hyperbaric chambers in the United States; they are primarily used in association with hospitals and clinics.

Hyperbaric oxygen is used medically to treat carbon monoxide poisoning, smoke inhalation, deep-compression sickness from diving (also called the bends), traumatic injuries, poorly healing wounds, and radiation tissue damage. It is also used as a therapy for stroke victims, for individuals with multiple sclerosis, and as a complementary therapy for the treatment of AIDS. If you are interested in finding a clinic in your area that administers hyperbaric oxygen, please refer to the appendix of this book.

LIQUID OXYGEN

Liquid oxygen refers to products containing oxygen, chlorine, chloride, or chloride ions. The term *liquid oxygen* is a misnomer, since it implies that oxygen has been turned into a liquid for therapeutic use. These products are actually manufactured as stabilized oxygen electrolytes and are sold either in health food stores or through multilevel marketing companies. Liquid oxygen is normally administered in dosages of ten to twelve drops in 8 oz. of water. The oxygen contained within the solution is said to be released upon coming in contact with stomach acid. This oxygen can then be absorbed into the general circulation, where it acts as both a minor oxygenating agent and an antibacterial, antiviral, antifungal, and anti-inflammatory substance. These formulations also release trace amounts of sodium and chlorine dioxide gas into the circulation.

While research studies are lacking on the use of liquid oxygen products, there is an abundance of anecdotal information from people who use these products for a variety of purposes such as the treatment of colds, flus, and allergies. Despite the lack of scientific evidence for their use, many individuals who use these products have found them to be quite helpful. These products are nontoxic and are essentially without any significant side effects. As a result, they are sold as over-the-counter products without any health claims made for their use on the label.

PART 2:
ANTIOXIDANTS

ANTIOXIDANT NUTRITIONAL SUPPLEMENTS should be used concurrently with oxygen therapies. Antioxidants allow oxygen therapies to be used safely and without concern about potential negative side effects. One of the major concerns about the use of oxygen therapies like ozone and hydrogen peroxide is that they can cause the production of free radicals within the body. Ozone reverts to stable oxygen and a singlet oxygen, while hydrogen peroxide breaks down into water and a singlet oxygen. A singlet oxygen is a free radical. In other words, it possesses an unpaired electron and will search for another electron that it can pull from any nearby cells or tissues to allow it to restabilize itself as O_2.

While free radicals can cause damage to healthy cells and tissues, some of the benefit that we derive from oxygen therapies is actually due to their free-radical activity. Free radicals are also produced within the body and are necessary for the maintenance of our health. For example, free radicals, including the hydroxyl and superoxide radicals, are produced by the body to destroy bacteria, fungi, and viruses. However, when produced in excessive amounts, they can be harmful to healthy cells and tissues. As a result, free radicals, whether produced by the body or generated through the use of oxygen therapies, need to be neutralized by antioxidants.

The body produces its own antioxidants, which include enzymes such as glutathione peroxidase, superoxide dismutase, and catalase. These enzymes protect our cells from free-radical damage by chemically changing the free radicals into harmless substances like water. Antioxidants protect our healthy cells and tissues by donating their own electrons to the free-radical compounds. When using oxygen therapies, you must supplement your natural antioxidant enzymes with nutritional antioxidants such as vitamin C, vitamin E, vitamin A (taken in its water-soluble form as beta-carotene), and the minerals selenium and zinc. The use of these nutritional antioxidants will allow you to use oxygen therapies safely and benefit from their tremendous range of therapeutic effects. Furthermore, numerous research studies have found that the use of antioxidants can reduce the risk of heart attack, strokes, cancer, rheumatoid arthritis, and even tissue damage caused by strenuous exercise.

The following daily dosages of antioxidants should be used with ozone and hydrogen peroxide therapies:

Vitamin A (as beta-carotene): 10,000 to 100,000 IU.

Vitamin C: 3,000 to 10,000 mg.

Vitamin E (as d-alpha-tocopherol): 400 to 2,000 IU.

Selenium: 200 to 400 mcg.

Zinc: 15 to 60 mg.

PART 3:
OTHER NUTRITIONAL SUPPLEMENTS

RESEARCH STUDIES HAVE found that a number of nutrients work synergistically with oxygen to support a variety of physiological functions within the body. These nutrients include vasodilators, which promote good blood flow and healthy oxygenation of all our cells and tissues. Certain other nutritional supplements can be used in conjunction with oxygen therapies to help increase energy production within the body. Several herbs can also be used with oxygen therapies to improve immune function in individuals with respiratory infections such as colds and flus. Finally, some individuals, such as menstruating women with iron-deficiency anemia and athletes participating in anaerobic or endurance sports, may need other nutrients such as iron or sodium phosphate. Iron is necessary to insure the transport of sufficient oxygen by the red blood cells, while sodium phosphate assists in the release of oxygen from the red blood cells into the muscles.

VASODILATORS THAT IMPROVE OXYGENATION

Several substances called vasodilators promote greatly improved oxygenation of all the cells and tissues of the body. Unlike oxygen therapies, which actually supplement the level of oxygen contained within the body, these substances act, in part, to improve circulation. As a result, oxygen is better able to reach areas of the body that have been devitalized either by poor circulation due to hardening of the arteries, or by vasoconstriction (narrowing of the blood vessels) due to stress, cold, or other environmental factors, hormonal imbalances, or disease. These substances include nitric oxide, a potent vasodilator produced within our bodies, and gingko biloba, a powerful circulation-enhancing herb.

Nitric oxide

Nitric oxide is a substance produced by our bodies that helps to optimize the flow of blood through the arteries and veins. As a potent vasodilator, it enhances the flow of blood and the transport of oxygen to all the cells and tissues of the body. Research studies suggest that nitric oxide may actually be one of the most important chemicals that our bodies produce.

Nitric oxide is a gaseous molecule produced in the body from the amino acid arginine. Extensive research conducted in the 1990s shows that nitric oxide is involved in regulating a wide variety of physiologic functions. In fact, some of these studies suggest that nitric oxide may even increase the level of oxygen within the body. For example, in patients with chronic lung diseases such as chronic obtrusive lung disease and adult respiratory distress syndrome, inhalation of nitric oxide improved oxygenation. Insufficient levels of nitric oxide are associated with many disease conditions, most of which relate to poor circulation and insufficient oxygenation. These include diseases of the heart and lungs and of the neuroendocrine, immune, reproductive, and other systems. Insufficient nitric oxide production can also greatly hamper one's level of performance in many important areas of life, leading to diminished physical and mental energy and immune function, erectile dysfunction (in men), diminished sexual responsiveness (in women), poor recovery from exertion and injury, and impaired wound healing. Nitric oxide production enhances sports performance in activities such as body building, football, swimming, and bicycle riding, where good muscular development and healthy circulation provide a competitive edge. It is also known that levels of nitric oxide tend to decrease with age.

Not only does optimal production of nitric oxide increase performance capability, but it also contributes to the "look of success" that many peak performers have, because it enhances peripheral circulation. High nitric oxide producers typically have healthy skin and hair, and well-developed muscles. In contrast, elderly individuals (and even younger individuals with diminished nitric oxide production) often have thinner hair and paler, thinner skin.

Nitric oxide production levels can be increased through nutritional supplementation, thereby improving vasodilation and oxygenation. This can greatly improve both health and performance capability. Research studies have shown that intravenous administration of the amino acid arginine can increase nitric oxide production in humans. Attempts to increase nitric oxide production in humans through oral administration of arginine have met with limited success. Interestingly, a Southern California nutraceutical research and development company has developed a product able to orally administer small amounts of arginine combined with other nutrients, which allows the body to increase its production of nitric oxide. This unique technology offers an effective oral supplement to support production of nitric oxide.

Ginkgo biloba

The ginkgo biloba tree species originated about 250 million years ago, and a single tree can live as long as 1000 years. This handsome tree is often planted in urban settings, as it resists disease, insects, and pollution. Modern science is finding that this ancient plant can also help slow the aging of the brain, alleviate depression, and, perhaps most importantly, improve circulation and oxygenation throughout the body. Ginkgo leaf extracts are used by individuals throughout the world for their circulatory and oxygenation benefits. The chemicals found in ginkgo have powerful vasodilating effects: They act by stimulating the release of prostacyclin (a prostaglandin hormone) and a vascular relaxing substance. These chemicals also improve the tone of blood vessels and reduce the stickiness of red blood cells, so that they flow more smoothly through the blood vessels as they carry oxygen throughout the body.

Numerous research studies confirm the benefits of ginkgo extracts on all parts of the circulatory system, improving blood flow and oxygenation to the brain, heart, and other vital organs and the extremities. It is useful for many conditions including coronary-artery disease, cerebral vascular insufficiency, peripheral vascular disease, Alzheimer's disease, Reynaud's disease (vasoconstriction of the extremities), impotence due to diminished blood flow, diseases of the eye due to diabetes mellitus or poor circulation, cyclic edema due to PMS, and even clinical depression (gingko acts as a potent mood elevator). Many important performance traits are enhanced by the improvement in the oxygenation of the body that occurs when using ginkgo. These include improvements in physical energy, mental clarity, cognitive function, mood, and ability to socialize. Side effects are rare; however, women should be aware that the flavanoid quercitin, which is found in ginkgo, may lower estrogen production within the body.

SUGGESTED DOSAGE: Only standardized extracts should be used (standardized to 24 percent flavonoid glycosides and 6 percent terpene lactones). Dosages may vary between 40 to 60 mg, two to three times a day.

NUTRIENTS THAT IMPROVE ENERGY PRODUCTION

The following nutrients are necessary for optimal energy production within the body. Susan highly recommends the use of these nutrients, including coenzyme Q-10, magnesium, potassium, and vitamin B complex, for individuals who are past midlife and are using oxygen therapies to improve their physical and mental energy, for antiaging purposes, or even to improve cardiovascular function. (These supplements are helpful for these conditions even without the use of oxygen therapies.)

Coenzyme Q-10

Along with oxygen, coenzyme Q-10 helps to maximize the amount of energy that can be produced within the body as adenosine triphosphate (ATP), the main energy currency of the body. Coenzyme Q-10 belongs to a family of brightly colored substances called quinones, which occur widely in nature. Good dietary sources of coenzyme Q-10 include whole grains, fish, organ meats, soybean oil, walnuts, and sesame seeds. It is also produced within our bodies, where it acts as an electron carrier in the energy cycles that take place within the cell that lead to the production of ATP. It is also a powerful antioxidant. Coenzyme Q-10 works in conjunction with vitamin E to scavenge free radicals, thereby protecting the tissues of the body from oxidative damage.

Unfortunately, our production of coenzyme Q-10 diminishes with age, which can have a limiting effect on the amount of energy we are able to produce. Many individuals who are middle-aged and older can benefit from the use of supplemental coenzyme Q-10. Not only does it increase the level of energy production within the body, but it has also been found to act as a mild metabolic stimulant. Research studies have also found that it improves cardiac function. Its usefulness in treating individuals with heart failure is probably due to its ability to improve energy production within the heart muscle cells. Coenzyme Q-10 has been found to enhance both the pumping and electrical functions of the heart. It is also used by some endurance athletes who may have an increased need for coenzyme Q-10, as well as individuals on antiaging programs.

SUGGESTED DOSAGE: The dosage of coenzyme Q-10 ranges from 50 to 100 mg a day. Physicians may recommend that patients with specific health conditions take even higher dosages. Other antioxidants—

such as vitamin E, vitamin C, vitamin A (as beta-carotene), selenium, and zinc—should be used in conjunction with coenzyme Q-10.

Magnesium

The body requires adequate levels of magnesium in order to maintain energy and vitality. The process of aerobic metabolism requires magnesium to produce ATP. When magnesium is deficient, ATP production falls and the body forms lactic acid. Accumulation of lactic acid can lead to acidosis and a drop in energy levels. Therefore, having sufficient amounts of magnesium helps to maintain a high level of physical energy. This has been confirmed in a number of studies. For example, a study reported at a conference on magnesium in 1976 described that when 200 individuals were given magnesium supplements, 198 of them experienced relief from fatigue, a remarkably high result.

SUGGESTED DOSAGE: Magnesium is given in divided doses, 400 to 1000 mg daily. There is a possible laxative effect at higher dosages. It is important to maintain a healthy calcium to magnesium ratio. Optimal levels are considered to be in a 2:1 or 10:4 ratio with calcium predominating over magnesium.

Potassium

Like magnesium, potassium has a powerful enhancing effect on energy and vitality. Potassium deficiency has been associated with fatigue and muscular weakness. One form of potassium, in particular—called potassium aspartate—has been found to be particularly useful for restoring the level of energy in individuals with chronic fatigue. It has been combined with magnesium aspartate in a number of clinical studies on fatigue. Aspartic acid plays a vital role in aerobic (oxygen-dependent) energy production within the cells and helps transport both potassium and magnesium into the cells. Potassium aspartate has been shown in a number of clinical trials to reduce fatigue after five or six weeks of constant use. Even within ten days, many volunteers began to feel better. The benefits of potassium were seen in 90 percent of the people tested. Magnesium aspartate also has the same effects.

SUGGESTED DOSAGE: The recommended dosage for potassium and/or potassium aspartate is 100 to 300 mg per day. Potassium supplements can cause intestinal irritation in susceptible individuals, particularly those with preexisting intestinal disease.

Vitamin B complex

Vitamin B complex consists of a group of eleven separate nutrients: thiamine, riboflavin, niacin, pantothenic acid, pyridoxine (vitamin B_6), folic acid, biotin, para-aminobenzoic acid (PABA), vitamin B_{12}, choline, and inositol. In many cases they participate in the same chemical reactions in the body; therefore, they need to be taken together for best results. The B vitamins play a critical role in the conversion of carbohydrates into energy. When carbohydrates are "burned" within the cells in the presence of oxygen, much more energy is released to fuel the needs of the body than can be produced in the absence of oxygen. Various B vitamins are necessary for this conversion to progress efficiently.

SUGGESTED DOSAGE: B-complex vitamins may be taken in a dosage of 25 to 100 mg a day, as a single dose or in divided dosages. It is best to take the B vitamins during the day, rather than at night, as they can be stimulating and can cause some people to have difficulty falling asleep.

Herbs That Improve Immune Function

Several different herbs assist the use of oxygen therapies for the treatment of infectious disease by improving the immune function of the body.

Echinacea

Echinacea root has long been used in traditional botanical medicine for its immunity-enhancing properties. In recent years, a number of studies have confirmed the beneficial effects that echinacea has on immune response, particularly against respiratory conditions like colds and flus. Research studies have found that using echinacea increases phagocytosis (the process by which cells of the immune system engulf and destroy pathogenic organisms), activates macrophages to destroy pathogenic organisms, and stimulates both T lymphocytes and B lymphocytes. In a review article published in 1997 in the *European Journal of Herbal Medicine*, the author summarized the findings of six clinical trials using echinacea for the treatment of colds and flus as well as six trials that evaluated echinacea for its preventive benefits. The results of these trials confirmed that echinacea improves immune function when used for the treatment of respiratory infections.

SUGGESTED DOSAGE: Take two capsules three times per day (125 mg capsules that have been standardized to 3.2 percent to 4.8 percent echinacosides), or take ten to thirty drops of liquid extract three times per day standardized for 1 percent echinacosides.

Ginseng

Ginseng root has been used as a tonic to improve resistance to disease in traditional Asian medicine for several thousand years. Research studies have confirmed that ginseng root improves immune function by stimulating the activity of natural killer cells and increasing the production of lymphocytes. An article published in 1996 in *Drugs Under Experimental and Clinical Research* discussed the results of a study in which the ability of ginseng to improve immune response to the influenza vaccine was evaluated versus a placebo. Two hundred twenty-seven adult volunteers were given either 100 mg of a standardized extract of ginseng root or a placebo daily over a twelve-week period. All of the volunteers were given an influenza vaccine at week four. The volunteers taking the ginseng root showed a significantly greater immune response to the influenza vaccine than did the placebo group. In addition, the individuals in the treatment group experienced fewer cases of influenza and fewer colds than those in the placebo group.

SUGGESTED DOSAGE: For maximum benefit, take a high-quality preparation, an extract of the main root of a plant that is four to six years old, standardized for ginsenoside content and ratio. Twice a day, take a 100 mg capsule. If this is too stimulating, especially before bedtime, take the second dose midafternoon, or take only the morning dose.

NUTRIENTS THAT SUPPORT OXYGEN-CARRYING CAPABILITY AND pH BALANCE

Several nutrients are needed to promote the healthy functioning of red blood cells. Red blood cells carry oxygen to the cells and tissues throughout the body.

Iron

Iron is an important mineral that exists in the body in combination with protein. In the bloodstream, iron combines with copper and protein to form hemoglobin, which provides the coloration of the red blood cell. Hemoglobin binds with oxygen, enabling it to be transported from the lungs to all the cells of the body via the circulation. Iron is also used by the body to produce myoglobin, which is found in muscle tissue. Myoglobin also acts as a transporter of oxygen, but only to muscle cells. Since oxygen plays such an important role in the production of energy within the cells, iron is needed in sufficient amounts if one is to have the physical and mental energy necessary for peak performance.

Women are at particular risk of iron-deficiency anemia because of menstruation. Anemia is associated with a diminished capacity to do physical activity, due, in part, to poor oxygenation. In an controlled study published in 1977 in the *American Journal of Clinical Nutrition*, seventy-five women were given a treadmill test. Those with the most severe iron-deficiency anemias were able to stay on the treadmill an average of eight minutes less than the women without anemia. Further, none of the anemic women were able to perform under the highest workload conditions, while all of the women with adequate iron levels could.

Some athletes, both males and females, have been found to have low iron stores, despite normal blood profiles. Low iron stores can significantly affect athletic performance. Athletes tend to be at higher risk of iron deficiency than the rest of the population for several reasons. Iron is lost through perspiration while performing physically demanding exercise. Physically demanding exercise can also cause hemolysis or the breaking apart of blood cells. Iron lost from the blood cells through hemolysis is excreted from the body. In addition, acidosis and small amounts of intestinal bleeding can occur during heavy training, further depleting the body's store of iron.

SUGGESTED DOSAGE: Dosage depends on gender and age. An average dosage is 15 mg per day, but a menstruating women who is anemic may need as much as 30 to 70 mg a day until her iron reserves have been restored and her blood count has returned to normal. Athletes who are engaged in heavy training may need as much as 25 mg of supplemental iron each day to maintain their reserves. Other supplemental nutrients such as folic acid, vitamin B_{12}, vitamin B_6, vitamin E, vitamin C, and zinc may also be necessary to restore and maintain a healthy blood profile in anemic individuals. Postmenopausal women, who are no longer menstruating, will not have high requirements, and recent studies have indicated that high levels of iron are associated with an increased risk of heart disease in men.

Phosphorus (sodium phosphate)

Iron is not the only mineral necessary for the healthy functioning of red blood cells. Phosphorus is needed for the production of an enzyme called 2,3-diphosphoglycerate (2,3-DPG), which is found in red blood cells. Red blood cells transport oxygen in the blood to the tissues; 2,3-DPG insures that oxygen, an important alkalinizing agent, is delivered to the muscles. It reduces the affinity that hemoglobin has for oxygen, so oxygen is more available to the tissues. Along with oxygen, phosphorus also promotes energy production within the cells. In addition, it improves the production and use of glycogen, a sugar that is a ready source of energy in the muscles.

Because the typical American diet contains plentiful amounts of meat and dairy products, which contain large amounts of phosphorus, most people are far from deficient. However, athletes may need especially high amounts of this mineral, since research studies have shown that muscles lose phosphorus into the bloodstream during periods of intense physical exertion. The more a person exercises, the more phosphorus is needed by the body. Endurance athletes such as marathon runners will have low levels of phosphorus immediately after participating in an athletic event. Loss of phosphorus can impair buffering within the muscle tissue and limit the amount of oxygen delivered to the muscle cells.

SUGGESTED DOSAGE: Phosphorus is given to athletes in a buffered form as sodium phosphate. It is used as an aid to improve sports performance. A typical dosage is 4 g a day, taken for three days prior to participating in an event. This has been found to improve both anaerobic and endurance performance. Sodium phosphate is nontoxic in normal amounts. However, taking large doses can lead to calcium loss, as phosphorus interacts with calcium metabolism.

PART 4:
OXYGEN-HEALTHY HABITS

MANY ASPECTS OF our lives have a direct impact on our oxygen levels. Our diet, our exercise habits, and how we manage stress all have an effect on the amount of oxygen that we take into the body as well as how efficiently it is transported into our tissues and cells.

EAT A DIET HIGH IN OXYGEN

Individuals who wish to follow a diet to help support and maintain the level of oxygen within their body need to follow an alkaline, mostly vegetarian diet. This is discussed in detail in chapter 2. If you have not already read that chapter, we strongly recommend that you review it at this time. Oxygen is one of the most energy-enhancing and alkalinizing substances within our bodies. It is best maintained by eating lots of raw, fresh fruits (except citrus fruits and berries, which tend to be highly acidic), vegetables, sprouted seeds, grains, beans, and green-food supplements such as spirulina, chlorella, wheat grass, and barley grass. These foods should be eaten in concert with other high-nutrient foods, some of which may require cooking, such as starches, whole grains, legumes, seeds and nuts, fish, and free-range poultry.

Fresh fruits and vegetables, in particular, tend to be high in oxygen content. This is because they are largely composed of water, which is made up of hydrogen and oxygen, and is mostly oxygen by weight. These foods are also excellent sources of alkaline minerals such as magnesium and potassium, which are needed, along with adequate oxygen, for the production of energy within our cells. They are also rich in antioxidants such as beta-carotene and vitamin C, which protect our cells from free-radical damage.

In contrast, a highly acidic diet will make you more prone to oxygen-depleting acidosis. Acidic foods are also discussed in chapter 2 and include foods high in refined sugar, saturated fat, and animal protein, such as red meat and dairy products. Stimulants, such as caffeine found in coffee, black tea, and cola drinks (which are also acidic), can provide a rapid pick-me-up, but this is often followed by a drop in energy. This is because these foods destabilize our blood sugar level as well as stress the adrenal glands. These kinds of foods, as well as the others described in chapter 2, will reduce the level of energy, deplete the stores of oxygen, and increase the level of acidic waste products within the body. The only individuals who can tolerate a highly acidic diet are naturally strong oxygenators who have exceptional lung capacity or people who are very alkaline in constitution. In addition, you should avoid food that is heavily processed, fried, boiled, or breaded, since this type of preparation either causes food to lose essential energy-enhancing nutrients or produces free radicals in the cooking process, thereby increasing oxidative stress in the body. Lightly steamed food is preferable, as more essential nutrients are retained.

Following a diet that helps to maintain high levels of oxygen in the body is absolutely crucial to good health and peak performance. Many people notice a significant increase in their level of energy and zest for life when switching from an oxygen-depleting, highly acidic diet to an oxygen-enhancing, mostly vegetarian diet. In addition, there is usually a significant improvement in health, as colds, flus, aches and pains, indigestion, and fatigue begin to diminish.

ENGAGE IN REGULAR AEROBIC EXERCISE

Aerobic exercise refers to any type of exercise that increases the amount of oxygen contained in the body. This type of exercise includes walking, swimming, bicycling, dancing, and tennis. All of these activities require a pumping action of the muscles that helps to move oxygen, blood, and nutrients throughout the body. With regular aerobic exercise, skeletal muscles become energized and toned, making every movement—from lifting objects to walking—more easily accomplished. The heart muscle also works more efficiently. As the heart becomes conditioned, it is able to pump more blood with each stroke. Thus, it can circulate the same volume of blood with fewer strokes and doesn't have to work as hard.

Aerobic exercise also causes vasodilation of the blood vessels and allows blood and oxygen to reach chronically contracted areas of muscle tension. By improving circulation, exercise also facilitates proper nutrient flow throughout the body. Removal of waste products such as carbon dioxide, lactic acid, and other products of metabolism becomes more efficient. With aerobic exercise, the production of energy by the cells in the form of ATP becomes more efficient. This is important since optimal energy production is needed to run the body's many chemical and physiological functions.

Exercise can help improve posture, which increases oxygenation through structural realignment. There are also important beneficial psychological effects to exercise. By improving blood flow and oxygenation to the brain, exercise has a beneficial effect on brain chemistry, promoting a feeling of peace, relaxation, and positive mood states due to an increase in the brain's natural opiates.

Most physicians recommend that individuals engage in moderate, regular aerobic exercise three to five times a week for thirty to sixty minutes per session. Doing this on a regular basis will not only improve your physical and mental energy, but will also help to reduce the risk of heart attack, cancer, and depression as well as other health problems.

PRACTICE DEEP BREATHING

Breathing slowly and deeply allows you take in large amounts of oxygen from the environmental air. Full expansion of the lungs in a relaxed, rhythmic way facilitates maximal oxygen uptake by the body. It is important to allow both the stomach and the rib cage to relax while breathing so that air can fill the entire lungs. This type of breathing strengthens the muscles in the abdomen and chest, relaxes the body, and allows for the most efficient oxygenation. (Two deep-breathing exercises are described on page 520.)

The oxygen that we breathe in enters the bloodstream, where it binds to the red blood cells. Oxygen is then transported to our cells and tissues. When present in sufficient amounts, it allows the cells to produce and use energy and to help remove waste products through the production of carbon dioxide. These waste products are cleared by the lungs through exhalation. Thus, the whole body needs optimal levels of oxygen for its normal cycle of building, repair, and elimination.

When you are stressed or anxious, your oxygen levels will decrease. Stress causes breathing to become erratic and shallow. You may find yourself breathing too fast, or you may even stop breathing altogether and hold your breath for prolonged periods of time without realizing it. None of these breathing patterns is healthful. Anxious breathing is often linked to other unhealthy physiological reactions that reflect your body's state of stress. When you are upset and emotionally stressed, you tend to tense and tighten your muscles, constrict blood flow, elevate your pulse rate and heartbeat, and stimulate the output of stressful chemicals from your glands. This further decreases oxygenation to your tissues and allows waste products such as carbon dioxide and lactic acid to accumulate in your muscles and other tissues. Aging also causes a decrease in the elasticity of our lungs as well as a decline in our forced vital capacity, further reducing the oxygen levels within the body. Practicing deep breathing helps to break this pattern, slows down the natural decline of the lungs, and helps the mind and body return to a state of peaceful equilibrium.

PRACTICE STRESS REDUCTION TECHNIQUES

Many individuals are easily made anxious by the small stresses of daily life. Situations that may seem insignificant to one person may be highly upsetting or irritating to another. Sensitivity to stress can cause an overreaction of the sympathetic nervous system (the part of the nervous system that regulates our internal physiological responses). This can cause the muscles to tense, the blood vessels to constrict, the adrenal glands to pump out stress hormones, and the heart and pulse rate to speed up so an individual can react to a perceived emergency.

If you have an especially stressful life, your sympathetic nervous system may always be poised to react to a crisis. This puts you in a state of constant tension, with your fight-or-flight response always turned on. In this mode, you tend to react to small stresses the same way you would react to real emergencies. (This is discussed in more detail in chapters 9 and 10.) The end result of the fight-or-flight reaction is the depletion of your oxygen stores, which can eventually result in a decline in physical and mental energy.

The practice of stress reduction techniques like meditation, visualization, and yoga can break the pattern of stress and improve oxygenation. Yoga deserves a special mention in this regard. When you practice a series of yoga exercises, or postures, you gently stretch every muscle in your body. In addition, yoga postures are meant to be accompanied by deep breathing, which helps to improve oxygenation. These postures relax tense muscles and improve their suppleness and flexibility. They also promote better circulation and oxygenation to tense and contracted areas throughout the body. As a result, general metabolism of the muscles and organ systems is improved. Both the stress reduction effects and the physiological effects of yoga benefit all body systems, including digestive and eliminative functions, the endocrine (glandular) system, the nervous system, and the immune system.

Other relaxation practices—like soaking in a tub of warm water, listening to classical music, and having a therapeutic massage—can also help increase the level of oxygen within the body. Soaking in a hot tub or bathtub filled with warm water is a great way to unwind after a busy day or before going to sleep at night. Many people find that a tub soak helps them sleep better. The warm water also loosens tight, constricted muscles and promotes better circulation and thereby better oxygenation of the muscles and skin. The healthy flush of the skin after a warm soak means that the small blood vessels, or capillaries, have relaxed, so more oxygen is able to reach all the tissues.

Listening to classical music can have a pronounced beneficial effect on your physiological functions. It can slow your pulse and heart rate, lower your blood pressure, improve your oxygenation through deeper and slower breathing, and decrease your levels of stress hormones. It promotes peace and relaxation and helps to induce sleep. Nature sounds, such as ocean waves and rainfall, can also induce a sense of peace and relaxation. Susan has patients who keep tapes of nature sounds in their cars and at home for use when they feel particularly stressed.

Massage or gentle touching, whether by a trained massage therapist, your spouse or partner, or even yourself, can be very relaxing. Tension usually fades away relatively quickly with gentle, relaxed touching. The kneading and stroking movement of a good massage relaxes tight muscles and improves circulation and oxygenation throughout the body.

SUMMARY OF TREATMENT OPTIONS
FOR RESTORING YOUR OXYGEN LEVELS

Oxygen therapies
> Pure oxygen
> Ozone therapy
> Hydrogen peroxide
> Hyperbaric oxygen
> Liquid oxygen

Antioxidants
> Vitamin A (as beta-carotene)
> Vitamin C
> Vitamin E
> Selenium
> Zinc

Vasodilators to improve oxygenation
> Nitric oxide
> Ginkgo biloba

Nutrients that improve energy production
> Coenzyme Q-10
> Magnesium
> Potassium
> Vitamin B complex

Herbs that improve immune-system function
> Echinacea
> Ginseng

Nutrients that support oxygen-carrying capability and pH balance
> Iron
> Phosphorus (sodium phosphate)

Oxygen-healthy habits
> Eat a diet of oxygen-rich foods
> Engage in regular aerobic exercise
> Practice deep breathing
> Practice stress reduction techniques

9

HOW THE ABILITY TO MANAGE STRESS
BENEFITS PEAK PERFORMANCE AND HEALTH

MORE THAN EVER, it is essential to do everything possible to maintain the body's stamina and resilience in order to be able to recover quickly from the many work-related, environmental, physical, and emotional stresses that we are exposed to regularly. The rewards for maintaining such inner fitness can be enormous. In the workplace, people who have the Chemistry of Success in terms of their ability to cope with stress have a much better chance of rising to the top of their professions. For these people, a stressful situation is simply a stimulating challenge that sharpens thinking and inspires determination. Individuals who manage a household and children and who know how to buffer and diffuse everyday stress are able to remain calm and compassionate in the middle of chaos and help hold their family together. Athletes who handle the stress of competition with equanimity are able to keep their mind on the game and play their best. For a list of the specific benefits of good stress management on both peak performance and optimal health, see the chart on page 436.

Stress is defined as a demand on physical or mental energy as well as the distress this demand causes. Stress can be emotional, psychological, social, chemical, and/or physical in origin. It can be acute and sudden, as when a car cuts in front of you on the freeway. There are also persistent, chronic forms of stress, such as loneliness or the demands of raising children. Changes in the weather can cause stress, as can changing jobs, getting a parking ticket, meeting new people, going away on vacation, competing in a tennis match, or giving a speech. Physical stresses include a poor diet and environmental pollution and toxins.

What we perceive as stress is purely subjective. A situation that one person considers manageable, another person may see as dangerous or threatening. People's perception of stress depends on their attitude toward challenges and change, their emotional and psychological coping skills, and their physical capability to respond to stress and recover quickly.

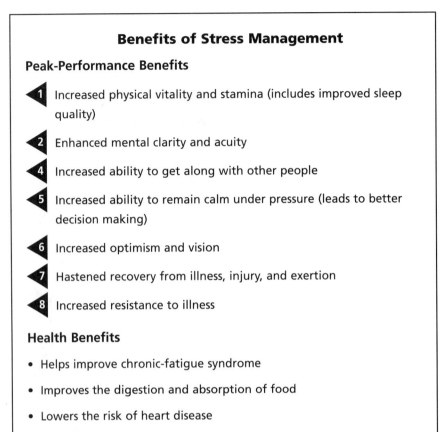

Benefits of Stress Management

Peak-Performance Benefits

1. Increased physical vitality and stamina (includes improved sleep quality)

2. Enhanced mental clarity and acuity

4. Increased ability to get along with other people

5. Increased ability to remain calm under pressure (leads to better decision making)

6. Increased optimism and vision

7. Hastened recovery from illness, injury, and exertion

8. Increased resistance to illness

Health Benefits

- Helps improve chronic-fatigue syndrome
- Improves the digestion and absorption of food
- Lowers the risk of heart disease
- Boosts immune system function
- Helps prevent and heal many other health conditions, including respiratory disease, arthritis, diabetes, and skin problems

Because we live in a period of great technological and social change, a person's success depends, in part, on their ability to manage the inevitable stresses of modern life. Successful stress management depends as much on the chemical makeup of the body as it does on emotional and mental programming. Much of life is centered around the workplace, with its attendant demands on our time and energy. With the corporate downsizing that has taken place during the past decade, both employees and executives are expected to work longer hours and are given tasks that used to be the responsibility of more than one person. The situation is no different for people who own their own business or do freelance consulting.

Work requirements often take up valuable morning and evening hours that might otherwise be spent on leisure pursuits or with the family, and even weekends are no longer sacred. As a consequence, most people experience a significant amount of stress in their daily lives. This can be particularly true for the many women who assume the dual responsibility of caring for their home and family while also managing a career.

Unfortunately, millions of people lack the Chemistry of Success for dealing with stress and, as a result, may feel incapable of meeting the demands of challenging situations. Such individuals tend to overreact to stressful situations, whether real or imagined, by triggering the output of chemicals within their bodies meant to help cope with stress. These chemicals have a profound effect on our physiology, affecting how we breathe, how blood circulates throughout the body, and even our level of muscular tension. If these stress chemicals are triggered only occasionally, the body does not suffer physical damage from their release. However, when triggered repeatedly, these chemicals may exhaust the body, causing unpleasant symptoms and, eventually, physical breakdown and disease.

Specific physical symptoms of stress include fatigue, insomnia, shortness of breath, heart palpitations, sweating, light-headedness, a craving for sweets, alternating constipation and diarrhea, low blood pressure, and blood sugar disturbances. Emotional signs of stress include anxiety, nervousness, and mood swings. Symptoms related to stress are very common in most physicians' practices. In fact, it is the most common complaint Susan hears.

Stress-related symptoms may occasionally be so intense that they can interfere with a person's ability to function. For example, anxiety disorders such as claustrophobia (fear of closed or narrow spaces) and agoraphobia (fear of open or public places) may actually cause affected individuals to avoid social and work situations that can trigger their fears. Susan has had patients who reported having panic episodes when driving their car on a freeway or when presenting a speech before a large audience. Obviously, performance is greatly hampered by such crippling emotional responses. It is estimated that 10 percent of the U.S. population, or 20 to 30 million people, have experienced phobias, panic attacks, and other anxiety disorders in the past year.

Checklist: Do You Have the Stress Management Abilities Needed for Peak Performance and Optimal Health?

Susan has found that a person's own evaluation of his or her susceptibility to stress can be a powerful motivator for making the changes in diet and lifestyle necessary to manage stress more effectively. Be sure to follow the nutritional, exercise, and stress management guidelines covered in the next chapter if you have any of the symptoms and risk factors for stress listed here. Work through the following checklist (you can photocopy it if you don't want to write in the book), and refer to it as you read through the chapter. Doing so will help you to evaluate your ability to deal with stress. For laboratory tests of adrenal function and for health conditions that increase susceptibility to stress, see page 479.

Lifestyle/environmental factors

Put a check mark beside those statements that are true for you.

- ❑ I have a history of drug or alcohol addiction.
- ❑ I use drugs recreationally.
- ❑ I frequently consume caffeine-containing beverages (such as coffee, tea, and colas) and/or chocolate.
- ❑ I frequently consume sugar-containing foods, fruit, and fruit juice.
- ❑ I do not eat foods high in calcium, magnesium, or potassium, nor do I use multimineral supplements containing these nutrients.

Performance indicators

- ❑ I often have difficulty concentrating (my mind goes blank).
- ❑ I have a poor memory.
- ❑ I often experience exhaustion at the end of the workday.
- ❑ I am susceptible to inappropriate outbursts of anger.
- ❑ I am easily deterred from my goals or easily frustrated by obstacles and setbacks.
- ❑ I am often afraid of saying something foolish.
- ❑ I often experience fatigue.

❏ I frequently have insomnia.

❏ I am often irritable and angry.

❏ I am often anxious.

❏ I avoid certain places or situations because I'm afraid of having a panic reaction.

Physical indicators

❏ I often experience shortness of breath or a smothering sensation.

❏ I frequently experience heart palpitations or a rapid heartbeat.

❏ I often experience bouts of trembling or shaking.

❏ I often sweat excessively.

❏ I am jumpy or easily startled.

❏ I have frequent bouts of alternating constipation and diarrhea.

❏ I have low blood pressure.

Psychological/medical history

❏ I have relatives with a history of anxiety disorders.

❏ I had or have overly critical parents.

❏ I had or have overly cautious parents.

❏ I lacked emotional nurturing in my childhood.

❏ I have a history of separation anxiety.

❏ I experienced a significant life stress (such as death, illness, or divorce) followed by excessive anxiety.

❏ I suffer from PMS.

❏ I am undergoing a stressful menopause.

❏ I use estrogen-containing medication.

❏ I have a history of hyperthyroidism or hypothyroidism.

❏ I have a history of hypoglycemia.

❏ I have a history of mitral-valve prolapse.

❏ I have a history of food allergies.

C Now that you have a preliminary understanding of the importance of stress management to peak performance and optimal health, as well as some idea from the checklist of your own abilities in this area, you are ready to decide what to read next. To learn more about the chemistry of stress, read the following section. To learn how diet, lifestyle, and aging affect stress levels, read section 2, on page 443. For a detailed discussion of how stress affects peak performance, read section 3, on page 458. For a detailed discussion of how stress affects general health, including specific conditions caused or exacerbated by stress, read section 4, on page 472. (Ideally, these latter two sections should be read consecutively, as the effects of stress on peak performance and health are intricately intertwined.) Finally, for information on how to restore and strengthen your ability to manage stress, read chapter 10.

SECTION 1:
THE CHEMISTRY OF STRESS MANAGEMENT

BECAUSE STRESS CAN have such a profound effect on performance and health, it is important to understand how the stress response develops within the body. When we sense serious danger, a sequence of biological events called the "fight-or-flight response" occurs. This response is a cascade of chemical and electrical processes meant to increase our ability to survive in the natural world. The fight-or-flight response occurs with any perceived threat, whether it is physically real, psychologically upsetting, or even imaginary; it can even occur simply when we are excited by a positive event.

The fight-or-flight response occurs first in the nervous system, beginning in the brain, moving down the spinal cord, and then to the peripheral nerves. The nervous system is divided into two parts: the voluntary nervous system and the involuntary, or autonomic, nervous system (ANS). The voluntary nervous system manages activity in the conscious domain, such as when you touch a hot stove and quickly pull your hand away. In contrast, the ANS regulates functions of which most people are unaware, such as pulse rate, circulation, and glandular function.

The ANS is also divided into two parts, which oppose and complement each other: the sympathetic and the parasympathetic nervous systems (SNS and PNS, respectively). The sympathetic nervous system tends to speed up the responses to our muscular and internal organs to help us deal with stressful situations. In contrast, the parasympathetic nervous system helps to slow our physiological responses down. For example, if excitement speeds up the heart rate too much, it is the parasympathetic nervous system's job to act as a control circuit and slow it down. But if the heart slows down too much, then it is the sympathetic nervous system's job to speed it back up.

In response to a stressful situation, the sympathetic nerves secrete a chemical called norepinephrine, which directly enters into the target tissues of organs such as the heart, the abdominal organs, the sweat glands, and the pupils of the eyes. Stimulation by norepinephrine causes an excitatory response within these tissues, which allows the body to react and protect itself from a stressful situation. For example, sympathetic stimulation increases blood flow to vital organs and the muscles. The end results are such stress-relieving and performance-enhancing qualities as increased muscular strength and enhanced mental alertness. However, the effect on the target tissues of norepinephrine from the sympathetic nerves is short-lived, lasting only a few seconds, because its reuptake and diffusion away from the tissues is rapid.

The adrenal glands work in tandem with the SNS as part of our stress response system. The adrenals are triangular-shaped organs resting on top of each kidney. Each gland consists of two parts, the medulla, or central section, and the cortex, or outer section. The SNS sends nerve impulses into the adrenal medulla causing it to secrete the same type of chemicals as the sympathetic nerves themselves: the hormones epinephrine (commonly referred to as adrenaline) and norepinephrine (or noradrenaline). However, while the SNS secretes these chemicals directly into the tissues, the adrenal medulla secretes them into the bloodstream, which transports them to various target tissues, also in response to stressful situations. Thus, the body has two overlapping systems to manage stress: the production of epinephrine and norepinephrine by both the SNS and the adrenal medulla.

However, while only a small percentage of cells in the body are stimulated by the epinephrine and norepinephrine produced by the sympathetic nerves, these same chemicals, when secreted by the adrenal medulla (especially epinephrine) are carried in the bloodstream to tissues and organs throughout the body. Even the time that these chemicals remain active in the tissues differs, depending on their source. The norepineph-rine secreted by the sympathetic nerves is active for only a few seconds, while the same chemical, when secreted by the adrenal medulla, remains active in the tissues for one to several minutes.

When the alarm response is triggered, epinephrine increases arterial pressure as well as blood flow to specific muscles needed for vigorous activity. It also increases the rate of metabolism, the concentration of glu-cose in the blood, the conversion of sugar to energy in muscles, muscle strength, and mental activity. All of these physiological responses are nec-essary for an individual to perform effectively in a challenging situation.

The adrenal cortex, or outer portion of the adrenal gland, also pro-duces hormones that help us to manage stress, called glucocorticoids and mineralocorticoids. (The adrenal cortex also produces a third class of hor-mones, the sex steroids, particularly dehydroepiandrosterone, or DHEA, which is discussed in chapter 11.) Adrenal hormones are primarily pro-duced from acetyl Coenzyme A (acetyl CoA) and cholesterol. Acetyl CoA is a chemical produced in the liver, made from fatty acids and amino acids. It provides an important source of energy for the body as well as being a building block from which hormones are made. Cholesterol is a waxy, white, fatty material, widely distributed in all body cells. The cholesterol in the body is supplied by animal foods in the diet, such as eggs and organ meats, and the liver also produces a certain amount of cholesterol.

Glucocorticoids are especially important in allowing an individual to withstand various kinds of stress. The secretion of cortisol accounts for at least 95 percent of adrenal-glucocorticoid activity. Cortisol is the primary stress hormone. In an attempt to buffer the effects of stress, cortisol is released when the body is threatened by extreme conditions such as infec-tion, intense heat or cold, surgery, and any kind of trauma. Cortisol acts as a natural anti-inflammatory when the body is assaulted by infection, a sports injury, arthritis, or allergy. Cortisol also affects carbohydrate and fat metabolism, promoting the conversion of stored sugars and fat into energy.

The mineralocorticoid aldosterone, also produced in the adrenal cor-tex, has an important role in protecting a person from stress by regulating fluid and electrolyte balance in the body. There must be a correct ratio of sodium and potassium ions inside and outside the cells to maintain nor-mal blood pressure and fluid volume.

SUMMARY

Perceived threats activate the fight-or-flight response in the nervous system, which causes the release of chemicals throughout the body. A series of complex physiological responses then take place to prepare the body to immediately defend itself. Thus, any kind of stress, whether emotional or physical, triggers an excited physical state that puts the entire body on alert.

SECTION 2:
HOW DIET, LIFESTYLE, AND AGING
AFFECT STRESS MANAGEMENT

EACH PERSON HAS his or her own level of stress tolerance. Some individuals can withstand an enormous amount of change and turmoil in their lives. They tend to thrive in high-pressure jobs and enjoy intense relationships and high-risk activities. However, the majority of individuals are unable to handle such stressful lifestyles. Over time, their ability to manage stress effectively can be hampered by a variety of chemical, emotional, and social factors as well as certain medical conditions.

A healthy body is constantly readjusting its internal chemistry and physiology so that it can remain in a balanced and basically unchanging state called homeostasis. For example, the body must maintain the pH of the blood at a slightly alkaline level and sustain a certain level of oxygen within the tissues to remain healthy. However, the fight-or-flight response tends to disrupt homeostasis. When the body is healthy, it is able to return to a state of balance after the perceived emergency has passed. The body's ability to maintain homeostasis allows us to live dynamic, challenging lives. When our bodies are in balance, stress can be exhilarating rather than debilitating. In fact, the fight-or-flight response can actually give us a surge of energy and causes no lasting harm, if triggered only occasionally. However, for many of us, the stress of our hectic world is an everyday occurrence, causing the body to remain in a nearly constant state of alarm. This results in exhaustion of the adrenal glands and nervous system and even lowered resistance to disease.

THE GENERAL ADAPTATION SYNDROME

In the mid-1930s, the various stages of the stress response were mapped out by Canadian physiologist Hans Selye. Selye called his model of how the body copes with stress the general adaptation syndrome (GAS). He divided the process into three stages. The first is the alarm stage. In this stage, there is an immediate, acute reaction to an irritant or stress. Such reactions can take the form of nervousness, restlessness, and agitation. When the body is in a state of balance and health, it is able to recover quickly from this stage.

Second is the resistance stage. In this stage, the stress occurs over a prolonged period of time, ranging from days to years. However, the body is still able to function, adapting to the ongoing stress through various mechanisms. Successful adaptation lasts as long as the body's resources and reserves will allow. This depends on factors such as the severity of the stress and the individual's genetic makeup, medical history, and reserves of vitamins and minerals. In this stage, the central nervous system and adrenal glands begin to overproduce the chemicals needed to mobilize the body to handle stress. People in this stage race through the day, running from task to task and meeting to meeting, giving the appearance of having too much to do and not enough time to fulfill all the demands of their lives. However, the body cannot maintain this degree of stress adaptation indefinitely.

As the ability to resist stress declines, a person enters the third and final stage, the exhaustion stage. In this stage, the mechanisms for stress adaptation begin to fail. When the body has reached the exhaustion stage, the glands and organs involved in stress management are weakened to the point where they are no longer able to cope. At this point, stress may lead to illness and actual disease such as high blood pressure, water retention, enlarged heart, strokes, arthritis, ulcers, kidney disease, allergies, neurological problems, diabetes, and cancer.

OTHER BODILY CHEMICALS THAT AFFECT OUR SUSCEPTIBILITY TO STRESS

Besides those chemicals produced by the adrenal glands and sympathetic nerves that create the stress response described above, there are a myriad of other substances produced by the body that affect our susceptibility to stress. These include serotonin, dopamine, beta-endorphins, estrogen and progesterone, digestive enzymes, and nitric oxide. When the normal balance of these substances within the body is upset, one's susceptibility to stress increases. Acid/alkaline balance is also a determining factor in resistance to stress.

Serotonin and dopamine

Serotonin and dopamine are neurotransmitters, substances that are released when a nerve cell is stimulated. The neurotransmitter travels across a synapse (the space between the junction of two nerve cells) to act on a target cell to either inhibit or excite it. Imbalances in these two neurochemicals can make a person more sensitive to everyday stress than someone who is able to produce these neurochemicals in appropriate amounts.

Serotonin is one of the brain's principal neurotransmitters. Its action on the nerves is inhibitory, relieving stress and calming the mind. Serotonin also regulates rapid eye movement (REM) sleep and appetite and influences mood. Because serotonin converts to melatonin (a hormone that influences the sleep/waking cycles), serotonin promotes sleep. Such peak-performance characteristics as the ability to get along with other people, to remain calm under pressure, and to have physical vitality and stamina are, in part, dependent on adequate serotonin production. Serotonin is made from tryptophan, an essential amino acid that must be supplied by the diet. Good sources of tryptophan are beef, pork, turkey, pumpkin seeds, and almonds. Some foods that contain tryptophan should regularly be included in meals, since it undergoes rapid turnover and must be replenished daily.

Dopamine is a neurotransmitter that stimulates and energizes the body. In fact, dopamine is actually a precursor to the chemicals, made by the adrenal medulla and sympathetic nervous system, that regulate the stress response within the body. High levels of dopamine have been linked to such traits as mental alertness, physical energy, and vitality. Dopamine production also supports other traits linked to a high level of physical energy, such as aggressive drive and libido. Dopamine is synthesized by the adrenal glands and is converted by the body into the stress hormones epinephrine and norepinephrine, which stimulate the body to action. Before ages forty to forty-five, dopamine levels remain fairly stable, but they then decrease by about 13 percent per decade. Phenylalanine is the precursor amino acid from which dopamine is made. Phenylalanine can be supplied in foods such as white chicken meat, fish, and Swiss cheese or even taken as a nutritional supplement.

Both serotonin and dopamine are needed to help us cope with stress. However, the need for adequate production of serotonin is particularly acute during the early stages of the stress response. In terms of Selye's three stages, sufficient serotonin is needed in the first two stages (alarm and resistance), when a person tends to have too much energy and is over-stimulated and agitated. These individuals can really benefit from the calming effects of serotonin. In contrast, excitatory dopamine is particularly important in the exhaustion stage, when energy is depleted and needs a boost. Stressed-out and depleted individuals need plenty of dopamine, which the body then converts to epinephrine and norepinephrine, both of which are necessary for physical energy and alertness.

As levels of these neurotransmitters begin to decline with age, the body's ability to handle stressful events can change. Depressed serotonin levels can trigger mood imbalances, sleeplessness, and food cravings. Individuals with low serotonin levels are more prone toward conditions like PMS and, in extreme cases, even aggressive and violent behavior. Women with PMS often respond to stressful events in an exaggerated manner. Irritability, anger, tension, and upset are common responses in the second half of the menstrual cycle to such usually small stresses as a nagging child, a minor disagreement with a spouse, or a work deadline. Women who suffer from a serotonin imbalance often feel like a firecracker about to explode for one to two weeks out of each month.

In contrast, when levels of the stimulatory neurotransmitter dopamine are depressed, epinephrine and norepinephrine production is also diminished. Individuals in this condition become fatigued, lethargic, and even depressed, as is typically seen in Hans Selye's exhaustion phase. These individuals may be too tired and de-energized to respond to stressful events with any vigor. In extreme cases, lack of dopamine can even cause an individual to become suicidal.

Beta-endorphins

Some researchers suggest that, in women, the symptoms of anxiety and mood swings characteristic of PMS are caused by a heightened sensitivity to fluctuations in the body's level of beta-endorphins. These substances are the body's natural opiates, producing a sense of well-being and even elation when present in large amounts. They are, in part, responsible for the elevated mood known as "runner's high" that people experience after long-distance running or another extended aerobic activity.

Beta-endorphin levels increase soon after ovulation and may decline with the approach of menstruation. A fall in beta-endorphin levels, like opiate withdrawal, causes symptoms such as anxiety and irritability in women who are very sensitive to the effects of these chemicals or who produce large amounts of them.

Estrogen and progesterone

Women produce two major sex hormones, estrogen and progesterone. These hormones regulate the menstrual cycle, with estrogen reaching a peak during the first half of the cycle, while progesterone output occurs after midcycle, when ovulation has already occurred. Estrogen causes the growth of the sexual organs at puberty and thickening of the lining of the uterus before it receives a fertilized egg. Estrogen also causes fluid and salt retention in the tissues, which helps to plump up the skin. In contrast, progesterone has a maturing and growth-limiting effect on the tissues of the body, including the uterus, and functions as a diuretic, preventing retention of excess fluid in body tissue.

These two hormones also help to keep in balance the various functions of the nervous systems, and they can have a strong impact on how a woman responds to stress. For example, estrogen tends to act as a natural mood elevator, whereas progesterone has a sedative or calming effect. When these hormones are out of balance in relation to one another, stress symptoms can be aggravated. When estrogen is elevated, it can cause anxiety and stress symptoms; progesterone dominance can cause depression and fatigue.

ACID/ALKALINE BALANCE

Both overacidity and overalkalinity can affect the way that we respond to stress. People who are naturally alkaline tend to be emotionally resilient and quite resistant to stress of any type. When we deviate from our normal, healthful pH range, our moods and emotions begin to fluctuate, creating either anxiety and panic or depression and fatigue. In either case, one's ability to handle stress is greatly compromised. See chapter 1, on acid/alkaline balance, for a more complete discussion of this topic.

DIGESTIVE-ENZYME PRODUCTION

Digestive enzymes, particularly those produced by the pancreas, have potent anti-inflammatory effects. Like the glucocorticoids secreted by the adrenal cortex, pancreatic digestive enzymes act as a natural anti-inflammatory when the body is assaulted by injuries, infection, and inflammation that occur in sites as disparate as the joints and sinuses. Pancreatic-enzyme production diminishes with age. This process is accelerated by the highly stressed and difficult-to-digest diet that many Americans eat, which puts additional wear and tear on this overworked organ.

NITRIC OXIDE

Nitric oxide is a substance our bodies produce that helps to optimize the flow of blood through the arteries and veins. As a potent vasodilator, it enhances the flow of blood and the transport of oxygen to all the cells and tissues of the body. Research studies suggest that nitric oxide may actually be one of the most important chemicals that our bodies produce.

Nitric oxide is a gaseous molecule produced in the body from the amino acid arginine. Extensive research conducted in the 1990s shows that nitric oxide is involved in regulating a wide variety of physiologic functions. Sufficient production of nitric oxide is needed to support the healthy function of many of our vital internal organs. Recent research has also found that nitric oxide may even play an important role in allowing us to adapt effectively to stressful situations of any type. For example, a research study published in 1998 in the journal *Biochemistry* describes the mechanism of how nitric oxide may help protect us against the physiological changes caused by stress. Nitric oxide may even enhance our ability to handle stress more effectively. In contrast, insufficient levels of nitric oxide are associated with many disease conditions, most of which relate to poor circulation and insufficient oxygenation. These include diseases of the heart and lungs and the neuroendocrine, immune, and reproductive systems, as well as our resistance to and ability to handle stress of any type. Research studies have shown that intravenous administration of the amino acid arginine can increase nitric oxide production. Attempts to increase nitric oxide production through oral supplementation with arginine have only met with limited success. However, a nutraceutical research company has created products which combine small amounts of arginine with other nutrients to successfully increase nitric oxide production.

DIET

Many men and women are unaware of the important role that food selection can play in either intensifying or reducing symptoms of anxiety, panic, and excessive stress. Medical research in the areas of diet and nutrition over the past twenty years has shown that many foods, beverages, and food additives can worsen and even trigger feelings of anxiety. This is true in emotionally based, as well as chemically or hormonally based, cases of anxiety and panic. At the same time, studies have found certain foods to be beneficial for their mood-stabilizing and calming effects.

Over the years, Susan has seen thousands of patients suffering from anxiety symptoms due to a variety of emotional and/or physical causes. Dietary modification is often the primary treatment for anxiety caused by PMS, hypoglycemia, and food allergies. In fact, Susan has found that continuing stressful eating habits actually works against other therapeutic measures a patient may institute, such as counseling or the use of antianxiety medication. Thus, the importance of healthful dietary practices in the treatment of anxiety should not be underestimated.

Caffeine

While overconsumption of caffeine can be highly stressful to the body, most people use caffeine-containing beverages and foods to counteract stress. Caffeine in small doses promotes quick, clear thinking and decreases fatigue and reaction time, all valued qualities in our achievement-oriented society. Caffeine stimulates the adrenals to send a signal for the release of glucose to flood the body with energy. However, even a dose of as low as 200 mg, or one cup of coffee, can cause nervousness in people who are under stress.

Of course, not everyone who is under stress develops a coffee habit. Type A personalities, who have an abundance of energy, may not feel they need a coffee fix every morning. People in the first two stages of stress (as defined by Selye), who are already running on adrenaline, also may not crave coffee. But by the time a person reaches Selye's exhaustion stage, caffeine will probably have become their drug of choice. The recent proliferation of cafés and chain-owned coffee shops may well be a sign of the large numbers of people in our society who are in the exhaustion stage and often need a quick lift to help them function.

Unfortunately, habitual overuse of caffeine weakens the adrenal stress response, leading to eventual exhaustion. Caffeine also stimulates the release of stress hormones from the adrenal glands, further intensifying nervousness, especially in persons with anxiety disorders. In a study published in 1984 in the *Psychopharmacy Bulletin*, plasma cortisol levels rose in response to a caffeine challenge. This study included eight patients suffering from panic disorder and two who were not. Anxiety increased in the panic disorder patients, but the two normal (control) subjects also experienced panic attacks, accompanied by a fivefold increase in plasma cortisol after a dose of caffeine equivalent to about six cups of coffee.

Sugar

Sugar is one of the most overused foods in the Western world. Present almost universally in desserts and sweet snacks, sugar is also an ingredient in condiments such as salad dressings, ketchup, and relish. In addition, foods such as pasta and bread, when made with white flour, act as simple sugars in the body.

Eating large amounts of sugar, especially in a short period of time, can trigger an episode of hypoglycemia (low blood sugar). The mechanism is as follows: Sugar is rapidly absorbed from the digestive tract into the circulation. In response to these elevated blood sugar levels, the pancreas secretes insulin to enable the sugar to be cleared from the bloodstream and be taken up by the cells, where it is used as a source of energy. In response to large amounts of ingested sugar, the pancreas often overproduces insulin, which causes the blood sugar to fall too low. As a result, hypoglycemia occurs, causing an individual to feel anxious, tremulous, and jittery; in addition, thinking can become confused because the brain is deprived of necessary fuel. To remedy this situation, the adrenal glands release hormones, which cause the liver to pump stored sugar into the bloodstream. However, while the adrenal hormones boost the blood sugar level, they also increase arousal symptoms and anxiety. Both the initial brain deprivation of glucose and the adrenal glands' attempt to restore the glucose levels can intensify symptoms of anxiety and panic in susceptible people. Studies confirm that people who are anxiety-prone are especially sensitive to the emotional effects of a drop in blood sugar.

Women with PMS may have hypoglycemia related to their menstrual cycles. It is known that women with PMS crave more simple carbohydrates, such as refined sugar and flour. Research shows that 80 to 90 percent of women who eat this way report stress, anxiety, moodiness, and irritability during the week or two preceding menstruation. Susan's clinical experience is that many of these symptoms can be reversed with dietary changes. An extensive review article on the role of low blood sugar and personality, reported in 1994 in *Complementary Therapies in Medicine*, provided evidence that low blood sugar is almost always accompanied by personality disorders and that improvement or complete remission is possible with nutritional therapy.

Alcohol

People with moderate to severe anxiety and mood swings should avoid alcohol entirely or limit its use to only occasional small amounts. Alcohol is a simple sugar and, like sucrose, is rapidly absorbed by the body, potentially causing symptoms of hypoglycemia. The nervous system is also subject to the deleterious effects of alcohol, which can lead to irrational anger and emotional outbursts. Alcohol can also increase anxiety and mood swings indirectly by hampering the liver's ability to detoxify substances such as estrogen, drugs, and pesticides (see chapter 5). As toxic levels of these chemicals build up in the body, anxiety can worsen. In a study reported in 1990 in the *Journal of Clinical Psychiatry*, ninety healthy male volunteers received separate administrations of ethanol and a placebo. Significant increases in anxiety were noted after administration of the ethanol, while a significant decrease in feelings of tension took place after administration of the placebo. Alcohol withdrawal also can cause anxiety.

Food allergies

The symptoms of an allergic reaction occur when the body overreacts to the ingestion of a foreign, usually harmless, substance. The two most common allergens in the American diet are (1) wheat and (2) milk and other dairy products. However, many people are also allergic to chocolate, alcohol, soy products, eggs, shellfish, tomatoes, corn, citrus fruits, strawberries, peanuts, and yeast. One of the most reliable signs of a food allergy is a food addiction, as we tend to crave the foods we are allergic to. In the test section of this chapter, we describe how you can test yourself for food allergies (see page 480).

Symptoms often occur immediately after exposure to the allergen and may include wheezing, tearing of the eyes, itching, nasal congestion, and hives. However, a person may also have a delayed reaction, with symptoms such as anxiety, irritability, depression or mood swings, insomnia, fatigue, spaciness, dizziness, confusion and disorientation, headaches, and aching joints. Food allergies can affect digestive function, causing inflammation of the intestinal lining and pain in the abdominal area, as well as bloating, gas, and bowel changes. For women with PMS, a food they are allergic to can worsen emotional symptoms and fatigue. Because allergens stress the adrenals, triggering the output of anti-inflammatory hormones, repeated allergic reactions can weaken the adrenals over time. This can greatly increase our susceptibility to stress of all types.

Food additives

Several thousand chemical additives are currently used in commercial food manufacturing. Some of the most popular, including the artificial sweetener aspartame (NutraSweet) and the flavor enhancer monosodium glutamate (MSG), produce anxiety-like symptoms in many people. Susan has had patients complain that the use of the artificial sweetener aspartame precipitated panic symptoms, such as rapid heartbeat, shallow breathing, headaches, anxiety, spaciness, and dizziness. Many patients with PMS or generalized anxiety find that aspartame worsens their nervous tension.

NUTRITIONAL DEFICIENCIES

The fight-or-flight response stimulates the nervous system to produce and regulate neurotransmitters, triggers the production of stress-modulating hormones, especially by the adrenals, increases our rate of metabolism, and draws on energy reserves. These processes depend on the presence of various nutrients. Other chemical pathways, such as those that regulate the production of estrogen, progesterone, serotonin, and dopamine and those that regulate blood sugar levels (as well as a myriad of chemical reactions that can affect our response to stress), also require specific vitamins and minerals to proceed. These nutrients include vitamin B complex, vitamins C and E, and the minerals magnesium, calcium, potassium, iron, zinc, chromium, manganese, and selenium. Unfortunately, many individuals are deficient in these nutrients, either because of inadequate intake or because stress itself can accelerate the loss of these nutrients from the body.

EXPOSURE TO TOXIC CHEMICALS

The toxic chemicals that are part of our contemporary environment are risk factors for anxiety and other symptoms of stress. There is evidence that exposure to environmental toxins can cause emotional stress and behavioral changes. In a study published in 1981 in *Biological Psychiatry*, researchers worked with ten male and twenty female patients, aged seventeen to fifty-six, who had complaints of anxiety or other psychological symptoms. When the volunteers were exposed to common pollutants such as auto exhaust and chlorine, they reported experiencing brain fog and generalized anger, and that their nervousness and depression increased.

A study published in 1992 in the *Southern Medical Journal* evaluated symptoms and psychological responses of members of thirty households located near a toxic-waste site who were drinking polluted water. As compared with persons not exposed to the chemicals, members of these households had significantly greater personal problems with their spouses and their extended families. They also reported high levels of depression and anxiety.

EMOTIONAL FACTORS

Many emotional factors can also trigger the stress response in susceptible individuals. These can include current or past events as well as early family programming.

Cumulative stress

Unremitting major life stresses are likely to cause wear and tear on the nervous system and, over time, can cause a person to become anxious or tense. Any change or dislocation, good or bad, can cause stress, because these changes throw people into entirely new situations for which they may have little or no preparation. Cumulative stress can be a risk factor for disease, as we will discuss later in the chapter. A person who has withstood stresses peaceably for years may one day suddenly have a panic attack over a single event when his or her resistance finally gives way.

A person can feel bombarded by stress at any age, but this is particularly common with people in midlife. People in their late forties and fifties are often in the most productive and responsible phase of their careers. Many are also raising teenage children, who are testing their parents as they try to find their own identity. These same midlife people may also have parents who are aging and need attention or are seriously ill or dying, so they have to find the time to give their parents custodial care as well.

Negative emotional programming

Children, up to the age of four or five, are completely dependent on adult caretakers, especially their mothers. When children receive excessive criticism from their parents and are asked to meet perfectionist standards, excessive dependency and clinging can develop. In adulthood, criticism can become a source of insecurity and even anxiety disorders, causing acute fear of trying new experiences for fear of failing.

Youngsters who are subjected to abuse, neglect, or abandonment through divorce, death, or sexual abuse also tend to have anxiety later in life, as do children of alcoholic parents. Separation anxiety can continue into adulthood. A threatened child may feel afraid leaving the house for school or when falling asleep. As adults, these same people may experience anxiety when separated from a safe person or place.

Many people in their adult lives continue to give themselves negative messages left over from childhood when they perceive certain situations or people as threatening or dangerous. Negative self-talk can do much to perpetuate anxiety disorders, so it is very important that our constant inner dialogue be positive and constructive.

An Inherited Predisposition to Stress

Genetics may also play a role in the development of anxiety disorders. For example, in studies of identical twins, the likelihood of both twins having an anxiety disorder if one is afflicted is statistically significant (greater than 30 percent). Fraternal twins, who do not have the same genetic makeup, are also at a higher risk of developing an anxiety disorder if their sibling is affected, although they do not have nearly the risk of identical twins. Agoraphobia (the fear of open or public places), the most common anxiety disorder, also seems to show a familial predisposition. While 5 percent of the entire population suffers from this condition, the rate of agoraphobia in people with one parent who had this diagnosis is 15 to 20 percent.

The Aging of the Autonomic Nervous System

Over time, all of the regulatory systems in the body age. While a healthy autonomic nervous system plays a crucial role in maintaining homeostasis and an appropriate response to stress, this system inevitably begins to become less efficient as a person grows older. There is a reduction in the synthesis of neurotransmitters, which are an essential part of this system, as well as changes in the functioning of higher stress-related regulatory centers within the brain. Sympathetic nerves must receive more intense stimulation in order to affect an end organ, and there is a reduction in the maximum frequency with which impulses can be transmitted. There are also parallel changes in the endocrine regulation of the stress response.

During midlife, changes in the structure of the adrenal glands begin to become apparent, with a slight loss of weight in the glands as well as an increase of connective tissue in proportion to a decline in function. However, plasma levels of glucocorticoids, chemicals that help the body withstand stress, do not significantly change with age. While there is a lower rate of secretion, this is matched with a lower rate of disposal.

Further, in older people, the pituitary release of adrenocorticotrophin, or ACTH (a chemical that promotes the manufacture and secretion of adrenal hormones), in response to stress as well as the reaction of the adrenal cortex to ACTH remain normal.

MEDICAL CONDITIONS

Sometimes feelings of anxiety and increased vulnerability to stress can be the consequence of certain ailments and diseases not associated with any psychological disorder. For example, mitral-valve prolapse, hyperthyroidism, and premenstrual syndrome can cause anxiety-like symptoms even though they may not have an emotional trigger.

Mitral-valve prolapse

Mitral-valve prolapse is a heart condition that can cause episodes of palpitations, chest pain, shortness of breath, and fatigue. Research studies have shown that this condition occurs more frequently in people with anxiety and panic episodes than in the general population. It is caused by a mild defect in the mitral valve, which is located between the upper and lower chambers on the left side of the heart. Normally, blood flows unimpeded between the two chambers. However, with mitral-valve prolapse, the valve doesn't close completely. As a result, the heart is put under stress and beats either too fast or erratically. Undue stress and stimulants such as caffeinated beverages should be eliminated in order to avoid triggering episodes of rapid heartbeat. Calcium, magnesium, and potassium supplements should also be taken, since these essential minerals help to regulate and reduce cardiac irritability.

Hyperthyroidism and hypothyroidism

When the thyroid gland excretes an excessive amount of thyroid hormone, hyperthyroidism occurs. This is a potentially serious problem if not diagnosed and treated right away. Symptoms of hyperthyroidism can mimic those of anxiety attacks and include generalized anxiety, insomnia, fatigue, rapid heartbeat, profuse sweating, heat intolerance, and loose bowel movements. In fact, the correct diagnosis is often missed initially if the symptoms are thought to be due to stress. However, individuals with hyperthyroidism may also present other symptoms, including ravenous appetite, quick movements, trembling of hands, and difficulty focusing the eyes. Conversely, decreased production of thyroid hormone, or hypothyroidism, is linked to fatigue and depression and other symptoms of sluggish metabolic function. Individuals with hypothyroidism, if untreated, often have poor resistance to stress and illness.

PMS

As mentioned earlier in the chapter, anxiety and mood swings are the hallmarks of premenstrual syndrome (PMS). These symptoms occur only in the second half of the menstrual cycle and last anywhere from one to two weeks. Medical researchers now believe that various hormonal and chemical imbalances can trigger PMS symptoms, especially an imbalance in the body's estrogen and progesterone levels. These symptoms can involve almost every system in the body. Women are especially at risk when they are under significant emotional stress, have poor nutritional habits, and do not exercise regularly—lifestyle habits that in themselves are stressful.

Women typically go through a transition period called peri-menopause in the years leading up to the cessation of menses. This transition period can be as short as one to two years or as long as seven to ten years, depending on an individual's chemistry. During this period, women may begin to experience imbalances in estrogen and progesterone production due to the aging of the ovaries, resulting in PMS-like symptoms.

SUMMARY

A healthy body constantly works to maintain itself in the balanced state called homeostasis. Too much stress can weaken our ability to return to this balanced state, leaving the body in a state of constant alarm. Many factors affect our ability to deal with stress. The body produces several substances to help it recover from stress, but the aging process can weaken their production. Other factors, such as acid/alkaline balance, diet, environmental toxins, emotional factors, and certain health conditions can also negatively affect the body's stress-relieving systems.

SECTION 3:
STRESS MANAGEMENT AND PEAK PERFORMANCE

THE WAY AN individual responds to stress varies from person to person. How capable a person is of responding appropriately to stressful events is primarily determined by the reactivity of his or her nervous system.

Some people tend to be parasympathetic-dominant in their nervous system response, which allows them to evaluate and react to stress in a calmer and more relaxed fashion. These type B personalities are able to accurately gauge the seriousness of the stresses they encounter and do not react with a fight-or-flight response unless they face a truly dangerous or upsetting situation. This type of person performs well under stress.

Other people are sympathetic-dominant in their response pattern and tend to react in an exaggerated manner to even the smallest events. Sympathetic-dominant people are frequently edgy and nervous and tend to exhibit anger and hostility for no apparent reason. These are the bosses who become enraged if dissatisfied by an employee's work performance or the tennis players who throw their racket after netting an easy shot. For these type A personalities, sleeping beyond the ring of the alarm clock can be almost as upsetting as having someone crash into their car.

Stress can disrupt performance, usually affecting a person's weakest and therefore most vulnerable skills. For example, people who can talk and charm their way through any problem, but who make poor decisions under pressure, will lose their reasoning powers first, not their gift of gab. These susceptibilities are determined by what skills a person has acquired and emphasized over the years, and what personality traits and talents they have inherited. The following sections describe some of the peak-performance traits that stress can undermine.

1 PHYSICAL VITALITY AND STAMINA

The excitatory chemicals produced within both the nervous system and the adrenal medulla—such as dopamine, epinephrine, and norepinephrine—not only help us to cope with stress but also assist in creating the alertness, physical energy, and vitality that are necessary for peak performance in every area of life. These chemicals are the spark plugs that ignite our libido, aggressive drive, and all-around zest for life. Having an abundance of these chemicals provides us with the physical energy necessary to cope with any stressful situation that we encounter. They also give us the stamina to participate in a wide variety of work and social activities, maintain a hectic schedule when necessary, party into the late hours, and wake up the next morning with enough energy to go out and engage in strenuous physical activity.

Peak performers in all walks of life produce an abundance of these valuable stress-coping and energy-sustaining chemicals. Individuals with superfunctioning adrenals and nervous systems can maintain this demanding pace well into old age. Other individuals, with less innate strength and reserve in these crucial systems, may find that, over time, their stress-coping abilities as well as their stamina and endurance begin to weaken. This is particularly true in modern society, where the stresses of day-to-day living are manifold and the outlets to discharge them are not readily available. In addition, the standard American diet and the thousands of toxic chemicals to which we are exposed take their toll on everyone except those who have superfunctioning adrenals and nervous systems.

Constant triggering of the stress response through dietary indiscretion, emotional and lifestyle strains, and exposure to toxic chemicals gradually leads to adrenal and ANS exhaustion. The glands and organs involved with our response to stress become so overworked and weakened that they are unable to produce enough of the chemicals and hormones that we need to create an energetic response to any of our life stresses.

When a person finally reaches this stage of physical exhaustion, fatigue and lack of vitality become the norm. In modern societies, fatigue is surprisingly common. In fact, it is one of the most common issues that patients complain about to their physicians. While many cases of fatigue can be traced to treatable, organic conditions such as anemia and hypothyroidism, many other cases have their origin in lifestyle and emotional stresses. For this type of exhaustion, doctors have no magic pills or panaceas.

Early-warning signs of stress-induced fatigue

There are many early-warning signs that you are at risk of adrenal and nervous-system exhaustion and are beginning to lose your ability to handle common life stresses. As our production of stress-coping chemicals begins to diminish, we lose our ability to deal with life's daily challenges with vitality, confidence, and optimism. Instead, people begin to react to stressful situations with exhaustion, depression, and a lack of resilience.

One of the early signals of adrenal-gland and nervous-system exhaustion is the need to use stimulants such as coffee and caffeinated soft drinks to help maintain energy levels. Another early-warning sign is lowered resistance to minor stressful events. Where previously you might have reacted to a minor stress with an appropriately calm response, you might now find yourself losing your temper and snapping at people. In addition, many people begin to worry excessively about minor or easily solvable problems. Molehills become mountains when day-to-day coping mechanisms become stretched. As the adrenal glands and nervous system begin to weaken, periods of fatigue become more frequent. You have less of the physical energy needed to maintain your usual complement of responsibilities and activities. You may then begin to abandon normally pleasurable activities such as sports, parties, social gatherings, and weekend trips, preferring instead to rest. Finally, restlessness at night and insomnia may further erode your energy. This is often due to worry and concern over your condition, as well as the depletion of your stress-coping chemicals.

There are a growing number of Americans who are severely sleep-deprived, which suggests that the stress-coping hormones and chemicals are being depleted in a large number of people. Studies show that stress is one of the most common causes of chronic insomnia and disturbed sleep patterns, whether the stress is caused by short-term events like spending an hour in traffic or anticipating having a root canal, or by long-term demands such as raising a teenager. A study conducted by the National Sleep Foundation (NSF), as reported in 1997 in the *Medical Tribune*, found that 47 percent of workers in the United States have trouble sleeping, and 48 percent of these individuals reported sleep loss due primarily to some form of stress or anxiety. Furthermore, the study found that of those workers with sleep problems, two-thirds felt that their insomnia had a negative effect on their job performance. This reduced productivity has a significant impact on the American economy. According to the NSF survey, poor performance related to sleep deprivation costs U.S. businesses $92.5 to $107.5 billion in absenteeism, medical costs, and decreased productivity.

Over the years, Susan has treated many patients with stress-related exhaustion. These are people of all ages and from all walks of life. They include professionals who had to abandon careers because of fatigue, to college students who had to drop out of school and go home and rest. Some individuals still maintain enough energy to continue to be hardworking and productive, but may be working fewer hours. They may be able to continue functioning only with the use of stimulants or because they have already curtailed their social and recreational activities. Other, more compromised individuals may be too fatigued to work at all.

The law of diminishing expectations

Fatigued people cope by following the law of diminishing expectations: As their energy levels drop, they begin to restrict their activities commensurate with their diminished energy reserves. They usually maintain survival activities like work, but the joy-of-living activities are eliminated. If they were previously exercising five times a week, they may reduce that to twice a week and finally cease exercising entirely. They begin to reduce their participation in social activities and finally stop going out altogether. They adopt sedentary activities like watching TV instead of participatory ones like woodworking or gardening. Most of the joy of living disappears, and life becomes dedicated to survival and earning a living. Other patients are farther along the fatigue continuum. They reach a point where they cannot even maintain their survival activities. These patients can no longer earn a living. They often go on disability or let family and friends provide for them. They go from independence to dependence.

Anna was a college student in her early twenties who, because of chronic fatigue and tiredness, had to drop out of school several times as she did not have the energy to keep up with the demands of her studies. Eventually, she dropped out for good and went home to live with her parents. She traded her independence so she could survive on her greatly reduced energy levels. After one year of living at home, she began to consult with Susan.

Rachel, a thirty-four-year-old travel agent, had for the two and one-half years prior to seeing Susan reduced her workload to half days, working in the mornings while she still had enough energy to handle the demands of her job. In the afternoons she would leave work to go home and rest. Finally, for Rachel, the law of diminishing expectations completed its cycle, and for six months prior to consulting Susan, she was unable to work at all.

George is an example of a person whose chronic stress was brought about by outside events. He was a forty-eight-year-old small business owner who had been quite successful for a number of years. However, problems with his business created extreme financial stress, culminating with an IRS foreclosure proceeding against his home. After several years of intense stress, this previously highly energetic man began to notice signs of extreme fatigue. He started getting frequent sore throats, colds, sinus conditions, and swollen glands in his neck. He survived on coffee and colas. By the time he saw Susan, even these stimulants could not maintain his energy level.

Restoring energy levels through stress management

To help restore the physical energy of her patients with stress-related fatigue and help them to return to their prior level of performance, Susan has found that a variety of therapeutic techniques must be implemented. To strengthen and restore adrenal-gland and autonomic-nervous-system function, all "energy leaks" must be eliminated from their lives. These include the use of energy-depleting foods, such as stimulants like caffeinated beverages, refined-sugar or white-flour products, and chocolate. Other foods such as saturated fats, red meat, and alcohol should also be eliminated because of their tendency to worsen fatigue. Any foods to which a patient is allergic should be avoided (wheat and dairy products are common offenders), as should common environmental toxins. Susan also helps to support and restore her patients with adrenal and nervous-system exhaustion through the use of nutritional-supplement programs, such as those discussed in the following chapter.

Many of her patients have also found it helpful to carefully examine their career and personal stresses to see if they need to institute lifestyle changes to reduce their sources of stress. They must either eliminate these factors or learn to modify their effects through stress management techniques such as meditation and biofeedback.

Be aware of the early-warning signs and symptoms of stress-related fatigue. Recognize these signs for what they represent, and act on them right away. Be sure to check with your doctor to make sure that there is no organic and easily treatable cause such as anemia or low thyroid production. Identify the stress factors in your life. Then begin lifestyle changes, implement stress reduction techniques, and initiate a restorative program for the adrenals and the nervous system to rebuild your store of stress-coping chemicals.

▲ To restore your physical energy, frequent physical activity is necessary; dietary supplementation alone is not enough. Physical activities, particularly those done outdoors, such as walking, golfing, swimming, and even gardening, help to restore our reserves of stress-coping chemicals because they improve oxygenation and blood flow to all the cells of the body. The oxygen provided through physical activity promotes the efficient conversion of food into energy as well as the excretion of the waste products of metabolism. Exercise is also a natural mood elevator, helping to promote the production of excitatory chemicals in the brain. Individuals with fatigue should make a point of getting outdoors as often as possible and begin a program of physical activity at a leisurely and relaxed pace, never going beyond their tolerance level. Over time, ten to fifteen minutes of activity a day will extend to a half hour to an hour a day as the health of the adrenal glands and nervous system is restored.

2 MENTAL CLARITY AND ACUITY

The abilities to assimilate and evaluate information through intensive, prolonged periods of reading and writing are necessary requirements of many careers. Individuals in technical fields—such as research scientists, physicians, software developers, and engineers—are required to regularly read technical journals and manuals to keep abreast of their fields, write reports, or, in the case of physicians, write up detailed and technically accurate records on thousands of patients each year. Teachers working at all educational levels spend a great deal of their time reading material relevant to the courses they teach to keep up with new information in their field and prepare class lectures, as well as reading and grading student tests and papers. Book editors, journalists, screenwriters, and other individuals in the media also spend most of their time creating their own or reviewing other people's written material.

Constant demands on one's mental faculties, combined with tight deadlines, tend to trigger the stress response. In the early stages of their careers, many of these people have an abundance of the stress-coping chemicals and hormones to meet these rigorous mental demands, and they are able to function as peak performers. However, as the years progress, the constant triggering of these stress-coping mechanisms begins to take its toll on performance and health.

Unfortunately, those who do intense mental work on a daily basis are often unaware of the strain that such demanding work places on their bodies. When people work intensely at their desks for hours at a time, they tend to lock their bodies into habitual positions. The tightening of muscles, shallow breathing, and overfocusing (the habit of concentrating and focusing on a subject or task too intently) are common stress responses during periods of intense mental concentration. Over time, such habits can cause chronic tension in the neck and shoulders, eyestrain, and diminished blood flow and oxygenation to the brain and eyes. The end result is mental fatigue, diminished cognitive abilities, and eventual career burnout.

▲▲ In order to maintain your cognitive functions and to continue to perform at peak levels in your career for many decades, pacing is crucial. To avoid overfocusing and habitual patterns of muscle tension that can lead to the triggering of the stress response, it is helpful to interrupt intense mental work with frequent breaks. Stand up, walk around, stretch, do isometric exercises, walk up and down a flight of steps, and look out the window at distant objects to rest your eyes. Try not to read or write for more than a half hour without taking one of these breaks. Frequent breaks will allow the brain, nervous system, and muscles to relax and recover, greatly reducing the negative effects of stress due to prolonged mental effort.

Besides the restorative benefits of frequent breaks, many research studies have found that the learning process itself is greatly enhanced in a calm, relaxed environment. A number of researchers have found that optimal learning occurs when the brain and nervous system are in a relaxed state. The original research that validated and developed these concepts was conducted by Bulgarian psychiatrist Georgi Lozanov in the 1960s.

He found that when information was given verbally in a rhythmic pattern while Baroque music was played in the background, people were able to retain and recall significantly higher amounts of information than by other learning methods. He found that the Baroque music, which is played at about 60 beats per minute, relaxed the brain and nervous system. The brain was then better able to absorb and assimilate new information. Lozanov found that retention rates for rote-memory work—such as learning a foreign language, expanding your current vocabulary, remembering anatomical parts in medicine, or memorizing lines in a play—were greatly enhanced. In addition, the material was retained by the brain in long-term storage and could be recalled when needed.

Another pioneer in this area is Paul Scheele, a developer of many advanced learning techniques based on neurolinguistic programming. Scheele found that when a person is put into a relaxed state and uses a "soft-focus" eye technique, printed information can be absorbed and recalled at rates exceeding 25,000 words per minute. Like Lozanov, Scheele found that when the brain is in a relaxed state, the brain can take in, assimilate, and store for future recall enormous amounts of information.

An entire industry has been built up around these techniques because they provide three benefits simultaneously: deep relaxation and stress reduction combined with the ability to learn, assimilate, and recall enormous amounts of information, either spoken or written. Today, these accelerated or superlearning techniques are available on cassette tapes, compact discs, and sophisticated light-and-sound devices.

▲▲ If your job or career requires you to constantly absorb, assimilate, and be able to recall large amounts of information, be sure to explore the many tools and techniques for accelerated or superlearning. The dual benefit of stress reduction and the ability to take in information at speeds not possible by any other method will allow you to mentally perform at peak levels for decades.

Stress may also negatively affect cognitive function by accelerating the progression of certain diseases such as hypertension and chronic lung disease in cigarette smokers. Over time, these conditions can reduce blood flow and oxygenation to the brain, causing diminished cognitive abilities. In a study reported in 1997 in *Stroke*, researchers from the National

Institute on Aging, in Bethesda, Maryland, employed magnetic-resonance imaging of the brain and a battery of tests that measured memory to assess cognitive function in patients aged fifty-six to eighty-four. The group was divided into twenty-seven volunteers with high blood pressure and twenty volunteers with normal blood pressure. The study found that the volunteers with high blood pressure had diminished cognitive function, with memory loss and evidence of brain atrophy, in contrast to the normal patients. A reduction in memory and cognition was apparent even in patients who were being treated for hypertension.

Winston S. Churchill: A Master of Stress Management

Many important political leaders have exemplified the benefits of being able to manage stress while required to do strenuous mental work throughout their careers. Heads of state have to take in, analyze, and act upon data and information in a variety of areas vital to the well-being and security of the countries they lead. Winston S. Churchill, throughout his long and distinguished career, was a master of stress management. He was effective, in part, because he frequently took breaks from the protracted and highly stressful mental work he was required to do. Besides all the day-to-day mental activity that his political office required, he was a prodigious reader and writer. A recipient in 1953 of a Nobel Prize in Literature, he is today remembered as much for his wit, wisdom, and way with words as for his political accomplishments.

During World War II, Churchill operated under incredible stress and pressure. In the early years of the war, there were constant defeats, shortages of troops and material, and the omnipresence of the militarily superior German war machine. The pressure on Churchill was everywhere, from mobilizing the British army as well as the British people to reading and dictating enormous numbers of military and government briefs and directives, and his intense involvement with the strategic planning and coordinating of the war effort with Roosevelt and Stalin. As Prime Minister of Great Britain, he had the ultimate responsibility for defending and preserving that nation.

Churchill relieved the constant mental stress and pressure under which he operated by taking a long bath every day and a nap every afternoon. He did this regardless of his physical surroundings or the urgency of the decisions he was forced to make regarding the war effort. Whether he was at his own home, the Prime Minister's residence, his country estate, in hotels, or on a ship, he always took a break from his hectic and strenuous daily schedule by dictating to his secretary while still in bed. These regular breaks relaxed and reinvigorated him. The baths started Churchill's day in a relaxed fashion, and the naps allowed him to work far into the evening with the same intense concentration and mental faculties that many people have only in the morning.

Churchill's work also required him to be physically active and constantly on the go: giving speeches in Parliament, walking the streets of London giving courage to the British people, or traveling to meet with the allies or his generals. Churchill also broke up his workday by attending social events where he would relax and enjoy good food, participate in stimulating conversation, and linger over his favorite cigars and brandy. Churchill's habit of constantly breaking up prolonged periods of strenuous mental and physical activity was one of the major factors in his being truly one of the peak performers of the twentieth century.

4 THE ABILITY TO GET ALONG WITH OTHER PEOPLE

When people are unable to cope with stress, they often become upset and irritable. As a result, their interpersonal relationships inevitably suffer. Family members bicker and fight instead of working out conflicts in a calm and rational manner. Many individuals who visit doctors complain about the poor quality of their relationships but may not be aware that this problem originates not only in poor stress-coping mechanisms but also in chemical imbalances. Women with PMS, for example, often have imbalances in the stress-coping chemicals such as serotonin and dopamine, as well as imbalances in the major female sex hormones, estrogen and progesterone. The stressful symptoms of PMS, including anxiety and irritability, can be an enormously disruptive factor in a woman's life and in her relationships, both personal and professional. Many studies confirm that women who experience PMS tend to have more marital conflict and a greater tendency to inflict verbal or physical abuse on children. Women with PMS also have a higher incidence of suicide. During certain days of the month, some women often become so agitated and emotionally fragile that they lose all concentration and are unable to do their household chores or function well at work.

Maria, a thirty-seven-year-old teacher and mother, has had severe PMS symptoms since her mid-twenties, particularly irritability and anger during the two weeks before the onset of her menstrual period. She was very quick to fly off the handle, but had no insight into the cause of her problem. When Susan met her, Maria was on her second marriage. Maria's husband had given her Susan's book on PMS after reading it himself, suspecting that this could be the cause of his wife's moodiness and sensitivity to stress. Maria and her husband had discussed this issue, and after some resistance, she finally promised that she would come to Susan for counseling. At the initial visit, Maria did concede that her PMS had probably played a role in the breakup of her earlier marriage and that she was now worried that the same pattern was repeating itself. Maria was especially concerned because she had two children and really did love her husband. In taking her medical history, Susan learned that Maria had a habit of eating lots of sugary foods on the days she was most upset. She would also drink several cocktails or wine with dinner and binge on chocolate for dessert. All of these foods worsened her blood sugar imbalance and fueled her irritability and sensitivity to stress. After a session of diet counseling, Maria began to make significant changes in her nutritional habits and quickly eliminated the offending foods. Within just one menstrual cycle, she noticed that she was feeling calmer and more relaxed during the week before her menstrual cycle began. At the same time, Maria and her husband began to repair their relationship and enjoy each other's company again. Maria's PMS symptoms continued to improve, and she was pleased with the greatly improved relationship she and her husband were now enjoying.

Men can, of course, also suffer from imbalances in their stress-coping chemicals. Imbalances in the level of chemicals that affect our response to stress, such as serotonin, dopamine, epinephrine, or norepinephrine, can lead to mood disorders. Such individuals may feel either too depressed or overly agitated and upset. Their response to life situations that would not normally cause such an intense emotional response may be inappropriately strong. This can wreak havoc in both one's personal and business relationships. Many relationships among families, friends, and coworkers have been wrecked by emotional upsets that are due more to imbalances in stress chemicals than to the poor emotional programming of the individuals involved.

5 THE ABILITY TO REMAIN CALM UNDER PRESSURE

In business, being able to remain calm under fire is essential. This is as true for the person at the top of an organization as it is for the new recruit in the mailroom. Giving as well as following directions both require that a person be able to control their thoughts and emotions when the going gets tough.

Many successful executives profit from their ability to have a measured and balanced response to stress. Not only do they make better decisions, but they are more pleasant to work with and earn the loyalty of their staff and, consequently, more job security. An executive we know says, half-jokingly, that calm people may not make better decisions, but they are the ones who get hired and promoted, as people tend to want to be around them. As he says, no one wants to have a boss who explodes and reacts inappropriately when events do not unfold as expected.

Many individuals who work in the stock and bond markets are often subject to the volatility and instability of these markets. Brokers and traders often suffer from early burnout, as young as forty years old or even younger. Stress-related conditions such as peptic ulcer disease and insomnia are reasonably common among these individuals. Similarly, private investors and professional money managers are also subject to these same stresses and may suffer from stress-related symptoms. A striking exception is Warren Buffett, acknowledged to be one of the wealthiest and most successful investors in the world. He has demonstrated the Chemistry of Success in his legendary ability to maintain a measured and rational response while making decisions involving billions of investment dollars, even under adverse conditions. His calm and relaxed demeanor has, without doubt, contributed greatly to his success in this field.

Being able to remain calm under pressure is equally crucial in sports. An athlete who loses his cool often loses the game. Jim has observed this frequently in golf and tennis tournaments. A few years ago, Jim was playing a match-play golf tournament, in which each hole is either won, lost, or tied, and the player who wins the most individual holes wins the match. In most golf tournaments, the player with the lowest number of overall strokes wins, so a very high score on any one hole can cause you to lose the tournament. In match play, a poor score on any one hole will not cause you to lose the tournament. However, the psychological tension and stress that players experience in match play is very high. A golfer's emotions can yo-yo dramatically depending on how well both they and their opponents are playing. In this particular tournament, Jim's opponent won the first five holes, giving him a tremendous real and psychological advantage. During this streak of winning holes, his opponent was obviously relaxed and confident, chatting cordially, giving Jim encouragement that his unsatisfactory performance would improve. Jim remained calm even though his play was awful, staying focused only on the current shot.

As often happens, Jim's game began to improve at the same time his opponent's game deteriorated. Jim won the next five holes, and the abrupt turnaround completely unnerved and devastated his opponent. He lost his ability to focus on his shots. He missed several easy putts. His drives, which had previously all been in the fairway, now went into the trees lining the fairways. His previous calm and collected demeanor disappeared. The rise in his stress hormones was obvious by the tensing of his face and the angry, jerky body motions he now displayed after missing shots. He simply went to pieces, cursing himself, his game, and the golf course. By the end of the match, Jim's opponent was so disturbed that he did not shake hands and walked away muttering and cursing to himself.

6 Optimism and Vision

The excitatory chemicals like dopamine, epinephrine, and norepinephrine not only help us to cope with the stresses of life but are crucial in their effect on mood and attitude. The production of these chemicals is responsible, in part, for the optimism, vision, and creativity that the most energetic and productive people in our society demonstrate no matter what their fields of endeavor. It is virtually impossible to be productive and able to carry out your vision and creative dreams without the power that these chemicals confer when produced by our bodies at levels compatible with good health. Possessing an open and optimistic state of mind makes it possible for a person to envision new goals and then work out solutions to achieve them. Such a person can achieve great things. These people become the entrepreneurs of American business, or are major players in movements such as fighting for women's rights or ending world hunger, or are the parents who help their family to survive against all odds.

Many counseling and support groups, self-improvement programs, and spiritual practices not only acknowledge the wonderful creative potential of such a state of mind and emotions, but help people to achieve this state by protecting and restoring their stress-coping mechanisms. Meditation and focusing techniques that have their origins in Buddhism or martial arts teach people to still their thoughts. Affirmations, which are positive statements about oneself and the world, help to generate positive thinking. Visualization techniques, in which a person holds a mental image of his or her goal as if it were fully accomplished, help create a desired reality through changes in thought and attitude. These techniques do much to reduce the deleterious effects of stress on the adrenal glands and nervous system so that people can use their mind creatively. However, because these practices fall outside the field of Western medicine, their practitioners are not always aware of how these techniques restore the chemistry of the brain, nervous system, and adrenal glands.

Many creative writers and artists of the twentieth century searched for ways to expand their brain chemistry to enhance their creativity and vision. Besides meditation and the practice of Eastern spiritual techniques, visionary authors like Aldous Huxley; Richard Alpert, a psychologist who subsequently metamorphosed into the spiritual guru Ram Das; and Carlos Castaneda all wrote about their use of mind-expanding chemicals like LSD and psilocybin (the "magic mushroom") to increase their vision, creativity, and even productivity. Individuals with superfunctioning stress-coping systems, who produce their own mind-enhancing excitatory chemicals, are able to lead lives of incredible productivity, vision, and creativity without such mind-expanding chemicals or mood-enhancing drugs such as Prozac and Zoloft. For individuals who want to maintain and increase their optimism and vision, the practice of stress management techniques is crucial.

7 Speedy Recovery from Illness, Injury, and Exertion

8 Resistance to Illness

An excessive level of stress in one's life, either perceived or actual, can have very harmful effects on health. Stress can affect one's resistance to illness as well as the ability to recovery rapidly from illness, injury, and exertion.

In fact, the negative effects of stress can be so pronounced that they can affect the course of virtually any illness. The role that stress can play in bringing about disease has been examined in thousands of research studies. Conversely, strengthening one's ability to handle stress can increase one's resistance to disease. Because of this link, the topics of speedy recovery from illness and resistance to illness are covered in the following section on health.

SUMMARY

People vary in their ability to deal with stress, but the fact that this ability is one of the most important factors in peak performance does not change. Stress can undermine a number of peak-performance traits, including physical vitality and stamina. Stress is an important factor in many cases of fatigue, for example. Other performance traits affected by stress are mental clarity and acuity, the ability to get along with people, the ability to remain calm under pressure, and optimism and vision.

SECTION 4:
STRESS MANAGEMENT AND HEALTH

THOUSANDS OF RESEARCH studies have confirmed the effect that stress has on the development of disease. Stress can exacerbate the symptoms and increase the risk of developing most health conditions. Many of the patients that Susan has worked with over the past two and a half decades have complained of a worsening of their symptoms during times of extreme personal stress. Stress also slows down the rate of recovery from and increases the likelihood of recurrence of most illnesses. This was illustrated in two studies reported in 1994 in *World Health*. In the first study, 400 air traffic controllers in the United States were evaluated for the effect that stress had on the frequency with which they became ill. The controllers with the highest stress scores had an average of 69 percent more episodes of illness over the following twenty-seven months than those whose stress scores were in the lowest quartile. The second study focused on 500 men and women who had undergone coronary-artery-bypass or cardiac-valve surgery. These individuals were analyzed for their level of stress as well as their attitudes toward life. Seventy percent of the patients who reported a low level of stress in their lives prior to their operation were free of symptoms six months after surgery. In contrast, only 42 percent of the patients who reported a high level of stress in their lives were symptom-free at this same juncture. In addition, 66 percent of the patients who were generally hopeful about their lives were free of postoperative heart symptoms, compared with only 37 percent of the least hopeful patients.

In this section, we will look at how stress can negatively affect a number of the major health conditions most commonly experienced by people in our society.

DIGESTIVE PROBLEMS

Stressful situations can frequently trigger intestinal problems. A child may complain of having a stomachache before going on stage to perform in a play or before taking a test. An executive may feel tension in the pit of his stomach as he prepares to enter the boardroom to present his version of next year's marketing plan. But stress can also increase the likelihood of developing more serious gastrointestinal complaints.

An article that appeared in 1991 in the *Journal of the Royal Society of Medicine* reported on sixty women, aged seventeen to seventy-one, who had functional bowel disorders of the colon and rectum. The onset of symptoms of bowel disorder or a worsening of symptoms was more likely to occur during times when the women subjectively experienced stress. Their health problems were associated with such life events as engagements, marriages, divorces, pregnancy, childbirth, and miscarriages. These women described themselves as having difficulty in relationships with men and found sexual relationships usually unsatisfactory. In addition, of those women who gave birth, 40 percent experienced abdominal symptoms around this time. Three-fourths of the women in the study also had a history of emotional trauma in infancy and childhood. Traumas included the death of a sibling, sexual abuse, a broken home, emotional instability within the family, depression, and life-threatening events.

In another study of patients with irritable-bowel syndrome (IBS), eighteen of twenty patients had a history of psychiatric illness during their lifetimes. Half of the patients with psychiatric problems had panic disorder, and another half had social phobia. Common problems included substance abuse, depression, and somatization disorder (a condition in which patients experience physical symptoms for which no underlying medical cause has been found). In addition, among the closest relatives of patients with IBS, 55 percent had a history of psychiatric illness.

Studies have confirmed that practicing stress reduction techniques can greatly improve symptoms of irritable-bowel syndrome. For example, a study of 102 patients with IBS, published in 1991 in *Gastroenterology*, found that a combination of relaxation, psychotherapy, and standard medical care resulted in a lessening of diarrhea and abdominal pain. In contrast, the patients who were only given standard medical care did not show the same degree of improvement.

CARDIOVASCULAR DISEASE

Many studies confirm that stress is an important risk factor for heart disease. Stress can cause spasm of the coronary artery, accelerate the formation of plaque, and increase platelet aggregation as well as clotting, all of which are risk factors for heart disease. A study published in 1997 in the *British Medical Journal* found that government workers who felt they had little or no control over their jobs had a greater likelihood of developing coronary-artery disease. The researchers followed the health of 10,308 civil servants, aged thirty-five to fifty-five, over an average of 5.3 years. These workers were assessed for new cases of angina, ischemic heart disease, and severe chest pain, as well as coronary events. Furthermore, the development of heart disease could not be attributed to one's grade of employment or the usual coronary risk factors.

Like powerlessness, anger appears to be an important risk factor in the development of cardiovascular disease. An article published in 1994 in *Heart Disease and Stroke* noted that, for a type A personality, anger can be the most important factor in the development of ischemia (which is a lack of blood in an area of the body due to a mechanical obstruction or constriction of a blood vessel). In fact, anger can be as strong a risk factor for cardiovascular disease as hypertension. Even less intense emotions, when they are negative, can also be a risk factor for cardiovascular disease.

According to a study published in 1997 in the *Journal of the American Medical Association*, researchers found that negative emotions can trigger myocardial ischemia, a reduction in blood flow to the heart. Researchers began with a group of 132 outpatients with coronary-artery disease who went about their daily life for forty-eight hours while being electrically monitored for their response to mental stress. Of this group, fifty-eight patients experienced myocardial ischemia and were included in the analysis of stress response. Results of the study showed that emotions such as sadness, frustration, and tension can more than double an individual's risk of myocardial ischemia in the hour after stress has occurred.

In addition, being habitually defensive can cause elevations in blood pressure, according to a study of forty-eight patients with heart disease, published in 1997 in the *American Journal of Cardiology*. Patients were given a standard true-false personality test to assess their reactions to various statements, such as "I'm always willing to admit it when I make a mistake." At the same time, researchers monitored the changes that occurred in the patients' blood pressure when giving their responses. Patients who were defensive in their responses showed the greatest elevation in their blood pressure readings.

Assertiveness in women can also be a risk factor for heart disease. A study of 809 male and 783 female participants, published in 1997 in the *Lancet*, found that women who had a more submissive personality were three times less likely to have a heart attack when compared with the more assertive women in the study. However, at the other end of the spectrum, powerlessness in the workplace actually increases the risk of vascular disease. This issue was examined in a study, published in *Circulation* in 1997, that followed the health of 940 Finnish men. The men in this study who had low-paying but highly demanding jobs had a significantly greater four-year progression of carotid atherosclerosis and plaque buildup than men with high-paying jobs that placed relatively low demands on them. This study suggests that millions of Americans who are stuck in similar types of low-paying, highly demanding jobs may also have a greater risk of vascular disease. Many articles have chronicled the frustration felt by individuals who have little control over their work setting, schedule, and the pace at which they must work. Such frustration can have extremely negative effects on one's health.

Further evidence of the deleterious effect that stress has on the heart comes from a 1997 study done in Japan and published in the *Lancet*. In this study, the researchers found that commuting and working overtime may cause more pronounced variations in heart rate than are normally seen, eventually leading to the onset of heart disease. Men who traveled at least ninety minutes to work by train, bus, or both had overstimulation of their stress-coping mechanisms, with evidence of increased sympathetic nervous system activity related to cardiovascular function, compared with subjects whose commute times were shorter.

While stress can worsen cardiovascular function, many studies have confirmed the benefit of practicing a variety of stress reduction techniques to help prevent frequent elevations in blood pressure as well as a worsening of cardiovascular function that can be triggered by stressful events in people with these conditions. Douglas, a business associate of Jim's, exemplifies how practicing stress reduction techniques can improve an underlying tendency toward vascular disease. A successful and hardworking businessman, he found himself in an acrimonious divorce and custody battle over his two young children after five years of a difficult and stress-filled marriage. Douglas had previously been diagnosed with mild hypertension. However, when faced with these additional personal stresses, his blood pressure soared to high levels. His doctor prescribed medication to lower his blood pressure and also recommended that he begin stress management training so that his stress levels would stop triggering such an exaggerated response in his blood pressure. Douglas enrolled in a series of biofeedback classes. Biofeedback is a technique that enables patients to learn how to regulate normally unconscious bodily functions, such as breathing, heart rate, and blood pressure. Regularly practicing this technique eventually allowed Douglas to regulate his own blood pressure without the use of medication.

INFECTIOUS DISEASES

The risk of developing infectious diseases is also increased by stress. The negative effect that stress can have on lowering resistance to infectious diseases has been confirmed in various studies. For example, one British study, published in 1991 in the *British Journal of Medical Psychology*, found that a period of feeling angry, tense, and skeptical, even for a few days, tended to precede the onset of a cold. Susan has seen this pattern for years, particularly in her patients who are prone toward common respiratory infections such as colds, flus, bronchitis, and pneumonia. These individuals are much more likely to become ill during periods of stress. She has also found that recurrences of genital herpes and bladder infections were also much more likely to happen during times of personal stress. There is also some evidence that stress may be a risk factor for cancer. A letter to the editor, published in 1993 in the *New Zealand Medical Journal*, refers to a German study that followed the health of over 2000 subjects over a thirteen-year period. The researchers concluded that there is a particularly cancer-prone personality. Emotional factors such as suppressing emotions, being unable to cope with interpersonal stress, and feeling helpless, hopeless, and depressed are six times more predictive of the development of cancer than a physical factor such as smoking. In another study, individuals with a cancer-prone personality type were trained in how to manage interpersonal stress. As a result, cancer deaths in this group were reduced by half over the next ten years.

In another study, published in 1993 in *Epidemiology*, individuals who were noted to have had job-related problems in the preceding ten years were five times as likely to develop colorectal cancer as people who reported being less troubled by stress.

In contrast, experiencing positive emotions can enhance immune function. This was illustrated by a study that compared the effect that positive emotional states had on immune function. Published in 1995 in the *Journal of Advancement in Medicine*, this study examined the effects that both anger and compassion had on IgA (immunoglobulin A) levels. IgA is an antibody found in the secretions of the lungs, digestive tract, and urinary tract as well as in saliva. It is one of the body's first lines of defense against common problems like colds, flus, and bladder infections. In this study, thirty individuals were asked to recall feelings of either compassion or anger. They were then monitored over a six-hour period for the levels of IgA in their saliva. Researchers observed that feelings of anger depressed immune function, inhibiting salivary IgA for up to five hours, while the positive emotional state of compassion caused a significant increase in IgA levels.

ASTHMA

Asthma symptoms occur when the airways become inflamed and a subsequent contraction of the airway causes difficulty in breathing. While environmental factors such as outdoor air pollutants, dust mites, and tobacco smoke can trigger asthmatic episodes, emotional stress is also a powerful trigger in some individuals. Asthma is a relatively common disease in children, affecting between 5 and 6 million youngsters in the United States. The link between emotional stress and asthmatic episodes in children was examined in a study reported in 1996 in *Family Practice*

News. Emotional stress was found to increase the risk of a fatal asthmatic episode. The researchers studied twelve asthmatic children who died suddenly after a severe asthma attack and compared their history of stress with that of twelve asthmatic children who survived a severe attack. They found that, of the children who died, ten had undergone stress due to separation or loss, while only two of the surviving children had experienced similar stress. Furthermore, eight of those who died were known to have had feelings of hopelessness or despair, compared with only three of the survivors. In another study, described in the same article, twenty-four children between the ages of eight and seventeen who had asthma were given methacholine (a drug used to treat this condition). They were then shown the movie *E.T.* Researchers noted that those children with the greatest tendency to be asthmatic also had the greatest emotional as well as physiological response to the movie, supporting the thesis that emotionally sensitive children are more susceptible to stress-mediated asthma.

ARTHRITIS

Stress management can also help relieve the symptoms of rheumatoid arthritis, a progressive inflammatory disease of the joints characterized by pain, stiffness, and joint deformity. A 1996 article in the *Medical Tribune* reported on a study of 141 rheumatoid arthritis patients who were given counseling in stress management and taught various stress-coping skills. After two months, the patients reported less pain and greater mobility as compared with patients who had no counseling.

SKIN DISEASES

The effects of stress often manifest as skin problems. In a study published in 1993 in the *International Journal of Dermatology*, thirty-four patients with atopic dermatitis (an inflammatory condition of the skin) and twenty-eight patients with psoriasis (a chronic skin disease characterized by reddish patches covered with silvery scales, occurring mostly on the knees, elbows, scalp, and trunk) were examined to determine if a relationship existed between certain emotional states and the presence of skin disease. The researchers found that those persons who felt angry but tended not to express this anger were more likely to develop these skin problems. In particular, individuals with atopic dermatitis were more anxious as well as less assertive. Another study, published in 1994 in *ACTA Dermatologica Venereol*, found that a stressful event can cause a relapse of psoriasis. Researchers observed eighty psoriasis patients, the majority of whom frequently experienced panic disorders. Some patients also had either personality disorders, moodiness, anxiety, or schizophrenia. When a stressful event occurred, nearly 90 percent of the patients had a recurrence of their psoriatic lesions.

SUMMARY

Stress can exacerbate the symptoms of and increase the risk of developing almost every health condition, including digestive problems, cardiovascular disease, infectious diseases, asthma, and arthritis.

LABORATORY TESTS FOR ADRENAL FUNCTION AND HEALTH CONDITIONS THAT INCREASE SUSCEPTIBILITY TO STRESS

Laboratory testing can be used to assess levels of adrenal stress hormones as well as to diagnose diseases that can produce anxiety-like conditions such as food allergies and hypoglycemia. If you suspect that you have any of these conditions, you should consult with a physician to have the appropriate diagnostic testing done.

TESTING FOR ADRENAL-GLAND FUNCTION

The measurement of blood pressure can provide a simple test of adrenal function. To assess adrenal function, a person will rest for five minutes lying down before having their blood pressure taken. The person then stands up, and their blood pressure is immediately taken again. Normally, the blood pressure is approximately 10 mm higher when going from a reclining to a standing position. If, instead, your blood pressure is lower after standing up, this can indicate weak adrenal-gland function.

Adrenal function can also be tested by measuring the level of cortisol and other adrenal hormones in the saliva, blood, or urine. The saliva test, in particular, is thought to accurately reflect the day-to-day functional status of the adrenals.

TESTING FOR FOOD ALLERGIES

Food allergies can cause symptoms of anxiety and stress. Allergens can be detected through various types of testing, such as skin testing, blood testing of antibodies to specific foods, and sublingual testing, in which symptoms are monitored after a potentially allergenic substance is placed under the tongue.

Food allergies can also be detected by the elimination method. If you suspect that you are allergic to a particular food, avoid eating this food for four weeks. At the end of the four weeks, reintroduce this food into your diet and monitor your symptoms. If you are allergic, you may experience any of a large number of symptoms, including nasal congestion, fatigue, brain fog, irritability, and anxiety. Once you discover the foods that you are allergic to, it may not be necessary to avoid these foods indefinitely. Many people find that after several months of avoiding a particular food, they are able to reintroduce it if they eat it only once or twice a week. For example, they may not be able to have wheat toast for breakfast every day, but they may be able to enjoy it once or twice a week.

TESTING FOR BLOOD SUGAR IMBALANCES

The symptoms of low blood sugar can mimic the symptoms of stress, causing shakiness, jitteriness, dizziness, and anxiety. A standard test for diagnosing hypoglycemia is the glucose tolerance test (GTT). After the patient fasts for twelve hours, a baseline measurement of blood glucose is made. A person is then given a glucose challenge, which is a very sweet-tasting drink. The blood sugar is checked again after thirty minutes and then hourly for up to five hours. Individuals with hypoglycemia will show an initial elevation and then a rapid decline in their blood sugar levels, at which point anxiety-like symptoms can occur.

10

RESTORING YOUR ABILITY TO MANAGE STRESS

A WEALTH OF dietary and nutritional therapies, stress reduction techniques, and new and effective stress management technologies can eliminate your susceptibility to stress and help to strengthen your stress-coping mechanisms. This chapter, which is divided into four parts, discusses many of these therapies and tells how to use them most effectively.

Our four-part plan for restoring and strengthening your body's natural ability to manage stress includes the following components: (1) following a stress reduction diet, (2) supplementing that diet with stress-reducing vitamins, minerals, and other nutrients,* (3) incorporating stress management techniques into your daily routine, and (4) using modern technology to help reduce the stress in your life.

Everyday challenges are inevitable, and the stress response is automatic and instinctive. However, by making the nutritional and lifestyle changes described in this chapter, you can dramatically alter your own response to stress and eliminate the accumulated negative effects that stress causes in your body. When a stressful situation occurs, these habits and techniques, when practiced over time, will help you to modulate and balance your response in virtually any potentially difficult or upsetting situation.

---

* Anyone beginning a nutritional supplement program should begin at one-quarter to one-half the recommended dosages given in this book. They can then increase their dosages slowly over the course of several weeks until they have reached either the full recommended dosage or a dosage that is therapeutic for them—whichever level comes first. Some individuals will experience therapeutic benefits at doses that are well below the doses recommended in this book. Also, while the dosages provided in this chapter are appropriate for most people, there are certain groups who should continue to use less than the recommended dosages. Children, the elderly, and individuals with a frail constitution or who are extremely sensitive to drugs and nutritional supplements usually do best at therapeutic dosages of no more than half the recommended levels. Consult your physician or nutritional consultant if you have any questions about the advisability of using a particular nutritional supplement or to determine the dosage most appropriate for you.

PART 1:
THE ANTISTRESS DIET

THE ANTISTRESS DIET emphasizes nutrient-rich foods that promote resistance to stress and eliminates foods that weaken the stress-coping capability.

NUTRIENT-RICH FOODS

When people experience significant levels of stress in their lives, following a nutrient-rich, easy-to-digest diet is crucial. When the body undergoes stress, cellular activity increases, which leads to an accelerated use of nutrients. Fortunately, a wide range of foods can support the nervous system and the endocrine glands involved in the stress response.

An optimal antistress diet provides a wide variety of essential vitamins and minerals. One of the best ways to make sure you are eating nutrient-rich food is to shop for and cook whole foods; that is, foods that are unprocessed and unrefined. These are foods with all their parts, such as an unpeeled apple or potato. The skin provides fiber and nutrients that are concentrated just below it. Whole grains such as brown rice and buckwheat should be used instead of refined grains like white rice and white flour. Whole grains provide a complex mixture of protein, carbohydrates, fiber, fats, vitamins such as B and E complexes, and many minerals like calcium, magnesium, potassium, iron, copper, and manganese. In contrast, refined grains, such as those found in white bread and most pasta, primarily supply starch, with relatively few nutrients. In the refining process, the nutrient-rich germ and bran are removed, along with most of the vitamins and minerals. If the flour is then "enriched," only about four or five of the approximately twenty nutrients in the original grain are added, resulting in lower amounts of the B vitamins and zinc needed for stress.

Many research studies have investigated the effect of various foods on energy levels, mood, and resistance to stress. These studies have tended to confirm the important role that diet can play in the stress response. For example, meals that are high in carbohydrates tend to increase the body's production of serotonin, a substance that has a calming effect, while meals high in protein promote the creation of dopamine, a chemical linked to increased alertness as well as physical and mental energy. One such study, conducted in Britain and published in 1994 in *Physiology and Behavior*, involved eighteen volunteers who were given three different lunches over three days. One lunch contained high amounts of carbohydrates, a second was high in fat, and a third contained evenly distributed amounts of each. Volunteers eating the high-carbohydrate and high-fat meals were reportedly more drowsy and less cheerful, felt less certain, and reacted more slowly than after eating the balanced-diet lunch. People who are required to be alert in the afternoon to meet career demands need to remember that what they choose at the local restaurant or company cafeteria will directly affect how they feel for the rest of the day.

▲▲ If your mornings and afternoons tend to be your most productive times of the day, be sure to eat a high-protein breakfast and lunch. The protein can be of either vegetable or animal origin. To slow down in the evening and produce more serotonin, which is necessary for a good night's sleep, eat a lighter meal with more emphasis on carbohydrates for dinner.

When determining which foods to include in your antistress diet, be sure to review chapters 1 and 2, regarding acid/alkaline balance. Depending on whether you have an overly acidic or more alkaline constitution, the specific foods that provide energy and support your ability to respond effectively to stress will vary. Overly acidic individuals tend to be much more susceptible to stress, because of their more nervous and high-strung constitution. These individuals tend to feel much calmer and stronger on a less acid, more alkaline, mostly vegetarian diet. In contrast, naturally alkaline individuals tend to handle stressful situations, emergencies, and even dangerous activities with greater equanimity. In fact, naturally alkaline people often prefer excitement and stressful situations, because these enable them to produce the acids needed to combat their tendency toward overalkalinity. In addition, the strength of your digestive organs also determines which foods can be optimally digested and used by your body. You should also review the chapters on digestive enzymes to see if a diet of mostly cooked or raw foods is most desirable in your case.

FOODS TO AVOID

Certain foods weaken the stress-coping mechanisms of all individuals. As discussed in the previous chapter, these include caffeinated beverages, sugar, foods made with white flour, and alcohol. While many individuals can benefit from eating whole fruit because of its high vitamin, mineral, and fiber content, individuals who are experiencing significant stress should avoid large amounts of fruit juice. Because fruit juice lacks fiber, it is rapidly absorbed from the digestive tract into the bloodstream, where it acts as a simple sugar, just like the sugar in candy. A glass of orange juice, if taken without other food, can actually destabilize the blood sugar level, worsening the symptoms of stress. Some twelve-ounce servings of commercial fruit juices contain up to twelve teaspoons of sugar, which is more than the sugar contained in a can of cola. Susan has had patients who have bought juicers thinking this would be a good way to consume a lot of nutrients easily and quickly; however, after drinking at least one large glassful or more of fruit and vegetable juices a day, they experienced a worsening of their stress symptoms, including mood swings, fatigue, and shakiness.

When under stress, some people actually forget or neglect to eat, depriving themselves of energy and nutrients. However, it is at these times that it is especially important to remember to feed yourself. Meals should be taken in a calm atmosphere. A few minutes of relaxation before and after meals can improve digestion and turn the time spent eating into a peaceful retreat from the day's activities. Dashing into a crowded luncheonette and gulping food down while sitting at the counter is not the way to refresh yourself if you want to have optimal mental clarity and function efficiently in the afternoon.

▲▲ Virtually every medium- to large-sized business in the United States has vending machines loaded with soft drinks, fruit juice, candy bars, and cookies. Employees also frequently bring in treats to share with their coworkers. Given the toll that these foods take on employees' physical and mental energy, their frequent use over time can only undermine productivity. Since corporations spend an enormous amount of money on the health needs of their employees, it would make more sense to eliminate these success saboteurs from the workplace. Businesses would be better served to provide their employees with snacks like air-popped popcorn, baked corn chips, low-fat bean dips, salsa, bottled waters, fruit, vegetables with dips, and energizing teas like peppermint, ginger, and ginseng. These types of snacks help to preserve energy by boosting the blood sugar level in a slow, controlled manner and provide stimulants for brain function that do not stress the adrenals and nervous system. Only the very small percentage of people who tend to be naturally alkaline can handle the stress that sugar, caffeine, and other highly acidic chemicals place on the body's stress-coping mechanisms.

PART 2:
ANTISTRESS VITAMINS, MINERALS, AND OTHER NUTRIENTS

NUMEROUS RESEARCH STUDIES support the importance of taking certain nutritional supplements to help maintain stamina and a balanced mood. Antistress nutrients include the B-complex vitamins, vitamin C, vitamin E, magnesium, calcium, potassium, chromium, manganese, selenium, and iron. While these nutrients play a significant role in healthy adrenal and nervous-system functioning, none works in isolation; adequate levels of all of these vitamins and minerals must be present for optimal performance. This is evidenced in a study involving alcoholics published in 1989 in the *Journal of Orthomolecular Medicine*, in whom anxiety was reduced by using a combination of vitamin C, niacin, vitamin B_6, and vitamin E. In another study, PMS-related mood swings were associated with low stores of vitamins A, B_2 and B_6, folic acid, copper, and zinc.

Most people have difficulty increasing their nutritional intake up to the levels needed for optimal healing and stress management through diet alone, given the depletion of nutrients in the soil in which our food is grown. Supplements can help make up this deficiency so a person can feel better as rapidly as possible. But the importance of following a good diet along with the use of supplements cannot be overemphasized. Supplements should never be used as an excuse to continue poor dietary habits.

The following section will provide you with information on the beneficial effects that many vitamins, minerals, herbs, and other nutrients have on reducing stress-related symptoms. Many of these nutrients also help to restore the stress-coping hormones and neurochemicals.

VITAMINS

There are a number of vitamins that play an essential role in improving our resistance to stress. These include the B vitamins, vitamin C, and vitamin E.

Vitamin B complex

Vitamin B complex is a group of eleven separate nutrients: thiamine, riboflavin, niacin, pantothenic acid, pyridoxine, folic acid, biotin, paba-aminobenzoic acid (PABA), vitamin B_{12}, choline, and inositol. In many cases they participate in the same chemical reactions in the body; therefore, they need to be taken together for the best results. The B vitamins play an important role in healthy nervous-system function. When one or more of these vitamins are deficient, symptoms of nerve impairment as well as anxiety, stress, and fatigue can result. Conversely, adequate intake of these nutrients can help to calm the mood and provide important components of a stable and constant source of energy.

Deficiencies of vitamin B complex have been associated with anxiety in both human and animal studies, and supplementation has been shown to be beneficial in reducing anxiety. In a study published in 1982 in the *Journal of Orthomolecular Psychiatry*, twenty-three agoraphobic patients received dietary counseling, high-potency, broad-spectrum nutritional supplementation, and additional megavitamin supplementation for deficiencies found on lab testing, including B complex when indicated. After three months, nineteen of the twenty-three patients showed dramatic improvement, and eleven of nineteen patients were free of panic attacks.

As the B vitamins play a critical role in the conversion of sugars into energy, it follows that a deficiency of these vitamins can lead to fatigue, a hallmark of the exhaustion stage of Selye's stress model. An article appearing in 1985 in *Sports Medicine* stated that poor intake of B-complex vitamins, individually and in combination, of approximately less than 35 to 45 percent of the RDA, may lead to a drop in endurance within a few weeks. Various studies, on both animals and humans, show that deprivation of specific B vitamins, such as folic acid, pantothenic acid, pyridoxine, and vitamin B_{12}, are associated with feeling listless and tiring easily. Addition of these nutrients restored energy levels.

SUGGESTED DOSAGE: B-complex vitamins may be taken in a dosage of 25 to 100 mg a day, as a single dose or in divided dosages. It is best to take the B vitamins during the day, rather than at night, as they can be too stimulating. While the B vitamins need to be taken together as B complex, certain B vitamins may also be taken separately, usually in higher dosages, for specific health indications.

Thiamine

A study published in 1943 in *Archives of Internal Medicine* links thiamine deficiency with fearfulness progressing to agitation, as well as with emotional instability and psychosomatic complaints. Thiamine is the coenzyme for pyruvate dehydrogenase, the enzyme that converts pyruvate into acetyl CoA. If too much pyruvic acid accumulates in the blood, it can cause a decrease in mental alertness and damage to the heart.

SUGGESTED DOSAGE: A standard dosage is 25 to 100 mg per day. This can be taken as a single dose or in divided dosages.

Pantothenic acid (vitamin B$_5$)

Pantothenic acid is perhaps the most important B vitamin for preventing symptoms of stress because it, along with folic acid and vitamin C, is essential for the proper function of the adrenal glands. Vitamin B$_5$ stimulates the adrenal cortex to produce cortisone. It is widely distributed in our food supply and is especially abundant in egg yolks, brewer's yeast, organ meats, and whole-grain cereals.

SUGGESTED DOSAGE: 250 to 500 mg once or twice per day.

Niacin

For those individuals who fall asleep easily but can't return to sleep after awakening in the middle of the night, niacin (B$_3$) may be helpful. Research studies have shown that niacinamide, a form of niacin, has a mild tranquilizing effect.

SUGGESTED DOSAGE: A standard dosage is 25 to 100 mg per day. This can be taken as a single dose or in divided dosages. Niacin may cause a "niacin flush" in the first few minutes after taking it, consisting of overheating, reddening of the face, and uncomfortable itching sensations.

If this occurs, the dosage should be lowered until this effect is minimized or no longer occurs.

Pyridoxine (vitamin B₆)

Pyridoxine affects mood through its important role in the conversion of linolenic acid to gamma linolenic acid (GLA) during the production of the beneficial series I prostaglandins. These prostaglandins have a relaxant effect on both mood and smooth muscle tissue. Lack of these has been linked to PMS-related anxiety as well as stress-related problems like irritable-bowel syndrome and migraine headaches. A deficiency of series I prostaglandins can also increase neuroendocrine responses to hypoglycemia.

Women on birth control pills and menopausal women on estrogen replacement therapy are at risk of B_6 deficiency. Anxiety symptoms can occur as a side effect of hormone use in both groups of women, in part because of vitamin B_6 deficiency. Vitamin B_6 is also helpful in counteracting anxiety associated with PMS. It can promote active transport of magnesium across cell membranes, reducing this symptom.

The brain's role in managing stress depends on having sufficient amounts of vitamin B_6. A deficit may be linked to brain neurotransmitter abnormalities. Vitamin B_6 also acts as a coenzyme in the final steps of dopamine and serotonin synthesis, the neurochemicals important for counteracting stress.

In particular, a deficiency of pyridoxine may impair the conversion of tryptophan to serotonin, a relaxant, causing anxiety due to serotonin depletion. In an article published in 1981 in the *Journal of Orthomolecular Psychiatry*, scientists reported studying thirteen patients who were experiencing at least two attacks of hyperventilation (a sign of anxiety) per week for the preceding six months to two years. They were treated with a combination of pyridoxine (125 mg three times daily) and L-tryptophan (2 g daily). After three weeks, nine patients were free of attacks, and after four weeks, all responders had no further hyperventilation (during three months of follow-up) without further pyridoxine or tryptophan.

SUGGESTED DOSAGE: Vitamin B_6 is safe in doses up to 300 mg. Above this level, it can be neurotoxic.

Inositol

Inositol, part of the vitamin B complex, is closely associated with choline, from which the neurotransmitter acetylcholine is made. Inositol nourishes the brain cells, and large amounts are found in the spinal-cord nerves, the brain, and the cerebrospinal fluid. Observations of its use indicate that inositol may have a calming effect. Its effect on the brain waves studied by electroencephalography (EEG) was similar to changes induced by mild tranquilizers. In studies, inositol has been used to treat panic disorder.

SUGGESTED DOSAGE: No RDA for inositol has been established, but the daily consumption in food is about 1 g. The human body contains more inositol than any other vitamin except niacin. Therapeutic dosages range from 500 to 1000 mg per day. There is no known toxicity.

Vitamin C

Vitamin C is an extremely important antistress nutrient that can help decrease the fatigue symptoms that often accompany excessive levels of anxiety and stress. It is needed for the production of adrenal cortisone and epinephrine. Stress can deplete vitamin C, as shown in a study that found that horses going through the rigors of training for a race had lowered levels of vitamin C. Vitamin C is critical for the structural support of the small arteries and veins in the adrenal glands, especially when the adrenals are overstimulated from stress. As an antioxidant, vitamin C also protects against free-radical deterioration of the antistress B vitamins and vitamin E. People with low vitamin C intake tend to have elevated levels of histamine, a chemical that triggers allergy symptoms. Allergy attacks can in turn, be the cause of emotional symptoms like anxiety.

Some epidemiological surveys have suggested a link between decreased capacity for aerobic physical activity and a deficiency of vitamin C. In an article published in 1976 in the *Journal of the American Geriatric Society*, 411 dentists and their spouses were surveyed for vitamin C intake and fatigue. There was a significant inverse relationship between the two, with the mean number of fatigue symptoms among those with low vitamin C intake double that of those with relatively high vitamin C intake. Stress quickly depletes the body of vitamin C. For example, an unexpected confrontational phone call can quickly use up the body's supply.

SUGGESTED DOSAGE: A standard recommendation is 1 to 2 g per day. However, during periods of high stress, a person may need as much as 8 to 10 g. As much vitamin C may be taken as your bowels will tolerate, with gas and diarrhea an indication to cut back on the dosage. Vitamin C is best taken several times throughout the day, because maximum blood levels are reached rapidly, and as a water-soluble vitamin, it is readily excreted from the body. Unlike fat-soluble vitamins such as vitamin A and D, vitamin C is not stored within the body.

It is extremely important when taking vitamin C to know whether you tend to be an overly acidic or naturally alkaline person (see the checklist in chapter 1). Most of the vitamin C sold in the United States is in the acidic form, ascorbic acid, which has a pH of 2.1. Most people who are highly stressed or who are suffering from fatigue due to stress are already in an overly acidic state. To receive the positive benefits of vitamin C without adding to your overly acidic condition, be sure to take a buffered form. Vitamin C buffered with alkaline minerals such as calcium, magnesium, potassium, sodium, and zinc has a higher pH than ascorbic acid. It is available in health food stores in tablets, capsules, and powders. Another benefit of buffered vitamin C is that it usually does not cause stomach burning or upset as ascorbic acid often does. If you are taking large doses of vitamin C buffered with calcium, be sure to take enough magnesium to keep your calcium/magnesium ratio in balance.

Vitamin E

Supplementing with vitamin E can reduce mood swings and anxiety. Much of the research on these benefits focuses on how vitamin E affects these conditions as they relate, in particular, to PMS and menopause. A study appearing in 1987 in the *Journal of Reproductive Medicine* reported that forty-one women were treated for PMS with daily supplements of 400 IU of vitamin E (as d-alpha-tocopherol) or a placebo, administered during the second half, or luteal phase, of their menstrual cycles. The study ran for the duration of three cycles. The results showed that the women on the vitamin E therapy experienced less irritability, tension, moodiness, and social impairment than women on the placebo. Vitamin

E therapy also produced the added benefit of better motor coordination and cognition. The authors of the article hypothesized that d-alpha-tocopherol acts, either directly or indirectly, through a prostaglandin-mediated mechanism, normalizing the level of central-nervous-system neurotransmitters that worsen PMS symptoms.

In the case of anxiety and menopause, depending on the study, between 66 and 85 percent of women tested found that vitamin E is as effective as supplemental estrogen in reducing these symptoms. This is of great benefit for women who for various reasons are not on hormone replacement therapy but need treatment for anxiety. Vitamin E is an essential part of a supplement program for women executives in their fifties, at the peak of their careers, who cannot afford to have their days disrupted by unstable emotions as they pursue their work.

SUGGESTED DOSAGE: Susan recommends using natural vitamin E. If you are using natural vitamin E, the bottle will read "d-alpha," not "d'l-alpha," which is the synthetic form. Natural vitamin E is better absorbed and used by the body than other forms. Women with PMS may take 400 to 1600 IU daily. For women with menopause-related anxiety and mood swings, Susan recommends between 400 and 2000 IU of vitamin E per day. However, women with hypertension, diabetes, or bleeding problems should start on a much lower dose (100 IU per day) and increase the dosage gradually. If you have any of these conditions, ask your physician about the advisability of these supplements. Any increase in dosage should be made slowly and monitored carefully. In general, vitamin E tends to be extremely safe and is commonly used.

MINERALS

Many minerals help to reduce our reactivity to stress by their beneficial effect on our nervous, muscular, and endocrine systems.

Magnesium

The body requires adequate levels of magnesium in order to maintain energy and vitality. The process of aerobic metabolism (occurring in the presence of oxygen) needs magnesium in order to produce ATP, the energy currency of the body's cells. When magnesium is deficient, ATP production falls, and the body forms lactic acid. Therefore, having sufficient amounts of magnesium helps to maintain a high level of physical energy and prevent fatigue. This has been confirmed in a number of studies. For example, a study reported at a scientific conference on magnesium in 1976 reported that magnesium supplements relieved fatigue in 198 out of 200 volunteers, a remarkably high result.

A deficiency of magnesium is also associated with nervousness and insomnia, and supplementation is especially useful when coupled with calcium. Low levels are associated with migraine headaches, and research in women with PMS found deficiencies of magnesium in the red blood cells. In one study of 192 women, magnesium nitrate was given for one week, premenstrually, and during the first two days of menstruation. It was found that nervous tension was relieved in 89 percent of the women in the study. They noted relief of breast tenderness, headaches, and weight gain.

Stress promotes the urinary excretion of magnesium, which can also lead to magnesium deficiency. Magnesium deficiency itself can also cause mood swings and anxiety, as it can lead to depletion of dopamine. Magnesium is also needed for conversion of the essential fatty acid linoleic acid to gamma linolenic acid, which in turn can be converted to series I and II prostaglandins, which promote relaxation. Low levels of magnesium are also associated with PMS and agoraphobia.

SUGGESTED DOSAGE: Magnesium is given in divided doses, 400 to 1000 mg daily. There is a possible laxative effect at higher dosages. It is important to maintain a healthy calcium/magnesium ratio. Optimal levels are considered to be in a 2:1 or 10:4 ratio with calcium predominating over magnesium. Adequate magnesium allows calcium to be better absorbed within the body and helps to prevent the formation of calcium-containing kidney stones. Research studies have used magnesium aspartate in a variety of doses, ranging from 100 to 1000 mg. All of these dosages have been found to be relatively free of side effects except for a mild dryness of the mucosal membranes at higher dosage levels. Susan usually recommends between 100 and 300 mg of magnesium aspartate per day.

Calcium

Calcium helps combat stress, nervous tension, and anxiety. A calcium deficiency increases not only emotional irritability but also muscular irritability and cramps. Calcium can be taken at night along with magnesium for its calming effect and to induce restful sleep. This is particularly helpful for women with menopause-related anxiety, mood swings, and insomnia. Calcium is also essential for the release of neurotransmitters such as norepinephrine. Case studies document that a deficiency is often linked to an acute onset of anxiety in older patients.

Low levels of calcium (a condition called hypocalcemia) are sometimes associated with mental disorders and organic anxiety syndrome. A paper published in 1986 in the *Journal of Clinical Psychiatry* discussed a patient with acute organic anxiety (without a personal or family history of anxiety) coupled with low calcium levels. When the patient's blood calcium level was corrected, the anxiety and emotional instability resolved.

SUGGESTED DOSAGE: Optimal dosages vary from 800 to 1500 mg per day, depending on the person's age. Postmenopausal women and older men will need 1000 to 1500 mg per day to help prevent osteoporosis. The higher dosage is also needed if a person consumes large amounts of protein, caffeine, sugar, and alcohol, all risk factors for osteoporosis as they promote the loss of calcium from the body. If there is chronic stress and stomach acidity is low, it is better to take calcium before bedtime.

▲▲ If you are using both buffered vitamin C and calcium supplements, be sure to add up the total amount of calcium that you are taking in from both sources. You may find that you need to increase your level of magnesium supplementation to maintain calcium/magnesium balance at an optimal 2:1 or 10:4 ratio.

Potassium

Like magnesium, potassium has a powerful enhancing effect on energy and vitality. Potassium deficiency has been associated with fatigue and muscular weakness. For example, a study published in 1971 in *Gerontologia Clinica* showed that older people deficient in potassium had weak grip strength. In a number of studies of chronic fatigue, potassium aspartate combined with magnesium aspartate significantly restored energy levels. This combination may be useful for people suffering from excessive fatigue and depression. Potassium aspartate has been shown to reduce fatigue after five or six weeks of constant use. Even within ten days, many volunteers began to feel better. The benefits of potassium were seen in

90 percent of the people tested. Magnesium aspartate also has the same effect. Aspartic acid plays a vital role in energy production and helps transport both potassium and magnesium into the cells.

Potassium has many other important roles in the body. It regulates the transfer of nutrients to the cells and works with sodium to maintain the body's water balance. Potassium aids proper muscle contraction and, important for treating stress, the transmission of electrochemical impulses. It helps maintain nervous-system function and a healthy heart rate. Potassium can be lost through chronic diarrhea or the overuse of diuretics. In addition, the excessive use of coffee and alcohol, both of which can magnify anxiety and emotional stress symptoms, increases the loss of potassium through the urinary tract.

SUGGESTED DOSAGE: The recommended dosage for potassium and/or potassium aspartate is 100 to 300 mg per day. Potassium supplements can cause intestinal irritation in susceptible individuals.

Zinc

Zinc plays an important role in combating fatigue. Supplementation with zinc improves muscle strength and endurance. It reduces fatigue by enhancing immune-system function, acting as an immunity stimulant and triggering the reproduction of lymphocytes in test tube environments. Zinc is an essential trace mineral necessary for the absorption and action of vitamins, especially the anxiety and stress-combating B vitamins. Zinc also helps reduce anxiety due to blood sugar imbalances since it plays a role in normal carbohydrate digestion. However, the stress of heavy exercise can increase the loss of zinc from the body, and some athletes, especially females, may be zinc deficient. In one study, after supplementation with 135 mg of zinc daily for fifteen days, the isokinetic strength and isometric endurance of the subjects' leg muscles significantly improved.

SUGGESTED DOSAGE: The recommended dosage for zinc is 15 to 30 mg per day.

Chromium

Chromium is an essential mineral and an active ingredient in glucose tolerance factor (GTF). Through its action in GTF, chromium helps maintain stable blood sugar levels, stimulating the enzymes involved in glucose metabolism. Chromium may also enhance the effectiveness of insulin, which allows glucose to be removed from the blood and stored in cells, preventing hypoglycemia (low blood sugar) and diabetes characterized by high blood sugar. Fluctuating levels of blood sugar often trigger mood swings and anxiety, which adequate chromium can help keep in check.

SUGGESTED DOSAGE: There is no RDA for chromium, but daily intake ranges from 80 to 100 mcg. A therapeutic dosage is 150 mcg. A patient with hypoglycemia may need as much as 200 to 400 mg several times a day.

Manganese

Manganese nourishes the nerves and brain. It also facilitates the use of choline, a precursor to the neurotransmitter acetylcholine, which is necessary for cognitive function. Manganese (along with chromium) also helps prevent the mood swings and anxiety caused by fluctuating blood sugar levels. Manganese also activates enzymes necessary for the use of thiamine and vitamin C.

SUGGESTED DOSAGE: A standard dosage is 20 mcg per day.

Selenium

Selenium is an essential mineral, present in the body in minute quantities. It is often taken along with vitamin E, as it works closely in some of its functions, enhancing the action of vitamin E. Selenium has been shown in medical trials to improve mood. In a study published in 1990 in *Psychopharmacology*, seventeen males and thirty-three females, aged fourteen to seventy-four and in good health, were given either a placebo of brewer's yeast, with minimal selenium, or organically bound selenium in a yeast base containing 100 mcg daily for five weeks. After six months, this was followed by a second five-week course of selenium. There was a significant improvement in mood at two and a half and five weeks with selenium. The researchers proposed that selenium's effect on mood may occur because selenium has an effect on brain chemistry (selenium is found in brain tissue).

SUGGESTED DOSAGE: Selenium supplementation may range from 50 to 150 mcg per day. High levels of selenium in soil have caused toxicity, but normal supplemental dosages do not.

Iron

Iron is an important mineral that exists in the body in combination with protein. In the bloodstream, iron combines with copper and protein to form hemoglobin, which provides the coloration in the red blood cell. Hemoglobin binds with oxygen, enabling it to be transported from the lungs to all the cells of the body as it is carried in the circulation. Since oxygen plays such an important role in the production of energy within the cells, it is needed in sufficient amounts if one is to have the energy to respond rapidly to stressful situations.

Anemia occurs when there is a deficiency of iron. This can cause fatigue and greatly exacerbate symptoms in the exhaustion stage of stress. Women are at particular risk of anemia because of menstruation. Low reserves of iron can also worsen the emotional symptoms of PMS. According to an article published in 1993 in the *Journal of the Federation of American Societies for Experimental Biology*, women who are low in iron are more susceptible to mood disturbances in the premenstrual and menstrual phases of their monthly cycle. Iron-deficiency anemia is also associated with a diminished capacity to do physical activity. In a controlled study published in 1977 in the *American Journal of Clinical Nutrition*, seventy-five women were given a treadmill test. Those with the most severe iron-deficiency anemias were able to stay on the treadmill an average of eight minutes less than the women without anemia. Further, none of the anemic women were able to perform under the highest workload conditions, while all of the women with adequate iron levels could.

SUGGESTED DOSAGE: Dosage depends on gender and age. An average dosage is 15 mg per day, but a person who is anemic may need as much as 30 to 70 mg a day. Postmenopausal women who are no longer menstruating will not have high requirements, and recent studies have indicated that high levels of iron are associated with an increased risk of heart disease in men.

FLAVONOIDS

There are two classes of flavonoids that are helpful in reducing the symptoms of stress in women due to hormonal causes such as menopause. These include isoflavones (found in soybeans) and flavones (found in citrus fruit and buckwheat). These flavonoids have weak estrogenlike activity and are helpful for reducing stress due to menopause-related estrogen deficiency. Since estrogen has a stimulant effect on the brain, the weakly estrogenic activity of the bioflavonoids can act as a mild mood elevator in hormonally deficient women. (For an in-depth discussion of the role of hormones in peak performance and health, see chapters 11 and 12.)

ESSENTIAL FATTY ACIDS

Essential fatty acids (EFAs) are important structural components of the brain and nerves and are needed for healthy nervous-system function. They make up 50 percent of the brain by weight and 60 percent of the myelin sheaths of the nerves. Stress increases the body's need for these oils, which are taken into the body through our diet, and an imbalance of essential fatty acids in the body can increase susceptibility to stress. This change occurs through the prostaglandin pathway. Prostaglandins are hormonelike, short-lived chemicals that regulate cell function. They are made from essential fatty acids and consist of three families, or series. Series I prostaglandins, among other functions, improve nerve function and produce a sense of well-being. Series II prostaglandins promote water retention and high blood pressure and are relied on in the fight-or-flight response. Series III prostaglandins help prevent the series II prostaglandins from being made.

Having sufficient levels of series I and III prostaglandins is an important part of stress management. However, various factors, including poor nutrition and aging, can interfere with the body's ability to produce them. Series I prostaglandins are made from the essential fatty acid linoleic acid (LA), an omega-6 EFA. The body converts LA to gamma linolenic acid (GLA), but at this point, if the conversion does not occur, the production of the series I prostaglandins is blocked. Supplementing with evening primrose oil, borage oil, or black currant oil, which contain GLA, can bypass this block.

The series III prostaglandins are made from alpha linolenic acid (LNA), an omega-3 EFA found in walnuts and flaxseeds, and docosahexaenoic acid (DHA), which is common in fish oils. DHA appears to be important to brain chemistry, playing a role in the maturation of brain cells during the development of the fetus and during infancy.

Supplementation with these oils, as well as eating foods that contain them, is an important adjunct to any antistress nutrition program. The effectiveness of these oils is documented in various controlled studies focusing on emotional and mental disorders.

An article appearing in 1997 in *Nutrition Science News* cites two such studies. The first, published in 1989 in the *Journal of Human Hypertension*, involved the administration of either borage oil capsules containing 1.3 g per day of GLA or an olive oil placebo. Each student received a standard psychological stress test before and after twenty-eight days of supplements. Unlike the students taking the placebo, those on the high-GLA borage oil evidenced a reduction in their vulnerability to stress. In the second study, published in 1996 in the *Journal of Clinical Investigation*, forty-one healthy fourth-year medical students were given either fish oil capsules containing 1.5 to 1.8 g of DHA daily or a placebo. The students were given psychological tests during summer vacation, and again three months later during final exams. In the control group, feelings of aggression were higher at exam time, but the students taking the DHA showed a modest decrease in anger and hostility during finals as compared with when they were tested during summer vacation.

There is also substantial documentation of the beneficial effect of GLA in reducing the depression and irritability associated with PMS. An article appearing in 1983 in the *Journal of Reproductive Medicine* reported on a study conducted at St. Thomas's Hospital Medical School, in London, in which sixty-eight women with severe PMS were given a formulation of GLA (Efamol). Of these patients, 61 percent experienced total remission of all symptoms, and another 23 percent had partial remission. Some of the women continued to be treated for up to eighteen months and showed a sustained response, but with a relapse of symptoms if the GLA administration was stopped. In another study quoted in the same article, GLA reduced irritability in 77 percent, and depression in 74 percent, of a group of PMS patients.

Serious mental illness and common phobias can also be treated with essential fatty acids. A deficiency of niacin, a condition known as pellagra, has long been known to eventually cause dementia. Pellagra was part of the vitamin B–deficiency epidemic observed in the poor and undernourished in America 50 to 100 years ago. Today, niacin-deficiency pellagra is rare, but there are cases of another type of pellagra that is caused by a deficiency of omega-3 essential fatty acids, which are a necessary substrate on which niacin, along with other B vitamins, acts to form series III prostaglandins. In a review of twelve case studies of patients with major psychoses and neuroses, eight of the patients showed substantial improvement in mental status and behavior while taking supplements of linseed oil, which is high in the omega-3s. Patients using linseed oil showed remarkable long-term amelioration of schizophrenia, with accompanying reduction of physical signs and psychomotor epilepsy. Several of the patients who had had agoraphobia for ten years or more experienced definite improvement, being able to travel farther from home and with less anxiety. Agoraphobia is the fear of open or busy public places (the *agora* was the marketplace in ancient Greece).

SUGGESTED DOSAGE: A normal dosage of essential fatty acids is 1 to 2 tbsp. per day, taken as flaxseed oil. This highly nutritious oil has a flavor similar to butter. It is important to be aware, however, that flaxseed oil must never be heated while using it in a recipe. It degrades easily when exposed to light, oxygen, or heat, generating toxic free radicals. Flaxseed oil should be added to foods, such as pastas and cooked vegetables, just before eating them, and also must never be stored as part of a leftover.

If EFAs are supplied by borage oil, two to four capsules per day is a standard recommendation. Borage oil is preferable to primrose oil, as it is necessary to take eight to thirteen capsules per day of the latter to produce a therapeutic effect.

AMINO ACIDS

Amino acids, the building blocks of protein, are converted within the brain to neurotransmitters. Having the proper balance of neurotransmitters is a prerequisite for the Chemistry of Success. These important substances directly affect such important success traits as physical and mental energy, perseverance and drive, the ability to get along with other people, and the ability to make sensible decisions in a calm and rational manner. Neurotransmitters either energize us and elevate our mood, if they are excitatory, or have a calming and relaxant effect if they are inhibitory. A good balance of excitatory and inhibitory neurotransmitters is needed for success in virtually all areas of life. For example, the amino acid tryptophan is converted into serotonin, a relaxant, while the amino acids phenylalanine and tyrosine are converted into dopamine, which is an energizer. Having appropriate amounts of these neurotransmitters produces a dynamic equilibrium of health. A person with balanced amounts of serotonin and dopamine is at the same time alert and relaxed. The following amino acids feed into the biochemical pathways that produce these two complementary substances.

Tryptophan

Tryptophan is an essential amino acid that can be used to promote relaxation and treat depression because it is a precursor to the neurotransmitter serotonin. Tryptophan is converted to a compound, 5-hydroxytryptophan, which is in turn converted to serotonin. The conversion of tryptophan occurs within the brain, but in order for this to happen, the tryptophan must cross the blood-brain barrier. Eating a meal high in carbohydrates promotes this crossing. The carbohydrates trigger the release of insulin, and the insulin permits various free amino acids to be removed from circulation and taken into the cells. However, tryptophan is not in this form and remains unaffected by the insulin.

Various studies show a decrease in psychological complaints with the use of tryptophan, especially complaints associated with aggressiveness and compulsion. Persons low in serotonin may be predisposed to certain excessive behaviors such as impulsive violence, alcoholism, and compulsive gambling. Such impulsiveness would be a great liability in business if it showed up as inappropriate behavior in the workplace.

In a study appearing in 1996 in *Psychopharmacology*, 25 g and 100 g of a tryptophan-free amino acid mixture were given to ten healthy male subjects after they ate a low-tryptophan diet for twenty-four hours. The researchers observed that when brain serotonin levels were lower due to tryptophan deprivation, the subjects exhibited a significant increase in aggressiveness. This occurred five hours after the 100 g tryptophan-free mixture was administered, and six hours after the 25 g mixture was given. In another study, appearing in 1994 in *Archives of General Psychiatry*, that looked at twenty-four males who had preexisting aggressive traits with tryptophan depletion, the subjects gave themselves higher scores in anger, aggression, annoyance, quarrelsome tendencies, and hostility. A third study, appearing in 1981 in the *Journal of Orthomolecular Psychiatry*, involved thirteen patients with hyperventilation syndrome, a function syndrome caused by stress. Patients had experienced hyperventilation from six months to three years prior to the study, and in the preceding two months had at least two attacks per week. After three weeks of treatment with a combination of 125 mg of pyridoxine three times a day and 2 g of tryptophan, nine of the patients were symptom-free.

At one time, tryptophan was available widely through health and natural-food stores. However, because of serious side effects traced to one tainted shipment of tryptophan imported from Japan, in 1988 the FDA pulled tryptophan off the market. It is currently only available by prescription. Fortunately, certain foods contain large amounts, including cottage cheese, beef, liver, lamb, turkey, fish, lentils, sesame and pumpkin seeds, peanuts, and soy protein.

SUGGESTED DOSAGE: It is thought that the human body needs a range of tryptophan between 80 and 250 mg per day. To optimize the benefits, supplemental tryptophan should be taken with a carbohydrate snack or meal, but it should not be taken with a protein meal. Combining tryptophan with vitamin B_6 and magnesium also enhances its effect.

5-hydroxytryptophan

While supplemental tryptophan is not readily available without a physician's prescription, 5-hydroxytryptophan (5-HTP) is becoming more so, and is available over the counter from several mail-order sources. (See the appendix for information on where to find 5-HTP.) The intermediary step in the conversion of tryptophan to serotonin yields 5-HTP, serotonin's metabolic precursor. 5-HTP produces all the benefits of tryptophan, reducing feelings of stress and anxiety. In clinical trials, 5-HTP has been shown to be even more effective than tryptophan in reducing depression. Researchers in France and Japan have used it successfully to treat various forms of depression. Research studies in France also demonstrated that mild insomnia can be treated with 5-HTP.

SUGGESTED DOSAGE: 5-HTP is available in 50 mg capsules. Dosage ranges from one to four capsules per day.

Melatonin

Melatonin is a hormone that is produced by the pineal gland (a pea-sized gland at the base of the brain) and other tissues, including those of the gastrointestinal tract. Melatonin sets and regulates the timing of natural rhythms of body function, including patterns of waking and sleeping.

Darkness stimulates the release of melatonin, and light suppresses its release. Melatonin is made from serotonin but is also present in a variety of common foods. These include bananas, tomatoes, cucumbers, and beets; it is also present in human milk. Because melatonin is fat soluble, unlike serotonin, it easily crosses membranes and enters the brain and other tissues, even those without melatonin receptors.

Melatonin can help reduce the fatigue associated with stress, especially in the exhaustion stage, by promoting a good night's sleep. People taking melatonin also report feeling emotionally balanced, with a sense of well-being on waking. An Israeli study, published in 1993 in the *Medical Tribune*, reported on individuals who were not able to fall asleep until 5:00 A.M. and then not able to wake until noon. They were given dosages of 1 to 2 mg of melatonin per day, taken before a desired bedtime, which restored their sleep to a normal cycle. In another Israeli study, melatonin shortened the time it took elderly patients to fall asleep.

For travel that involves crossing time zones, melatonin reduces jet lag. Studies suggest that for maximum benefit, serotonin should be taken for several days, starting when a person reaches his or her destination (see Lamson's Layover Law, on page 503). This can be useful for people whose careers demand that they sleep irregular and unusual hours, such as airline pilots, flight attendants, night-shift workers, and businesspeople who need to be bright-eyed at a breakfast in Cleveland after taking the red-eye flight from the West Coast.

Melatonin has been used to treat sleep disorders in children who are hyperactive or have neurological problems, resulting in improved mood and disposition and a significant reduction in age-inappropriate temper tantrums. In older people, melatonin production is greatly reduced, and supplementation helps improve sleep problems. Unfortunately, many older people take beta-receptor blocker medications for high blood pressure, and these further depress melatonin secretion. Melatonin is also helpful for blind people, whose sleep patterns may be disrupted because of the lack of sight.

Much epidemiological evidence links low melatonin levels with mood disorders. Melatonin levels are lower in individuals with panic disorder and other major depressive disorders. One theory is that this reduction is caused by low levels of norepinephrine, which is needed to stimulate melatonin production. Brain serotonin levels also increase with supplemental melatonin, reducing anxiety and elevating mood.

Melatonin has also been used to treat cancer, especially breast cancer, and it is a very potent antioxidant.

SUGGESTED DOSAGE: Melatonin supplements are commonly available in 1 to 3 mg dosages, in tablets, capsules, and tinctures. Physicians often recommend beginning with minimal amounts and then increasing the dose slowly until you begin to experience benefits. Current research suggests that using as little as 1 mg can improve sleep. Dosages as low as 0.1 mg have been shown to have a sedative effect in persons with low melatonin levels. It should be noted that melatonin produces no sedative effects in persons with normal production. Melatonin should be taken at bedtime, as taking it during the day may cause fatigue, confusion, and sleepiness.

The following program was developed by our good friend Bob Lamson. He is a businessman who travels frequently and truly embodies the Chemistry of Success. He has found this program to be very helpful and effective, particularly for cross-country and international flights.

Lamson's Layover Law: Reducing Jet Lag

1. If possible, schedule your flight so that at the time of takeoff, it is time to go to sleep at your destination.
2. On the plane, drink no alcoholic or caffeinated beverages.
3. Drink plenty of water—at least eight ounces every two hours.
4. Eat more protein than fats or carbohydrates. When eating carbohydrates, emphasize fruits and vegetables and avoid refined-flour products such as bread, pasta, and cakes.
5. Always know the time at your destination. When it is time to go to sleep (somewhere between 10:00 P.M. and 2:00 A.M.) in the time zone you're traveling to, take 1 to 3 mg of melatonin, put on your eye mask, put in your earplugs, and go to sleep. Every time you wake up, drink more water.
6. After arriving at your destination, take a ten- to twenty-minute walk as soon as possible, and eat a light snack. If you have time and feel the need, take a short nap—no more than one hour.
7. For the first two or three nights at your destination, take 1 to 3 mg of melatonin again each night before going to sleep.

Phenylalanine

Phenylalanine is an essential amino acid found in relative abundance in a number of foods, including meat, poultry, fish, cottage cheese, soybeans, lentils, garbanzo beans, sesame and pumpkin seeds, pecans, Brazil nuts, and almonds. It is converted within the body to several excitatory neurotransmitters. Phenylalanine is converted into tyrosine, which in turn is converted into dopamine, and finally into norepinephrine and epinephrine, the adrenal stress hormones that initiate the fight-or-flight response. When this sequence of chemical events is hampered, a wide variety of psychological problems can result.

Phenylalanine functions as an antidepressant, improving memory and mental alertness and increasing sexual interest. In animal trials, low phenylalanine levels were associated with depression. When the body lacks the enzyme to convert phenylalanine to tyrosine, the condition causes psychotic behavior in children and schizophrenic behavior in adults.

Many of Susan's chronic-fatigue patients, who suffer from symptoms of exhaustion, depression, and a decreased ability to think and react quickly, find that phenylalanine supplementation can be quite helpful. Nancy is a good example. She is a thirty-four-year-old woman who runs a busy day care center. She also has two young children of her own, both under the age of five. Her days are filled with overseeing children, interacting with parents, organizing games and activities, and getting snacks for the children. After she had her first child, it took Nancy three months to return to her normal level of energy. The postpartum depression she felt at this time passed quickly. But after Nancy had her second child, her fatigue lingered and she was unable to snap out of her depression. She was also troubled by anxiety and mood swings that were not PMS-related. She began a nutrition program that emphasized phenylalanine and other nutrients that support brain function. After taking these supplements for one or two months, Nancy found that she had more energy, her moodiness improved, and she was able again to make decisions quickly and handle the many details required in her work at the center.

SUGGESTED DOSAGE: Phenylalanine is available in 500 mg capsules. Standard dosages range from 500 to 2000 mg per day. It is recommended that phenylalanine be taken on an empty stomach, usually on arising and again in the afternoon. Anyone with high blood pressure should begin with the lowest dosage and have their blood pressure levels regularly monitored.

▲▲ If you find that you are slow to get started in the morning, suffer from brain fog, or feel that you are not as mentally alert as you used to be, you may be low in dopamine. Try supplementing with phenylalanine, as it may be able to restore your levels of dopamine and give you back much of the spark that you need to perform at peak levels and enjoy life to its fullest.

HERBS

Herbs have long been the province of traditional and folk medicine, but many Western doctors are now turning their attention to their many uses. In the last few years, several universities, including UCLA and Columbia, have hosted conferences on how to incorporate both European and Chinese herbs into standard treatment protocols. Many herbs can help relieve the symptoms and treat the causes of anxiety and stress. Susan has used anxiety- and stress-relieving herbs in her practice for many years, and many of her patients have found them to be effective remedies. Susan uses them to extend the nutrition of a healthy diet and to balance and expand the diet while optimizing nutritional intake. Some herbs, the adaptogens and natural sedatives, can relax tension and ease anxiety. Others, the relax-ant herbs and antispasmodics, relieve the muscle tension and spasm that often accompany stress. Certain herbs are also effective in relieving stress-related indigestion and intestinal gas.

Adaptogenic Herbs

Adaptogenic herbs support the adrenals and other glands, thereby pre-venting the long-term adrenal burnout and exhaustion that occurs with chronic stress. (An adaptogen is a substance that is innocuous, is able to increase resistance to a wide range of adverse physical, chemical, and bio-chemical factors, and promotes a normalization between extremes.) These herbs also contain a wide variety of chemicals that help the body recover more quickly from hard physical labor, athletic exertion, and even convalescence from surgery.

Panax ginseng. Panax ginseng is an ivylike ground cover originating in the wild, damp woodlands of northern China and Korea. Its use in Chinese herbal medicine dates back more than 4000 years. In colonial North America, ginseng was a major export product. The wild form is now rare, but panax ginseng is a widely cultivated plant.

Ginseng has a legendary status among herbs. While extravagant claims have been made about its many uses, scientific research has yielded inconsistent results in verifying its therapeutic properties. However, enough good research does exist to demonstrate ginseng's activity, especially when high-quality extracts, standardized for active components, are used.

Ginseng has a balancing, tonic effect on the systems and organs of the body involved in the stress response. It contains at least thirteen different saponins, a class of chemicals found in many plants, especially legumes, which take their name from their ability to form a soaplike froth when shaken with water. These compounds (triterpene glycosides) are the most pharmaceutically active constituents of ginseng. Saponins benefit cardiovascular function, immunity, hormone production, and the central nervous system.

During times of stress, ginseng acts as a general stimulant, delaying the alarm phase in Selye's classic model of stress. The saponins in the ginseng act on the hypothalamus and pituitary glands, increasing the release of adrenocorticotrophin, or ACTH (a hormone produced by the pituitary that promotes the manufacture and secretion of adrenal hormones). As a result, ginseng increases the release of adrenal cortisone and other adrenal hormones, and prevents their depletion from stress. Other substances associated with the pituitary are also released, such as endorphins. Ginseng is used to prevent adrenal atrophy, which can be a side effect of cortisone drug treatment.

In a double-blind study published in 1996 in *Drugs Under Experimental and Clinical Research*, two groups of volunteers suffering from fatigue due to physical or mental stress were given nutritional supplementation over a twelve-week period. One hundred sixty-three volunteers were given a multivitamin and multimineral complex, and 338 volunteers received the same product plus a standardized Chinese ginseng extract. Once a month, the volunteers were asked to fill out a questionnaire during a scheduled visit with a physician. This questionnaire contained eleven questions that asked them to describe their current level of perceived physical energy, stamina, sense of well-being, libido, and quality of sleep.

While both groups experienced similar improvement in their quality of life by the second visit, the group using the ginseng extract almost doubled their improvement, based on their questionnaire responses, by the third and fourth visits. Thus, ginseng, when added to a multivitamin and multimineral complex, appears to improve many parameters of well-being in individuals experiencing significant physical and emotional stress.

Many of Susan's patients have used ginseng and have found it to have energizing effects, especially Korean red ginseng, which is considered to be hotter (more "yang") and stronger than other forms of ginseng, including Chinese and American, which are more cooling (more "yin") and calming in their effects. While Korean ginseng is well suited to men, women may find the effects of this form of ginseng too extreme for the female body. Some women experience extremely heightened levels of libido with the use of Korean ginseng, as well as tremendous surges of energy. However, it can also disrupt the menstrual cycle, causing a decrease in normal menstrual flow and dryness of the skin and mucous membranes. As a result, women tend to do better with Chinese or American ginseng.

There is evidence in animal and human studies that ginseng increases stamina and endurance. Studies show that ginseng prevents fatigue, lengthening the time it takes to reach exhaustion. Ginseng also enhances mental capacity, as demonstrated in both animal studies and clinical trials in humans. Improvements in logical deduction, reaction time, mental arithmetic, alertness, and accuracy have been observed. ACTH (the hormone that stimulates the adrenal cortex) and adrenal hormones, which ginseng stimulates, are known to bind to brain tissue, increasing mental activity during stress.

SUGGESTED DOSAGE: For maximum benefit, take a high-quality preparation, an extract of the main root of a plant that is six to eight years old, standardized for ginsenoside content and ratio. Companies manufacturing ginseng products may mention the age of the plants used in their products as a testimony to their products' quality. Take a 100 mg capsule twice a day. If this is too stimulating, especially before bedtime, take the second dose midafternoon, or take only the morning dose.

Siberian ginseng. Siberian ginseng (*Eleutherococcus senticosus*) belongs to the same family as panax ginseng, but the exact composition differs considerably. The most pharmacologically active constituents in Siberian ginseng are eleutherosides, some of which are similar in structure to the saponins contained in Asian ginseng. Siberian ginseng has been used in Asia for nearly 2000 years to combat fatigue and increase endurance. The medicinal properties of this plant have been studied in Russia, with a number of clinical and experimental studies demonstrating that eleutherosides are adaptogenic, increasing resistance to stress and fatigue. According to a review of clinical trials of more than 2100 healthy human subjects, ranging in age from nineteen to seventy-two, published in 1985 in *Economic Medicinal Plant Research*, Siberian ginseng reduces activation of the adrenal cortex in response to stress, an action useful in the alarm stage of the fight-or-flight response. It also helps lower blood pressure. In this same study, data indicated that the eleutherosides increased the subjects' ability to withstand adverse physical conditions including heat, noise, motion, an increase in workload, and exercise. There was also improved quality of work under stressful work conditions and improved athletic performance. Siberian ginseng can be of benefit to athletes and also to a person working hard to meet a deadline. Ginseng may help a person push beyond their normal capacity when the only way to finish a job is to pull an all-nighter. Herbalists have also long prescribed Siberian ginseng for chronic-fatigue syndrome.

One way in which ginseng may increase energy reserves is through its ability to facilitate the conversion of fat into energy, in both intense and moderate physical activity, sparing carbohydrates and postponing the point at which a runner, for instance, may "hit the wall." This occurs when stored glucose is depleted and can no longer serve as a source of energy. Siberian ginseng is also used to treat a variety of psychological disturbances, including insomnia, hypochondriasis, and various neuroses. The reason ginseng is effective may be its ability to balance stress hormones and neurotransmitters such as epinephrine, serotonin, and dopamine.

SUGGESTED DOSAGE: Siberian ginseng has virtually no toxicity, although individuals with fever, hypertonic crisis, or myocardial infarction are advised not to use it. A standard dosage of the fluid extract (33 percent ethanol) ranges from 2.0 to 4.0 ml, one to three times a day, for periods of up to sixty consecutive days. An equivalent dosage of dry powdered extract concentrated at a ratio of 20:1 is 100 to 200 mg. Take in multiple-dose regimens with two to three weeks between courses.

▲▲ Susan has had a number of patients over the years who have bought inexpensive ginseng, either as a root or in capsule form, expecting miraculous results, given ginseng's venerable reputation. Unfortunately, these cheaper grades of ginseng rarely, if ever, deliver the punch that individuals expect—that is, the chemical equivalent of an auxiliary set of adrenal glands, testicles, or ovaries. Susan has, however, seen some remarkable results with high-grade ginseng purchased from reputable Chinese pharmacists that sell top-of-the-line herbs or American companies selling herbs of equivalent quality. Given that the potency of the therapeutic chemicals takes many years to develop within the ginseng root, it is no surprise that, with ginseng, you get what you pay for. Individuals with a serious interest in using ginseng for its adaptogenic properties should search out the reputable dealers.

Licorice root. Licorice has been enjoyed over the centuries as a candy, but it is also an herb with medicinal properties, featured in the great recorded herbals for 4000 years. Respected by the ancient Egyptians, licorice was among the treasured items archaeologists discovered (in great quantities) when they opened King Tut's tomb. Sometime around the year 1600, John Josselyn of Boston listed licorice as one of the "precious herbs" brought from England to colonial America.

Licorice is used to treat respiratory conditions, urinary and kidney problems, fatty liver, hepatitis, the inflammation of arthritis, and ulcers. The herb also exhibits hormonelike activity. Licorice root increases the half-life of cortisol (the adrenal stress hormone), inhibiting the breakdown of adrenal hormones by the liver. As a result, licorice is useful in reversing low cortisol conditions and helping the adrenal glands rest and restore function.

Licorice also contains potent estrogenlike chemicals. Since estrogen has profound mood-elevating effects, licorice has antidepressant properties. For a person under a variety of stresses, licorice may be the needed antidote because of its energizing and antidepressant actions.

SUGGESTED DOSAGE: A standard dosage is 1 to 2 g of powdered root administered at three separate times per day. Licorice has activity similar to aldosterone, the adrenal hormone responsible for regulating water and electrolytes within the body. As a result, taking large doses of licorice (10 to 14 g of the crude herb) can lead to high blood pressure, water retention, and sodium and potassium imbalances. Licorice should not be taken by children under age two. Caution should be used with older children, pregnant and nursing women, and people over sixty-five. Start with low dosages and increase the strength only if necessary.

Gotu kola. Gotu kola (*Centella asiatica*), also called centella, has been used since prehistoric times in India. It has been used both internally and externally, based on its ability to heal wounds and treat skin conditions such as eczema, varicose ulcers, and leprosy. In the 1880s, gotu kola was incorporated into the French pharmacopoeia. (American consumers sometimes confuse gotu kola and its rejuvenating activity with kola nuts, which are stimulating because they contain caffeine.) Gotu kola has an action similar to Siberian ginseng, acting as a potent antifatigue nutrient. People who are experiencing excessive levels of anxiety may find the energy-supporting qualities of gotu kola quite helpful.

Gotu kola was used in China to delay senility. Modern studies are beginning to confirm its effectiveness in improving mental function. It has been used to increase the mental abilities of disabled children. The primary active components of gotu kola are triterpene compounds. These are asiatic acid, madecassic acid, asiaticoside, and madecassoside. These triterpenes liberate the neurotransmitter acetylcholine, which is important for cognitive function. And it is assumed that because of this, mental capacity often improves. Gotu kola also has a tranquilizing effect and counteracts stress.

SUGGESTED DOSAGE: If using a standardized extract, take 60 to 120 mg per day. If taking the crude dried plant leaves, take 2 to 4 g per day.

Mood-balancing herbs

There are a number of mood-balancing herbs that calm and relax the nervous system. The herbs described below have a notable relaxant effect and help to promote a sense of well-being.

Kava root. The kava plant is native to the Pacific Islands and is a member of the black pepper family. It thrives in warm, moist climates, where it grows abundantly, reaching a height of fifteen to eighteen feet. As a medicinal plant, herbal preparations are made from the root. It has been used for centuries during social and tribal ceremonies to encourage a greater sense of well-being and relaxation. Pacific Islanders also used kava to relieve pain and enhance mental clarity. Modern research has identified kava lactones, or pyrones, as the active ingredients in the plant that are most responsible for its potent antianxiety and sedative effects. Kava root contains between 3 and 9 percent kava lactones. European extracts of kava are standardized to contain as much as 70 percent kava lactones for medicinal use. Kava is used to reduce pain (when first swallowed, it produces a numbing sensation within the mouth). It is also used to reduce anxiety and relax tense muscles. One small study even found it to be useful in controlling epileptic seizures.

SUGGESTED DOSAGE: The standard dosage is 140 to 210 mg of the herbal extract of kava lactones per day to reduce anxiety and nervous tension. Kava should be taken with meals. It may also be taken before bedtime for the treatment of insomnia. It should not be used for more than four- to eight-week periods without consulting your health care practitioner.

A Caution on Using Kava

As with prescription antianxiety medications, kava may cause drowsiness. Individuals experiencing this side effect should avoid driving while using kava. It may also cause mild intestinal symptoms in some individuals. Rarely, kava has been known to cause a yellowing of the skin or a skin rash. Kava should be avoided by pregnant and lactating women. Finally, kava should not be used with other medications that affect the central nervous system, such as barbiturates, antidepressants, and alcohol or even other sedative herbs like valerian root.

St. John's wort. St. John's wort has been used for centuries in Europe as a remedy for lung, kidney, and skin conditions as well as a treatment for depression. It also grows in the United States, particularly in northern California and southern Oregon. St. John's wort is currently much in vogue as a natural antidepressant and has been researched for its mood-elevating effects. Its most important active ingredient is hypericin, which is thought to have antidepressant and antiviral effects. Other substances contained in St. John's wort, such as flavonoids and xanthones, are also thought to have antidepressant effects, thereby increasing the efficacy of the herb for the treatment of depression.

SUGGESTED DOSAGE: Extracts of St. John's wort are normally standardized to 0.3 percent hypericin. This should be taken three times daily, with meals. Herbal tinctures of St. John's wort may also be used in dosages of 1 to 2 ml, three times a day.

A Caution on Using St. John's Wort

Do not use St. John's wort with prescription antidepressants. Pregnant or lactating women should also avoid its use. St. John's wort has few side effects, but it may make the skin more light-sensitive. Individuals using St. John's wort may therefore need to avoid exposure to strong sunlight.

Valerian root. Valerian is a perennial plant widely distributed in the temperate regions of North America, Europe, and Asia. It is most often cultivated for medicinal purposes. The dried root has a distinctive odor now thought offensive, but in the sixteenth century, it was considered fragrant and laid among clothes as a perfume. In World War I, valerian was used to prevent frontline troops from developing shell shock, and in World War II, it was used to reduce anxiety among civilians exposed to air raids.

Valerian is listed in the French, German, and Swiss pharmacopoeias as a sedative and is traditionally used for relief from insomnia, hysteria, fatigue, intestinal cramps, and other nervous conditions. In herbal terms, valerian is a calmative (a sedative, or depressant), a carminative (good for upset stomach and digestion), a nervine (a tranquilizer), and an anodyne (a pain reliever). The volatile oils are perhaps the most active components. Valerian is especially beneficial because it normalizes the autonomic nervous system, acting as a sedative when a person is agitated and as a stimulant in the case of fatigue. It balances the opposing forces, the parasympathetic and sympathetic aspects of the nervous system, helping to maintain homeostasis.

While some sedatives may relax a person to the extent that reading a report or cooking dinner becomes an uphill struggle, valerian is known to actually increase concentration, reasoning powers, energy levels, and motor coordination. Herbalists recommend valerian for childhood behavior disorders and learning disabilities. There are no hypnotic or depressive side effects when taking appropriate amounts of valerian, and no morning sleepiness.

The therapeutic effects of valerian are well documented in scientific literature. In a study appearing in 1985 in the *Journal of Medicinal Plant Research*, eight volunteers received either a placebo or 450 or 900 mg of an aqueous extract of valerian root. The time it took volunteers to fall asleep was shorter with valerian than the placebo, but the higher dosage of valerian produced no further improvement. In another study, published in 1982 in *Pharmacology, Biochemistry and Behavior*, 128 people rated their quality of sleep, taking either a placebo, a valerian extract, or an over-the-counter valerian preparation. With valerian, individuals subjectively reported shorter sleep latency (the time they lie in bed before falling sleep) and a significant improvement in sleep quality, especially among people who considered themselves poor or irregular sleepers.

SUGGESTED DOSAGE: Because valerian has an unpleasant taste, it is more palatable in capsule form. The standardized extract of valerian (0.8 percent valeric acid content) is preferred to other forms, taken as a mild sedative. The standard dosage is 150 to 300 mg, taken thirty to forty-five minutes before retiring. Valerian is generally regarded as safe and is approved for food use by the FDA.

▲▲ Individuals who tend to have dryness of their tissues, such as menopausal women, may not like the drying effect that valerian root can have. Rather than abandoning the use of a natural sleeping aid altogether, try melatonin or 5-hydroxytryptophan instead. If one type of therapeutic agent doesn't work, another often will.

Passionflower. Spanish explorers discovered passionflower in Peru, where it was highly prized as an herb by the mountain people. The flower was introduced to Europe and eventually brought to North America by colonial settlers. Passionflower is considered a mild sedative or nervine that reduces nervous tension, anxiety, and blood pressure and also encourages deep, restful sleep, free from frequent wakening. Because it can allay general restlessness, it is recommended for schoolchildren who have difficulty concentrating.

Passionflower sedates the central nervous system due to the presence of small amounts of harmala alkaloids. This herb also has a particular effect on serotonin, a substance produced in the brain that promotes sleep. Passionflower maintains body levels of serotonin by inhibiting the breakdown or metabolism of the serotonin already present. The enzyme monoamine oxidase (MAO) normally converts serotonin to an acid. The class of medications known as MAO-inhibitors keeps this from happening, as does this MAO-active herb. An MAO-inhibitor can double the serotonin content of the brain in less than an hour, and even though passionflower is only a mild MAO-inhibitor, it can still have considerable effect.

SUGGESTED DOSAGE: Use 1 tsp. of dried leaves per one cup of boiling water to make tea. Let steep ten to fifteen minutes. For insomnia, drink a cup of tea before bed. Three cups a day may be taken for other uses. Passionflower is generally considered safe, but because the harmala compounds are uterine stimulants, it is suggested that pregnant women not use the herb.

Skullcap. Skullcap is a blue-helmeted flowering plant, traditionally used as a tonic for nervous tension and insomnia. Herbalists consider it one of the best nerve tonics ever discovered. It acts through the cerebrospinal centers, and its active components are its bitter principles and a volatile oil, scutellarin. Skullcap is used for insomnia, exhaustion, and lockjaw.

SUGGESTED DOSAGE: To take as a tea, pour one cup of boiling water onto 1 to 2 tsp. of dried herb and let infuse for ten to fifteen minutes. Drink once a day, or as needed. To be of benefit, skullcap needs to be taken regularly for a long period of time. Take one to two capsules before bedtime for its sedative effect.

Relaxant and antispasmodic herbs

Many people with anxiety suffer from the unpleasant physical symptoms of tight, tense muscles in vulnerable areas of their bodies (the neck, shoulders, jaw, and upper and lower back are common areas to store tension).

The following relaxant herbs help to relieve the muscle tension and spasm that often accompany stress. These are also often effective in relieving stress-related indigestion and intestinal gas.

Peppermint. Peppermint is a natural hybrid of the two mints, garden spearmint and water mint. Both peppermint and spearmint are used in herbal healing and have similar effects, but peppermint is somewhat tastier and more potent. Especially because it is a digestive, peppermint tea is enjoyed at the end of a meal, diffusing like alcohol and warming the entire body. The medicinal component of peppermint is a volatile oil. There are more than forty compounds in the oil; menthol, flavonoids, tocopherols, carotenes, and choline are just some of the substances that contribute to its therapeutic effect.

Peppermint has been used traditionally to cleanse and strengthen the entire system, including the nerves. A bath containing peppermint oil is said to be calming. Peppermint also has an antispasmodic effect on smooth muscle. Calcium in muscle cells causes the muscles to contract. Peppermint blocks this influx, which might explain why peppermint has relaxant properties. Peppermint is a suitable treatment for upset stomach and intestinal spasm. As a stomach sedative, it also helps relieve gas.

In a study appearing in 1996 in *Phytomedicine*, thirty patients (twelve female and eighteen male) received the herbal drug Lomatol, containing peppermint leaves, while sixteen males and fourteen females received metoclopramide hydrochloride drops. Each patient was instructed to take twenty-five drops of the preparation in water twenty minutes before each meal, three times a day for two weeks. By the seventh day, gastrospasms were eliminated in nearly 90 percent of the patients using Lomatol, compared with only 50 percent of the patients on the hydrochloride compound.

SUGGESTED DOSAGE: Peppermint is commonly taken as a tea, prepared with 1 to 2 tsp. of the dried leaves per one cup of water. Be sure to use the organic dried leaves that are available in bulk or organic leaves prepackaged in tea bags. Peppermint oil and menthol, when applied topically, can cause contact dermatitis in sensitive persons. Pregnant women are advised to use peppermint only in diluted, beverage-tea concentrations, not potent medicinal infusions. Moreover, the use of peppermint during pregnancy is discouraged for women with a history of miscarriage.

Chamomile. Chamomile is a time-honored herb, called "ground apple" by the ancient Greeks because of its pleasant applelike scent. Chamomile was used as a stewing herb during the Middle Ages, and today it is enjoyed as a tea by both adults and children throughout Europe and Latin America. Used medicinally as a relaxant, chamomile calms nerves and promotes sleep, a benefit documented scientifically since the 1950s. The active principles of chamomile include flavonoids, glycosides, a very important dicylic ether, and essential oils.

As a relaxant, chamomile depresses the central nervous system, reducing anxiety while not disrupting normal performance or function. Chamomile seems an ideal herb to have on hand, given the demands and pace of modern life. Anyone who is overwhelmed by the demands of running a household while also conducting a business from home might benefit from a chamomile tea break. A calming drink, rather than a cup of coffee, can sometimes better restore clear thinking and the ability to work efficiently. A cup of chamomile can also temper a child's restlessness.

Chamomile also acts as an antispasmodic, helping to relax muscles that can automatically tighten when the fight-or-flight response is activated. As a tonic, chamomile can help prevent stress-related stomach cramps, poor digestion, and irritable-bowel syndrome.

SUGGESTED DOSAGE: There are two types of chamomile, German (or Hungarian) and Roman (or English), both of which produce the same effects. To take as a tea, make an infusion of 2 to 3 heaping tsp. of chamomile flowers per one cup of boiling water. Let steep for ten to twenty minutes. Drink up to three cups a day. Children under the age of two may be given a weaker infusion. For a chamomile bath, tie a bunch of chamomile flowers into a cloth hung from the tub faucet, and run the bath water through it.

Gingerroot. Ginger has thick, underground stems (tuberous rhizomes), and it is these knotted and branched rhizomes, commonly called the "root," which are used in cooking and for medicinal purposes. Records of its use in China date to the fourth century B.C. As an antispasmodic, ginger is effective in relieving the nausea and vomiting associated with motion sickness and morning sickness in pregnancy. The most pharmacologically active compounds in ginger are the various "pungent" principles, aromatic ketones known collectively as gingerols.

As for its effects on stress management, the gingerroot helps stabilize blood sugar levels, preventing the mood swings that erratic highs and lows of blood glucose can trigger. Ginger also increases the efficiency of the digestive processes and thereby the availability of essential nutrients needed for proper maintenance of blood glucose.

SUGGESTED DOSAGE: Mix $1/2$ tsp. ground ginger or 1 to 2 tsp. grated fresh ginger with 1 tsp. honey. Add one cup of boiling water to make a cup of ginger tea.

AROMATHERAPY

The essential oils of plants may be used to counteract stress, an aspect of herbal medicine called aromatherapy. Essential oils are the subtle, volatile liquids that are distilled from a wide variety of plant material, including flowers, shrubs, trees, roots, and seeds.

Essential oils are known to contain trace elements of vitamins, minerals, enzymes, hormones, and substances with immunity-stimulating properties. However, much of the therapeutic effect of the oils is due to the specific chemistry of their aromatic compounds. Essential oils are also effective because of their ease of absorption, due to the small size of the molecules that make up the oils.

Essential oils may enter the body in one of two ways. The oils may be absorbed by inhaling the volatile, aromatic compounds through the olfactory system (hence the term *aromatherapy*), using vaporizers, steam inhalation, or a tissue dampened with a drop of oil that is held to the nose. When essential oils are inhaled, the aroma of the oil stimulates the olfactory bulb. The olfactory bulb is part of the limbic system, the section of the brain that controls stress levels as well as heart rate, blood pressure, and breathing, all of which can be affected by stress. A whiff of a particular essential oil alters the neurochemistry of the brain and can produce physiological or psychological changes, often in a few seconds.

Essential oils can also be absorbed through the skin via massage. Oils absorbed transdermally travel through the circulatory system and act on the adrenal glands and the thyroid, interacting with various branches of the nervous system.

Aromatherapy has long been used throughout Europe, where its practitioners have developed time-tested applications for certain essential oils. To calm emotions, Victorian ladies routinely sniffed a handkerchief daubed with oil of lavender. Now, according to a study cited in an article in the magazine *Country Living/Healthy Living*, scientists find that lavender increases the alpha brain waves associated with relaxation. Studies also confirm lavender's ability to induce restful sleep. In a study published in 1995 in the *Lancet*, researchers took nursing home patients off of sedating drugs for two weeks. They then infused the room with lavender oil. Three patients who had been taking sleeping medications had difficulty sleeping during the two weeks off medication, but with the infused lavender oil they slept as well as with the medication. A fourth patient, who had not been using a sleep medication, reported sleeping better with the lavender oil.

Other essential oils used to reduce nervous tension, fatigue, or mental stress include Roman chamomile, orange, tangerine, lemon, rose, spruce, and ylang-ylang, as well as the culinary flavorings spearmint, marjoram, and fennel. Jasmine, which is an energizing essence, and nutmeg are used in cases of nervous exhaustion, when the stress response is weak. These tonics can be diffused in the air or rubbed on the wrists, solar plexus, temples, or soles of the feet. Oils such as lavender are added to bath water or sprayed on bed linens.

Essential oils can be purchased in health food and beauty stores, and by mail order; however, the quality may vary. For the best-quality distillations, look for essential oils packaged in small dark blue or brown bottles. Prices within a particular product line will vary, as some essential oils are far more expensive than others. A product line with similar pricing throughout may be offering oils of inferior quality. Essential oils, provided they are used in the right quantities, are harmless; however, they can be toxic if taken orally.

PART 3:
STRESS MANAGEMENT TECHNIQUES

DURING THE PAST few decades, there has been a tremendous increase in awareness on the part of the American public about the performance and health benefits of stress management techniques. Like diet and nutrition, the regular practice of these techniques can literally change your body's chemical profile, helping to restore your stress-coping chemicals and hormones. These techniques can also create beneficial effects in your physiology, providing you with greater energy and vitality and enabling you to become more resistant to disease. In this section we will discuss many of these helpful techniques.

BRAIN-BASED STRESS REDUCTION TECHNIQUES

Cutting-edge investigations in medicine are exploring the relationship between an individual's mental state and physical health, the so-called mind/body connection. Traditional medicine in China and India has long noted details of what a patient has been feeling and thinking as part of the medical history used for diagnosis. Western medicine, with the help of advanced technology, is just now discovering specific chemicals and biological mechanisms that indicate that this link between the two realms really exists on a physical level. For instance, molecules once believed to be unique to the function of thinking have now also been found in the lymphatic system, which is involved with immunity.

Thoughts and feelings can also affect the stress response. Many studies have shown that our output of stress hormones and chemicals can be interrupted by changing the pattern of our thoughts. There are many brain-based mental techniques whose ability to reduce stress is well documented. These include deep-breathing exercises, yoga, self-hypnosis, focusing and meditation, grounding and centering techniques, relaxation exercises and techniques, erasure techniques (erasing old mental "programs"), visualizations, and positive affirmations. What all of these techniques have in common is their ability to interrupt the flow of emotions and thought patterns that trigger the fight-or-flight response.

Breathing exercises

Therapeutic breath work is remarkably effective in calming the mood. Taking deep, slow breaths, drawing air into the lungs and deep into the body, and expanding the abdomen can have a major impact on feelings of anxiety and upset. Breathing deeply can generate a feeling of internal peace and calm, as well as relaxing and loosening muscles.

Deep breathing brings oxygen to the cells and helps the body function optimally, while also eliminating waste products with every exhalation. However, when an individual feels stressed, breathing tends to become jagged, erratic, and shallow. A person may breathe too fast or even stop breathing and hold his or her breath for prolonged periods of time without realizing it, reducing the supply of oxygen to the body. Furthermore, when a person is upset, muscles tend to tense and tighten, blood flow becomes constricted, pulse rate and heartbeat elevate, and there is an increase in the output of stress chemicals from the glands. Autonomic-nervous-system function becomes imbalanced. However, taking longer breaths causes physiologic responses to slow down. Muscles relax, blood vessels dilate, and a state of equilibrium is restored.

Exercise: Deep Abdominal Breathing

Deep, slow abdominal breathing is a very important technique for the relief of anxiety and stress. It also improves energy and vitality. Abdominal breathing brings adequate oxygen, the fuel for metabolic activity, to all tissues of the body. In contrast, rapid, shallow breathing decreases oxygen supply and keeps you nervous and tense. Deep breathing helps to relax the entire body and strengthens muscles in the chest and abdomen. Do this exercise for three to five minutes:

- Lie flat on your back with your knees pulled up. Keep your feet slightly apart. Try to breathe in and out through your nose.

- Inhale deeply. As you breathe in, allow your stomach to relax so the air flows into your abdomen. Your stomach should balloon out as you breathe in. Visualize your lungs filling up with air so that your chest swells out.

- Imagine that the air you breathe is filling your body with energy.

- Exhale deeply. As you breathe out, let your stomach and chest collapse. Imagine the air being pushed out, first from your abdomen and then from your lungs.

Focusing

In this technique, the mind is allowed to rest on a single object with the purpose of stilling the everyday chatter that normally fills our thoughts. Select a small personal object that you like a great deal. It might be a decorative bowl or a single flower from the garden. Focus all your attention on this object as you inhale and exhale slowly and deeply for one to two minutes. While you are doing this exercise, try not to let any other thoughts or feelings enter your mind. If they do, just return your attention to the object. At the end of this exercise you will probably feel more peaceful and calm. Any tension or nervousness that you were feeling on starting the exercise should be diminished. Meditation, which is similar to focusing, has also been used to treat depression and panic disorder.

Visualization

This technique uses the ability to visualize a desired outcome in a person's life or health condition. These pleasant and positive internal pictures often realign the body's chemistry toward a state more consistent with health and well-being. A research study published in 1994 in the *Journal of the National Cancer Institute* stated that about 20 percent of the population has a facility for practicing this technique. Protocols using visualization techniques have been found to be beneficial in some cancer patients.

Spirituality and prayer

For many people, working with mind/body techniques borders on the spiritual. Disciplines such as meditation and guided imagery are also components of various religious practices. Whatever the context, these are effective tools for reducing stress. Countless people over the centuries have also turned to prayer for a sense of safety and calm. Many studies have examined the effect of spiritual practices on healing, and these show that when people pray or meditate, their heart rate and blood pressure are lowered.

Not only can prayer be effective in promoting self-healing, but it can also be used to foster healing in others. Larry Dossey, an internist and best-selling author, incorporates the use of prayer as therapy into his practice. An article in May 1997 in the magazine *Hippocrates* refers to various studies that show evidence of the ability of prayer to improve medical outcomes. In one study conducted at San Francisco General Hospital in 1988, of 393 cardiac patients, those who were prayed for did noticeably better than other patients. The therapeutic effects are all the more intriguing because neither the patients nor their physicians knew which patients were being prayed for. There are dozens of other studies showing similar results. According to this article, in the fall of 1996 nearly thirty medical schools offered courses exploring the role of spirituality in clinical practice.

People who develop the spiritual side of their nature sometimes acquire a sense of meaning in their lives that helps them to cope with anxiety. People with a clear sense of inner direction may be less prone to panic attacks or agoraphobia.

Laughter

When laughter is a person's automatic "stress response," trying times are less likely to diminish health and well-being. Dr. Norman Cousins introduced this concept to medicine after he was diagnosed with ankylosing spondylitis. He was determined to find a treatment for this disabling condition and essentially cured himself by listening to records of laughter and taking large doses of vitamin C. More recently, research studies have provided scientific confirmation of this phenomenon. Laughter has been shown to lower the stress hormone cortisol as well as blood pressure and heart rate, and to increase mood-elevating beta-endorphins. According to an article published in 1992 in *Family Practice News*, children laugh, on average, about 400 times a day, while adults laugh only about 15 times a day. Boosting our daily laughter is a great way to relax the tensions we are holding. One of the ways to increase the benefits that come from laughter is to follow the example of Cousins and listen to laugh recordings. At first, the process seems a bit silly, but after listening for a few minutes your brain and body stop resisting and you begin to laugh right along with the tape. Also, always try to see the humor in all situations, as this is one of the great diffusers of stress.

Everyone's idea of humor is different. Participate in or have available whatever is humorous to you. Rent your favorite comedy videos, get tickets to a local comedy club, or even adopt a pet. Some people find the antics and playfulness of their animal friends to be a source of continual delight. Always try to see the humor in the little frustrations and minor disasters that occur in everyone's life.

HEART-BASED STRESS REDUCTION TECHNIQUES

While the stress response is commonly discussed in terms of the effect of brain chemistry on the production of neurotransmitters and stress hormones, another way of looking at it has recently drawn attention. Thinking of the heart as the initiating organ of the sequence of chemical reactions involved in responding to the environment is a radically new idea, in terms of biology and physiology. However, a growing number of scientific studies are beginning to provide solid evidence of this relationship. The Institute of HeartMath, a research organization in Boulder Creek, California, is devoted to researching this hypothesis and has also developed a program for people to put this concept into practice.

The brain generates electrical activity in the form of brain waves. The heart, much more than a mechanical pump, also has electrical activity, similar to that of a radio transmitter, generating forty to sixty times more electrical power than the brain. Because the heart's electrical signal is so strong, these frequencies radiate throughout the body, affecting everything.

The heart responds to any stimulus the mind or brain processes, from thoughts and emotions to sensations of light and sound. This occurs through the baroreceptor system, a collection of neurons and nerves that transport impulses from the heart to the brain and back to the heart again. It regulates the cortex, the outer layer of gray matter of the brain and the part responsible for perception, organ function, and higher mental function.

Negative mental processes disrupt the natural rhythms of the heart, affecting heart rate and the heart's electrical signal. When this occurs, the brain's ability to process information declines. In this state, a person may have difficulty making a decision, being creative, or solving a problem.

At the Institute of HeartMath, through the use of specific techniques that the organization developed, people are taught how to stop a negative train of thought and convert it to a positive feeling or emotion. They learn to generate feelings of sincere love, caring, and appreciation. When this occurs, entrainment takes place; that is, the frequency of the heart pulse, respiration, and brain waves all synchronize. The result is a more harmonious functioning and efficiency of the cardiovascular, immune, and hormonal systems. People practiced in these techniques report dramatic increases in their ability to handle stresses such as conflict on the job, rush-hour traffic, and rebellious children. Problem solving becomes easier, and people report a greater sense of intuition. The exercises take only about a minute and are designed to be performed while a person is in a stressful situation.

Jim learned about HeartMath about five years ago from Hobart, a friend from business school. Hobart was born with a mild case of cerebral palsy, which had restricted movement on his left side, and he also had suffered from high blood pressure, which often reached daytime highs of 200–210/110. In 1990, he suffered a mild stroke and shortly thereafter discovered the HeartMath process. Since practicing the techniques, he has completely recovered from the effects of the stroke, has reduced his blood pressure to 140–160/75, and is now able to perform movements with the left side of his body that were never before possible. About the same time that Jim learned about HeartMath from Hobart, a laboratory located in the state of Washington contacted Susan. In addition to describing their facilities and services, they told Susan about the research they were doing with HeartMath and the impressive results they were seeing. Susan contacted HeartMath, sent for their literature, and was very impressed by the quality of their research.

The research suggests that the heart is a highly intelligent organ, having a far more central role in mental and emotional balance, perception, and stress than previously thought. Numerous studies exist that link a positive attitude to a good prognosis for heart disease. A research article in 1996 in *Alternative Therapies* reported on a study that suggests that emotional experiences affect cardiovascular function. The researchers concluded that positive emotions may be helpful in treating hypertension and reduce the likelihood of sudden death in patients with congestive heart failure and coronary-artery disease. Another study, published in 1995 in the *American Journal of Cardiology*, also showed that a positive emotional state may help hypertension and that anger significantly increases the sympathetic-nervous-system stress response.

Entrainment of heart and mind also strengthens the immune system. Studies show that feelings of happiness and joy are associated with an increase in white-blood-cell count. In a study appearing in 1995 in the *Journal of Advancement in Medicine*, thirty individuals who demonstrated feelings of caring significantly increased their levels of S-IgA, the body's first line of defense against bacteria and viruses. In contrast, anger produced an increase in mood disturbance and heart rate and a decrease in S-IgA that persisted for from one to five hours.

OTHER TECHNIQUES FOR REDUCING STRESS

Besides the brain- and heart-based stress reduction techniques described above, there are many other effective methods to reduce stress. We describe a few in this section.

Music

Many studies have examined the effect of music on mood and performance. For instance, a study published in 1994 in the *Journal of the American Medical Association* found that when surgeons listened to classical music, their autonomic reactivity was reduced and their performance improved. The volunteers were fifty male surgeons, aged thirty-one to sixty-one, with an average age of fifty-two. The volunteers were all self-described music enthusiasts who regularly listened to music during surgery. The setting for the experiment was a soundproof hospital research laboratory. Researchers measured skin conductivity, blood pressure, and pulse. To generate a stress response, surgeons performed mental arithmetic calculations (serial subtractions). Their performance was measured for speed and accuracy. All of the volunteers were able to do the mathematical calculations with more speed and accuracy when listening to music as compared to having no music. Furthermore, the researchers investigated which type of music was most effective: the surgeon's personal taste in music (forty-six classical, two jazz, and two Irish folk) or soothing music typically used for stress reduction—specifically, Pachelbel. In every case, the volunteers performed with notably greater speed and accuracy when listening to music of their own choice.

The Institute of HeartMath makes use of music to alter mental and emotional states. In a study conducted by the Research Division of the Institute, presented at the Eighth International Congress on Stress in Montreux, Switzerland, in 1996, various types of music were compared for their effects. A total of 144 persons listened for fifteen minutes to four kinds of music and completed a feelings-state profile. The results with classical and New Age music were mixed, a particularly interesting result because New Age music is generally thought to soothe the emotions. Grunge music significantly increased negative mood and tension while decreasing mental clarity and positive mood. However, "designer music," specifically created by the research facility to reduce stress and increase energy, produced significant reduction in tension and negative moods while increasing positive moods and mental clarity. Music offers an inexpensive and readily available means of stress management for improved functioning. Tapes of the Institute's "designer music" are available by mail order (see the appendix).

Hydrotherapy

For centuries, people have used warm water as a way to calm moods and relax muscles. You can have your own spa at home by adding relaxing ingredients to bath water. Susan has found an alkaline bath (see page 160) to be extremely useful in relieving muscular discomfort and tension. Heat of any kind helps to release muscle tension. Many people find that saunas and baths also help to calm their moods.

Massage

Massage can be extremely therapeutic for men and women who feel anxious. Gentle touching either by a trained massage therapist, your relationship partner, or even yourself can be very relaxing. Tension usually fades away relatively quickly with gentle, relaxed physical contact. The kneading and stroking movement of a good massage relaxes tight muscles and improves circulation. If you can afford to do so, Susan recommends treating yourself to a massage by a trained professional, since they are skilled in locating areas of held tension in the body and are able to thoroughly massage the muscles and tendons affected so that a deep relaxation is achieved.

A review article appearing in 1995 in the journal *Presse Medicale* found that massage therapy had a beneficial effect on a wide range of physical and psychological problems in infants and children. These conditions included dermatitis, diabetes, and cancer as well as eating disorders, developmental delays, physical and sexual abuse, and post-traumatic stress disorder. With massage therapy, pediatric patients not only had lower levels of anxiety but even lower levels of stress hormones. Massage not only resulted in improved clinical outcomes for the patients, but the grandparents and parents giving the massage treatments also found that their own health was enhanced.

The experience of being touched can affect health in both the short and the long term. As reported in 1997 in *Science*, premature babies who are regularly touched have improved health and shorter hospital stays. In an animal study conducted at McGill University, in Montreal, two adult rats from each of nine litters were measured for hormone stress response. Those that had been licked and groomed by their mothers during their first ten days of life released smaller amounts of hormones in response to stress. These animals were also braver and less anxious than those handled less frequently.

For those who are unable to use massage services, there are many mechanical massage tools available—from small, simple handheld devices to sophisticated massage chairs. One moderately priced device that we have found to be extremely beneficial is a Canadian product called the Thumper (see the appendix). We both use it and find that it is excellent for relief of large muscle tension in the back, abdomen, and legs. A new addition to the line is designed for smaller muscles in the shoulders, arms, and neck.

Exercise

One of the best ways to reduce everyday stress is by exercising. This can be as simple and inexpensive as taking a walk and as immediate as deciding to clean out the garage or do some gardening. Regular exercise allows a discharge of physical and emotional tension, helping to prevent the accumulation of stress that can lead to a state of chronic anxiety and related health problems. Even a single round of exercise such as a dance class or jog through the park can be valuable short-term therapy for someone feeling distressed, according to a study appearing in 1996 in the *Journal of Psychosomatic Research*.

Physical exercise, particularly aerobic exercise, discharges fight-or-flight tension. Exercise conditions the heart, improving oxygenation and blood circulation to tight muscles. Research studies have shown that a conditioned heart reacts less dramatically during episodes of anxiety and stress. When anxiety causes the adrenal glands to pump out stress hormones, a conditioned heart will not experience a significant rise in heart rate. Further, a fit person will tend to stay calmer and more in control of emotions during a taxing situation, helping to maintain more harmonious relationships with coworkers and loved ones.

Improved cardiovascular function, according to an article in 1995 in *Sports Medicine*, leads to increases in blood flow, thereby sending more oxygen to the brain and nerves. The neurotransmitter norepinephrine is also made more available. More nutrients can flow into the brain and more waste products be removed, promoting the clearer and quicker thinking needed in moments of stress. Waste products such as excessive carbon dioxide accumulate in this physical environment and can worsen fight-or-flight symptoms.

Exercise also increases the brain's production of beta-endorphins, chemicals released from the pituitary gland that act as natural opiates. They are chemically similar to the pain reliever morphine but 200 times more potent. Brisk aerobic exercise can raise beta-endorphin levels fivefold, producing feelings of peace. Many studies show a general improvement in mood associated with exercise, even of low intensity, perhaps due to a variety of factors. This was shown in one study, published in 1995 in the *Medical Tribune*, of 220 women over the age of forty, of whom 127 were either menopausal or postmenopausal and 41 were on hormone replacement therapy. All the women who had started menopause and were exercising reported better moods and less depression and anxiety.

Exercise also promotes sound sleep, an antidote for chronic anxiety. The beneficial effects, according to an article published in 1996 in *Sports Medicine*, are more likely to be produced by mild to moderate exercise late in the afternoon rather than morning exercise or exercise close to bedtime, which can be too energizing. An article published in 1991 in *The Physician and Sports Medicine* suggests that isometric exercise may improve sleep latency (the amount of time between reclining in bed and the onset of sleep) than dynamic exercise.

Blood sugar imbalances often have a negative effect on mood. However, according to a study published in 1993 in *Diabetes Research and Clinical Practice*, yoga can effectively improve glucose tolerance, which can worsen symptoms of stress and anxiety. In this study, 149 noninsulin-dependent diabetes patients were evaluated for glucose tolerance. After forty days of yoga therapy, 104 patients showed fair to good improvement in their ability to regulate their blood sugar levels.

Exercise doesn't always reduce stress. Overexercising can actually be stressful. If exercise leaves you feeling even more tired and depleted, the form of exercise you've chosen may be too rigorous or you may be exercising for too long a period at each session. Monitor how you feel during an aerobics class, for instance. Give yourself permission to stop partway through the class if you need to. Gradually add to your exercise time as you are able. You should complete an exercise session feeling refreshed and enlivened. If exercise is leaving you tired after the recovery phase, reduce the intensity or the amount of time you exercise. If that doesn't work, then try other less strenuous or demanding forms of exercise, like walking or slow swimming. Experiment with different forms of exercise, different intensities, and different durations until you find the formula that reduces stress but does not overtire you.

Exercise can improve cognitive function. A study quoted in an article in *Total Health* concluded that adults who were aerobically fit tended to be better able to process information quickly and easily than those who were not notably fit. In another study, published in 1997 in the *British Journal of Sports Medicine*, sixty-three subjects were given standard tests to evaluate creative thinking after a twenty-five-minute aerobic workout or aerobic dance and after watching an emotionally neutral documentary for about the same period of time. Those individuals who exercised scored significantly better. There was also a significant increase in positive mood after the exercise, but a drop after watching the film.

PART 4:
STRESS REDUCTION THROUGH MODERN TECHNOLOGY

THOUSANDS OF RESEARCH studies have investigated the beneficial effects that a surprisingly wide variety of healing modalities can have on reducing stress and restoring our stress-coping mechanisms to a more optimal state of health. These modalities include light-and-sound devices, phototherapy units, and electrotherapy devices. Many of these devices have been developed for home use and are readily accessible to the public (see the appendix for a list of resources).

LIGHT-AND-SOUND DEVICES

The last twenty years has seen a revolution in the availability of tools that induce the brain and nervous system into deep states of relaxation for either short or long periods of time. These tools can not only "force" the brain and nervous system to relax at a given moment, but, used consistently, they can have a profound effect on reducing and eliminating the effects of accumulated stress. To understand why these tools are so powerful and have such a great effect on reducing stress and increasing performance, a short review of the physiology involved is needed.

During any twenty-four-hour period, we experience many different states of consciousness, from heightened awareness and activity to deep sleep. Each of these states has a particular brain wave pattern associated with it, and these waves can be detected by using a very sensitive amplifier called an electroencephalograph (EEG). These brain wave frequencies change depending on the neural activity within the brain. While British researcher Maxwell Cade found fifteen different wave patterns associated with human activity, we tend to group these patterns into four major categories:

1. Beta: Consists of rapid pulsations of between 14 and 30 cycles per second (measured as hertz, or Hz). This is our normal waking-state pattern and is used for problem solving and reacting to external stimulation. This pattern range allows us to respond quickly to events, do calculations, and process and create complex functions. Beta is increased under stress and anxiety in order to deal with immediate problems.

2. Alpha: This is the feel-good brain wave frequency that occurs in focused imagery, meditation, daydreaming, or in rhythmic athletic activity such as yoga or tai chi. Its frequency range is 9 to 13 Hz.

3. Theta: The theta pattern is from 4 to 8 Hz and tends to be produced during deep meditation and as a person becomes drowsy and near sleep. It allows for deep unconscious imagery, and often great creativity is experienced in this state. Theta patterns are evident during rapid eye movement (REM) sleep, when most dreaming occurs.

4. Delta: This is the slowest of the brain wave frequencies and is the rhythm of deep, dreamless sleep, during which the body accomplishes its physical restoration. The waves vary between 1 and 3 Hz in this state.

Controlled external-stimuli pulsed light, sound, or electromagnetic waves are able to dictate the level of activity of the brain through the process of entrainment. Entrainment occurs when the brain's activity level synchronizes with and tracks the pattern of an external source such as pulsed light or sound. The brain literally gets in lockstep with the external frequency pattern. Entrainment to sound is often accomplished by feeding signals of different Hz into each ear, such as 90 Hz in the left ear and 100 Hz in the right ear. The two brain hemispheres then work together to produce a brain wave pattern in the 10 Hz range (the difference between the two frequencies), which is the feel-good alpha state.

Since the brain is unable to resist getting into lockstep with the external stimulus, a highly stressed person can force the brain and the nervous system into any relaxed state that they desire and for any length of time. The opposite is also true, of course: The brain can entrain to high-frequency beta states with highly stimulating music and disruptive sounds. If you are in stress overload or fatigue, be very careful of the external stimulation you are exposed to so you do not unwittingly add to your stress level.

The primary technology that uses brain entrainment is light-and-sound equipment, where you put on a pair of glasses that have small lights installed and a set of earphones. When you turn the equipment on, you receive both pulsed light and sound signals predesigned to entrain the brain waves to certain target frequencies. The same process occurs when you listen to audiotapes or CDs designed to entrain the brain.

These advanced technologies offer tremendous stress reduction capability because they can be used almost anywhere at any time. Portable tape and CD players can fit in most briefcases. They can be used at home, in the office, while traveling, or at any time it is necessary or desirable to change your mental state or release stress. While these can be used while traveling, do not use this equipment while driving or operating dangerous or heavy equipment.

Besides stress reduction and relaxation, mind "software" has been developed to use brain wave entrainment for incredible advances in optimal learning, treating insomnia and sleep disorders, enhancing creativity and performance states, dealing with panic disorders and anxiety, controlling anger, augmenting self-esteem and confidence, and controlling psychophysiological disorders such as migraine headaches and chronic pain.

▲▲ Many overstressed people get caught on such a treadmill that they are in a constant excitatory state and are unable to sit still; or worse, they may fear that if they begin to relax, they may never wake up. If you are in a highly stressful state, work in a high-pressure job, or are just naturally nervous, brain wave entrainment technologies can have a profound impact on your ability to perform. Remember, good decisions, performance under pressure, and optimal learning occur when the brain wave patterns are controlled. If you have trouble controlling yours in critical situations or are trying to recover from accumulated stress and fatigue, you should explore the exciting possibilities of entrainment technologies.

PHOTOTHERAPY UNITS

Light is a nutrient for the body that is as important as vitamin C or magnesium. Visible light is only a small part of the electromagnetic spectrum, yet it is the only portion of the spectrum that our eyes can differentiate. Visible light is absorbed by the eye and strikes the photoreceptors of the retina, called the cones. The cones contain pigments that are sensitive to red, blue, and green light. They enable light rays to be translated into color vision. When all bands of the visible-light spectrum are present, a light source will appear white when illuminated. No one color bank predominates. This is called full-spectrum light.

Sunlight is full-spectrum lighting. It is well known that exposure to natural outdoor light, at specific hours and for a certain length of time, regulates our biorhythms of waking and sleeping. Light triggers the release of neurotransmitters such as serotonin that control these functions.

Exposure to sunlight has traditionally been used to regulate mood, treat fatigue, and reverse depression. There is a growing body of research, especially from the former Soviet Union, that suggests the benefits of natural sunlight for the adrenal glands. Exposure for one-half to two hours a day is recommended. Indirect as well as direct sunlight are both effective. As an activator of the adrenal glands, sunlight may enhance adrenal function, including its role in stimulating the body to respond to stress. This is particularly important during the winter months, when the radiant energy from the sun is its weakest. (Of course, overexposure to the sun's rays should be avoided because of the increased risk of skin cancer, skin damage, and cataracts.)

If it is not possible to spend time outdoors in natural light, a good alternative is to install bright incandescent or halogen lightbulbs in your home and place of work (see the appendix). It has also been reported that exposure to red light may also benefit the adrenals.

Many studies document the use of light as a successful treatment for seasonal affective disorder (SAD), a type of depression that occurs in the winter months. It is well known that our body's circadian (twenty-four-hour) rhythms of waking and sleeping coordinate with the rising and setting of the sun, affecting serotonin levels, which helps regulate sleep. But serotonin also regulates mood and can effect depression, a component of the exhaustion stage of stress. In a study appearing in 1990 in the *Archives of General Psychiatry*, eight patients with winter depression were compared with five who did not suffer from this disorder; the SAD patients showed significant improvement in depression when exposed to bright morning light. Evening light, which is not as bright, was not as effective. The researchers concluded that patients with winter depression have delayed circadian rhythms and that bright-light therapy benefits SAD by allowing an earlier secretion of melatonin. Another study, appearing in 1994 in *ACTA Psychiatrica Scandinavica*, also found that morning-light therapy counteracted depression. A total of fifty-four drug-free outpatients with SAD received 2500 lux cool-white fluorescent light exposure from 6:00 A.M. to 8:00 A.M. daily for two weeks. Researchers noted significant reduction in their depression scores.

For those who have been diagnosed with SAD or who seem to be mildly depressed during the winter months, light boxes that produce 10,000 lux are available. In contrast, sunshine produces 100,000 lux. Exposure for one-half hour per day, preferably in the morning, substitutes for the lack of sunlight and helps improve mood and reduce SAD. Dawn-simulator devices are also available that produce a gradual transition in the amount of indoor morning light that a person with SAD is exposed to. These devices help to reduce morning fatigue in susceptible individuals. Positive results are often noted within several days.

BIOFEEDBACK

Traditional relaxation techniques, such as yoga and meditation, have long been used to regulate bodily functions such as heart rate, blood pressure, and even brain waves. To provide more quantitative information regarding the ability of individuals to modify their stress response, biofeedback equipment was developed. This equipment enables people to measure their own physiological responses to stress. During a biofeedback session, an individual is fitted with sensors that monitor muscle tension, skin temperature, sweat activity, pulse, and respiration. The data is communicated back to the patient through computer graphics, lights that blink, and audible beeps.

Through the use of biofeedback, patients are taught to modify their response to stress. When a patient feels stressed, rapid feedback helps him or her to make a physical adjustment and relax more quickly. This technology is so successful that after using biofeedback, most patients are able to control their stress responses without the machines and can produce relaxation on their own.

Biofeedback is used in the treatment of various disorders including anxiety, headaches, and ringing in the ears (tinnitus), which is often associated with stress and hypertension. Biofeedback training can produce lasting results, as evidenced by a study published in 1991 in *Biofeedback and Self-Regulation*. Among forty hypertension patients, twenty-six successfully completed one year of biofeedback-assisted relaxation. Measured after one, two, and three years of follow-up, 31 percent, 38 percent, and 27 percent, respectively, continued to meet the criteria for success. Some of the patients were able to maintain lower levels of anxiety, cortisol, blood pressure, and muscle tension over a long period.

SOUND WAVE DEVICES

Sound wave devices consist of equipment that emits a modulated, very low frequency sound that is soothing and relaxing to the human body. This technology is based on research done by Lu Yan Fang, a senior scientist at the China National Institute of Electro-Acoustics, in Beijing, who observed that chi gong doctors in China (practitioners trained in this ancient healing art) emitted high levels of low-frequency sound waves from their hands. The sound wave emitted by these practitioners was 100 times higher than that of normal, healthy individuals and 1000 times higher than that of elderly and hospitalized patients. In 1983, she constructed a device that reproduced this low-frequency, infrasonic sound. When she directed the low-frequency sound into hospitalized patients, there was an immediate improvement in pain management, vitality, and recovery time.

This equipment is now available in the United States. It is used to relax muscle spasm as well as to increase local circulation and relieve pain. It uses modulated, very low frequency (8 to 14 Hz) sound waves. A small tabletop unit generates the frequency, which is emitted from a handheld transducer. This can be directed to any area of the body needing treatment. The gentle massage action of the frequency waves gives the sensation of bubbling water or light rain falling on the skin. While this agitation may seem mild, the inaudible sound is actually quite powerful and will travel easily through the body.

Chi gong equipment is also useful for individuals who have difficulty relaxing. The infrasonic sound is thought to synchronize alpha wave function throughout the brain and promote deep relaxation. A typical treatment lasts ten minutes, making this equipment well suited to the busy person who has no time to take a vacation but needs frequent relaxation breaks to maintain their ability to perform at a peak level.

MUSCLE-RELAXANT DEVICES

Another interesting device promotes a gentle, rocking motion of the body. It was developed by scientists in Asia who wanted to develop equipment to mimic the undulating, swimming motion of fish to promote greater flexibility of the spine. The device is used by lying down on a flat surface and placing your feet on top of the device. When turned on, the device moves the feet back and forth from left to right, causing the body to gently mimic the motion of a swimming fish. We have found this device to be very useful in loosening the muscles around the spine, lower back, shoulders, and neck. It appears to reduce muscle tension and relieve muscle fatigue as well as improve circulation.

This device can produce a profound effect and must be used for only short periods of time at first (only two sessions per day of no more than five minutes each). After the first few weeks, the use of the device may be gradually increased up to a maximum of fifteen minutes per session.

SUMMARY OF TREATMENT OPTIONS FOR RESTORING YOUR ABILITY TO MANAGE STRESS

The antistress diet

Antistress vitamins, minerals, and other nutrients

    Vitamins

        Vitamin B complex

        Vitamin C

        Vitamin E

    Minerals

        Magnesium

        Calcium

        Potassium

        Zinc

        Chromium

        Manganese

        Selenium

        Iron

    Flavonoids

    Essential fatty acids

    Amino acids

        Tryptophan

        5-hydroxytryptophan

        Melatonin

        Phenylalanine

    Herbs

        Adaptogenic herbs

        Mood-balancing herbs

        Aromatherapy

Stress reduction techniques

Brain-based stress reduction techniques
Heart-based stress reduction techniques
Other techniques for stress reduction

Stress reduction through modern technology

Light-and-sound devices
Phototherapy units
Biofeedback
Sound wave devices
Muscle-relaxant devices

11

HOW SEX HORMONES BENEFIT PEAK
PERFORMANCE AND HEALTH

MOST PEOPLE WANT to live into old age with strength, vitality, and vigor. We want to maintain a zest for life and be able to participate in our favorite activities, including sex. We also want to be able to think clearly and remember facts and events. No one relishes the idea of becoming infirm or losing the faculties needed to fully participate in favorite activities. The older we become, the more we dread the thought of losing our independence.

Luckily, there is a solution to these concerns. Thousands of research studies and decades of clinical experience have confirmed that the maintenance of sex hormones, both testosterone in men and estrogen and progesterone in women, can go a long way toward helping most people remain vital, strong, and healthy well into old age. Sustaining the levels of male or female sex hormones as well as pregnenolone and DHEA (the two precursor hormones from which all the other sex hormones are made) can help maintain virtually every aspect of performance. Research also suggests that the maintenance of sex hormone levels can play a major preventive role in such debilitating conditions as cardiovascular disease, osteoporosis, and even Alzheimer's disease. It can also play an important role in helping to sustain your productivity and physical vigor. Sufficient levels of sex hormones support the performance traits needed if you plan to extend your career well beyond the normal retirement age or fully participate in sports or maintain your sexual vigor.

Of the various steroid hormones made by the adrenal glands and the reproductive organs, five have a profound effect on the quality of a person's life: the two precursor hormones pregnenolone and DHEA and the three sex hormones testosterone (the primary male sex hormone) and estrogen and progesterone (the two primary female sex hormones). For peak performance and optimal health, a person needs adequate levels of all five. In this chapter and the next, we will be discussing in detail these important hormones and how to maintain them either through replacement therapy, nutritional therapies, or techniques that help to sustain your own hormone production.

C Now that you have a preliminary understanding of the important role sex hormones play in peak performance and health, you are ready to decide what to read next. To learn more about the chemistry of hormones in general, read the following section. The five major hormones are then discussed individually: To learn more about pregnenolone, read section 2, on page 544. To learn more about DHEA, read section 3, on page 556. To learn more about testosterone, read section 4, on page 572. To learn more about estrogen, read section 5, on page 592. To learn more about progesterone, read section 6, on page 613. Sections 1 through 4 apply to both men and women, while sections 5 and 6 apply primarily to women.

Sections 2 through 6 are each divided into the subjects that have organized the preceding chapters that describe chemical functions: the chemistry of the specific hormone, what factors affect the production of the hormone, how the hormone affects peak performance, and how the hormone affects health. Furthermore, sections 2 through 6 each include a chart listing that hormone's benefits for peak performance and health as well as a checklist to help you to begin to determine if your body is producing adequate amounts of the hormone. Finally, for information on how to restore your levels of these hormones, read the next chapter.

SECTION 1:
THE CHEMISTRY OF HORMONES

HORMONES ARE POWERFUL substances that function as the chemical messengers of the body. They are primarily secreted by our glands and released into the bloodstream, where they circulate either to a target gland or to various tissues of the body. Hormones either stimulate a target gland to release its own hormone or directly trigger chemical reactions in the tissues.

The glands of the body (also referred to as the endocrine system) secrete dozens of hormones, which have a multitude of physiological effects on target tissues. Working in concert, hormones initiate and coordinate cellular events, as well as balancing and pacing various physiological processes. As an integral part of many bodily functions, hormones enhance cognitive abilities, help stabilize mood, and are essential for health, promoting growth, healing, and repair. They play a crucial role in preventing the onset of many ailments, such as cardiovascular disease, Alzheimer's disease, and osteoporosis. Considering all the functions that hormones influence, it is no wonder that achieving excellence in any area of life is not possible without an optimally functioning endocrine system.

WHAT ARE SEX HORMONES?

Sex hormones belong to a classification called steroid hormones, which are all derived from cholesterol, a waxy, white, fatty material found in all cells of the body. Other steroid hormones are the stress hormones, the glucocorticoids, and the mineralocorticoids. The steroid hormones are made in the adrenal glands in both men and women. Women also produce steroid hormones in the ovaries (a pair of almond-sized glands nestled deep in a woman's pelvis), while men produce these hormones in the testes (two small oval glands located in the scrotum that are also responsible for producing sperm). Within these tissues, cholesterol is converted to hormones through a number of intermediary steps, leading to the final production of three major sex hormones—estrogen and progesterone in women and testosterone in men.

Both men and women produce the same three major sex hormones but in different proportions. In women, estrogen and progesterone predominate, supporting normal functioning of the reproductive tract and menstrual cycle. The ovaries and adrenals also make small amounts of male hormones, or androgens. Although they are only secreted in tiny amounts, androgens play a vital role in the female libido, or sex drive, as well as helping to maintain bone mass. In men, the reverse is true: The predominant hormone is testosterone, which controls sperm production as well as libido. However, men also produce tiny amounts of estrogen and progesterone.

The sex hormones help to determine the physical characteristics of both men and women, such as skin texture, muscle tone, and body shape. The effect of these hormones on appearance and body type will be covered in more detail later in this chapter.

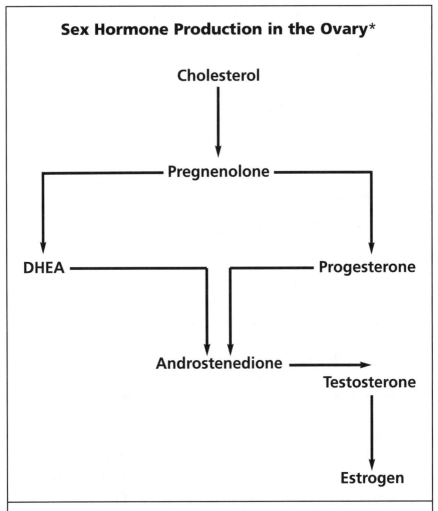

Sex Hormone Production in the Ovary*

Cholesterol

Pregnenolone

DHEA

Progesterone

Androstenedione → Testosterone

Estrogen

*For women in their active reproductive years, the DHEA pathway occurs during the first half of the menstrual cycle and the progesterone pathway normally occurs during the second half. Women in menopause normally go through only the DHEA pathway.

Sex hormone production in men occurs primarily in the testicles. The main male sex hormone, testosterone, is produced from cholesterol or acetyl coenzyme A. Male sex hormones are also produced by the adrenal glands.

HOW SEX HORMONES ARE PRODUCED WITHIN THE BODY

Sex hormones are produced through a series of chemical reactions, beginning with cholesterol (see the diagram above). Of the total cholesterol in the body, about 75 percent is produced in the liver. The remaining

25 percent is supplied in the diet by foods such as meat and dairy products. On average, a person's body contains about one-third of a pound of cholesterol (150 g), mostly as a component of cell membranes. There is also about 7 g of cholesterol that circulates in the blood.

Both the overproduction and the underproduction of cholesterol can lead to hormone imbalances. People who go on stringent low-fat diets may lower their levels of cholesterol to such a degree that they don't have enough to make sufficient amounts of hormones. For example, teenage girls who go on crash diets often have irregular menstrual cycles, as their body's production of estrogens and progesterones, which regulate the cycle, diminishes. At the other extreme, people who are obese and eat the high-fat foods of the standard American diet have the opposite risk: Their bodies make too much cholesterol, making them prone to diseases and disorders for which elevated levels of estrogen are a risk factor., including premenstrual syndrome (PMS), fibroid tumors, fibrocystic disease of the breast, heavy menstrual bleeding, and uterine cancer.

As shown in the diagram of the hormonal pathway, cholesterol is first converted into pregnenolone, a steroid hormone that is the precursor to all the other sex hormones. Because of its precursor role, pregnenolone is considered the mother sex hormone, thus inspiring its name. Pregnenolone is then converted into a variety of other hormones, following two pathways. By one route, pregnenolone leads to DHEA, which is then converted into testosterone and subsequently estrogen. This pathway is operative in women during the first half of the menstrual cycle, when estrogen is the dominant hormone. In the second pathway, pregnenolone is converted into progesterone. The progesterone is then converted into testosterone and, finally, into estrogen. In females, this second pathway predominates during the second half of the menstrual cycle, when progesterone and estrogen are dominant.

HOW HORMONES DELIVER THEIR MESSAGES

Each hormone is coded to bind only to certain tissues. The cells in these hormone-sensitive tissues contain specific receptors. When a hormone reaches its target tissue, it binds to these receptors like a key fitting into a lock. When binding occurs, the hormone then transmits its chemical message to the target tissue, causing a change in the tissue. For example, estrogen is a growth-stimulating hormone that causes tissues to grow and thicken, while progesterone is a growth-limiting hormone. Some hormones can cause rapid changes in a target tissue, occurring literally within seconds, while other reactions may take several days, but may then have a continuing influence for days or even years.

SUMMARY

Hormones, primarily secreted by the glands, or endocrine system, are the chemical messengers of the body. They perform myriad functions and are divided into several categories. The series of chemical reactions that produce the sex hormones begins with cholesterol. The three major sex hormones are testosterone, a primarily male hormone, and estrogen and progesterone, which are primarily female. The two precursor hormones, from which these and all other sex hormones are made, are pregnenolone and DHEA. An adequate supply of sex hormones and their precursors is necessary for peak performance and optimal health.

SECTION 2:
PREGNENOLONE

MANY PEOPLE HAVE never heard of the hormone pregnenolone. However, it is the most important of the five primary sex hormones, as it plays a pivotal role in the production of all the others. As a precursor to all the major sex hormones, pregnenolone has a widespread effect throughout the body. However, pregnenolone delivers peak-performance characteristics far beyond being a precursor to the other sex hormones. In animal and human studies, pregnenolone has been shown to increase energy, improve cognitive function, and stabilize moods. Other studies suggest that pregnenolone may be useful in reducing symptoms due to inflammation in cases of rheumatoid arthritis, spinal-cord injuries, and possibly Alzheimer's disease. For a list of the benefits of pregnenolone for peak performance and optimal health, see page 545.

Benefits of Pregnenolone

Peak-Performance Benefits

 1 Increased physical vitality and stamina

2 Enhanced mental clarity and acuity

4 Increased ability to get along with other people (balances mood)

Health Benefits

- May help to lessen symptoms of arthritis and other autoimmune diseases

- May be useful in speeding recovery from spinal-cord injuries

- May be helpful in the treatment of Alzheimer's disease and multiple sclerosis

---

Pregnenolone was first synthesized in Germany in 1934, and by the 1940s, researchers had begun to study its many uses, including reducing fatigue, increasing physical and mental endurance, and in treating various inflammatory conditions. However, this research came to a halt in the 1950s when synthetic cortisone became the therapy of choice for such diseases as rheumatoid arthritis. Cortisone relieved symptoms quickly, while pregnenolone sometimes required weeks to produce results. Furthermore, synthetic cortisone could be patented, turning it into a highly lucrative drug, so pharmaceutical companies were far more motivated to develop cortisone as a product, and research on pregnenolone was abandoned. Subsequently, patients on cortisone began to suffer its harmful side effects, including a weakening of the immune system and a deterioration of bone mass leading to osteoporosis. Unfortunately, by the time these side effects were fully known, cortisone was established as a widely accepted treatment, and pregnenolone therapy, although known to be nontoxic, was forgotten.

Today pregnenolone is again being studied, thanks to the widespread renewed interest in natural therapies. Researchers are investigating pregnenolone in relation to a wide range of topics, including memory, mood, enzyme activity, joint function, premenstrual syndrome, and the aging process. Given the exciting results of these studies, the potential benefits that pregnenolone can provide in the areas of peak performance and health deserve greater attention.

Pregnenolone is currently available as an over-the-counter supplement. Many people are self-medicating themselves with pregnenolone in an attempt to restore their sex hormone production. To begin to determine whether your body is producing the optimal amount of pregnenolone needed for peak performance and health, see the checklist below. For a description of laboratory tests of pregnenolone production, see page 628.

CHECKLIST: DO YOU PRODUCE THE PREGNENOLONE YOU NEED FOR PEAK PERFORMANCE AND HEALTH?

This checklist will give you a preliminary idea of whether you are experiencing the effects of inadequate pregnenolone production. Work through the following checklist (photocopy it if you don't want to write in the book) and refer to it as you read through this section of the chapter. If your responses suggest that your pregnenolone level is low, you can learn about ways to increase it in chapter 12.

Performance indicators

Put a check mark beside those statements that are true for you.

- ❏ I have low energy and lack stamina.
- ❏ I am unable to work efficiently and effectively under stress.
- ❏ My state of mind is negative.
- ❏ My sleep quality is poor; I tend to wake intermittently during the night.
- ❏ I am a man, and I have poor visual/spatial memory.
- ❏ I am a woman, and I have poor verbal recall.
- ❏ I have unstable moods, am irritable, and/or tend to be depressed.

Physical indicators

- ❏ I am over the age of fifty.

The Chemistry of Pregnenolone

Pregnenolone is made primarily in the adrenal glands, but it is also produced in the cells of the liver, skin, ovaries, testicles, and brain. It is manufactured in the mitochondria, the energy-producing factories of the cells. In the mitochondria, nutrients from our diet are converted into usable energy, and cholesterol is converted into pregnenolone. The pituitary gland regulates the amount of pregnenolone produced. A study published in 1991 in the *Journal of Steroid Biochemistry and Molecular Biology* found that pregnenolone accumulates in the brain, independent of sources in other areas of the body. This may have great significance, given the beneficial effects that pregnenolone seems to have on maintaining physical energy as well as stabilizing mood.

Pregnenolone levels are assayed by measuring the amount of pregnenolone sulfate in the blood. Pregnenolone sulfate is a more water-soluble than pregnenolone itself and is therefore more easily transported through the circulatory system. In adult men, blood levels of pregnenolone sulfate are about 10 mcg per 100 ml. Average daily production of pregnenolone is about 14 mg a day, a relatively small amount (30,000 mg equals about 1 oz.). However, these amounts may vary significantly among individuals.

A variety of factors can decrease pregnenolone production, as noted in a 1995 article published in *Biochemical Pharmacology*. Stress and disease can lower levels of pregnenolone throughout the body and in specific tissues. Pregnenolone production also naturally decreases with age. Blood serum levels of pregnenolone can drop as much as 60 percent between ages thirty-five and seventy-five. Obviously, as pregnenolone levels diminish, the production of all the other sex hormones arising from pregnenolone also declines.

How Health Affects Pregnenolone Production

In order to maintain adequate production of pregnenolone, many systems of the body must function properly. Good digestion is required so that hormone precursors such as amino acids (the smallest units of digested protein), protein fragments, and fat molecules can be absorbed and enter the system. Liver health also is important for pregnenolone production. When liver enzyme systems are impaired and the detoxification function is inadequate, hormone production can be affected. For instance, poor liver function can prevent the conversion of pregnenolone into DHEA. A person's cholesterol profile is another factor in pregnenolone production. When the level of HDL (high-density lipoproteins) is low, because it is a carrier molecule for hormones, pregnenolone production can become blocked.

PREGNENOLONE AND PEAK PERFORMANCE

Although much of the body's pregnenolone is converted into other sex hormones, a certain portion of it remains unchanged and can produce a variety of effects on both health and performance. Research studies have demonstrated that pregnenolone plays a role in increasing physical stamina and productivity when a person is working under stress, as well as enhancing mental acuity, concentration, and memory. Pregnenolone can increase a person's productivity on the job and improve leisure skills that require spatial thought, such as playing bridge or figuring out how to repair a dining room table. Pregnenolone has also been found to stabilize mood, thereby benefiting social relationships. Supplementing with this hormone may be of great benefit for those individuals who want to improve performance as well as for older people, whose body's production of pregnenolone is diminishing. The following subsections describe the peak-performance traits that are supported by an adequate supply of pregnenolone.

1 Physical vitality and stamina

Several breakthrough research studies done on pregnenolone in the 1940s have major implications for its use in maintaining physical energy and enhancing productivity. These studies were done to see if pregnenolone could improve work performance and productivity among people performing complex tasks and/or operating under stressful conditions. According to the studies, pregnenolone improved productivity under all of these conditions. Even though this research was conducted as part of the war effort and has been largely ignored for over fifty years, its implications are relevant for today's high-stress work environment.

Researchers conducted several experiments using pregnenolone in the 1940s, as reported in a 1944 article in *Aviation Medicine*. In one experiment, fourteen volunteers were trained to operate a machine designed to simulate airplane flight. The goal of the exercise was to operate the equipment properly in order to avoid obstacles and prevent crashes. Of the volunteers, seven were pilots, while the others had no flying experience. These volunteers were tested for their flying ability many times over several weeks. Before each test, a volunteer was either given a 50 mg capsule of pregnenolone or left untreated. The results of this test showed that pregnenolone improved performance for all the volunteers. The pilots participating in the experiment also reported that their actual flying on the job improved and that they felt less tired when taking the hormone.

In another experiment reported in the same article, the researchers measured levels of a stress hormone (17-ketosteroid) in the urine of pilots. The amount of 17-ketosteroid normally increased in direct relation to the number of flights completed by the pilots. However, pilots taking pregnenolone had only half the increase in stress hormone excretion as compared with pilots not receiving pregnenolone. Based on these results, the researchers suggested that pregnenolone can help sustain competent performance over a period of time, which could benefit anyone who must work long hours and perform tasks that require coordinated mental and physical activity.

The same research team conducted three other experiments, cited in a 1995 review article in *Biochemical Pharmacology*, in which they gave pregnenolone to three groups of skilled workers: leather cutters, lathe operators, and optical workers. The benefits of pregnenolone were assessed by monitoring units of work produced, wastage of material, and number of flaws in the finished product. They found that when workers received a fixed wage and the work was unhurried and stress-free, pregnenolone had no effect on productivity. But when workers were paid by the piece and worked under pressure, pregnenolone was associated with an increased output above their usual levels. Given the amount of stress in the contemporary workplace, having a sufficient amount of pregnenolone appears to be essential for peak performance. Of particular interest in this study is that some of the volunteers taking pregnenolone also reported a sense of well-being and felt better able to cope with the requirements of their jobs.

This research is as compelling and exciting in today's work environment as it was during World War II. In many ways the demands on employees are as strenuous today as they were during that period. The prevailing reality of today's business world is that of an economic war whose objectives are for constantly higher productivity with resultant lower costs. Most people work under constant stress, doing high-precision work. Think of technicians producing computer chips under sterile conditions or surgeons performing microscopic laser surgery. The requirements and complexity of modern economic life are extraordinarily stringent. Food and nutritional products must be processed and delivered free of disease-causing microorganisms, products must arrive at retailers at almost the same time the sale is made, and airplanes must operate perfectly. All of this economic complexity requires precision and great concentration. The stresses are found throughout the economy, from automobile and computer manufacture and repair to people performing stressful mental jobs such as physicians, accountants, and book editors. Many professions require after-hours reading just to keep up with new developments in the field. Given these stresses and the fact that the population is aging, it is exciting to know that pregnenolone can support productivity and stress, especially after midlife when the body's natural production begins to decline.

Not only does the job stress take its toll on productivity, but many individuals are engaged in work that causes them to be sleep deprived. Research studies have shown that sleep deprivation can lower productivity through the interruption of normal biological cycles. Pregnenolone may be beneficial for those individuals whose jobs require them to work swing or late shifts, such as police officers and firefighters, emergency room doctors and nurses, entertainers, casino employees, and quite often people engaged in manufacturing.

Pregnenolone not only offers promise in improving work productivity by increasing physical energy and mental alertness, but it may also help to improve productivity and maintain energy in workers who are sleep deprived. In a 1993 study published in *Brain Research*, twelve healthy male volunteers, aged twenty to thirty, who were given pregnenolone experienced improved sleep quality and were also somewhat less likely to wake intermittently during the sleep period. These results are particularly impressive since the effects seen in this study were achieved using a dosage of only 1 mg of pregnenolone, given orally before sleep. The normal range of dosage for pregnenolone is much greater, typically 5 to 50 mg per day.

2 Mental clarity and acuity

Pregnenolone has the potential of being of great benefit to individuals who have jobs that require them to learn and retain large quantities of new information. While most of the studies on pregnenolone and memory have been done on animals, several recent human studies are confirming pregnenolone's potential benefits in the area of cognitive function.

Researchers designed an animal study, published in 1992 in *Proceedings of the National Academy of Sciences, USA*, that assessed the effectiveness of pregnenolone in improving the memory of mice trained to avoid electric shock as they proceeded through a maze. Some of the mice were then given individual dosages of various steroid hormones, including pregnenolone, pregnenolone sulfate, DHEA, and testosterone. One week later, the mice were again placed in the maze to test if they remembered the correct way out. While all the hormones improved memory to some extent, pregnenolone and pregnenolone sulfate had the most potent effect.

This same team of researchers conducted another experiment, published in 1995 in *Proceedings of the National Academy of Sciences, USA*, that demonstrated that even remarkably small dosages of pregnenolone can improve memory. In this study, mice were given dosages containing fewer than 150 molecules of pregnenolone sulfate, and again posttraining memory processes improved. The investigators injected pregnenolone into various regions of the brain, with the amygdala (a portion of the brain believed to play an important role in arousal and alertness) proving the most sensitive. These researchers concluded that the effectiveness of pregnenolone treatment in improving memory, when given after learning trials, may indicate that the hormone has an effect on memory storage and retrieval processes.

In the arena of human cognitive research, several recent studies suggest that pregnenolone may also enhance memory in humans. Rahmawhati Sih, a specialist in geriatrics and currently an associate professor of medicine at Loyola University Medical School, in Chicago, conducted several trials to explore this possibility. In the fall of 1997, she presented her work at a meeting of the American Federation for Medical Research. In the study, thirteen healthy older adults—five men and eight women over the age of sixty-five—were given pregnenolone in randomly assigned quantities. Dosages were 10 mg, 50 mg, 200 mg, and 500 mg. Every fourteen days, volunteers received a single dose and were asked to complete a variety of memory tests. The results of this study were promising, with memory improving somewhat as the dosage increased.

In a second trial, the volunteers were again given a range of dosages between 10 and 500 mg and asked to complete a second set of memory tests. In general, the men showed more improvement in visual/spatial tasks, while the women showed improvement in verbal recall. Dr. Sih hypothesized that the difference in these results reflects the different metabolic pathways pregnenolone follows in men and women. In males, pregnenolone metabolizes to testosterone, which is associated with visual/spatial memory, whereas in women, pregnenolone metabolizes to estrogen, which is associated with verbal recall.

While more study is needed, these trials suggest that for older persons with diminished pregnenolone production, supplementation may prove an effective memory enhancer.

4 The ability to get along with other people

Mood is an important determinant of how well we handle our business and social relationships. When an individual is overwhelmed by feelings of either anxiety or depression, it is difficult for them to interact with other people and maintain healthy relationships. Pregnenolone's role as a mood stabilizer can help to support this performance trait.

Recent research has found that pregnenolone may play an important role in stabilizing mood due to its effect on balancing nervous-system function. A study reported in 1991 in the journal *Molecular Pharmacology* discusses the role pregnenolone plays in regulating the delicate balance between excitation and inhibition in the central nervous system. As discussed in the chapters on stress management, there needs to be a balance between the excitatory neurotransmitters, which increase nerve activity, and the inhibitory neurotransmitters, which decrease nerve activity. A person in the excitatory state will experience a heightened mood and feel energized. In contrast, in the inhibitory state, an individual will feel relaxed and calm. For normal human functioning, it is important that a balance exists between these two nervous states to avoid the extremes of anxiety and depression. And pregnenolone may play an important role in maintaining that balance.

A deficiency in pregnenolone has been linked to unstable moods in patients with emotional (affective) illness. In a 1994 study published in *Biological Psychiatry*, researchers analyzed the pregnenolone present in the cerebrospinal fluid (CSF) of twenty-seven mood-disordered patients and ten healthy volunteers as a way of measuring levels of pregnenolone. Pregnenolone normally circulates throughout the brain and spinal column and is seen as an indicator of changes in brain chemistry. The investigators found that those patients with affective illness had lower levels of pregnenolone in the CSF compared to the healthy volunteers. Levels were especially low among those patients who were depressed on the day the CSF was drawn.

Research studies estimate that about 5 to 10 percent of the population is affected by feelings of helplessness, low self-esteem, and poor motivation. Such a state of mind can act as an emotional barrier, preventing someone from even thinking about setting goals, let alone trying to reach them. When these feelings are caused by a deficiency of brain steroid hormones, pregnenolone supplementation may potentially help.

PREGNENOLONE AND HEALTH

Besides its possible benefits in supporting various aspects of performance, pregnenolone may also prove useful in the treatment of several diseases, including Alzheimer's disease, multiple sclerosis, rheumatoid arthritis, and other autoimmune diseases. It may also be helpful in the treatment of spinal-cord injuries.

Alzheimer's disease

A 1995 review article on pregnenolone in *Pergamon* suggested that pregnenolone may one day be proven useful in the treatment of Alzheimer's disease. This degenerative brain disease is characterized by loss of memory and other cognitive functions. The progression of the disease is believed to involve a low-grade inflammatory process that is self-perpetuating and interferes with the body's ability to repair itself. Pregnenolone may prove to be an effective anti-inflammatory therapy for the treatment of this disease. As pregnenolone is nontoxic and readily absorbed, it has great potential as a treatment and deserves further investigation in this capacity.

Multiple sclerosis

Multiple sclerosis is a disease of the central nervous system involving progressive destruction of the myelin sheath surrounding the nerves. This disease commonly affects young and middle-aged adults, causing symptoms such as weakness, loss of coordination, unsteady gait, and visual deterioration. In 1995, researchers found that both pregnenolone and the female hormone progesterone play a role in the healing of damaged nerves. Another study, published in 1995 in *Science*, confirmed these findings. This study found that when progesterone and pregnenolone were administered, myelin sheath development progressed normally. However, much more research on the use of pregnenolone as a treatment for multiple sclerosis remains to be done.

Arthritis and other autoimmune diseases

Early research studies suggest that pregnenolone may be effective in treating patients in the early stages of rheumatoid arthritis, lessening symptoms associated with inflammation. A study published in 1951 followed the results of pregnenolone treatment of eleven patients with rheumatoid arthritis. Of these men and women, ranging in age from thirty-four to sixty-five, six experienced moderate to marked improvement, and some of the others showed slight improvement. Furthermore, between the third and seventh day of therapy, patients noted a sense of well-being and improved appetite. And between the fourth and eighth days, patients reported a noticeable reduction in joint pain. This improvement allowed greater joint mobility and reduced muscular atrophy. In some of the patients, there was also less swelling in the joints.

Other studies have also suggested that pregnenolone has potential in the treatment of other inflammatory diseases such as systemic lupus erythematosus (an autoimmune condition), ankylosing spondylitis (a chronic inflammatory disease of the joints in the spine that causes back stiffening and pain), scleroderma (a rigidity and hardening of the skin and even fibrosis of internal organs), and psoriasis. While much more research needs to be done in this area, pregnenolone may eventually prove to be an exciting new and effective therapy for these disabling chronic conditions.

Spinal-cord injuries

Pregnenolone is useful in reducing the inflammation that occurs at the time of accident in spinal-cord injuries. The inflammation that occurs as a result of these injuries can cause tissue damage and may even lead to permanent functional impairment and paralysis. By reducing inflammation, pregnenolone speeds recovery and helps prevent further health problems. Because so many factors are involved in recovery from a spinal-cord injury, any single therapy is usually not effective in reversing this process.

Combining pregnenolone with other therapeutic agents may lead to improved recovery from this serious health issue. This was investigated in an animal study published in 1994 in the *Proceedings of the National Academy of Sciences, USA*. In this study, investigators combined several treatments including pregnenolone; dehydroepiandrosterone (DHEA); indomethacin (IM), an anti-inflammatory compound; and bacterial lipopolysaccharide (LPS), a substance that stimulates cytokine secretion (cytokines are intercellular messengers that regulate many cell functions, especially those related to immunologic and inflammatory responses). This combination of therapies was given to animals that had undergone injury. In twenty-one days after the injury, eleven of sixteen animals were able to stand and walk, four of the animals almost normally. Of all the therapies administered, the combination of IM, LPS, and pregnenolone produced notably significant improvements. This treatment was far more effective than any of the treatments given independently or in any combination of two.

SUMMARY

Pregnenolone is a crucial sex hormone as it plays a pivotal role in the production of all the others. Recent studies indicate that an adequate supply of pregnenolone benefits memory, mood, enzyme activity, and joint function and ameliorates the effects of premenstrual syndrome and the aging process. The production of this hormone is affected by general health, stress, and disease. Pregnenolone benefits a number of peak-performance traits and has great potential as a treatment for several major health conditions, including Alzheimer's disease and multiple sclerosis.

SECTION 3:
DHEA

SUSAN FIRST BECAME aware of DHEA as a medical student nearly 30 years ago while reading her textbooks on reproductive medicine. However, it was barely mentioned since no one seemed to know what it actually did. DHEA was always described as a hormone produced abundantly by the adrenal glands, the production of which appeared to diminish significantly with age. During her early years in the medical field, Susan thought it odd that the body would produce so much of a hormone that seemed to have no purpose. As subsequent research studies on DHEA began to receive attention, both in the medical literature and in the popular press, it became apparent that this hormone actually has great importance in maintaining many aspects of health and performance. See a list of these benefits below.

Benefits of DHEA

Peak-Performance Benefits

 1 Increased physical vitality and stamina

2 Enhanced mental clarity and acuity

3 Strengthened determination and perseverance in pursuing goals (includes enhanced assertiveness, aggressive drive, and possibly libido)

5 Increased ability to remain calm under pressure

6 Increased optimism and vision

Health Benefits

- Decreases the risk of heart disease
- Strengthens the immune system
- May be useful in the treatment of autoimmune diseases such as rheumatoid arthritis, lupus, ulcerative colitis, and multiple sclerosis
- May help prevent cancer
- Reduces body fat
- Lessens symptoms of menopause and osteoporosis in women
- May be useful in the treatment of diabetes, asthma, and burns

---

DHEA is produced in abundance in the body during youth, but its production slows markedly with time. To begin to determine whether your body's supply of this hormone has lessened enough to affect your ability to perform at your best and maintain optimal health, see the following checklist. For a description of laboratory tests of DHEA, see page 628.

Checklist: Do You Produce the DHEA You Need for Peak Performance and Health?

This checklist will give you a preliminary idea of whether your production of DHEA is inadequate. Work through the following checklist (photocopy it if you don't want to write in the book) and refer to it as you read through this section of the chapter. If your responses suggest that your DHEA level is low, you can learn about ways to increase it in chapter 12.

Performance indicators

Put a check mark beside those statements that are true for you.

❏ I am often unable to recall details of recent events.

❏ I am easily upset.

❏ I am unable to handle stress.

❏ I have a negative outlook on life.

❏ I tend to tire easily; my level of stamina is low.

Physical indicators and medical history

❏ I am over the age of fifty.

❏ I lack muscle mass and strength.

❏ I have a history of cardiovascular disease.

❏ I have a weak immune system or a history of autoimmune disease.

❏ I have significant excess body fat.

❏ I experience symptoms of menopause such as hot flashes.

❏ My bones fracture easily.

THE CHEMISTRY OF DHEA

DHEA is the abbreviation for dehydroepiandrosterone, one of the primary steroid sex hormones. Until about ten years ago, scientists thought that DHEA had little use beyond its role as a precursor for other hormones. Only recently have studies begun to reveal its many physiologic activities that benefit both performance and health. DHEA is produced mainly by the adrenal glands, but some is also made in the brain and skin tissue. As discussed in the previous section, pregnenolone is converted to many other hormones via two pathways; the first stage in one of these pathways is the creation of DHEA. Curiously, not all animals make DHEA in significant amounts. It is produced in abundance by just the primates, which include humans, monkeys, apes, and gorillas.

Once DHEA is produced by the adrenals, it travels through the bloodstream to cells throughout the body. Within the glands and sex organs, it is converted to testosterone and estrogen in both men and women. However, the conversion is predominantly to testosterone in males and to estrogen in females. Some DHEA is also converted in the liver to a sulfur compound when a molecule of sulfate, which is sulfur plus oxygen, is added to it. This new substance is referred to as DHEA-S. It is thought that DHEA is predominantly produced in the morning. This form of the hormone is rapidly excreted through the kidneys. In contrast, DHEA-S is eliminated slowly, so levels remain more constant in the body. Because of the two different rates of excretion, of the total amount of this hormone in the blood, 90 percent is DHEA-S.

HOW AGING AFFECTS DHEA PRODUCTION

Of all the steroid hormones in the human body, DHEA is the most prevalent and circulates in the bloodstream in the highest concentrations. Production in males is from 1 to 2 mg per day of DHEA, and 10 to 15 mg of DHEA-S. Women produce about 10 to 20 percent less. This production declines with age. A fetus has relatively high amounts of DHEA, which functions to ease the birth process. However, by the time an infant is six months old, DHEA production all but ceases, and only revives at age six to eight in preparation for puberty. Peak DHEA production is between the ages of twenty-five and thirty; after this, production declines by as much as 10 percent per year. A person may feel the effects of this by their mid-forties. At age eighty, we make only about 15 percent of what we produced in our twenties. A study appearing in 1994 in the journal of the New York Academy of Sciences documents this. Sixty-four volunteers, between the ages of twenty and forty, had four times the levels of DHEA-S as 138 volunteers over age eighty-five. Patients with major diseases such as atherosclerosis, cancer, and Alzheimer's also have significant deficiencies.

As explained in the section on pregnenolone, when various functions such as digestion and detoxification by the liver are impaired, or if a person has elevated levels of HDL cholesterol, this can have an impact on the production of precursor hormones such as DHEA. Levels of DHEA are also sensitive to a person's general state of health.

The physical and psychological well-being enjoyed in youth may well depend in part on having sufficient levels of DHEA. For many years, little attention was given to the effect of DHEA in humans, especially in terms of aging and the decline of performance functions. Most of the research on DHEA had been done on rodents and focused on disease. Then in 1994 a study by Morales et al. investigating the effects of DHEA in older individuals was published in the *Journal of Clinical Endocrinology and Metabolism*. Volunteers in the study described a list of benefits that made DHEA seem like a fountain of youth: They reported increased energy, improved mood, better sleep quality, and a greater ability to remain calm and handle stress. Since then, DHEA has become a popular over-the-counter supplement.

DHEA AND PEAK PERFORMANCE

A wealth of research on DHEA has begun to accumulate, particularly during the past decade. These studies have examined many of the different physiological effects that DHEA produces within the body. Some researchers have even focused on the performance benefits that DHEA production supports. In future years, DHEA may come to be regarded as an essential component for continued vitality and productivity. Following are the peak-performance traits supported by DHEA.

◀1 Physical vitality and stamina

DHEA helps increase physical strength by increasing stamina and muscle power. One study, published in 1990 in the *European Journal of Applied Physiology*, found that boys with higher levels of DHEA-S experienced earlier physical development and maturity. In this study, a comparison was made between 175 boys, ten to sixteen years old, who played football competitively and a second group of 224 boys who had no regular sporting activities. One comparison was made of the boys in each group in the prepubescent age range, and no significant differences were found in their bodily measurements. However, the prepubescent boys who exercised regularly did have higher levels of DHEA. A second comparison was made of the boys in each group in the pubescent age range. The pubescent boys who played football were taller and more advanced in physical development than their nonexercising counterparts. Indicators of development were pubic hair, testicular volume, and bone age. The boys who exercised also had higher levels of DHEA, testosterone, growth hormone, and cortisol.

These results are not surprising, since DHEA is directly converted within the body into testosterone in men, and first testosterone then estrogen in women. Testosterone is the hormone that directly influences muscle mass and strength. The more testosterone an individual has, the more likely he or she is to be well muscled. Teenage boys with high levels of DHEA and testosterone are more likely to have heavier beards, deeper voices, larger muscles, and even a higher sex drive than their less androgenized peers. At the other end of the spectrum, Susan's older male patients occasionally complain about a loss of muscle mass and muscle atrophy. These men have usually related these changes in their physical structure, often occurring with a decline in libido, to the aging process. Not surprisingly, these physical changes are often seen in their sixties and seventies, when DHEA as well as testosterone production normally declines in many men.

DHEA also plays a role in reducing fatigue by improving the quality of sleep. A study published in 1995 in the *American Journal of Physiology* demonstrated that a single 500 mg oral dose of DHEA significantly increased rapid eye movement (REM) sleep in ten healthy young men. This phase of sleep, when most dreaming occurs, is essential for a person to feel rested. While this is an enormous dose of DHEA, much greater than that normally used in clinical practice, the finding in this study may have important implications in the field of sleep physiology. Obviously, much more research needs to be done in this area before DHEA can be definitively recommended as a sleep-enhancing therapy.

Beyond these specific physical effects, DHEA also promotes a general sense of well-being. This was demonstrated in the 1994 Morales study noted above. In this study, thirteen men and seventeen women, ages forty to seventy, were given 50 mg of DHEA nightly for three months. At the end of the period, 67 percent of the men and 82 percent of the women reported an increase in perceived physical well-being.

2 Mental clarity and acuity

Having a good memory is one of the most fundamental skills required in all areas of life. And there is both anecdotal and scientific evidence that DHEA enhances memory. DHEA improves the brain's ability to process and store information. In a study published in 1997 in *Biological Psychiatry*, six middle-aged and elderly volunteers were monitored for the effects of DHEA supplementation on memory. For four weeks, the volunteers were given 30 to 90 mg a day of oral DHEA so that the hormone was restored to youthful levels. The researchers noted a significant improvement in memory performance.

The mechanism by which DHEA may benefit memory is not known. However, DHEA has been added to tissue cultures of brain cells from mice, which has stimulated the growth of certain structures that allow communication between nerves. Older mice injected with DHEA completed a memory test as easily as younger mice and retained this information at a second testing. In yet another study, various individual steroid hormones were administered to mice who were given a shock-avoidance test. In this instance, DHEA was able to enhance learning in doses 10 to 100 times lower than those of other steroid hormones.

People taking DHEA find that it aids two specific types of memory: (1) incidental memory, the ability to recall details of recent events, and (2) semantic memory, the ability to retrieve more general types of stored data. These two types of memory tend to decline with age and are the first aspects of memory to deteriorate in patients with Alzheimer's disease. Various studies have been conducted to discover whether DHEA may be useful in treating Alzheimer's. Current research is focusing on the most effective dosages and on whether DHEA is best used in the early stages of the disease.

▶3 Determination and perseverance in pursuing goals

Not only does DHEA, through its conversion to testosterone, help maintain physical energy and muscle mass, it also affects behavioral traits also linked to male hormone production, such as assertiveness and the maintenance of libido. For this reason, it is important in supporting the ability to pursue goals. The case of Russell exemplifies how DHEA deficiency can affect this trait. Over the past few years, Susan has worked with a couple, Russell and Sandra. Both in their mid-sixties, they are hardworking, lively, delightful people. For the past four years they have shared both their personal lives and business careers, having started a consulting business together. Both of them are also totally dedicated to preserving their health. Two years ago, Russell began to experience symptoms that turned out to be due, in part, to a decline in his DHEA level, such as fatigue, loss of initiative, and even a reduction in his sex drive. Supplementation with DHEA restored all of these qualities. Here is his story in Sandra's words:

> Two years ago, Russ was a physically active, energetic, and enthusiastic man, the one I fell in love with. Slowly his energy level began to drop. He began to tire easily, taking long naps in the afternoon and retiring early to bed, often requiring ten or eleven hours of sleep. His gait slowed, he forced himself to do chores like mowing the lawn, and he began to drag out his other business and personal responsibilities. His energy level decreased to the point where his favorite activity became going out on his boat to relax. I complained about his lack of assertiveness, to no avail. I began to have doubts about being able to depend on him.
>
> Then he began taking DHEA, and the change was amazing. His old assertiveness returned, and once again he became actively involved in our life together. He stopped taking naps and now needs only a normal seven or eight hours of sleep, and he goes out like a light. He finally finished projects he had started months before and got reinvolved with his business.

The energy in his voice returned and, fortunately for both of us, his interest in sex has come back! He even took a trip and bought some new clothes. All of this was not possible prior to taking the DHEA.

▲▲ The field of medicine is notoriously poor at restoring functional qualities such as physical energy, vitality, and stamina in individuals who may be losing these capabilities. Supplementation with DHEA should be considered for individuals who are losing these attributes. While Susan recommends seeing a physician before starting DHEA supplementation, this is not always possible, as many areas lack physicians who have any experience using the newer hormone therapies like DHEA. As a result, millions of units are currently being sold on a self-medication basis. If you elect to use DHEA without a physician's guidance, buy the lowest-dose products available in your health food store or pharmacy, begin to use it cautiously, and do not go above 25 mg on your own. Let your physician recommend dosages at higher levels, and be sure to carefully monitor the effects on your body.

Susan has found DHEA to be useful not only for men with loss of libido but also for women patients. Linda, a forty-eight-year-old office manager, consulted Susan for treatment of her premenopausal symptoms. As her periods began to be lighter and more irregular, she also found that her sex drive began to diminish. After using DHEA, her interest in sex returned, and she became a more enthusiastic participant in sexual activity with her husband. However, not all women are good candidates for DHEA therapy. Some of Susan's female patients have found that DHEA causes anxiety, nervousness, and other side effects. Women should approach DHEA therapy cautiously and begin supplementing at low-dosage levels.

5 The ability to remain calm under pressure

Animal studies suggest that DHEA may have a modulating effect on stress hormones, thereby lessening the impact of stress on the body. As discussed in the chapters on stress management, the stress response involves an increase in the production of stress hormones, or corticos-teroids. DHEA can lessen the strength of this stress response so that cor-ticosteroid levels do not increase as dramatically. This was found in a study on mice, published in 1994 in *Pharmacology, Biochemistry and Behavior*. The researchers concluded that DHEA has anxiety-reducing properties.

However, it appears that stress itself can lower levels of DHEA. This has been shown in several studies. In one notable study, appearing in 1994 in the *European Journal of Endocrinology*, a group of eighteen Norwegian cadets were give a five-day military training course. They participated in continuous heavy physical activities and had almost no food or sleep. DHEA-S blood levels were measured for ten of the cadets at the start of the test and at completion. During the five days, the normal hourly changes in DHEA output were diminished, and while DHEA levels did increase with continued stress, once the training was over, DHEA-S lev-els remained low during the recovery period. According to another study, appearing in 1992 in *Experimental and Clinical Endocrinology*, levels of DHEA in patients undergoing thyroid surgery continued to decline dur-ing the two days following the operation.

This decline in DHEA levels can lead to a situation in which stress hormones dominate. Older persons are more likely to experience this oversensitivity to stress hormones, as they are in a period of their lives where DHEA levels naturally decline. In a study appearing in 1996 in the *Journal of Clinical Endocrinology and Metabolism*, researchers measured DHEA and cortisol levels in sixty-two volunteers, aged three to eighty-five, and found that the ratio of cortisol to DHEA in the brain increased with age. High levels of cortisol are known to cause brain damage in ani-mals. This imbalance of cortisol to DHEA may permit normal levels of cortisol to become toxic.

6 Optimism and vision

Many individuals and studies report that DHEA has the ability to enhance psychological well-being, a state of mind in which all seems right with the world. A small but significant study cited in an article appearing in 1995 in the *Lancet* found that when volunteers were given 50 mg per day of DHEA, 70 percent of them reported an increase in feelings of well-being. At the same time, DHEA helps alleviate depression. A study appearing in 1997 in *Biological Psychiatry* observed the effects of DHEA on six older patients. The dosage was 30 to 60 mg a day of oral DHEA, given for four weeks. Ratings for depression significantly declined, but when treatment stopped, measurements of mood returned to pretreatment levels.

Having a sense of well-being predisposes a person to having an optimistic approach to life and encourages visionary thinking. Because DHEA fosters this general state of mind, having higher levels of DHEA may allow an individual to live a fuller life. This is indicated by a 1993 study published in the *Journal of Clinical Epidemiology*. In this study volunteers, aged seventy to seventy-nine, were assembled into three groups representing various levels of functioning. There were 1192 persons in the highest-functioning group, 80 in the medium-functioning group, and 82 in the low-functioning group. Values of DHEA-S increased with functional levels, from a value of forty-eight in the low group to sixty-nine in the top group. Persons in the highest-functioning group felt more effective, had a greater sense of mastery, and were more satisfied with life. Furthermore, these individuals also engaged in more productive activities, exercised more, and engaged more frequently in volunteer activities.

Russell, who was described on page 562, found that DHEA had a dramatic effect on his mood and outlook on life. As Sandra again explains:

> At the same time as Russell's physical energy began to diminish, his mood began to change. He had always been a bright, happy, flexible, and enthusiastic man. However, he began to become depressed easily, fighting with his mind not to. His thinking, which had always been sharp, began to be muddled. However, when he began taking the DHEA, all of these problems resolved. He is no longer depressed but actively involved in his personal and business affairs, and he is once again planning trips and events. His wonderful sense of humor has resurfaced, and it is fun to be with him again. His clarity and sharpness of thought have returned. I now feel he can be depended on, and I have all the confidence in him that I had when I first met him. It has been a joy to rediscover him all over again.

DHEA AND HEALTH

Maintaining DHEA at youthful levels can lower the risk of developing various health problems as a person ages. A review article on DHEA, appearing in 1996 in the *Journal of Clinical Endocrinology and Metabolism*, described a range of animal and human studies indicating that having an adequate level of DHEA may help prevent and heal various diseases. These include cardiovascular disease, autoimmune disease, cancer, diabetes, and degenerative diseases of the nervous system.

Cardiovascular disease

Heart disease is currently the leading cause of death among Americans. In younger women, coronary-heart disease (CHD) is rare, but by the time a woman reaches age sixty-five, her probability of having the disease is equal to that of a man.

Adequate levels of DHEA appear to be protective. The majority of research studies on this topic support the conclusion that maintaining adequate levels of DHEA can help prevent heart disease. A 1986 study reported in the *New England Journal of Medicine* studied 242 men, aged fifty to seventy-nine. Increases of DHEA-S levels by 100 μg per deciliter of blood were associated with a 48 percent reduction in death from cardiovascular disease. While another study contradicted this result, there is still considerable evidence that having higher levels of DHEA protects against heart disease, especially in men.

Conversely, depressed levels of DHEA can be a risk factor for heart disease. An article appearing in 1995 in the *Journal of Internal Medicine* referred to a study conducted in Poland in which women with CHD had significantly lower levels of DHEA-S than women with no heart disease. In another study, published in 1994 in *Circulation*, DHEA-S blood levels were measured in forty-nine men who had survived premature heart attacks and compared with an equal number of men who had not suffered heart attacks. DHEA-S levels were significantly depressed in the cardiac patients.

Many theories of how DHEA protects against heart disease are now being investigated. Both laboratory and human studies have indicated that DHEA helps prevent blood clots that can block an artery and trigger a heart attack or stroke. DHEA is known to reduce plaque on the walls of arteries, which can also limit blood flow. In an animal study published in 1988 in the *Journal of Clinical Investigation*, rabbits with severe atherosclerosis were treated with DHEA, and plaque size was reduced by almost 50 percent. It has also been observed that women taking DHEA experience a decline in cholesterol levels. DHEA may produce this effect by facilitating the breakdown of cholesterol in the liver.

In a healthy person, DHEA is able to counteract these risk factors for heart disease. But various conditions, such as stress, can lower DHEA levels and increase the probability of cardiac problems. A study appearing in 1992 in the *Journal of Psychosomatic Research* found that army officers who participated in a stress reduction program had a small increase in their DHEA-S levels, while those officers not participating had a marked reduction in DHEA.

High levels of the hormone insulin, which manages the metabolism and storage of sugars and starches, can also reduce DHEA levels. To maintain cardiovascular health, there needs to be a balance between these two powerful hormones. During the early stages of diabetes, insulin levels rise and DHEA activity is blocked. This was observed in a study published in 1992 in the *FASEB Journal*. The researchers observed that insulin lowers blood concentrations of DHEA and DHEA-S by decreasing production of these hormones and by increasing their breakdown and excretion. They suggested that the well-known association between high levels of insulin in the blood (hyperinsulemia) and heart disease may be through insulin's effect on DHEA. Gaining a great deal of weight, as well as normal aging, is also associated with increased insulin levels. In this way, both obesity and aging can also lower DHEA.

Weakened immune function

DHEA strengthens immune-system function, which can ward off a cold and help prevent diseases that can be life-threatening. A variety of laboratory studies, both animal and human, give evidence of DHEA's role in immunity. One such study, appearing in 1994 in the *Journal of Steroid Biochemistry and Molecular Biology*, analyzed the amount of DHEA by-products present in various tissues in mice. The results suggested that in tissues involved in the immune response, locally produced DHEA metabolites, or breakdown products, may participate in the regulation of the immune response.

Health care practitioners working with DHEA find that patients with adequate levels tend not to have colds or the flu. But there is also indication that DHEA may be a potent tool for combating diseases directly involved with the immune system itself. These include autoimmune diseases such as rheumatoid arthritis, lupus, multiple sclerosis, and ulcerative colitis. There is also evidence that DHEA can be of benefit in the treatment of AIDS (which is caused by human immunodeficiency virus).

A study published in 1992 in the *Journal of Infectious Diseases* measured levels of DHEA in forty-one men who were asymptomatic HIV-seropositive who subsequently progressed to AIDS. They also monitored DHEA in forty-one similar men who did not develop AIDS, and in an equal number of men who were HIV-1-seronegative. The researchers found that among the men who developed AIDS, DHEA levels were lower than in the other two groups five months before progression to AIDS.

How DHEA levels impact immunity involves changes that occur in the immune system with age. In the immune system, the fighter T cells identify and disarm invading substances that find their way into the body. One type of T cell is the suppressor cell, which detects which substances are foreign versus which ones are a natural part of body tissues. With age, suppressor cells perform these functions less efficiently. DHEA may help prevent this decline and even reverse it.

Another component of the immune system is cytokines. These are hormonelike substances, produced by immune cells, that determine how our cells respond. Cytokines can either trigger a reaction or inhibit one, and either promote or limit growth. They are the communication system between immune-system cells. With age, however, they begin to send the wrong messages. It appears that DHEA may restore their proper function.

Lastly, DHEA suppresses the stress response, which can weaken the immune system and cause a person to be vulnerable to disease. Low levels of stress hormones are associated with higher levels of DHEA.

Cancer

Research has shown that individuals who develop certain kinds of cancer have low levels of DHEA. A retrospective study, published in 1991 in

Cancer Research, compared thirty-five individuals who developed bladder cancer with sixty-nine others who remained cancer-free. The cancer patients had significantly lower levels of DHEA and DHEA-S. Another study, of thirty-seven male lung cancer patients at the Gujarat Cancer and Research Institute, in Ahmedabad, India, found that these patients also had lower levels of DHEA-S, as compared with the control group; the research was published in 1994 in *Neoplasma*. It is also known that levels of DHEA are significantly lower in patients with prostate cancer. This is particularly significant because prostate cancer accounts for 47 percent of all cancers in men, according to a 1995 report from the American Cancer Society. DHEA levels are also low in women with breast cancer.

Various laboratory and animal studies suggest that DHEA protects against a wide range of carcinogens and may inhibit the growth of tumors. Whether the initiating carcinogenic substance is cigarette smoke, heavy metals such as lead and cadmium, or radiation, DHEA may be able to block its activation. One theory is that DHEA blocks an enzyme required for certain cancer-promoting chemical reactions to occur. DHEA may also prevent the formation of free radicals, which are unstable atoms that easily bond to other atoms. Free radicals can damage cells and cause them to mutate, resulting in cancerous growth.

Excess weight

As people age, their weight can slowly increase to a condition of obesity. As the excess pounds and fat accumulate, self-esteem can plummet, and health problems such as heart disease and diabetes are more likely to occur. It appears that levels of DHEA influence the changes in weight and body composition that occur over time.

There is conflicting evidence about whether DHEA promotes weight loss, but certain animal studies indicate this is possible. In one such study, published in the *International Journal of Obesity*, nineteen dogs were given increasing doses of DHEA daily. Over the six months of the study, 68 percent of these animals lost an average of 3 percent of their total body weight each month, without any reduction in food intake. This suggests that DHEA may affect metabolism, the process by which food is turned into energy, causing more calories to be used.

There is even clearer evidence that DHEA causes fat to be replaced with muscle. One such study, published in 1988 in the *Journal of Clinical*

Endocrinology and Metabolism, monitored ten men for body fat. The men, in their early twenties and matched for weight, were divided into two groups. One group was treated with DHEA, a 400 mg dosage four times a day for twenty-eight days, and the other group was left untreated. The men reported no changes in their regular activities or diet. At the end of the treatment period, it was found that among the five men receiving DHEA, their average percentage of body fat dropped 31 percent. However, there was no drop in weight, suggesting that while there was a decline in fat, muscle mass increased. No change in these measurements occurred in the untreated men.

Some researchers suggest that DHEA may decrease body fat by blocking the synthesis of fatty acids, which eventually become body fat. Others have noted that DHEA can act as an appetite suppressant and dampen the desire for fatty foods. As the DHEA story unfolds, dieters may someday find that DHEA can help them toward the goal of having a fitter, healthier, slimmer body.

Menopausal symptoms and osteoporosis in women

As estrogen production declines in menopause, many women experience a variety of symptoms due to this deficiency. Supplementing with DHEA can help remedy these complaints. Once it is absorbed, DHEA is converted to estrone, a form of estrogen, so DHEA supplementation becomes a natural form of estrogen therapy. Women in menopause may experience a thinning of the vaginal tissue and a decline in vaginal secretions. And at this time in life, a woman's skin becomes drier. DHEA has been found to revive vaginal tissues; it also activates oil glands in the skin, restoring a youthful texture to the hands and face. Another possible consequence of menopause and low levels of estrogen is thinning bone. Animal studies have shown that DHEA increases bone mineral density. More relevant human studies need to be done before DHEA can be recommended as a routine part of osteoporosis therapy.

Diabetes

Blood sugar (glucose) is a source of energy used throughout the body. Normally, the pancreas produces a sufficient amount of insulin, the hormone that manages levels of glucose in the blood and enables the storage of glucose in the cells. The balance between insulin activity and cell uptake determines blood sugar levels. As a person ages, the cells become less responsive to insulin and do not store glucose as readily, a condition called insulin resistance. However, studies have shown that DHEA causes tissues to be more insulin sensitive. In this way, DHEA may one day become a useful treatment for diabetes (a disease characterized by high levels of insulin and glucose circulating in the blood, coupled with insulin resistance of the cells). In addition, as insulin levels increase, the amount of DHEA-S decreases, according to a study published in 1994 in the *Journal of Clinical Endocrinology*. This was observed in nondiabetic men who were treated with a medication that lowers circulating insulin.

Asthma

The use of DHEA for treating asthma is now being explored. Studies have found that persons with asthma have lower levels of DHEA. Various medications are used to treat the tightening and spasming of the lung tubes (bronchi). It has been noted that when a medication such as prednasone (a potent anti-inflammatory agent) is given to asthma patients, DHEA-S levels rise.

Burns

Animal studies indicate that DHEA has been found to help in the healing of burns. Giving DHEA to burn patients may be useful in stopping the progressive destruction of tissue that can occur when blood is unable to reach the damaged area.

SUMMARY

DHEA is the most prevalent steroid hormone in the human body, but its levels decline as the body ages. The physical and psychological well-being enjoyed in youth may well depend in part on having sufficient levels of DHEA. Studies of DHEA supplementation in older individuals have reported increased energy, improved mood, better sleep quality, and a greater ability to remain calm under pressure. Other studies indicate that DHEA may help prevent and heal such conditions as cancer, autoimmune disease, and cardiovascular disease.

Section 4:
Testosterone

THE ABILITY TO be a peak performer is closely associated with testosterone production. As the primary male sex hormone, testosterone is the physiological source of the drive and assertiveness associated with many successful males; however, it benefits peak performance and health in both men and women. See a list of these benefits, below.

Benefits of Testosterone

Peak-Performance Benefits for Men

 Increased physical vitality and stamina (helps build muscle mass and restore muscle strength and tone, enhancing athletic performance)

2 Enhanced mental clarity and acuity

3 Strengthened determination and perseverance in pursuing goals (includes enhanced assertiveness, aggressive drive, and libido)

4 Increased ability to get along with other people (balances mood)

6 Increased optimism and vision

Health Benefits for Men

• Protects against heart disease

• Helps prevent osteoporosis

Peak-Performance Benefits for Women

 Increased physical vitality and stamina (restores energy)

3 Strengthened determination and perseverance in pursuing goals (includes enhanced assertiveness and libido)

 Increased ability to get along with other people (balances mood)

Health Benefits for Women

• Relieves menopausal symptoms such as hot flashes, nervousness, and vaginal dryness

• Helps prevent osteoporosis

In this section, we explain how testosterone functions in men and women and discuss the many ways this important sex hormone influences energy, mental agility, mood, outlook on life, and sex drive. To begin to evaluate your own production of testosterone, see the following checklist. For a description of laboratory testing of testosterone levels, see page 629.

CHECKLIST: DO YOU PRODUCE THE TESTOSTERONE YOU NEED FOR PEAK PERFORMANCE AND HEALTH?

This checklist will give you a preliminary idea of whether you are experiencing the effects of inadequate testosterone production. Work through the following checklist (photocopy it if you don't want to write in the book), and refer to it as you read through this section of the chapter. If your responses suggest that your testosterone level is low, you can learn about a variety of ways to increase it in chapter 12.

Performance indicators

Put a check mark beside those statements that are true for you.

❏ I suffer from persistent fatigue.

❏ I lack stamina.

❏ I have experienced a decline in my level of assertiveness.

❏ I typically have little desire to take risks.

❏ I have less interest than I used to in launching new projects and attempting new activities.

❏ I am a man, and I have difficulty thinking in visual/spatial terms.

❏ I have a tendency toward depression.

❏ I often feel withdrawn.

Physical/emotional indicators and medical history

❏ I am a man, and I have poorly developed secondary sexual characteristics (such as facial hair and a low-pitched voice).

❏ I am over the age of fifty.

❑ I have poor muscle tone or weak muscles.

❑ I lack interest in sex.

❑ I have experienced a decline in the frequency of my sexual activity and orgasms.

❑ I am a man, and I am at high risk for heart disease.

❑ I have osteoporosis and suffer from frequent bone fractures.

❑ I experience menopausal symptoms such as hot flashes, mood swings, and vaginal dryness.

THE CHEMISTRY OF TESTOSTERONE

Testosterone is the predominant male sex hormone, or androgen, a substance that stimulates the development of male sexual characteristics. All androgens, including testosterone, are steroid compounds and share a similar structure. They can all be synthesized from cholesterol or made directly from acetyl Coenzyme A, a chemical produced in the liver and made from fatty acids and amino acids.

In men, testosterone is essential for normal sexual behavior; it also promotes the development of secondary sexual characteristics such as facial hair and the lower pitch of the male voice. But beyond its impact on sexuality and appearance, testosterone influences many metabolic activities that affect such fundamental performance factors as energy level and cognitive thinking. Women, who produce testosterone at much lower levels than men, also experience some of its performance benefits.

The use of testosterone as a male tonic has a long history. Traditional healers have used the sexual organs and glands of male animals to restore potency in men. These medicines probably contained small quantities of animal testosterone. The search for a male elixir continued into modern times. In France, in the late nineteenth century, physiologist Charles-Edouard Brown-Sequard injected himself with fluid extracted from animal testicles and pronounced the substance rejuvenating. The use of such substances to treat male impotence became a fad in the first decades of this century; however, it is questionable whether these contained active ingredients or only had a placebo effect. Then in 1934, scientists synthesized testosterone from cholesterol, preparing the way for the development of present-day testosterone replacement therapy.

The production of testosterone in men

The production of testosterone follows the hormone pathway outlined in the beginning of this chapter. Pregnenolone, the mother hormone, is converted to DHEA and progesterone, which combine to form a new substance, androstenedione, which is then converted to testosterone.

In men, testosterone is predominantly produced in the testes, the reproductive glands located in the scrotum, or pouch, that lies outside the male body in the groin area. The testes contain about 250 compartments, and within each of these are from one to four canals, or tubules. These tubules are surrounded by a web of loose connective tissue, nerves, and lymphatic and blood vessels, plus specialized cells called Leydig cells. It is these cells that produce and secrete testosterone. Leydig cells are plentiful and active in a newborn male infant but quickly decline in number and are virtually nonexistent during childhood. Then in adulthood, after puberty, these cells again become numerous, making up about 20 percent of the mass of the adult testes.

Small amounts of testosterone are also made in the adrenal glands, in the adrenal cortex. After testosterone is secreted from the glands, it circulates in the blood for fifteen to thirty minutes. It then either binds with target cells or is rapidly converted by the liver into breakdown products that can be readily excreted.

The availability of testosterone in men

The quantity of testosterone a male produces varies during different phases of life. A small quantity is produced by the male fetus beginning at about the second month of embryonic life, and production continues for a short time after birth. However, there is virtually no testosterone production during childhood until puberty, at about age ten to thirteen, when there is a rapid increase in testosterone production. In young men, total blood level of testosterone is normally 300 to 350 ng/dl.

By the time a man reaches age forty, testosterone production begins to gradually decline. At the same time, there is also a reduction in the number of Leydig cells, which are responsible for producing testosterone. The brain regulates testosterone secretion through the pituitary gland. The pituitary releases luteinizing hormone (LH), which then triggers the testes to secrete testosterone. With age, the testes become less sensitive to this stimulation.

The availability of testosterone also changes with age. Normally, there is only a small amount of testosterone that is actually free or unbound, about 4 percent of the total amount of testosterone produced by the testes and adrenals. However, as a man ages, the amount of free testosterone decreases, leaving less testosterone available for binding in the tissues to produce its masculinizing effects on the body.

A significant number of men over the age of sixty have an average blood level of total testosterone near the lower end of the normal range for an adult male. As production decreases, physiological changes also occur, but because the male transition is subtle—unlike the sudden drop in hormones women experience in menopause—these changes are often blamed on old age. By age eighty, a man may produce only one-fifth of the testosterone he had in his youth.

How testosterone affects the male body

Testosterone is carried by the blood to various target tissues throughout the body. When it reaches these tissues, it binds to special receptors and triggers various metabolic processes.

The primary function of testosterone is to control the characteristics that distinguish the male body. Even before a child is born, testosterone stimulates the development of male sexual characteristics. All fetuses are initially female, and it is not until the testes in the fetus produce testosterone that the male sexual apparatus develops. This includes the scrotum, penis, testes, prostate gland, and seminal vesicles, saclike structures that lie behind the bladder close to the prostate. The seminal vesicles secrete a thick alkaline fluid that comprises part of the semen.

In a young man, from puberty to about age twenty, testosterone causes the enlargement of the scrotum, testes, and penis, and there is also an increase in libido, the interest in and desire for sexual activity. During puberty, testosterone also stimulates the development of secondary male sexual characteristics. Hair begins to grow on the face, chest, and in the area of the genitals. (Testosterone also eventually decreases hair growth on the top of the head.) The larynx, the organ of the voice, at first enlarges, causing the voice to crack, then gradually causing it to deepen. The skin thickens and becomes more rugged, and typically young men begin to develop greater muscular mass. Testosterone increases the bone matrix, helping to retain calcium and increase bone mass. It is responsible for rapid bone growth in children, which consequently stimulates total body growth as well. Testosterone is also thought to be responsible for the greater number of red blood cells in men as compared with women. Testosterone causes these changes through its anabolic function, increasing the rate of protein formation in cells and the growth of tissue.

The production of testosterone in women

Women also make small amounts of testosterone in the ovaries and adrenal glands. As in men, the precursor to testosterone is androstenedione. Like estrogen and progesterone, the level of androstenedione varies throughout a woman's menstrual cycle. The level rises at midcycle, when androstenedione is secreted from the ovarian follicle (a structure in the ovary containing a female reproductive cell), and during the second half of the menstrual cycle, when it is produced by the corpus luteum (a structure that develops within the ruptured ovarian follicle after ovulation or the release of the egg from the ovary and that secretes progesterone and estrogen).

The availability of testosterone in women

A woman normally produces about 0.3 mg of testosterone per day. Total production is about one-tenth the amount produced by men. Production peaks around age twenty, and by the time a woman reaches age forty, it will have declined by about half. After menopause, testosterone production in women is minimal. Most circulating testosterone is bound to sex hormone–binding globulin (SHBG), with only a small percentage that is biologically active. Because estrogen increases the concentration of SHBG, natural fluctuations in estrogen levels, as well as estrogen replacement therapy, can further diminish available testosterone.

How testosterone affects the female body

As in men, testosterone in women plays an important role in normal female sexual development. The initiation of menstruation and puberty is, in part, triggered by testosterone production. As with men, testosterone stimulates libido in women. Levels of the hormone rise and decline during the menstrual cycle to insure that sexual desire increases just before ovulation, when a woman is fertile and chances are greatest for conception. Testosterone also impacts female performance. It restores vitality and energy levels, helps reduce depression, and, in part, engenders in women the attributes of assertiveness and aggressiveness usually associated with male behavior. Testosterone also benefits female health by helping to strengthen bones and minimize the symptoms of menopause.

HOW DIET, LIFESTYLE, AND HEALTH AFFECT TESTOSTERONE LEVELS

As we have just discussed, the aging process affects testosterone levels in both men and women, but testosterone levels are also sensitive to various environmental factors such as diet, alcohol use, lifestyle habits such as smoking, stress levels, and a person's general state of health. Poor lifestyle habits can negatively impact testosterone production as well as sperm count.

Eating a typical American high-fat diet can alter testosterone levels. This correlation was demonstrated in a study published in 1991 in *Modern Medicine*. Eight healthy men, ages twenty-three to thirty-five, were given a daily milk shake containing 800 calories, 57 percent of which was fat. The researchers found that following the high-fat meal, blood levels of testosterone dropped by about 30 percent. How much caffeine and alcohol a person consumes will also affect testosterone levels. The effect of caffeine on testosterone levels in women was investigated in a large study published in 1996 in the *American Journal of Epidemiology*. Women who had more than two cups of coffee or four cans of caffeinated soda per day experienced a decline in testosterone levels.

A noted decline in sperm count among men, thought to be related to hormonelike toxins, may also be linked to smoking. Researchers examined sperm density, motility, and morphologic abnormalities in smokers versus nonsmokers and published the results in 1985 in *Fertility and Sterility*. The volunteers consisted of 253 men, aged nineteen to thirty-two, 103 of whom were smokers. Analysis of sperm indicated that twice as many smokers as nonsmokers had a sperm count in the lower limit of normal, as well as lower motility. Stress is also associated with diminished hormone levels, as evidenced in a study appearing in 1995 in the *Journal of*

Internal Medicine. The study examined 439 men, all aged fifty-one, and found that chronic psychosocial stresses such as tense, difficult working conditions, painful thoughts, and sad feelings were associated with a low testosterone level. The researchers suggested that chronic stress contributed to premature aging.

Having a low level of HDL cholesterol, which performs the function of transporting hormones, can impair the body's ability to produce testosterone. Poor digestive function can also be a limiting factor. The ability of the body to absorb certain substances such as fat molecules and fragments of protein from which hormones are manufactured affects the quantity of testosterone that the body can produce. How well the liver is able to break down toxins and metabolize hormones will also impact testosterone levels.

TESTOSTERONE AND PEAK PERFORMANCE IN MEN

Having the stamina, desire, and drive needed to aim for the top depends in part on adequate production of sex hormones. Testosterone has been found to enhance problem-solving abilities that require the use of visual/spatial perception, and it also helps to maintain the upbeat and positive mood that is needed for launching projects and sustaining effort. While research into the relationship of testosterone to performance issues lags behind the study of estrogen, there is growing evidence to support its importance for peak performance for both men and women.

Physical vitality and stamina

Although there is a lack of studies specifically addressing the relationship between testosterone and physical stamina, men who use testosterone therapy for a variety of reasons often report that they have more vitality and an improved sense of well-being. Because testosterone plays an important role in promoting muscle development and physical strength, having sufficient levels of testosterone initiates an upward cycle of increasing energy and strength, as it promotes exercise, which in itself is vitalizing.

Testosterone's effect on muscle strength is well documented by the scientific literature. In one notable and highly controlled study, testosterone had the effect of increasing muscle size among participants who exercised and even among those who did not. As reported in 1996 in the *New England Journal of Medicine*, forty-three normal men were divided into two groups, one of which exercised and the other of which did not. Some of the men in each group were given high doses of a form of testosterone, 600 mg of testosterone enanthate, weekly for ten weeks; the others were given a placebo. Those volunteers who exercised participated in standard weight-lifting exercises three times a week. Researchers measured the size of the triceps and quadricep muscles, increase in fat-free mass, and strength assessed by bench-press and squatting exercises. They found that the men taking testosterone who did exercise had significantly higher scores in all categories than those men taking the placebo. However, the researchers also observed that those men not exercising but receiving testosterone also had markedly higher scores.

This study is not meant to be an argument for avoiding exercise, but it does demonstrate the powerful effect that testosterone can have on physical performance. Neither is it an endorsement for using large doses of testosterone to build strength and enhance performance. It is well known that anabolic steroids, such as testosterone, are sometimes abused by athletes trying to push themselves beyond their normal level of achievement. Many athletic competitions prohibit the use of steroids and screen participants for their use. Furthermore, the liberal use of testosterone has several unwanted side effects, such as extremely aggressive behavior and significant deterioration of liver function. However, the ability of testosterone to increase muscle size can be of great use to individuals who are at risk of muscle atrophy because of disabilities that prevent them from exercising, and for older people who have lost muscle mass through the normal aging process.

Maintenance of muscle strength is particularly crucial for the elderly. Loss of muscle can contribute to frailty and lead to impaired balance, loss of gait, and immobility. A study published in 1993 in the *Journal of the American Geriatric Society* assessed the effect of testosterone treatment in eight men with an average age of seventy-eight. They were given testosterone therapy of 200 mg/ml every two weeks for three months. Six men with abnormally low testosterone levels did not receive treatment. Those volunteers receiving testosterone demonstrated increased handgrip strength after treatment. The researchers also monitored hematocrit, the measurement of the concentration of red blood cells in the blood. Testosterone is known to increase the concentration of these cells, and this was observed in this study. This can affect physical energy since these cells transport oxygen throughout the body, which is essential for energy production and optimal muscle function.

▲▲ Testosterone therapy may be of great benefit to the man who has long anticipated a physically active retirement but finds himself not as strong as he would like to be due, in part, to diminished levels of testosterone. A man who has his career behind him and with time to spare may want to finally tackle projects around the house or become much more active in his favorite sport or hobby. Restoring testosterone to youthful levels may help make these plans a reality.

Testosterone therapy has traditionally been given to men in pill form; however, new technologies such as the testosterone patch allow testosterone to be absorbed directly into the body through the skin. Methods to improve testosterone absorption by the body are currently being researched. If you are interested in using testosterone replacement therapy, it is important to consult a physician with the most up-to-date technologies.

2 Mental clarity and acuity

Testosterone is associated with a specific aspect of cognitive function, the ability to conceptualize in visual/spatial terms. This is the type of thinking involved in map reading, throwing a basketball through a hoop, and being able to picture an object rotated a quarter turn. These are the skills required in engineering, architecture, many sports, and arts such as sculpture and dance. Though some women are skilled at this kind of thinking, men in particular, who produce far more testosterone than do women, excel at visual/spatial conceptualizing. Moreover, this conceptual ability is not the result of learning because this gender difference is observed even in infancy.

Many scientific studies, from the 1970s to the present, have confirmed gender differences in mental acuity, and many have examined the role that hormones play. A study published in 1991 in *Psychoneuroendocrinology* specifically looked at the relationship of visual/spatial skills and testosterone, which is known to be present in brain tissue. Researchers worked with eighty-eight men and women volunteers with an average age of twenty-one. They were individually given several tests to assess cognitive ability. The researchers then sampled the volunteers' saliva to determine testosterone concentration. The male volunteers, with naturally higher testosterone levels than women, had significantly better scores on tests involving mental rotations and paper folding than did the females in the study.

This association of testosterone and visual/spatial acuity holds the promise that one day a therapy will be found to help older persons who have lost their sense of balance. The coordination of physical and visual skills and the ability to think in three dimensions are very much involved in the ability to stand upright. Navigating through your own furniture-filled house or going shopping in a crowded store requires a good sense of balance. A person who cannot visually assess distances and the sizes of objects has a higher risk of falling and seriously injuring themselves.

Testosterone may also help prevent senility. Animal studies suggest that testosterone improves the ability to learn and retain new information. Recently, scientists have begun to gather evidence that testosterone may be useful in preventing Alzheimer's disease.

Testosterone therapy may potentially add years of productive activity to an older person's life. Having sufficient levels of testosterone may make it easier to continue hobbies, care for the home, and manage personal needs such as dressing and bathing.

3 Determination and perseverance in pursuing goals

The masculine aggressiveness that often takes men to the top of the corporate ladder and is necessary for success in contact sports has a basis in hormones, testosterone in particular. The drive for sexual conquest also depends on testosterone, as does libido.

In a study appearing in 1992 in the *Journal of Clinical Endocrinology and Metabolism*, thirteen men received testosterone injections of 100 mg/ml or a placebo weekly for two sequential three-month periods. While the purpose of the study was to monitor various physiological changes such as alterations in body fat, at the end of the study the researchers also asked the men if they had known when they were receiving hormone treatment. Twelve of the thirteen volunteers were able to identify the periods in which they were given testosterone and gave reasons that ranged from an increase in libido and a greater sense of well-being to a notable increase in assertiveness in business transactions.

In men with low testosterone production, testosterone supplementation has been used successfully to increase libido and sexual activity. In a study appearing in 1979 in the *Journal of Clinical Endocrinology and Metabolism*, six volunteers, married men between the ages of thirty-two and sixty-five, were given different doses of testosterone, which varied between 100 mg and 400 mg, administered by injection, every four weeks for approximately five months. The volunteers kept records of their sexual activity. The researchers found a significant dose-related correlation between frequency of erections and testosterone treatment, with the higher dosage having a greater impact, and concluded that the testosterone therapy had a stimulating effect on sexual activity that was rapid and reliable.

However, it is important to note that testosterone is not effective in treating impotence caused by certain physiological factors. Being able to have an erection requires healthy nerve function and blood circulation. The penis must be able to receive neural stimulation and blood flow. For example, men with diabetes who have impaired neural function, or men with generalized hardening of the arteries, which can impede blood circulation, may be impotent due to a mechanical dysfunction, not reduced testosterone.

As stated earlier, a natural decline in male testosterone begins to occur at midlife. At this time, there is also a parallel reduction in libido and sexual function. One study, appearing in 1983 in the *Journal of Clinical Endocrinology and Metabolism*, studied this relationship in 220 men, aged forty-one to ninety-three. Researchers monitored number of orgasms and morning erections as well as sexual thoughts, fantasies, and the enjoyment of sex. They found that, with age, there was a decline in all these measurements of sexuality.

Along with a decline in libido, some men tend to experience a general decline in drive, usually beginning in their fifties or sixties, both in the workplace and in private life. A man may no longer be interested in getting his supervisor's job, the thought of starting a new business may no longer appeal to him as it once did, and taking risks of all kinds may no longer seem fun. Less demanding goals, such as improving one's golf game, take the place of daredevil activities. A man accustomed to dating numerous partners may begin to wonder what drove him to do this when he was younger and regret that he never settled down with one of them. While this may be due, in part, to changes in a man's goals and values with age, it is also partly due to changes taking place within the body. As hormone production begins to decline, the chemical support for a man's physical energy, drive, and perseverance also begins to diminish. Male midlife and older patients have expressed this to Susan, saying they are slowing down and don't have quite the same drive and vigor that they had in earlier years.

Of course, there are exceptions. There are men in their eighties and nineties who have fathered children. The media regularly features well-known personalities who have continued living highly active and creative lives well into their later years. These men are able to maintain a greater involvement in life than many men much younger.

4 The ability to get along with other people

Although we tend to think of our relationships as strictly being determined by our emotional programming and belief systems, these are not the only determinants. The production of important sex hormones, like testosterone, can also strongly affect the ways in which we interact with other people. Men who suffer from extremes of emotion—either depression, anger, or extreme upset—due to a deficiency of testosterone, are less likely to enjoy positive and healthy social and business relationships. In contrast, the beneficial effect that testosterone has on mood is more likely to enable a person to be outgoing and extroverted.

While the relationship between male sex hormones such as testosterone and mood is unclear, there are several animal and human studies that indicate that testosterone does play a role in our moods and emotions. In one study, published in 1992 in the *Journal of Andrology*, six men with very low testosterone production (hypogonadal) were significantly more depressed and also felt more anger as compared with fourteen healthy, normal male volunteers. In another study, reported in 1985 in *Clinical Endocrinology*, treatment with testosterone improved mood. Eight men with low testosterone levels were given increasingly greater dosages of testosterone for one month each. Throughout the study, the men made daily records of their mood state. The researchers observed a dose-related response in improvement of mood and sense of well-being.

This same association is often noted in studies focusing on other benefits of testosterone. In a study on impotence published in 1991 in *Urology*, four men with low testosterone output were given transdermal testosterone patches, which they wore for twenty-two hours each day for four weeks. The patches supplied a dosage of either 2.4 or 3.4 mg of testosterone. The patches restored the men's ability to have erections and also seemed to have a positive effect on their mood. The researchers did not specify whether the improvement in mood was directly the result of the hormone supplementation or the consequence of restored sexual activity. However, a decline in sex drive is very troubling to most men and can easily lead to emotional withdrawal and depression.

◀ 6 Optimism and vision

There are certain men who are naturally ebullient, not prone to depression and low moods. Often they are creative types, such as painters, performers, and movie directors, with a robust libido. This sort of man lives life to the fullest, even into his eighties. We associate such vitality and male passion with having an abundance of male sex hormones—specifically, testosterone. Continued production of testosterone in significant amounts can allow people to go forward in life. They are able to take a step away from self-absorption, which can plague many people as they age, and move toward greater participation. In this state of physical health, failure seems less of a possibility. A man is more likely to simply get on with his life.

TESTOSTERONE AND PEAK PERFORMANCE IN WOMEN

Even the small amount of testosterone that a woman produces can have an effect on her performance and influence her quality of life. As in men, testosterone increases energy, enhances mood and imparts a sense of well-being, and stimulates assertiveness and libido in women. These effects have been observed in women who have taken testosterone replacement to restore natural levels of the hormone.

1 Physical vitality and stamina

Various studies have demonstrated that women taking a hormone replacement that includes estrogen *and* an androgen experience a greater level of energy than women on estrogen alone. In a study published in 1985 in the *American Journal of Obstetrics and Gynecology*, forty-three women had received a total hysterectomy, including removal of their ovaries. As the ovaries make one-third of the testosterone in the female body, their removal causes a significant decline in testosterone production. The women were divided into four groups and given combined estrogen and androgen, one or the other of the hormones alone, or a placebo. A treatment was administered for three months, followed by a differing treatment for another three months. There was also a control group of ten women who underwent hysterectomy but retained their ovaries. The women receiving androgen therapy, alone or with estrogen, and the women with ovarian function intact reported significantly higher ratings of energy level and well-being than those women not receiving androgens.

Regular exercise results in an increase in oxygen reaching the tissues and a greater production of beta-endorphins (natural mood elevators), both of which can potentially increase energy. Because higher testosterone levels can increase strength, such an increase in physical ability can mean that a person finds exercise easier to do and is more likely to spend time in energy-generating physical activity.

3 Determination and perseverance in pursuing goals

Testosterone levels in women, as in men, are associated with assertiveness and sexual drive. Women who report a higher libido are also more assertive in their behavior, often with a greater drive to achieve, and are usually busy, highly effective people. However, during menopause, testosterone levels decline. About 10 to 20 percent of menopausal women experience a drop in libido soon after ceasing menstruation, because the ovaries stop making testosterone as well as estrogen. For others, the decline may be less rapid. Many of Susan's patients say that they suddenly feel as if something is missing in their relationship with their sexual partner, and that their interest in sex just evaporated after menopause. For these women, supplementing with testosterone can be of great benefit.

Testosterone cream or the oral estrogen/testosterone combination therapy can significantly increase their sex drive. A study cited in a 1996 review article appearing in the *Journal of Clinical Endocrinology and Metabolism* verifies this conclusion. Women who had had their ovaries surgically removed were injected with testosterone enanthate and reported an increase in the intensity of sexual arousal, sexual interest, and frequency of sexual fantasies above the effect they experienced taking only estrogen.

Susan has had a number of women patients who have been placed on testosterone therapy after a total hysterectomy (in which both the uterus and the ovaries are removed) or for the treatment of certain gynecologic conditions. Many of these women found that their libido went into high gear. These women reported that they thought and fantasized about sex constantly and requested frequent sexual activity with their partner if they were currently in a relationship. Several of her patients told Susan that such intense sexual desire was a problem since their partners simply did not have the sexual stamina to keep up with their demands. This was particularly true for women in their fifties and sixties whose husband's libido was on the decline.

4 The ability to get along with other people

While estrogen therapy is often prescribed in postmenopausal women as a mood elevator, it is not the only hormone to produce this benefit. Research studies have shown that testosterone also has beneficial effects on emotional well-being, perhaps even more striking than those noted with estrogen replacement therapy (ERT). The 1985 *American Journal of Obstetrics and Gynecology* study cited above also examined the effect of androgens on a variety of psychological symptoms. Patients completed a daily questionnaire, rating such items as feeling blue and depressed, crying spells, needless worry, and loss of interest in most things. Those women receiving testosterone reported negative feelings significantly less frequently than women not receiving the hormone. If testosterone therapy is able to elevate mood in postmenopausal women, they are far more likely to get up in the morning with a seize-the-day attitude and participate fully in social and business activities.

TESTOSTERONE AND HEALTH IN MEN

Long-term health in men depends in part on having sufficient levels of testosterone. Recent research suggests that testosterone helps protect against the development of heart disease. There is also considerable evidence that testosterone is important for bone health and the prevention of osteoporosis. Of course, preventing such diseases can help insure a long and productive life. The following are some of the specific conditions that testosterone affects.

Heart disease

Each year, as many as 90,000 men between the ages of forty-five and sixty-four die of a heart attack or a related health problem, according to the American Heart Association. There is some evidence that testosterone may protect against coronary-artery disease, helping to prevent atherosclerosis (the narrowing of blood vessels by deposits of plaque) and heart attacks. However, other research contradicts these findings, and more investigation is needed. Various changes in lifestyle can reduce the risk of heart disease, including changing one's diet, consuming more antioxidants, exercising more regularly, and stopping smoking.

In a study published in 1994 in *Arteriosclerosis and Thrombosis*, researchers observed the relationship of testosterone levels and risk factors for heart attack in fifty-five men undergoing coronary angiography (diagnostic radiography of the heart and blood vessels) who had not had a heart attack. Lower levels of testosterone were clearly correlated with several risk factors, including abnormal levels of clotting factors such as fibrinogen and tissue plasminogen activator and high levels of insulin. Furthermore, the relationship persisted after controlling for age, body mass index, drug intake, and smoking.

Osteoporosis

Testosterone plays an important role in the growth and formation of bone in children and teenagers, and in adults it helps maintain bone mass and strength. Even as men begin to lose some bone mineral mass, testosterone helps keep bones strong. However, at about age forty, men begin to experience a decrease in bone strength and size, and there is approximately a 3 to 5 percent decline in bone mass per decade. Women also begin to lose bone at midlife as hormone production rapidly declines, but unlike women, men do not develop osteoporosis as quickly. There are two reasons for this: (1) Men have approximately 30 percent more bone mass than women do to begin with, and (2) males maintain testosterone levels well into old age, helping to preserve bone mass and strength. Like estrogen, testosterone helps control calcium absorption by the bones. It also prevents the resorption of calcium from the bones into the blood, where calcium can then be excreted from the body. These effects translate into fewer osteoporosis-related fractures for men than women: eight times fewer hip fractures and ten times fewer wrist fractures.

However, some men do eventually develop osteoporosis later in life. According to an article published in 1994 in *Clinical Andrology*, between the ages of sixty and eighty, the incidence in men of fracture of the hip bone increases significantly. It is estimated that 1.5 million American men have osteoporosis and that an additional 3.5 million are at risk, according to an article published in 1997 in *Family Practice News*. While a great deal of media attention has recently been given to osteoporosis in women and the role that estrogen deficiency plays in its development, the role of hormones and osteoporosis in men is often overlooked.

There are to date no long-term studies of the effect of testosterone on bone maintenance, but there are some preliminary studies that focus on the relationship of testosterone to bone health. In an animal study published in 1995 in the journal *Bone*, monkeys were used as subjects and divided into three groups and treated for two years. Researchers noted significant increases in bone elasticity and improvement in the ability of the bone to withstand force or pressure without fracturing.

Men who are hypogonadal (with low testosterone production) are especially at risk of osteoporosis. These men have a lower bone density as compared with men who have normal levels of testosterone. In fact, older men with hypogonadism have six and a half times greater risk of minimal-trauma hip fracture than men with normal testosterone production. Testosterone deficiency as a risk factor for hip fractures was also observed in a study conducted at an inpatient orthopedic service, published in 1992 in the *American Journal of Medical Sciences*. The volunteers included seventeen men who came to the clinic with a hip fracture, eleven men who had fractured their hip sometime in the preceding twenty-five months, and twenty-five men with no fracture of the hip. The volunteers had an average age of seventy-three. The researchers measured testosterone levels and found that 71 percent of the men with a hip fracture had testosterone deficiencies, as compared with only 32 percent of the men in the control group.

Furthermore, the ability of testosterone to increase stamina and vitality may indirectly strengthen bones. A man with an abundance of energy is more likely to exercise, and it is well known that sports that involve impact, such as tennis and horseback riding, or resistance, like weight lifting, can do much to strengthen and build bones.

TESTOSTERONE AND HEALTH IN WOMEN

Although studies on the benefits of testosterone for female health are scarce, there is evidence that testosterone relieves some of the symptoms of menopause and that it helps prevent osteoporosis. However, although testosterone seems to be protective of heart disease in men, high levels of this hormone may actually increase the risk in women. In clinical practice, testosterone is most often prescribed for women who complain that their libido seemed to evaporate with the onset of menopause. For these women, testosterone can restore their quality of life if they wish to remain sexually active. Following are some health conditions that testosterone affects in women.

Menopausal symptoms

As a woman passes through menopause, she may experience a variety of symptoms initiated by the drop in hormone production that occurs at this time, including hot flashes, mood swings, and vaginal dryness and atrophy. Estrogen replacement therapy (ERT) is successfully used to treat many of these symptoms; there is also a growing body of clinical and experimental research that indicates that testosterone may be of benefit in reversing some of these symptoms, especially when combined with estrogen therapy.

A small study, reported in 1996 in *American Family Physician* and presented at the sixth annual meeting of the North American Menopause Society, monitored two groups of women experiencing menopausal symptoms. One group of twelve women were each given 1.25 mg of estrogen daily, while a second group of thirteen women were each given the same dosage of estrogen and 2.5 mg of methyltestosterone. While both treatments had a positive effect on vaginal dryness and hot flashes, only the combined therapy helped relieve associated nervousness, irritability, fatigue, and insomnia. Other studies have shown that combined hormone therapy is also more effective in improving sleep quality and energy levels.

As stated above, many menopausal women experience a decline in libido, and estrogen treatment has not been found to be effective in reversing this decline. However, testosterone has proven to be of great use. A study appearing in 1996 in the *Journal of Clinical Endocrinology and Metabolism* cited several controlled studies documenting an increased intensity of sexual drive, sexual arousal, and frequency of sexual fantasies in women receiving testosterone supplementation. Susan has seen the benefits of testosterone therapy in her own patients, particularly when it is used in combination with the female hormones estrogen and progesterone. While replacement with estrogen and progesterone may be enough to control most menopause-related symptoms, it may not be effective in restoring libido. Susan, like other physicians, has found that nothing matches testosterone for its effectiveness in restoring libido.

Testosterone is available through most pharmacies in either pill or cream form. Testosterone creams are sometimes used as a treatment for vaginal atrophy. It must be used carefully, however, because side effects of excessive androgen use can include masculinization such as deepening of the voice or growth of excessive facial hair.

▲▲ A wide variety of testosterone products are available from compounding pharmacies. These are pharmacies that will take a hormone like testosterone and formulate it in a variety of ways, such as in creams, gels, ointments, and pills. This array of choices greatly increases the options that women have for treatment and allows them to choose the most effective way to administer testosterone into their bodies. If you are interested in using testosterone therapy, have your physician contact one of these compounding pharmacies (see the appendix for a selective list).

Osteoporosis

The importance of androgens in the development of the male skeleton is generally accepted, but scientists are now discovering that testosterone also plays a more important role in female bone health than was previously thought. The use of combined estrogen and testosterone therapy may be more effective at preventing osteoporosis than estrogen therapy alone. While estrogen slows down the rate of bone loss, testosterone helps promote formation of new bone. This can be of great benefit even for women in whom osteoporosis has already begun. In one study, appearing in 1995 in *Obstetrics and Gynecology*, sixty-six women who had undergone surgical menopause were given estrogen either alone or combined with testosterone. While both treatments prevented loss of bone in the spine and hip, only the combined therapy produced a significant increase in bone mineral density in the spine.

SUMMARY

Testosterone is the predominant male hormone. It is essential for normal sexual behavior in men, but it also supports peak-performance traits in both men and women. Several factors affect testosterone levels, including aging, diet, stress, and general health. Sufficient testosterone enhances physical energy, assertiveness, problem-solving abilities, and a positive outlook on life in both men and women. It also helps to protects against heart disease in men and osteoporosis in both men and women.

SECTION 5:
ESTROGEN

ESTROGEN IS ONE of the two major female sex hormones and is therefore an important factor in peak performance and health for women; for a list of the benefits of estrogen in women, see page 593. Men produce small amounts of estrogen in their adrenal glands; however, estrogen in men has not been shown to have the same importance as testosterone in women. A recent study does indicate that estrogen therapy may be valuable in preventing heart disease in men; see page 610.

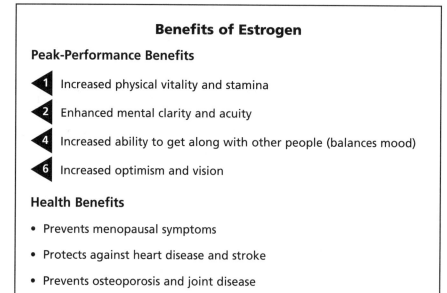

Benefits of Estrogen

Peak-Performance Benefits

1 Increased physical vitality and stamina

2 Enhanced mental clarity and acuity

4 Increased ability to get along with other people (balances mood)

6 Increased optimism and vision

Health Benefits

- Prevents menopausal symptoms

- Protects against heart disease and stroke

- Prevents osteoporosis and joint disease

When many women enter their menopausal years, it's as if they cross over an invisible line in their lives. As a result of the decline in their estrogen levels, these women find that many of the functions needed for peak performance, which had formerly been effortless, seem to evaporate or diminish. While women often do complain of menopausal symptoms that are strictly physical—such as vaginal dryness, more frequent bladder and vaginal infections, and dryness of the skin—just as often they complain about menopausal symptoms that impair their job performance, social relationships, and even their ability to take pleasure in day-to-day activities. To begin to determine whether or not your body is producing adequate estrogen, see the checklist below.

Many of the long-term consequences of estrogen deficiency during the menopausal years, such as osteoporosis and an increased risk of heart attacks and strokes, do not initially produce symptoms. It is important that women check their risk of these conditions at the time of menopause with tests such as lipid panels and bone density studies as well as routine blood counts and blood chemistry. Many of these tests provide sensitive and very helpful indicators of early risk and are particularly important for women who do not want to use conventional hormone replacement therapy. For a description of these laboratory tests of estrogen levels, see page 630.

CHECKLIST: DO YOU PRODUCE THE ESTROGEN YOU NEED FOR PEAK PERFORMANCE AND HEALTH?

This checklist will give you a preliminary idea of whether you have inadequate estrogen production. Work through the following checklist (photocopy it if you don't want to write in the book), and refer to it as you read through this section of the chapter. If your responses suggest that your estrogen level is low, you can learn about a variety of ways to increase it in chapter 12.

Performance factors

Put a check mark beside those statements that are true for you.

❏ I lack energy, stamina, and vitality.

❏ I have difficulty with my short-term memory.

❏ I have difficulty remembering names.

❏ I often experience feelings of anxiety, mood swings, and/or depression.

❏ I have a negative outlook on life.

Physical/emotional indicators and medical history

❏ I am over the age of fifty.

❏ My sleep quality is poor.

❏ I experience symptoms of menopause such as hot flashes, mood swings, vaginal dryness, loss of libido, and pain during intercourse.

❏ I have a history of heart disease, or there is a history of heart disease in my family.

❏ I have osteoporosis or bones that fracture or break easily.

Susan has always been amazed by the number of women patients she has worked with who reach menopause and begin to complain of forgetfulness and memory loss. Small details of life, such as remembering someone's name or where they put the car keys, suddenly become an issue. Competent performance at work is a real concern for some of these women. They report going from one office to another with no idea of why they went there. They may even complain about an inability to recall important work data. Virtually all of her patients who suffer from forgetfulness and memory loss are concerned about this problem. Some of them wonder if they are in the early stages of senility or even Alzheimer's disease. Fortunately, this is rarely the case. However, the brain is loaded with hormone receptors, and our normal mental and emotional functions depend, in part, on the abundant production of female sex hormones.

While memory loss can affect a woman's competence at work, frequent hot flashes can be downright embarrassing. As many as 85 percent of all menopausal women in the United States experience some degree of hot flashes. Women with more severe symptoms may have as many as ten, twenty, or even forty episodes a day. Hot flashes cause a woman to turn pink and either perspire profusely or simply generate a lot of heat within the body. In any case, women often feel like shedding clothes, which is often not possible in a professional setting.

Hot flashes are triggered by stress and often occur at the worst possible times. Some of Susan's patients report having hot flashes and starting to sweat profusely when presenting a report in front of a professional audience, in meetings with important customers, or when going for a job interview. Hot flashes also frequently occur at night, waking the woman, and sometimes even her bedmate, from a deep sleep. Frequently interrupted sleep can cause anyone to be tired, irritable, and relatively unproductive the next day.

In addition, the ability to experience joy in life can be blunted by the onset of menopause. The hormones produced within the ovaries as well as within the adrenal glands are crucial for maintaining sexual pleasure, a sense of emotional well-being, and optimism, and other qualities that many women regard as essential for an exciting and satisfying life.

The negative effects that the natural decline in female sex hormone production during menopause can have on a women's ability to perform at peak levels are not uncommon. Menopausal symptoms are so common in the United States that 80 to 85 percent of American women experience them to some degree. A small number of these women are lucky enough to have mild symptoms, such as occasional hot flashes over a period of a few months to a year. However, the majority of women have symptoms that are bothersome enough to cause them to seek the help of physicians or complementary health care practitioners, or to seek solutions on their own by reading books and articles and exploring the use of natural hormones, vitamins, and herbs to relieve their symptoms.

THE CHEMISTRY OF ESTROGEN

Estrogen, along with progesterone, is one of the two major hormones that support the functioning of the female reproductive organs and the menstrual cycle. The ovaries and adrenal glands produce substantial amounts of estrogen during a woman's active reproductive years and continue to produce small amounts after menopause. While we are accustomed to using the term *estrogen*, this term actually refers to several different types of estrogens made within the body. At least six types of estrogen have been identified and are classified according to their potency. The term *potency* refers to the time that estrogen is bound to the estrogen receptor within a specific tissue. The higher the estrogen potency, the more time it remains bound to the receptor and, therefore, the more pronounced are the physiological effects that estrogen promotes within that tissue. For example, estrogen is a growth-stimulating hormone, causing tissues to grow and thicken; it also causes water and salt to be retained within the tissues of the body. The more potent and powerful forms of estrogen cause these effects to occur in a more pronounced fashion.

The three main types of estrogen produced within the body are estradiol, estrone, and estriol. Estradiol is the most potent form of estrogen. It is the primary type of estrogen produced by the ovaries during a woman's reproductive years. Estrone is an intermediate-potency form of estrogen, twelve times weaker than estradiol. It is mainly produced within the fatty tissue of the body from precursor hormones made by the adrenal glands. Obviously, the more weight a woman carries, the more adrenal estrogen she is capable of making. Small amounts of estrone are also produced by the ovaries after menopause, when production of estradiol ceases. As estradiol and estrone circulate through the body, they pass through the liver. It is the liver's job to detoxify and metabolize these two estrogens to a weaker form, which can then be eliminated from the body. Since estrogen is constantly being produced by the ovaries and adrenal glands, the liver helps to prevent its accumulation to toxic levels. Estriol, the liver metabolite of the other two estrogens, is the weakest form of estrogen produced by the body. It is eighty times weaker than estradiol.

How estrogen affects the female body

The effect that estrogen has on a woman's body begins even before birth, since estrogen plays an important role in the development of female sexual characteristics. During childhood, a girl's body produces only small amounts of estrogen. Then, at puberty, when estrogen production increases twentyfold or more, these higher levels stimulate the female sexual organs of young girls to begin to mature into those of an adult woman.

Estrogen causes the uterus and vagina to increase in size. It stimulates the vagina and urinary tract linings to thicken and become more resistant to trauma and infection, thus preparing a woman to eventually become sexually active and bear children. In addition, estrogen causes an increase in overall body fat, contributing to the softly rounded female contours that we associate with sexual maturation. Firm, youthful-looking skin is also attributable to estrogen, which stimulates collagen, a protein that makes up 90 percent of the skin. Estrogen promotes the growth of pubic hair and coloration of the nipples and also stimulates bone growth. Beginning at puberty, when estrogen production soars, a young woman's height rapidly increases.

The various actions of estrogen are balanced by the complementary effects of progesterone. These two hormones, working together, help regulate a notably wide range of physiological processes. For instance, estrogen decreases the level of oxygen in cells, and progesterone restores oxygen to normal levels. While estrogen increases body fat, progesterone helps the body burn fat for energy. Estrogen also promotes salt and fluid retention, and progesterone is a natural diuretic, increasing the flow of urine. Estrogen promotes blood clotting, while progesterone normalizes clotting. Furthermore, progesterone normalizes blood sugar levels, and estrogen impairs blood sugar control. When these hormones are in balance, they provide a host of benefits affecting performance and health.

How aging affects estrogen production

The amount of estrogen a woman produces changes during her lifetime. The normal output of estradiol is 100 to 300 mcg a day. Estrogen is also produced in pregnancy by the placenta (a spongy structure in the uterus, from which the fetus derives oxygen and nourishment). The placenta produces estrogen in great quantity, as much as 100 times the amount normally made by the ovaries.

Levels of estrogen also fluctuate during the month because of menstruation, reaching peak levels during the first half of the menstrual cycle. During the second half of the cycle, both estrogen and progesterone predominate, though estrogen production does decline somewhat from its levels earlier in the month.

With the onset of menopause, after menstruation has ceased entirely, ovarian production of estrogen is greatly reduced, and levels of circulating estrogen decline by as much as 75 to 90 percent. However, after menopause, one-fourth to one-third of all American women continue to make enough ovarian and adrenal estrogen in its weaker form, estrone. While the quantity produced is not enough to cause a monthly menstrual cycle, it is sufficient to support the health of tissues such as bone, skin, and the vaginal lining. Although being overweight is a liability for many health conditions, those women who have more fatty tissue are better able to convert androgens to estrone after menopause. Consequently, they tend to have stronger bones and more youthful-looking skin. These women who maintain estrogen production after menopause probably do not need to consider hormone replacement therapy for ten to fifteen more years. The majority of women, however, have an abrupt decline in their estrogen production to the point that uncomfortable symptoms will lead these women to seek medical care.

HOW DIET, HEALTH, AND THE ENVIRONMENT AFFECT ESTROGEN LEVELS

While estrogen production declines with age, the amount of estrogen in the body will also be influenced by a range of other factors, including diet, digestive capabilities, liver function, enzyme levels, and exposure to environmental toxins, a topic that has not received sufficient attention to date.

Diet

Meat, poultry, and dairy foods contain estrogens that have been injected into the animals to fatten them for market. One of the synthetic estrogens routinely given to livestock was DES (diethylstilbestrol). DES was also given to women to prevent miscarriages and symptoms of menopause, until it was associated with birth defects in their offspring and was finally banned in 1979. However, today poultry and livestock, especially dairy cows, are still given other forms of estrogen compounds. Hormones such as estrogen accumulate in fatty tissue in the animals we eat as well as in us, and high-fat diets have been associated with changes in human estrogen levels.

Caffeine and alcohol consumption can also influence estrogen levels. Excessive alcohol intake can affect the liver's ability to break down estrogen for excretion, thereby elevating the body's blood estrogen levels, particularly of the more chemically active forms of estrogen. A three-year study appearing in 1996 in the *American Journal of Epidemiology*, involving 728 white, postmenopausal females aged forty-two to ninety, found that caffeine intake had an effect on estrogen levels. Having more than two cups of coffee or four cans of caffeinated soda per day increased blood levels of this hormone. Another research study suggested that a diet high in sugar may impair liver function, affecting its ability to metabolize estrogen. Even the public water supply may contain estrogens, if that water is recycled at treatment plants and still contains traces of excreted synthetic estrogens such as those contained in birth control pills and excreted from the bodies of women using these products.

Physiological factors

Poor digestive function can prevent hormone precursors such as fat molecules from being absorbed. Problems with the liver can also lead to low levels of hormones. Persons with functional disorders of the liver have been shown to have low levels of estrogen. When liver enzyme systems are impaired and the detoxification function is inadequate, the quantity and quality of hormone formation is reduced. Depressed levels of HDL cholesterol can also lead to lower levels of estrogen, as this deficiency blocks the biochemical pathway required for the production of the primary precursor hormone, pregnenolone, and all the consequent sex hormones.

Environmental estrogens

Pollutants that have estrogenlike activity when they are taken into the body (xenoestrogens) are found in an enormous range of products for the home and workplace. They are present in cosmetics, detergents and dishwashing liquids, and bug spray. Pesticides and industrial chemicals such as organochlorines, dioxins, and PCBs (polychlorinated biphenyls) also contain substances related to estrogen. A study from Stanford University, published in 1994 in the *Journal of the American Medical Association*, noted that when polycarbonate plastics are heated, they release bisphenol-A, a substance that is known to have estrogenic activity. Microwaving foods in plastic containers or using a plastic cup for hot coffee can cause estrogen substances to shed into the food.

There are many suspected health consequences of our wide exposure to xenoestrogens, including PMS, breast cancer, and low sperm count. According to a study published in 1992 in the *British Medical Journal*, there has been a clear decline in the average sperm count worldwide during the last fifty years. The researchers conducted an analysis of sixty-one papers published between 1938 and 1991, which involved a total of 14,947 men. When the results were compared, the researchers found that the average sperm count had decreased by nearly half from the late 1930s to the early 1990s. A further study, published in 1995 in the *Lancet*, found that the multiplication of Sertoli cells, which are responsible for sperm production, is inhibited by estrogen.

ESTROGEN AND PEAK PERFORMANCE

Estrogen affects a number of crucial performance factors, including energy level, memory, and emotional stability. Following are the peak-performance traits supported by estrogen.

1 Physical vitality and stamina

Estrogen appears to benefit physical energy and a sense of well-being. Women who produce sufficient amounts of this hormone during their active reproductive years tend to have more energy than menopausal women, who have experienced a significant decline in their production of this hormone. While there has been a lack of scientific studies investigating this association, many physicians have noted the important role that estrogen plays in maintaining the physical energy and stamina in certain women. In addition, many research articles on menopause make reference to estrogen's effect on vitality and well-being. This may occur, in part, because estrogen promotes good-quality sleep and reduces the number of hot flashes that may interrupt a women's sleep during the night. A number of studies have shown that estrogen decreases the frequency of awakenings during the night and increases the amount of REM sleep, the type of sleep that occurs when a person is dreaming, which is necessary for feeling rested the next day. When estrogen levels are deficient, a woman is likely to sleep more fitfully and for fewer hours. Lacking adequate sleep, she is more likely to feel tired during the day. Women who have had an abrupt decline in their estrogen levels by undergoing gynecological surgery, including the removal of their ovaries, may suffer most acutely from interrupted sleep.

Besides directly influencing sleep patterns, an estrogen deficiency can also trigger hot flashes, which are characterized by a rise in skin temperature and a flushing of the skin. Hot flashes in themselves can be physically draining, as the body loses fluids and minerals in the process of perspiring. When hot flashes occur at night, in the form of night sweats, a woman may go weeks without a good night's sleep, resulting in exhaustion. Fredi Kronenberg, a leading researcher on menopause, points out, in an article published in 1994 in *Experimental Gerontology*, that the consequences of hot flashes can also include strained family, work, and social relationships as well as poor concentration and the avoidance of close physical and sexual contact. Living with these stresses only adds to a woman's general feeling of fatigue.

2 Mental clarity and acuity

Maintaining one's ability to learn and having a good memory are essential if a woman decides to return to school or pursue further job training in her forties. More and more women are taking on this challenge as their children grow up and they no longer have full-time family responsibilities. Other women at midlife become bored and dissatisfied with their work and are ready to start a new career. Often, this may require additional training or taking and satisfactorily passing licensing examinations. For example, a woman who has been a teacher for many years and decides that working in real estate now holds more appeal must have the mental firepower to study for and pass a challenging licensing test. Some women, who are recently divorced or widowed, may return to school to acquire survival skills that allow them to return to the workforce and become financially self-sufficient. In all of these cases, learning new material can be a considerable challenge if a woman's short-term memory has begun to weaken due to the decline in her estrogen production and she is having difficulty concentrating.

The ability to concentrate and remember details depends, in part, on having adequate amounts of estrogen. As a woman's own estrogen production begins to diminish, cognitive function can decline. Susan regularly hears complaints from her menopausal patients of muddled thinking, brain fog, and poor memory, which can cause embarrassment and worse. When short-term memory fades, a person may misplace the car keys, forget a friend's name, or miss an appointment with a potential new client. When such mishaps begin to interfere with the ability to function at work and carry out personal responsibilities, a fickle memory can become a major performance issue.

As estrogen replacement therapy became more popular in the 1960s and 1970s, researchers began to study the effects of hormones on cognitive function in young and middle-aged women. In a review article on estrogen and memory done at McGill University and published in 1990, the researcher found that there is strong indication that estrogen does help maintain short- and long-term memory in women. However, these benefits are seen in verbal recall but not in visual/spatial memory. Another study investigated the effects of estrogen on memory function in women with surgical menopause; the results were published in 1992 in *Psychoneuroendocrinology*. Nineteen women who were scheduled for hysterectomy and removal of the ovaries were given verbal memory tests before surgery and again two months after their operation. Postoperatively, the women were treated with either 10 mg of estrogen or a placebo. Memory scores of those women treated with estrogen showed no decline after surgery, whereas the scores of those women who were untreated declined significantly.

Estrogen deficiency in menopause can make an educational challenge overwhelming, as in the case of Rachael, an old friend of Susan's. Rachael began the process of becoming a registered dietitian and earning a master's degree in science when she was forty-four. Because she was also self-supporting and had a full-time job, her professional education took nearly ten years to complete. At age forty-nine, Rachael had a hysterectomy and began to have typical menopausal symptoms that included fuzzy thinking and memory lapses. She did not consult with her gynecologist to have these symptoms evaluated, since she assumed that her symptoms were either due to low blood sugar or, even worse, that she was simply a failure and not qualified for the job. During her clinical internship at a local hospital, Rachael found that she could not remember patients' names and had great difficulty assessing their needs and planning her schedule each day. She began to rely on coffee, which cleared the mental fog for a half hour at best. In desperation, she finally consulted with her physician, a woman doctor who was herself also in menopause. Her doctor immediately diagnosed the problem and prescribed estrogen replacement therapy. Unfortunately, Rachael's boss at the hospital had already decided to terminate her internship, and she was forced to leave the program. This was a serious blow since Rachael had invested a significant amount of time and money pursuing this new career. During the following summer, Rachael began to investigate natural alternatives for prescription hormone replacement therapy, including estrogen-containing herbs and foods. She was then able to return to school, rested and clear-headed, although somewhat behind schedule.

Estrogen deficiency at midlife may increase the risk of developing Alzheimer's disease later in life. Recent studies indicate that the use of estrogen replacement therapy (ERT) reduces the risk of developing this disease. In a study conducted over eleven years and presented in 1993 at a meeting of the Society for Neuroscience, memory was assessed in 8879 women living at a retirement community in California. Those women receiving ERT were 40 percent less likely to develop Alzheimer's than those women not taking estrogen.

4 The ability to get along with other people

The emotions a woman experiences are determined in part by her estrogen levels. Because estrogen is a natural stimulant, with a mood-elevating effect, fluctuating estrogen levels can cause emotions to go haywire, affecting a woman's ability to work with others and her personal relationships as well. When estrogen levels are elevated, a woman may experience anxiety and irritability, while a deficiency of estrogen can lead to depression. To sustain an even mood, estrogen levels must also be in balance with progesterone, which has a sedative or depressant effect on the nervous system. The balance between estrogen and progesterone can have a profound effect on psychological well-being.

Estrogen and emotions in premenopausal women. Mood-altering changes in estrogen levels can occur at various stages of a woman's life. For women in their twenties and thirties, estrogen and progesterone are usually in balance with one another, allowing for healthy childbearing and regular menstrual cycles. However, when the levels of these hormones become unbalanced during the monthly cycle, the result is premenstrual syndrome (PMS), which affects one-third to one-half of American women between the ages of twenty and fifty. PMS is a common cause of anxiety and other emotional symptoms like depression and fatigue.

In Susan's practice, more than 90 percent of women with PMS complain of heightened anxiety and irritability that increases in intensity the week or two prior to menstruation. Many PMS patients describe severe personality changes, a Dr. Jekyll and Mr. Hyde scenario. Some say they spend the rest of the month repairing the emotional damage done to their personal and work relationships while in the throes of PMS.

Though it is not entirely known what causes the anxiety symptoms, it is known that both estrogen and progesterone levels increase during the second half of the menstrual cycle and that their chemical actions affect the function of almost every organ system in the body. When properly balanced, estrogen and progesterone promote healthy and balanced emotions. However, PMS mood symptoms may occur if the balance between these hormones is abnormal, because they have an opposing effect on the chemistry of the brain.

Furthermore, this hormone imbalance is aggravated during perimenopause, the period in a woman's life leading up to menopause, when the number of menstrual cycles diminishes until they finally stop completely, and a natural state of hormone imbalance develops in which estrogen dominates and less progesterone is produced. These women can easily become anxious and upset.

About 5 percent of women with PMS actually have the opposite problem: Their estrogen levels diminish while progesterone production continues. In such cases, the depressant effects of progesterone are not counterbalanced by estrogen. According to Dr. Guy Abraham, former clinical professor of obstetrics and gynecology at UCLA and an authority on PMS, this type of PMS is potentially the most serious because the women affected can be suicidal in severe cases. In milder cases, women may become introverted and will tend to pull away from relationships at certain times of the month, which can be counterproductive for a woman whose job is an area of business that requires her to be outgoing, such as sales.

Premenstrual depression can be treated with hormone therapy, and some physicians also treat postnatal depression with estrogen for its mood-elevating effect. A letter to the editor, published in 1992 in the *Lancet*, noted that women with postnatal depression have been effectively treated with estrogen therapy using high dosages administered through transdermal estrogen patches. The author termed estrogen a "mental tonic."

Estrogen and emotions in menopausal women. With the decline in estrogen production that occurs during menopause, many women notice that their moods may fluctuate. Some of Susan's patients have complained about mood swings varying between increased anxiety and irritability to depression and fatigue. They have reported being bad tempered toward family, friends, and coworkers and responding to daily-life stresses in a more irritable fashion, similar to the emotional ups and downs of PMS. A woman who has had PMS during her active reproductive years may be particularly distressed to experience similar emotional fluctuations during menopause. Often, the expectation is that PMS symptoms will stop, rather than become worse, during the transition into menopause. Luckily, not every woman experiences such pronounced emotional swings (in fact, some women go through menopause with no mood changes at all).

Because menopause signals the loss of reproductive capability, some women experience this change as an end to their usefulness. For other women, menopause is a time when children leave home and move away, major career changes are made, or a marriage ends in divorce. The combination of hormonal/biochemical changes plus lifestyle changes can be quite difficult for many women to handle, especially if they find themselves alone, without their familiar support systems. Other women find that they have to cope with a husband's midlife crisis, engendered by the loss of a job or job dissatisfaction, health problems, or other issues that are common for men around midlife.

Although menopause does not inevitably cause depression, some women do become despondent and gloomy as hormone production declines. These effects of low estrogen are most pronounced in women who have undergone surgical menopause. The authors of a long-term survey of 2500 middle-aged women in Massachusetts, published in 1987 in the *Journal of Health and Social Behavior*, observed that women in natural menopause were not depressed, but those women with hysterectomies had clinically significant depression.

Other research studies have shown that supplemental estrogen, prescribed by physicians as replacement therapy, has a mood-elevating effect. Women on hormone replacement therapy may perceive this effect as an enhanced sense of well-being and overall mental balance, which contributes to the relief of other menopausal symptoms such as hot flashes and vaginal dryness. In a study published in 1977 in *Clinical Obstetrics and Gynecology*, volunteers were given 1.25 mg daily of either conjugated equine estrogen or a placebo for a period of two months. The women were assessed for their degree of irritability and anxiety. Those volunteers receiving estrogen treatment reported calmer and more even moods with longer periods of well-being. Susan's patient Nora, a fifty-year-old homemaker, reported lashing out at her husband with little provocation. Janice, a fifty-one-year-old lawyer, complained of her overreactivity to the small stresses and irritations in her life. Both of these women noticed an improvement in their family and social relationships as well as being less sensitive to stress once they started estrogen replacement therapy.

However, some women do experience side effects on estrogen replacement therapy, about 10 to 15 percent of all women who try it. Paradoxically, ERT medication can aggravate preexisting menopausal symptoms such as hot flashes, jittery nerves, and mood swings. These women may find that they are better candidates for various types of alternative therapies.

6 Optimism and vision

A positive attitude depends in part on having the right balance of hormones to stimulate the brain and promote creativity. Because estrogen is a natural mood elevator, during the phase of their menstrual cycle when estrogen levels are higher, many women will experience this lift as an increase in their enthusiasm for living. They are more outgoing and have a more positive attitude. Potential problems are seen as opportunities instead. This positive attitude opens doors and increases the likelihood of finding solutions. Furthermore, a woman who is able to maintain a certain buoyancy while dealing with the complexities of everyday life is far more able to sustain friendships and workable partnerships.

Studies confirm this effect of estrogen. In a special report on menopause, assembled in 1993 by Harvard Medical School, the authors refer to an investigation of postmenopausal women who received estrogen replacement therapy for three months. These women, who had no significant emotional symptoms of menopause, reported that when taking supplemental estrogen they experienced an improvement in mood, confidence, and optimism.

ESTROGEN AND HEALTH

Producing sufficient estrogen plays a key role in maintaining health and preventing certain diseases that can develop as a component of aging. Having an adequate supply of estrogen can mean that a woman will remain active and productive into her seventies and eighties.

Estrogen acts directly on various body tissues, including the uterus, vaginal tissue, heart, and bones. As estrogen production decreases, there can be significant changes in the function and appearance of these organs. These effects can be felt immediately, as low estrogen triggers symptoms of menopause, and in the long term, as estrogen deficiency increases the risk of heart disease and osteoporosis. Estrogen therapy has been proven very successful in preventing and reversing these conditions, which are discussed below.

Menopausal symptoms

While some women experience virtually no annoying signs of menopause, the great majority of women in Western countries are afflicted by a wide range of symptoms, ranging from those that impact performance, such as fatigue and poor memory, to physiological changes such as thinning of the vaginal walls, reduced sex drive, and an inability to regulate body temperature, resulting in hot flashes.

Hot flashes. Hot flashes affect at least 80 to 85 percent of American women who are going through menopause. While their exact cause is not known, it is agreed that hot flashes are related to fluctuating estrogen levels, which cause blood vessels to enlarge and narrow unpredictably. As a consequence, blood flow to the brain, organs, and skin increases, causing a woman to feel suddenly warm, the sensation of heat usually beginning in the face and neck and then proceeding into the chest. Her face may become bright red, and she may begin to perspire. This heating may then be followed by chills. Most hot flashes last two to three minutes.

Dr. Fredi Kronenberg, a leading menopause researcher, in a comprehensive article on hot flashes published in 1994 in *Experimental Gerontology*, states that estrogen supplementation is an unsurpassed therapy in treating hot flashes. However, estrogen is not a permanent cure. Hot flashes may return when replacement therapy is discontinued.

Vaginal changes. Without adequate estrogen, the vaginal walls gradually lose their elasticity and actually shrink and become thinner. This means that during sexual arousal, the interior end of the vagina will no longer increase in size, and there can be a decrease in vaginal lubrication, making sexual intercourse uncomfortable and even painful. ERT, given either systemically or as a vaginal cream, is very effective in rebuilding the vaginal lining and improving lubrication and resistance to friction. With the use of ERT, sexual intercourse can become more enjoyable and comfortable. The use of ERT can also help prevent repeated vaginal and bladder infections.

Estriol, the weakest form of estrogen produced by the body, is a very effective form of supplemental estrogen for women with vaginal atrophy. Several research studies have found estriol to be as or even more effective than the stronger and more potent estrogens for the treatment of vaginal atrophy, hot flashes, and mood swings. Unlike the more potent estrogens, estriol does not stimulate the uterine lining, nor does it bind to estrogen receptors in the breast. Thus, estriol does not increase the risk of either uterine or breast cancer. Susan has found it to be an excellent option for women who either do not need or cannot handle the more potent forms of estrogen therapy. Estriol is currently available by prescription through compounding pharmacies throughout the United States.

Lack of libido. While it is true that many women experience a marked lessening of their sexual drive as they go through menopause, many women experience no reduction in their interest in sex (libido). Some even notice an increased level of desire, since the possibility of pregnancy has passed and their grown children have moved out of the house, allowing greater privacy.

Studies show that estrogen supplementation increases libido either because it has a direct effect on sexual desire or because it reduces troublesome symptoms, such as hot flashes and mood swings, that can leave a woman feeling uninterested in sexual intimacy.

Heart disease and strokes

Women and estrogen therapy. Coronary-heart disease claims the lives of more than a quarter of a million American women each year, more than die from all forms of cancer. Although younger women also die of heart disease, it occurs less frequently in women during the active reproductive years. The incidence of heart disease escalates as women age and estrogen production declines. Estrogen is known to help keep the arteries clear of plaque. From age thirty to sixty, cancer is the main cause of death in women, with heart disease the second-leading cause from age forty to sixty. Over age sixty, however, heart disease becomes the leading cause of death in American women.

The use of estrogen replacement therapy (ERT) has been found to have a beneficial effect on the blood lipid profile, a major determining factor in assessing the risk of cardiovascular disease. ERT increases the level of HDL, the "good" cholesterol, and decreases the level of LDL, the "bad" cholesterol linked to coronary-artery disease. Estrogen also has a relaxant effect on blood vessels and improves arterial blood flow throughout the body.

ERT does, however, have one negative side effect: Its use can cause a moderate increase in the triglyceride level, and elevated triglycerides are a minor risk factor for the development of heart disease. However, on balance, given the mostly positive effects that ERT has on blood lipids, many physicians prescribe ERT to women for its long-term cardiovascular benefits. ERT prescribed for postmenopausal use does not appear to significantly affect blood pressure, carbohydrate metabolism, or blood coagulation.

Research has found that ERT not only protects women from death due to heart attacks, but it also appears to reduce the likelihood of developing a heart attack by 50 percent. An important study, published in 1991 in the *New England Journal of Medicine*, indicated that the heart benefits of estrogen far outweigh any risks. Almost 50,000 nurses were studied for ten years, and the results showed that those taking estrogen after menopause were half as likely to develop or die from cardiovascular disease. Moreover, this protection appears to extend to women who have undergone surgical removal of the ovaries and use ERT.

Every year, 86,000 American women die of strokes. A stroke is a sudden and severe loss of blood flow in the brain caused by a blocked blood vessel. The medical term for stroke is cerebral vascular accident, or CVA. This condition may be caused by hemorrhage, thrombosis, or a clot and is associated with hypertension. The event may result in tragic, often irreversible brain damage. Small strokes may cause dementia, also an irreversible condition.

Another benefit of estrogen therapy may be to reduce the incidence of strokes. While some estrogen studies have shown no protective effects against strokes, current research appears to support the theory that using estrogen results in fewer strokes. A 1993 study of almost 2000 white postmenopausal women, published in the *Archives of Internal Medicine*, found that when women used estrogen there was a 31 percent reduction in the incidence of strokes. When strokes did occur, estrogen users were less likely to die, with the study showing a 63 percent reduction in the death rate from strokes.

In 1991, over 8000 women in a retirement home in California were monitored: Those still taking ERT after at least fifteen years on the medication suffered 40 percent fewer deaths from heart disease and stroke than those who had never used estrogen.

Men and estrogen therapy. There has been a consensus that while estrogen therapy lowers the risk of heart disease in women, it does not do so for men. However, a recent study, published in 1997 in the *American Journal of Cardiology*, suggests that estrogen supplementation may one day become an accepted method of preventing heart disease in men as well. Twenty male volunteers with heart disease, aged fifty-one to sixty-one, were studied. Twelve of the men were given a single injection of conjugated estrogens, while the remaining men were given a placebo. Fifteen minutes after the injections, the men receiving estrogen therapy had an average increase in blood flow to the heart of 32 percent, while there was no change in blood flow for those volunteers who remained untreated. Earlier studies had examined the effects of using only one form of estrogen, estradiol, and it is thought that the benefits noted in this study were due to the use of conjugated estrogens. As the use of estrogen can be feminizing, causing breast enlargement and redistribution of body fat from the abdominal area to the hips and thighs, researchers are now focused on developing a type of estrogen that helps prevent heart disease but does not have these undesired side effects.

Osteoporosis and joint disease

Osteoporosis is a major health problem affecting more than 25 million older Americans, 90 percent of them women. One out of three American women will develop osteoporosis, most after menopause. The statistics on osteoporosis are astounding. According to the National Osteoporosis Foundation, more than 1.5 million fractures occur each year as a result of this condition. Eighty percent of the 300,000 hip fractures in the United States each year occur in women over age sixty-five as a result of osteo-porosis. About one-quarter of these women die within one year from complications, such as blood clots and pneumonia, caused by their conva-lescence. Another one-third never regain the ability to function physically or socially on their own, spending the rest of their lives requiring long-term care in nursing facilities. Osteoporosis is also responsible for loss of bone in the jaw, gum recession (both of which are early signs of this con-dition), dowager's hump, loss of height, back pain due to compression and fractures of the vertebrae, and fractures of the wrist. Often these fractures occur when only mild stress is put on the bone, such as missing a step and falling down, or lifting a heavy object, or even without any preceding trauma.

Certain eating habits can predispose a woman toward osteoporosis, including a high intake of caffeine, high alcohol use (more than five ounces per day), a diet low in calcium and vitamin D, and smoking. Certain phys-ical characteristics also predispose a person to developing osteoporosis, such as being short and thin; having fair, pale skin; belonging to a non-black ethnic group; and having female relatives with osteoporosis.

Many medical studies show that estrogen therapy not only helps prevent osteoporosis but also protects women against further bone loss. Estrogen reduces urinary calcium and hydroxyproline excretion, which suggests that it inhibits the function of osteoclasts, the cells that break down bone tissue. Current research suggests that estrogen may even have a stimulatory effect on osteoblast cells, the cells that build up new bone. Estrogen also facilitates calcium absorption from the intestinal tract and increases parathyroid hormones and calcitonin production. The parathyroid hormone facilitates calcium absorption, while calcitonin stimulates bone formation. Estrogen appears to be critical to bone remodeling; therefore, it may well be the most essential component of prevention for osteoporosis.

In addition to protecting the bones, ERT has been shown to help reduce symptoms of osteoarthritis, a type of arthritis marked by progressive cartilage deterioration in joints and vertebrae. Joint pain tends to become worse in early menopause. Many women with muscle and joint pain, including low-back and pelvic pain, note relief of these symptoms within two weeks of beginning ERT. In a study published in 1997 in the *Annals of the Rheumatic Diseases*, researchers assessed the risk of osteoarthritis in 606 women, aged forty-five to sixty-five, who had used ERT for a period of more than twelve months. They found that those women taking ERT were three times less likely to have osteoarthritis in their knees than women not receiving hormones.

SUMMARY

Estrogen, one of the two major female hormones, plays an important role in the development of female sexual characteristics. Estrogen levels are affected by age, diet, health, and the environment. This hormone benefits a number of crucial performance factors in women, including energy level, memory, and emotional stability. The natural deficiency of estrogen after menopause can cause a variety of health conditions, such as depression, hot flashes, heart disease, and osteoporosis. Supplementation with estrogen can alleviate or improve these conditions.

SECTION 6:
PROGESTERONE

PROGESTERONE IS ONE of the two major female sex hormones. It is produced in the ovaries in women, and both men and women produce some progesterone in the adrenals. During pregnancy, as the fetus matures, the placenta produces large amounts of progesterone (the name actually means "for gestation"). Men produce a small but significant amount throughout life, comparable to how much a woman makes after age forty-five or fifty. In women, progesterone works in tandem with estrogen, in many cases acting to balance the effects of that hormone. See the list of progesterone's peak-performance and health benefits for women below. In men, the main function of progesterone seems to be helping to maintain libido.

Benefits of Progesterone

Peak-Performance Benefits

1. Increased physical vitality and stamina (improves sleep patterns)

2. Enhanced mental clarity and acuity

4. Increased ability to get along with other people (balances mood)

5. Increased ability to remain calm under pressure

Health Benefits

- Helps control excessive and irregular menstrual bleeding during perimenopause

- Helps prevent health problems related to high estrogen levels, such as endometrial hyperplasia and uterine fibroids

- Reduces hot flashes

- Helps prevent uterine cancer

- Helps prevent osteoporosis

- Increases libido

- Aids in the healing of certain types of nerve disease

Low levels of progesterone in women can contribute to a number of health conditions and can negatively affect one's outlook on life, energy level, and emotions. To begin to determine whether your progesterone production is adequate for peak performance and health, see the checklist below. For a description of laboratory tests of progesterone levels, see page 631.

CHECKLIST: DO YOU PRODUCE THE PROGESTERONE YOU NEED FOR PEAK PERFORMANCE AND HEALTH?

This checklist will give you a preliminary idea of whether you have a deficiency of progesterone. Work through the following checklist (photocopy it if you don't want to write in the book), and refer to it as you read through this section of the chapter. If your responses suggest that your progesterone level is low, you can learn about many ways to increase it in chapter 12.

Performance indicators

Put a check mark beside those statements that are true for you.

 My sleep quality is poor.

 I am often unable to concentrate.

☐ I am unable to remain calm under stress.

☐ I suffer from premenstrual fatigue and depression.

Physical indicators and medical history

☐ I am over the age of fifty.

☐ I am in perimenopause.

 I have experienced a decreased interest in sex.

☐ I get hot flashes.

 I experience heavy, irregular menstrual bleeding.

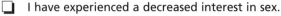 I often get menstrual migraine headaches.

☐ I experience premenstrual edema or swollen breasts.

❑ I have a history of endometrial hyperplasia.

❑ I have a history of fibroid tumors.

❑ I have a history of endometrial cancer.

❑ I have osteoporosis.

❑ I have a history of nerve damage.

THE CHEMISTRY OF PROGESTERONE

The chemical structure of progesterone is similar to that of the other sex hormones, such as estrogen and testosterone, and like the other sex hormones, it is converted from the precursor hormone pregnenolone.

The progesterone used in replacement therapy today, whether described as synthetic or natural, is all produced by commercial laboratories. The terms *natural* and *synthetic* refer to the actual structure of the progesterone molecule. Progesterone that is natural has the same structure as the hormone the body produces. In contrast, while synthetic progesterone has the same function as the progesterone produced by the body, its structure differs slightly. In the United States, most prescriptions are for the synthetic form, called a progestin. The most common progestin is Provera, or medroxyprogesterone.

Natural progesterone became available in the early 1980s but initially only as a rectal or vaginal suppository. Although many women found the use of natural progesterone to be helpful, using it as a suppository was messy, since it tended to leak from the rectum or vagina. Progestin remained the preferred form because it was easy to take as a pill and also more absorbable. However, a natural progesterone was subsequently developed in a micronized form (pulverized into tiny particles) that is readily absorbed and is taken orally. In the last seven to ten years, oral micronized estrogen has also become available as an over-the-counter cream. Today, many women prefer using natural progesterone, as it produces fewer side effects.

The role of progesterone in menstruation and pregnancy

The purpose of the menstrual cycle is to prepare the female body for conception and possible pregnancy. The process depends on the balanced interaction of several hormones, especially estrogen and progesterone. Working together, they prepare the lining of the uterus (the endometrium) to receive a fertilized egg, should pregnancy occur. The surge of progesterone after an egg is released from the ovarian follicle greatly stimulates the libido, which increases the likelihood that a sperm will enter the female and unite with the egg.

The increase in production of progesterone at midcycle causes a rise in body temperature of about 0.5° to 1°F, which many women monitor to identify when ovulation is most likely to occur and therefore the days when they are fertile. If the egg does not unite with a sperm, progesterone output declines. This stimulates the cells of the uterine lining to slough off and be excreted, which is experienced as menstruation. A rapid decline in progesterone triggers the monthly menstrual bleeding.

During a woman's monthly cycle, the level of progesterone rises and falls dramatically, from 2 to 3 mg per day in the first half of the month, to 22 mg per day in the second half of the month. Production in some women a week after ovulation may be as high as 30 mg per day.

Should pregnancy occur, the placenta also begins to produce progesterone, greatly adding to the amount in circulation. By the fourth month of gestation, a woman produces ten times her normal amount. During the last months of pregnancy, daily production can be as high as 300 to 400 mg a day. To appreciate the significance of this quantity, consider that the various hormones produced within the body are usually measured in micrograms (a thousandfold less).

How progesterone affects the female body

While estrogen causes tissues to grow and thicken, progesterone has a maturing and growth-limiting effect on these tissues. For example, progesterone prevents the uterine lining from becoming too thick during the second half of the menstrual cycle and even, over time, from becoming cancerous. Progesterone also prevents menstrual bleeding from becoming too profuse or long lasting.

Progesterone and estrogen have a balancing effect in other ways as well, affecting many physical and chemical functions in the body. For example, progesterone acts as a sedative on the nervous system, and high levels of progesterone can cause depression and fatigue. In contrast, estrogen has a stimulatory effect on the nervous system. In fact, levels of estrogen can trigger anxiety, irritability, and mood swings. Progesterone tends to elevate the blood sugar level, while estrogen lowers it. Thus, the healthy balance between these two female sex hormones is crucial.

HOW LIFESTYLE, HEALTH, AND AGING AFFECT PROGESTERONE LEVELS

Progesterone production diminishes with age, but its output is influenced by lifestyle factors as well. Digestive capability and liver function will also influence progesterone levels. Following is a discussion of how all these factors affect progesterone production.

Exercise

Women who exercise a great deal and consequently have low levels of body fat may eventually no longer ovulate once a month. In this event, the body does not have sufficient levels of cholesterol to manufacture the hormones needed to cause ovulation to occur. And when a women is anovulatory, the ovaries cease making progesterone.

Stress

Physical, emotional, and mental stress can inhibit the production of progesterone. When the body is put through long-term physical stress, as is true of athletes, the daily rhythms of hormone production, including progesterone, can be disrupted.

Physiological factors

People with poor digestion are unable to absorb certain hormone precursors, which limits hormone production. Poor liver function, with reduced activity of liver enzyme systems, can also lead to lower levels of progesterone, as the conversion of pregnenolone to DHEA and progesterone is impaired. Elevated levels of HDL can also block this conversion pathway.

Aging

Unfortunately, the balance between estrogen and progesterone does not remain intact as a woman ages. By the time a woman is in her thirties, progesterone production begins to decline. Having an irregular menstrual cycle can also affect progesterone production. This decline continues in perimenopause, when changes occur in both the length of the menstrual cycle and the amount of blood lost. Often, this occurs during a woman's mid to late forties, although the age can vary greatly. Women can begin this process as young as their thirties and as late as their late fifties, and it can last as briefly as one year or as long as five or six years.

In the early stages of menopause, the ovarian follicles begin to atrophy, reducing the ability to produce estrogen. Women ovulate less frequently, thereby producing less progesterone, or no progesterone at all during certain months. In an attempt to force the ovaries to manufacture more hormones, the levels of the pituitary hormone FSH (follicle-stimulating hormone) become elevated. FSH is the hormone that triggers follicular function in the ovaries. Paradoxically, the ovaries may go into overdrive in response to the pituitary stimulation. In fact, for a time the ovaries may produce high levels of estrogen until they are finally exhausted. (When this occurs, estrogen levels may drop permanently, and menstruation ceases.) As a result, hormonal levels may fluctuate during this time, and the balance between estrogen and progesterone is disrupted.

Although both estrogen and progesterone stimulation are needed for healthy menstruation, the overabundance of estrogen and lack of progesterone can cause changes in the menstrual cycle. Too much estrogen causes the uterine lining to grow and thicken excessively. Without the addition of progesterone during the second half of the cycle, the lining continues to thicken and proliferate until it finally outgrows its blood supply and begins to shed. Heavy, irregular bleeding can be the unfortunate result for many women.

At menopause, the production of progesterone declines more than that of estrogen. While estrogen production can fall 75 to 90 percent, progesterone production declines to negligible levels in postmenopausal women. Levels of progesterone in women can be even lower than those in men.

PROGESTERONE AND PEAK PERFORMANCE

As one of the major female sex hormones, progesterone affects many body systems and tissues. Optimal levels of progesterone within the body can provide important support for the following peak-performance traits.

1 Physical vitality and stamina

Progesterone therapy during perimenopause and the postmenopausal years can potentially reduce fatigue and increase energy by improving sleep quality. An often-noted side effect of progesterone therapy is that it causes sleepiness. In fact, this hormone is thought to restore normal sleep patterns. Various reasons for this have been suggested, related to its ability to calm and act as a tranquilizer; see page 621.

2 Mental clarity and acuity

Mental acuity and the ability to concentrate depend on adequate progesterone levels within the body. After menopause, when ovarian progesterone production has ceased, maintaining youthful amounts can be crucial for continuing to meet job requirements. A person working as a lawyer or an accountant for forty years needs to think as quickly and accurately at the end of his or her career as when it began.

Progesterone treatment has been shown to increase mental ability. A study published in 1985 in the *British Medical Journal* followed twenty-three women for four months. Each woman received 300 mg of oral progesterone daily for two continuous months. Those women receiving treatment had a clear improvement in concentration. Similar increases in mental acuity and the ability to remain focused on a subject have also be found in premenopausal and postmenopausal women. Progesterone has also been effective in elderly people who have become senile, helping them to regain some degree of mental alertness. This effect of progesterone may be due to several factors involving brain function. Relatively large amounts of progesterone are present in brain cells, twenty times greater than in the blood. It is thought that progesterone enhances the amount of oxygen in the cells of the brain, thereby increasing mental acuity.

◀4 The ability to get along with other people

Progesterone has a significant effect on mood, thereby affecting how women relate to others both at home and in work situations. For example, pregnant women, who produce great quantities of progesterone, tend to have an exceptional sense of well-being. Conversely, after birth, when progesterone production suddenly plummets, women may develop post-partum depression. Low progesterone levels also contribute to the emotional symptoms associated with PMS, including anxiety, irritability, and depression. Treatment with progesterone has been found to relieve these symptoms. In a study published in 1995 in the *Journal of Assisted Reproduction and Genetics,* twenty-five women with severe PMS and seventeen reproductive-age females participated in a controlled trial. Treatment consisted of a 200 mg vaginal progesterone suppository, taken twice daily. The researchers observed that the women receiving the progesterone reported significant improvement in nervous symptoms.

The association of progesterone with mood swings is evident when considering the years in a woman's life in which they most commonly occur. About 60 percent of women have mild to moderate PMS in their late thirties and forties. These are the perimenopausal years, when hormone production becomes irregular. An additional 15 to 20 percent of women will have symptoms severe enough to disrupt functioning both at home and at work. However, with the onset of menopause, when the ovarian production of progesterone, as well as estrogen, virtually ceases, these symptoms permanently subside. Furthermore, cross-cultural epidemiological studies worldwide show that anxiety disorders and depression are two to three times more common in women than they are in men.

One way in which progesterone may influence mood is through its direct affect on neurotransmitters. According to an article appearing in 1987 in the *International Journal of Fertility,* changes in levels of progesterone have been shown to influence the production and breakdown of brain chemicals that modulate mood. These include the central-nervous-system neurotransmitters dopamine, norepinephrine, acetylcholine, and serotonin. Both the peripheral and the central nervous systems have hormone receptors and react to changes in the level of progesterone. It is thought that the ability of progesterone to generate a sense of well-being depends on this brain-related activity.

▲▲▲ Any woman considering taking progesterone for its performance as well as health benefits should consider using natural progesterone rather than the progestins. Susan has been recommending natural progesterone since the early 1980s and was one of the first physicians to have clinical experience in using it. She has found it to be better tolerated and cause less detrimental effects on such important performance traits as physical energy and mood than the synthetic forms. Research studies are beginning to confirm its benefits. Be sure to consult with a physician who is knowledgeable about how to use natural progesterone.

◄5 The ability to remain calm under pressure

Being able to remain calm under stress is a capability rarely listed on a resume but a prerequisite for many jobs nonetheless. Progesterone helps promote this natural calm. It is sometimes referred to as a natural tranquilizer, as it has a calming and even mildly sedating effect. Taken in high dosages, it has been used as an anesthetic. It is thought that this calming effect is due to the conversion of progesterone into substances that slow activity at GABA (gamma-aminobutyric acid) receptors. GABA is an amino acid that inhibits neurotransmitters (chemicals that relay information from one part of the brain to another) and has a calming effect. While progesterone has a sedating effect on its own, having a balance between estrogen and progesterone levels is crucial for remaining even-tempered under pressure.

A Caution on Using Progesterone

Some women are extremely sensitive to the depressant and sedative effects of progesterone. Progesterone, when prescribed during menopause to these women, may actually cause a form of clinical depression. This is particularly true for the synthetic progestins. Many menopausal women have mistakenly been prescribed antidepressants like Prozac when the real culprit is their progesterone therapy. Check with your physician if you are concerned that your symptoms of depression may be related to hormone therapy.

PROGESTERONE AND HEALTH

Besides its role in the menstrual cycle, progesterone participates in several other vital functions. These other metabolic actions are especially important because they help women to maintain general good health and also help prevent disease. For instance, progesterone helps keep blood sugar levels normal, aids the activity of the thyroid, and functions as a natural diuretic. It also normalizes zinc and copper levels, promotes the metabolic conversion of fat into energy, and normalizes blood clotting. Having sufficient levels of progesterone also helps to prevent the development of a variety of diseases. Progesterone deficiency is a risk factor for menopause symptoms, endometrial cancer, osteoporosis, and certain nerve diseases.

Excessive production of estrogen

During the years preceding menopause, a woman will sometimes produce elevated levels of estrogen as compared with progesterone, which is more likely to be produced in normal or low amounts. This imbalance can lead to health problems such as headaches, fluid retention in the tissues, irregular or heavy menstrual bleeding, and swelling of the breasts premenstrually. Progesterone therapy can help keep these conditions in check.

Elevated levels of estrogen can also overstimulate the growth of the uterine lining and the outer muscular tissue of the uterus, causing the growth of benign tumors called fibroids. Both of these conditions can cause heavy menstrual bleeding, which can, if untreated, lead to severe anemia. Elevated estrogen levels can also stimulate a potentially precancerous condition called endometrial hyperplasia. According to a study published in 1993 in Fertility and Sterility, low doses of progesterone are able to control this growth. The study group was comprised of 157 symptomatic postmenopausal women, who were given from 1.5 to 3 mg of estrogen along with 200 to 300 mg of progesterone. Treatment was monitored for a minimum of five years. Cell division was consistently reduced after nine or more days of progesterone use.

Symptoms of menopause

Between 15 and 20 percent of women who are making the transition into menopause experience hot flashes even while they're still having fairly regular menstrual periods. They may also experience heavy bleeding and premenstrual tension. Unfortunately, estrogen replacement therapy (ERT) cannot be used to suppress hot flashes because many of these women have higher than normal levels of estrogen and often are not ovulating regularly. Thus, ERT used alone could actually intensify the preexisting state of hormonal imbalance. However, progesterone used alone can relieve hot flashes and other vasomotor symptoms in about 60 to 80 percent of women. Because of its sedative and calming effects, progesterone is also useful in treating menopausal mood swings. Unfortunately, progesterone is not particularly useful for the treatment of vaginal atrophy or vaginal and bladder infections due to thinning of the mucous membranes—these symptoms are related to estrogen deficiency.

Endometrial cancer

Prevention of endometrial cancer is the primary reason physicians prescribe progesterone during menopause. This became evident several decades ago when the incidence of uterine cancer increased in American women who were prescribed unopposed estrogen. Estrogen use fell into decline among the menopausal female population until studies showed that combined estrogen therapy could protect women from the development of this cancer. Without the addition of progesterone to an estrogen treatment regimen, the incidence of endometrial (uterine) cancer increases four- to eightfold in women with an intact uterus. The importance of progesterone therapy has been emphasized in a number of important medical studies. In one such study, cited in a review article in the *American Family Physician*, 5563 postmenopausal women were followed for nine years. In women using estrogen alone, the incidence of endometrial cancer was 390.6 cases per 100,000 women per year. In contrast, with combined estrogen and progesterone therapy, the incidence was only 99 cases per 100,000 women per year. Not only does progesterone confer protection in women using ERT, but it actually appears to protect against the development of endometrial cancer in all postmenopausal women. In the same study, women using no ERT at all were at higher risk than those on progesterone because of their own endogenous estrogen. These women developed 245.5 cases of endometrial cancer per 100,000 women per year. Not only has the rate of this cancer declined with the use of progesterone, but those women who develop it tend to do so at a later age.

Heart disease

Various studies suggest that estrogen replacement therapy significantly reduces the incidence of heart disease. However, as just discussed, estrogen increases the risk of uterine cancer. When researchers discovered that adding progesterone to the treatment lowered this risk, combined therapy became a preferred treatment. But a question remained: Does the addition of progesterone eliminate the benefits of estrogen for the heart? This issue has been a concern of physicians and researchers for many years because progesterone has the opposite effect on blood lipids that estrogen does. Progesterone increases low-density lipoproteins (LDLs) and decreases the HDLs. As a result, researchers were concerned that the addition of progestins, although necessary for protection against uterine cancer, would negate the beneficial effects of estrogen on the cardiovascular system.

Several studies have been done to compare the risks and benefits of estrogen alone versus estrogen/progestin therapy. To date, studies lasting more than twelve months do not suggest that progestins used in ERT affect blood lipid levels adversely. Early studies suggest that oral micronized progesterone may have even fewer adverse side effects than the synthetic form of progesterone commonly used. This was confirmed in a study published in 1995 in the *Journal of the American Medical Association*. Regimens of estrogen and progesterone (both progestins and oral micronized progesterone) were studied as to their effect on blood lipids. The researchers found that estrogen used in combination with oral micronized progesterone had more beneficial effects on blood lipids than regimens using synthetic progestins.

Osteoporosis

A woman reaches peak bone mass in her early to mid-thirties, after which bone loss slowly begins, accelerating after menopause. A woman can lose 3 to 5 percent of bone mass per year for the first five years after menopause, and 1 to 1.5 percent per year in subsequent years.

Although there has recently been a great deal of media attention on the role of estrogen in bone health, the benefits of progesterone have received far less attention. Nevertheless, as cited in a review article published in 1990 in *Endocrine Reviews*, a variety of clinical, experimental, and epidemiological data indicate that progesterone plays an important role in bone metabolism. While estrogen does help to prevent osteoporosis by inhibiting calcium loss from the bone and facilitating calcium absorption from the intestinal tract, the addition of progesterone to a treatment regimen may provide even greater benefits. A number of medical studies have confirmed that progesterone therapy increases bone mass by promoting new bone formation. Recent research has led to the conclusion that progesterone acts directly to stimulate new bone by attaching to the osteoblast cell receptors. (These are the cells from which new bone tissue is created.) Most of these studies have examined estrogen/progestin therapy and found it to be beneficial.

In one study, reported in 1988 in the *British Medical Journal*, women using combined progesterone and estrogen therapy had a 5 to 6 percent increase in vertebral bone density per year (the gain was slightly greater percentagewise in women on continuous therapy versus cyclical therapy). In another study, published in 1990 in the *Journal of Gynecological Health*, progesterone and estrogen used in combination increased the bone mineral content significantly, even in women starting the therapy after age sixty. As a result, the addition of progesterone to ERT provides more complete, as well as more effective, treatment for osteoporosis than ERT alone.

A few studies have also suggested that natural progesterone may be effective in protecting women from osteoporosis. John R. Lee, a physician in California, has done much research into the use of progesterone to reverse osteoporosis. The results of one of his studies were published in 1990 in the *International Clinical Nutrition Review*. Dr. Lee selected 100 patients, white postmenopausal women between the ages of thirty-eight and eighty-three. The average age was 65.2 at the beginning of the study. The majority of the women had already experienced some loss of height due to osteoporosis. They were instructed to use conjugated estrogen, 0.3 to 0.625 mg per day for three weeks each month, and progesterone, a 3 percent topical cream, applied daily to the skin for twelve days each month or during the last two weeks of estrogen use. They were also given a dietary and exercise program to follow, plus vitamin and mineral supplements. Alcohol consumption was limited, and no smoking was allowed. The bone health of the women was followed for at least three years.

All the women in the study experienced some degree of progressive increase in bone mineral density, as well as improvement in such clinical symptoms as height stabilization, pain relief, and an increase in physical activity. During the course of the study, there were also no fractures due to osteoporosis per se. These improvements occurred independent of the woman's age. The women commonly had an increase in the density of vertebral bone of 10 percent in the first six to twelve months of treatment. This increase was purportedly followed by additional yearly increases of 3 to 5 percent. This degree of bone remineralization over a relatively short period of time constitutes an exceptionally good therapeutic response.

Susan has worked with patients who have been found to have decreased bone density but have refused conventional estrogen/progestin therapy. One such woman, Honda, chose instead to use natural progesterone cream along with a variety of dietary and plant-based estrogens. She also adopted a vegetarian diet and started performing resistance exercises with weights. Although she had a higher than normal risk of osteoporosis given a 20 percent loss of bone mass by age fifty, she showed a steady improvement in her bone density in the years after initiating this program.

Lowered libido

Progesterone level is an important component of both men's and women's ability to maintain their libido, or sex drive. This was observed in one study by John Lee that was primarily designed to assess the benefit of progesterone on bone health. In conducting a study of 100 post-menopausal women for three years, Dr. Lee found that one of the effects of treatment was a restoration of libido to normal levels. This is thought to occur through progesterone's effect on the brain, as libido is primarily a brain function. Animal studies have demonstrated that while estrogen readies the brain cells involved with libido, progesterone is the hormone that activates them. Certainly for most people, continuing to have fulfilling sexual activity is an essential part of life. Progesterone offers one way to restore this ability in those women who have experienced a decline in this function.

Nerve damage

Progesterone helps to maintain the health of the nervous system. Nerves extend throughout the body and are coated with a protective covering, the myelin sheaths. These help protect the nerves from injury caused by trauma and chemical damage, and prevent the electrical impulses from being short-circuited. Myelin is produced by specialized cells called Schwann cells. These cells also produce progesterone, which makes the manufacture of myelin possible.

Besides helping to maintain healthy nerves, progesterone may also be of use in repairing nerve damage. Animal studies have shown that progesterone levels near the site of a nerve injury are far more concentrated than they normally are in the blood, and when the animals receive additional progesterone, the myelin sheaths surrounding the nerves thicken. This association suggests the possibility that progesterone may one day be useful in the treatment of diseases involving nerve damage, such as multiple sclerosis, which involves a loss of myelin and a resulting impairment of communication functions of the nerves.

SUMMARY

Progesterone, the other major female sex hormone, acts together with estrogen to facilitate menstruation and pregnancy. A healthy balance of these two hormones is important for health and mood in women. Sufficient progesterone is necessary to support physical energy, the ability to concentrate, the ability to remain calm under pressure, and an even emotional state. Aging, excess exercise, stress, and poor health cause the production of progesterone to diminish, affecting health as well as performance. Health conditions caused by a lack of progesterone include elevated levels of estrogen, hot flashes, endometrial cancer, heart disease, and osteoporosis. Supplementation with progesterone, whether natural or synthetic, helps to prevent and correct these conditions.

LABORATORY TESTS FOR HORMONE LEVELS

Laboratory testing is currently available to assess the levels of all the major sex hormones.

TESTS TO EVALUATE THE PRODUCTION OF PREGNENOLONE

Levels of pregnenolone can be measured in the blood and the saliva. Tests can be ordered to assess the quantity present of pregnenolone, pregnenolone-sulfate, and 17-hydroxy-pregnenolone. The latter is the intermediary hormone in the conversion of pregnenolone to DHEA. Health care practitioners who place patients on pregnenolone therapy recommend especially close monitoring of levels, since taking this hormone as a supplement is somewhat new.

Experts caution on the usefulness of such tests. There is not a lot of information on what consists of a normal reading in different age groups. It is also not known how accurately blood levels represent tissue levels of the hormone. Various tissues may also make use of pregnenolone in different ways, so that a blood reading would tell little about its eventual activity level. Taking these questions into consideration, the following ranges for blood levels of pregnenolone are currently used by several labs:

Range of pregnenolone production in adult men: 0 to 200 ng/dl

Range of pregnenolone production in adult women: 10 to 230 ng/dl

Range of pregnenolone production in postmenopausal women:
5 to 100 ng/dl

TESTS TO EVALUATE THE PRODUCTION OF DHEA

The DHEA in the blood is a combination of DHEA sulfate (DHEA-S) and unbound, or free, DHEA. It is generally thought that unbound DHEA is most active and that DHEA-S is not fully metabolically active. Therefore, it is important that any lab assessment distinguish between the two. When a physician is assessing a patient's DHEA levels in relation to specific illnesses, this differentiation takes on special meaning. For instance, research has shown that DHEA levels, but not levels of DHEA-S, can be predictive of the progression of HIV to AIDS.

Levels of DHEA are routinely assessed using a blood test, but salivary testing is also thought to be accurate. DHEA can also be assessed using a twenty-four-hour urine test.

A person taking DHEA supplementation needs to have initial levels tested and then be tested again every few months, to keep the amount in the upper normal range typical of a young person. As supplementing with DHEA is a relatively new practice, it is a particularly good idea to have levels monitored regularly. However, some physicians believe that this is unnecessary when the dosages used are low. A cautious approach is also advised to monitor metabolites of DHEA such as androsterone and etiocholanolone, as well as hormone metabolites such as testosterone. This can be done using a twenty-four-hour urine test.

Some practitioners also think it is important to monitor DHEA levels if an individual has a significant illness, and that at age forty, all people should obtain a baseline reading.

Range of DHEA blood levels in adult men:	180 to 250 ng/dl
Range of DHEA blood levels in adult women:	130 to 980 ng/dl
Ranges of DHEA-S blood levels in adult men:	
Aged 31 to 50	59 to 452 µg/dl
Aged 51 to 60	20 to 413 µg/dl
Aged 61 to 83	0 to 283 µg/dl
Ranges of DHEA-S blood levels in adult women:	
Aged 31 to 50	2 to 379 µg/dl
Postmenopausal	30 to 260 µg/dl
Range of DHEA salivary levels in men:	50 to 200 pg/ml
Range of DHEA salivary levels in women:	40 to 140 pg/ml

TESTS TO EVALUATE THE PRODUCTION OF TESTOSTERONE

Total testosterone production in men is somewhat difficult to assess, as the amount varies during the day, with higher levels occurring in the morning; there are also seasonal variations. Furthermore, a normal testosterone reading may mask a testosterone deficiency because the majority of testosterone in the bloodstream is bound to the protein SHBG and the protein carrier albumin. Only about 4 percent of testosterone in the bloodstream is free and unbound and available to body tissues, where it can perform its functions. As a person ages, an increasing amount of testosterone remains bound, so in an older person, a normal reading of circulating testosterone does not necessarily indicate that adequate amounts of testosterone are bioavailable. Routine laboratory testing measures total hormone concentration, so special assays are required to measure the amount of active free testosterone.

One useful method of measurement is saliva testing, since the testosterone in the saliva is the type that is unbound. From 2 to 5 ml of saliva is needed. Samples remain viable for up to seven days but must be analyzed within that time. A person submitting a saliva sample must note the time of day it was taken, as hourly levels vary. Persons using testosterone creams applied to the skin may have very high readings. Although testosterone blood levels can be tested through hospital and clinical laboratory facilities, saliva testing is currently being done by only a few specialized laboratories. Most of these laboratories require a physician's prescription in order to have testing done; for a laboratory that will allow consumers to request their own sex hormone testing, see the appendix.

Ranges of testosterone levels in women:

A.M.:   20 to 40 pg/ml

P.M.:   10 to 20 pg/ml

Ranges of testosterone levels in men:

A.M.:   75 to 150 pg/ml

P.M.:   50 to 100 pg/ml

TESTS TO EVALUATE THE PRODUCTION OF ESTROGEN

Testing is available to assess blood levels of two forms of estrogen, estradiol and estriol. A measurement can be taken indirectly by sampling the saliva for the presence of these hormones. Salivary levels are approximately 1 percent of the total blood concentration.

Levels of estradiol normally fluctuate during the menstrual cycle and decline significantly with menopause. Variability is rather broad among individuals. The use of estrogen creams results in much higher readings, while women taking oral hormone replacement therapy show the same pattern of ranges as those not supplementing. Estriol production is uniformly low throughout a woman's life, except in pregnancy, when high levels occur. Men also have consistently low levels of estriol.

Ranges of estradiol in women:

Follicular phase:	< 2 to 4 pg/ml
Early luteal phase:	4 to 10 pg/ml
Mid luteal (peak) phase:	2 to 4 pg/ml
Postmenopausal women:	1 to 2 pg/ml
Women taking oral contraceptives:	< 1 pg/ml
Range of estradiol in men:	< 1 pg/ml

Ranges of estriol:

Nonpregnant women:	< 15 pg/ml
Men:	< 15 pg/ml
With estriol supplementation:	20 to 500 pg/ml

TESTS TO EVALUATE THE PRODUCTION OF PROGESTERONE

Progesterone levels are commonly assessed through blood testing; however, newer testing methods use saliva. The level of progesterone measured in the saliva represents about 1 percent of the total blood concentration. This test is thought to be representative of the free versus the bound progesterone within the body. Peak levels with supplemental progesterone use, whether taken orally or as a cream, occur about three hours after use. The lowest levels occur just prior to the next scheduled dose. Readings of progesterone levels help detect luteal insufficiency in the early stages of pregnancy. Progesterone levels are also monitored in women on replacement therapy.

Ranges of salivary progesterone without supplementation in women:

Follicular phase:	0.05 to 0.1 ng/ml
Luteal phase:	0.05 to 0.3 ng/ml

Range of salivary progesterone in men: 0.02 to 0.05 ng/ml

Ranges in saliva with progesterone supplementation:

Transdermal cream users: > 0.5 ng/ml (peak levels to 100 ng/ml)

Oral micronized progesterone users: 0.05 to 0.5 ng/ml

Ranges of blood progesterone in women:

Menstruating women, luteal phase (midcycle): 7 to 28 ng/ml

Normal, untreated, postmenopausal women: 0.03 to 0.3 ng/ml

After three months' treatment with transdermal progesterone: 3 to 4 ng/ml

12

RESTORING YOUR SEX HORMONES

WHEN SUSAN BEGAN her medical training, nearly thirty years ago, hormone replacement therapy (HRT) was available only through a doctor's prescription or administered by injection in a medical office. Very few types of hormone replacement therapy were available, and the use of precursor hormones like DHEA and pregnenolone was virtually unknown. Consumers were uninformed about the benefits (and risks) of hormone therapy, and few sources of information were available. This situation has changed dramatically over the last three decades. Books and articles on this subject have proliferated, and hormone therapy is now discussed constantly in the media. The types of hormones and their availability in many types of delivery systems—from pills, creams, and patches to sprays and tinctures—offer a vast and potentially confusing choice of products. While certain hormones, such as testosterone and estrogen, must still be obtained through a physician's prescription, others such as progesterone, DHEA, and pregnenolone can be purchased freely from health food stores and pharmacies. Many people today are self-diagnosing and self-medicating themselves with these readily available nonprescription hormones.

Although there is much consumer interest in hormone therapy, many men and women are confused or uninformed about their choices of hormonal therapy. They don't know what to ask at medical visits to determine which hormonal regimens, if any, would suit them best; and they are often unaware of, or do not understand, the possible side effects or long-term risks of HRT. To compound this confusion, there are a wide variety of herbs, vitamins, and foods available that can also be used for their hormonal properties, providing much of the benefits of the hormones themselves.

This chapter provides information about and guidelines for the use of the many available types of hormone therapies. This information will enable you to obtain the best results when using hormones to enhance both performance and health.

CUSTOMIZING YOUR HORMONE REPLACEMENT PROGRAM

As we discussed in the previous chapter, there are many different hormone replacement therapies available. These include conventional hormone replacement therapy and natural hormones synthesized in the laboratory from plant sources, as well as a variety of nutrients such as herbs, vitamins, essential fatty acids, and foods that offer sex hormone–like activity.

Your choice of hormone therapy should be based, in part, on your own philosophy of health care. Some individuals prefer to use nonprescription self-care treatment options that can be acquired in natural-food stores and pharmacies without a doctor's prescription. Others prefer to use conventional HRT prescribed and monitored by their physician. Both of these options can be effective, depending on your predilection. If you suspect or are concerned that you might have a medical condition that makes the correct choice of a particular hormone replacement therapy crucial for your health and well-being, it is important to consult a physician before making a decision. For example, there are medical conditions, such as breast or prostate cancer, that conventional HRT such as estrogen and testosterone therapy can actually worsen. In contrast, conventional HRT may be entirely appropriate for women with severe osteoporosis or high risk for heart attack or stroke.

However, the use of hormones should not be treated in an offhand or casual manner. Serious consequences can occur from overdosing with any sex hormone, as has been explained in chapter 11. To enjoy the therapeutic benefits and avoid the potential negative side effects of hormone use, it is important to start at the lowest therapeutic dosages. If these dosages are not sufficient, continue to gradually increase them until the desired therapeutic response is obtained. If side effects begin to occur, cut your dosage back immediately.

Furthermore, if you decide, after having begun a regimen of HRT, that it is not for you, begin to taper your usage of these hormones gradually over a several-month period, going from daily to every other day to every third day until your intake tapers off to zero. Individuals who go "cold turkey" are likely to have rebound symptoms more severe than the ones they originally took the hormones to relieve.

Taking hormones in combination

It is often beneficial to combine several types of hormonal therapies. For example, men may choose to take both pregnenolone and DHEA for their effects on both cognitive function and memory, as well as to increase their level of testosterone within the body. Women may take estrogen and progesterone in combination, both to restore bone mass and to prevent cancer of the uterus. In addition, some women take estrogen and testosterone together to restore their libido after menopause. It is best to consult a physician before taking various hormones in combination. In fact, some of these combinations are available through a physician's prescription.

PREGNENOLONE

As described in the preceding chapter, pregnenolone is the precursor hormone from which all other sex hormones are made. In the last few years, this powerful compound has become available over the counter and is sold in pharmacies and natural-food stores. It can also be ordered by a physician from a compounding pharmacy (see the appendix).

The Mexican wild yam contains the raw material from which pregnenolone is made. The plant belongs to the *Dioscorea* species, and the active steroid compound used in manufacture is diosgenin, which has a chemical structure closely related to the structure of the hormones in our own body. (The Mexican wild yam is not related to the yams and sweet potatoes found in the supermarket, and eating these does not increase hormone levels.) To make pregnenolone, diosgenin must be converted in a laboratory. For this reason, when purchasing pregnenolone, it is important to note if the container specifically states that the product contains pregnenolone, rather than just an unprocessed extract of wild yam.

Many people take pregnenolone rather than DHEA, which is also a powerful precursor hormone, because a much lower dose of pregnenolone can enhance the central-nervous-system function. Other advantages of pregnenolone are that it has more potent anti-inflammatory effects and is less likely than DHEA to cause side effects such as skin problems and facial hair.

Methods of Administration

Pregnenolone is available as an oral pill or capsule, in a micronized form, as a sublingual tablet, as an ointment or cream, and in a liposome-based oral spray. The degree to which pregnenolone is absorbed and the amount that eventually enters the general circulation depends on which route of delivery is used. Pregnenolone in capsule form, taken orally, first travels to the liver, which metabolizes it into other hormones. As a result, the amount of pregnenolone in circulation will be less than what was consumed. In contrast, micronized pregnenolone—in the form of tiny particles, taken as a capsule—is absorbed from the intestines directly into the lymphatic system, with most of it initially bypassing the liver. Another way to bypass the liver is by taking a sublingual tablet, which is absorbed through the tissue under the tongue. There is also a topical cream, a spray, a chewing gum, and a liquid, all of which can deliver pregnenolone through the mouth.

In retail stores, pregnenolone is available in capsule form in various dosages, including 10, 15, 25, 30, and 50 mg. It can also be found in combination with DHEA, vitamin C, vitamin E, and herbs such as ginkgo biloba. Compounding pharmacies working with physicians can prepare pregnenolone in doses from 2 to 100 mg. These pharmacies offer pregnenolone as a pill, a sublingual tablet, a cream, and a micronized capsule. Different delivery systems produce markedly different rates of assimilation and absorption. Be careful not to overdose if you switch from one method to another. Also, most dosages you will read about are based on pregnenolone in capsule form. Use the information below as a guideline for using a different delivery system. This information was supplied by VitalSource Nutrition.

Capsules. The assimilation and absorption rate is between 30 and 50 percent, because the pregnenolone is first processed through the liver before going into the bloodstream. Higher absorption rates may be attained by opening a capsule and releasing the contents under the tongue; hold this for a minute or two before swallowing.

Liquid sublinguals. Assimilation and absorption rates run as high as 90 to 95 percent. This is because these are held under the tongue and the absorption is directly into the bloodstream, avoiding the liver. Sublinguals usually provide 5 mg of pregnenolone per drop, while liposome sprays usually contain 7.5 mg per spray.

Creams. The assimilation and absorption rate is between 50 and 85 percent. Absorption is also directly into the bloodstream, again avoiding the liver. The absorption rate depends on the quality of the cream, what carriers are present, where on the body the cream is applied (areas where skin is thinner or areas of fatty tissue), the cleanliness of the skin, and the humidity.

SUGGESTED DOSAGES

When pregnenolone is used for hormone replacement therapy, the dosage depends on sex and age. In general, any regimen of pregnenolone supplementation should begin at the lower end of the dosage range. To achieve a general improvement in mood and well-being, the recommended dosage is 10 mg per day to start (individuals who are sensitive to the use of supplements may want to start at 5 mg per day). If you notice an immediate therapeutic effect, then stay at this dosage. If, on the other hand, you do not notice any effect from the use of pregnenolone at this dosage, increase your dosage by 10 mg on a weekly basis until the desired result has been achieved. Take pregnenolone in the morning, before or with breakfast. Do not take it in the evening, as it can increase your level of alertness and interfere with sleep.

When pregnenolone is used to treat chronic health problems such as rheumatoid arthritis, effective dosages used in studies range from 100 to 200 mg. However, a dosage this high should be taken only under the supervision of a physician.

For men

For men in their forties, suggested dosages are from 5 to 10 mg, taken in the morning. For men aged fifty to sixty-five, the dose is 10 to 15 mg, also taken in the morning. Men over sixty-five may require from 10 to 30 mg daily.

For women

The range of dosages for women in their forties is 5 to 10 mg, taken in the morning. For postmenopausal women, dosages range from 10 to 15 mg, taken in the morning. If a woman is also taking progesterone as part of her hormone replacement program, the dosage may need to be reduced, as pregnenolone is converted into progesterone, adding to the overall supply of the body. Women over sixty-five may need from 10 to 20 mg daily, taken in the morning.

SIDE EFFECTS

While animal and human studies have shown that pregnenolone is nontoxic, this powerful hormone should be used carefully, preferably under the supervision of a health care professional. There has been no formal assessment of its safety when used for years, and research on its side effects is only in the early stages. For instance, it is not known with certainty whether it is safe to allow pregnenolone to enter the general circulation without first passing through the liver, where it can be partially broken down.

If a person is taking more pregnenolone than their system can handle, side effects such as irritability, anxiety, and anger may be experienced. Although there are no studies available, physicians who prescribe hormones suggest that pregnenolone and DHEA be taken in the morning as the body appears to have its highest concentrations of these hormones at that time. If, however, pregnenolone is taken later in the day, it can cause overactivity and heightened alertness in sensitive individuals and may prevent them from falling asleep.

If you are taking any prescription or over-the-counter drugs, you should check with your physician for any possible negative interactions or dosage changes.

A Caution on Taking Pregnenolone

Individuals under forty, who normally produce sufficient levels of sex hormones, should not take pregnenolone. It is also not recommended during pregnancy, for people with cardiac problems, or for those who are taking multiple medications. Also, men and women who are using conventional HRT must consult with their prescribing physician before supplementing with pregnenolone, as it may effect the HRT dosages. Pregnenolone is a powerful hormone and should be treated as such.

DHEA

DHEA is a powerful precursor hormone from which the body produces testosterone, estrogen, and progesterone. Until 1996, DHEA was regulated by the FDA and required a doctor's prescription. Now DHEA can be purchased in health food stores, most drugstores, and by mail order. While DHEA has gained great popularity as its availability has increased, it continues to be considered an alternative therapy.

The majority of DHEA is produced in laboratories from diosgenin. Research on DHEA is far behind that of other sex hormones such as estrogen and testosterone. Much still needs to be learned about optimal dosage, timing, and how the hormone is best administered. There is a question of whether it is appropriate to raise DHEA to youthful levels or simply to a level that is adequate, given a person's age. Clinical trials are under way; in the meantime, clinicians who regularly prescribe DHEA generally agree on a certain range of starting dosages and recommend a gradual increase if needed.

A Caution on Taking DHEA

Before starting DHEA supplementation, it is imperative to measure the amount of DHEA in the blood, and during the course of treatment, DHEA levels should continue to be monitored as regularly as every month. In fact, we strongly recommend that any individual considering taking DHEA consult an informed health care professional before starting a regimen. Taking more than 50 mg of DHEA definitely requires supervision.

METHODS OF ADMINISTRATION

Various preparations of DHEA are on the market, as well as yam extract, and it is important to understand the differences between these products. The conversion of the extract to DHEA can be achieved only in the laboratory, not in the human body. Therefore, natural yam extract, while it does have some benefits, does not increase blood levels of DHEA. This was confirmed in a study published in 1996 in *Life Science*. Seven men and women, aged sixty-five to eighty-two, were given yam extract for three weeks with no change in their DHEA level. In contrast, when the same group received 85 mg of DHEA a day, their blood levels of DHEA doubled.

Different delivery systems produce markedly different rates of assimilation and absorption of DHEA. Be careful not to overdose if you switch from one method to another. Also, most dosages you will read about are based on DHEA in capsule form. Use the information below as a guideline for using a different delivery system. This information was supplied by VitalSource Nutrition.

Capsules. The assimilation and absorption rate is between 30 and 50 percent, because the DHEA is first processed through the liver before going into the bloodstream. Higher absorption rates may be attained by opening a capsule and pouring the contents under the tongue; hold this for a minute or two before swallowing it.

Liquid sublinguals. Assimilation and absorption rates run as high as 90 to 95 percent. This is because these are held under the tongue and the absorption is directly into the bloodstream, avoiding the liver. Sublinguals usually provide 5 mg of DHEA per drop, while liposome sprays usually contain 7.5 mg per spray.

Note: In this method of delivery, the hormone bypasses the liver, and a significant amount of DHEA is able to enter the general circulation. Be sure to adjust your dose for the different absorption rate that sublinguals have from capsules.

Creams. The assimilation and absorption rate is between 50 and 85 percent. Absorption is also directly into the bloodstream, again avoiding the liver. The absorption rate depends on the quality of the cream, what carriers are present, where on the body the cream is applied (areas where skin is thinner or areas of fatty tissue), the cleanliness of the skin, and the humidity.

SUGGESTED DOSAGES

DHEA is most often taken in the form of capsules, which come in 5 mg, 10 mg, 25 mg, and 50 mg dosages. Once absorbed, the DHEA travels to the liver, where much of it is converted into androgens and estrogen. Because of this, not all the DHEA ingested enters the general circulation. Micronized DHEA (the hormone broken into tiny particles) is more efficiently absorbed by the body because the small size of the particles allows them to enter first the lymphatic system and then the general circulation, initially bypassing the liver. Since DHEA is a fat-soluble hormone, it is better absorbed when taken with food. DHEA taken orally is quickly absorbed, and blood levels rise within one hour.

Some physicians recommend taking DHEA in the morning to reflect the body's own production of the hormone by the adrenal glands. Taken later in the day, DHEA can have a stimulating effect and sometimes causes insomnia; however, for a person suffering from a condition such as chronic-fatigue syndrome, this energizing effect could be of benefit.

For men

It is appropriate for men to supplement with DHEA if blood levels of the hormone are depressed. Starting dosages should range from 10 to 25 mg per day. This can be increased weekly, adding 5 to 10 mg to a maximum dosage of 50 mg per day, if the smaller dosage does not produce the desired results or if blood levels of DHEA do not rise sufficiently. Many physicians who recommend the use of DHEA in their practice often do baseline testing and only recommend this hormone if the levels are low. Testing can be done through blood, saliva, or a twenty-four-hour urine test. Once DHEA therapy is started, hormone levels can be rechecked every month or two until therapeutic levels are reached.

Note: To insure complete safety, since DHEA is converted into testosterone, a prostate-specific antigen (PSA) test should also be done, as testosterone can stimulate the growth of a preexisting prostate cancer.

For women

DHEA levels begin to decline significantly in women after menopause, so supplementation with DHEA may be helpful in this age group. Beginning dosages should range from 5 to 15 mg a day, then be increased by 5 to 10 mg a day, as needed. DHEA dosages in women should not exceed 25 mg per day. Susan has found that women tend to be much more sensitive to DHEA than men and may have side effects when using this hormone. Thus, dosages should normally be kept lower than in men.

There is no reason for women who have not reached menopause or perimenopause to consider taking DHEA replacement therapy. Women with normal menstrual cycles have no need for supplementing with DHEA since their bodies are making sufficient amounts of this hormone. Susan occasionally has younger women patients who do so, and she strongly recommends against it.

Note: Women should have a mammogram and pap smear test done before beginning DHEA supplementation to avoid the risk of stimulating a preexisting cancer of the reproductive tract, since DHEA will increase the levels of the major sex hormones.

SIDE EFFECTS

DHEA is generally considered safe when taken in recommended dosages of 25 mg or less. While some sensitive people may experience side effects with dosages as low as 5 mg, side effects usually occur only when DHEA is taken in much higher amounts. Anyone taking over 50 mg a day of DHEA should be under a physician's supervision. Elevated doses of DHEA can actually prevent the adrenal glands from making the quantity of DHEA they normally produce.

As DHEA is a precursor hormone, which side effects occur in women depends on whether DHEA is being converted to male or female sex hormones. This varies from woman to woman depending on her genetic predisposition. Side effects of DHEA supplementation can include emotional symptoms such as irritability and depression, headaches, menstrual irregularity, and fatigue. DHEA may also have a slight masculinizing effect, especially in older women, who may develop mild acne and, even more rarely, facial hair.

There may also be long-term side effects from using high doses of DHEA. If a person has a family history of certain cancers that are hormone dependent, such as prostate cancer in men and cancers of the ovary, uterus, and breast in women, DHEA supplementation may increase the risk of developing these types of cancer. DHEA may also affect reproduction; therefore, taking the hormone is not recommended for women who are pregnant or breast-feeding.

Physicians who prescribe hormones suggest that DHEA be taken in the morning, as the body appears to have its highest concentrations at that time. If you are taking any prescription or over-the-counter drugs, you should check with your physician for any possible negative interactions or dosage changes.

Recent reports indicate that some individuals who have taken dosages of between 25 and 50 mg for only three to four weeks have experienced irregularities in heart rhythm. This information reinforces the advice that, if you are self-medicating, you should start at very low doses and only attempt higher doses under the supervision of a medical doctor who specializes in hormone therapy.

NATURAL TECHNIQUES FOR ENHANCING DHEA PRODUCTION

If a person has healthy glands that are capable of producing hormones, DHEA production can also be increased through exercise and by practicing stress reduction techniques and meditation. In one study, people who meditate were found to have DHEA levels comparable to nonmeditators who were five to ten years younger.

TESTOSTERONE

Although testosterone is a major male sex hormone, it benefits both men and women (see the preceding chapter), and supplementation can support both peak performance and health.

TESTOSTERONE THERAPY FOR MEN

Testosterone therapy has traditionally been used to treat a condition called hypogonadism, in which the sexual organs of young males do not develop properly due to an abnormally low production of testosterone. However, older men in greater numbers are also using testosterone replacement therapy to combat the signs and symptoms of aging.

As midlife women are turning to hormone replacement therapy, midlife and older men are realizing that they may also need to supplement with hormones. Although males do not experience the abrupt decline in sex hormone production that women do in menopause, their production of testosterone does diminish with age. Physicians are prescribing testosterone for men over forty to increase their sexual drive, overall assertiveness, vitality, and well-being.

Testosterone is available as a synthetic compound and is also derived from natural sources. Each type has its own means of administration.

Synthetic testosterone

The two primary ways that synthetic testosterone is delivered to the body are by injection or through the use of a transdermal (skin) patch. Subdermal pellets are also used.

Injections. Injection is the form of delivery longest in use. Injections contain testosterone cypionate, testosterone enanthate, or testosterone propionate. The form of testosterone women normally take, methyl testosterone, is not recommended for men, as men who have used this have had a higher incidence of liver tumors.

The dosage for injections of testosterone to increase sperm count ranges from 100 to 200 mg/ml, given every four to six weeks. Some men prefer injection delivery to the patch because an injection has a surge effect, providing a high level of hormones. However, the trade-off is that this peak is followed by an abrupt decline, so there is no consistent level of testosterone in the body.

Transdermal patches. Until recent years, the only synthetic testosterone patch available on the market had to be applied to the scrotum, delivering from 4 to 6 mg of testosterone. But now patches have been developed that can be worn on the chest, abdomen, thighs, arms, or upper back. The benefit of the new patches, according to SmithKline Beecham, the manufacturer of Androderm, is that testosterone is supplied throughout the day in quantities that mirror a man's natural rhythm of production.

The patch is applied at 10 P.M. and left on for twenty-four hours before being replaced, resulting in a peak of testosterone in the early-morning hours, followed by a steady level of the hormone throughout the rest of the day.

It is important to rotate where the patches are placed on the body from day to day. They must not be applied to bony areas or any place on the body that receives pressure, as while a person is sleeping in bed. Such continuous pressure can result in skin irritation from the patch or the adhesive.

Androderm is available in a 2.5 mg dose, to be used twice a day, or in a newer version that supplies 5 mg and is used once a day. Androderm supplies testosterone as testosterone USP, which has the exact form of the testosterone that the body makes.

There is also a more recently introduced patch product, from Alza Corporation, called Testoderm TTS. This is a thin, clear patch that can be worn on the arm, back, or upper buttocks. It contains 5 mg of testosterone and is worn for a twenty-four-hour period. According to Alza, their patch is an improvement over others on the market in that it can be removed for activities such as bathing and swimming and later reapplied. Placement of their patch does not need to be rotated, and in a clinical study of 457 men, done over a period of six weeks, there was a low incidence of skin irritation.

As the patch delivers a considerable amount of testosterone, it is not suitable for women, for men with a history of breast or prostate cancer, or for geriatric patients, who may develop prostatic hyperplasia (enlargement of the prostate gland) or carcinoma (new cancerous growth that occurs in skin tissue).

Subdermal administration. Pellets containing testosterone can be implanted beneath the skin. These contain 75 mg of testosterone USP and provide sustained release of the hormone. Treatment consists of implanting two such pellets, providing a total of 150 mg of testosterone over a period of four to six months.

Natural testosterone

Natural testosterone is made from either the Mexican wild yam or soy. While this type of testosterone is not readily available through most pharmacies, it may be obtained from compounding pharmacies. These pharmacies typically offer hormone therapies, like testosterone, that are produced in the laboratory from preformed steroid molecules found within plants. Some individuals prefer this type of hormone since it more closely replicates the hormones made by our own body.

Some men prefer the use of topical natural testosterone, applied as a cream rather than taken as an oral pill. An average dosage is 50 mg a day. Once the cream is absorbed, its duration of action is brief, and it is rapidly excreted within a twenty-four-hour period.

Side effects

When testosterone therapy is administered to younger men, the side effects can include too frequent or persistent erections. The effect of the hormone on bone maturation must be monitored by assessing bone age of the wrist and hand every six months. In boys, testosterone may accelerate the maturation of bone without appropriate linear growth, preventing the child from reaching his final mature height.

In mature men, a side effect of testosterone is an elevation in the level of red blood cells, which if they become too high, can increase the risk of blood clots. Red blood cell levels should be checked routinely. Testosterone may also stimulate the growth of an existing prostate cancer.

Note: If you are considering testosterone therapy, make sure that your physician performs a prostate-specific antigen (PSA) test before initiating treatment. This is particularly important if you are fifty years of age or older, since most cases of prostate cancer are diagnosed in older men.

TESTOSTERONE THERAPY FOR WOMEN

Now that hormone replacement therapy has become more generally accepted, more women also are beginning to consider supplementing with testosterone. At about age twenty, a woman produces peak levels of estrogen, progesterone, and testosterone, but by the time she reaches midlife and passes through menopause, production of these hormones is greatly diminished. To remedy this, estrogen and progesterone are routinely prescribed to restore a woman to youthful hormone status. However, testosterone, which was very much a part of her original hormonal makeup, is rarely added into the mix. It is estimated that less than

5 percent of menopausal women who are taking estrogen also supplement with testosterone.

Among those women who do decide to take this hormone, the most common reasons are its ability to help prevent vaginal discomfort and soreness while increasing sex drive. In her practice, Susan has seen testosterone rapidly restore libido, which is an issue for many of her patients as it affects the pleasurable aspects of intimate relationships. Testosterone is also prescribed for postmenopausal women who are troubled by abnormally low body weight, poor musculature, poor coordination, and osteoporosis.

Physicians who practice conventional medicine prescribe testosterone in the form of capsules. However, there are other forms of testosterone that are considered alternative in that the average pharmacy does not stock them. These include testosterone creams and gels.

Synthetic testosterone

The two forms of synthetic-testosterone administration for women are by capsule and subdermally.

Capsules. The synthetic androgen methyltestosterone has been used clinically for many years. Taken orally as a capsule, the product name is Android, from ICN Pharmaceuticals. Each capsule contains 10 mg of the hormone. Replacement therapy starts at 10 mg a day and can be gradually increased to a limit of 50 mg per day.

Testosterone is also marketed combined with estrogen, in a product called Estratest. The full-strength capsule contains 1.25 mg of esterified estrogen and 2.5 mg of methyltestosterone. There is also a half-strength capsule. Combined estrogen/testosterone therapy is not appropriate for all women. It is probably most useful in women who have undergone surgical removal of their ovaries (oophorectomy) or whose ovaries have stopped producing even small amounts of testosterone and estrogen soon after menopause. Estratest is recommended for short-term use only, to treat moderate to severe hot flashes associated with menopause. The hormone replacement should be taken for three weeks on and one week off. Medication should be stopped or reduced at three- to six-month intervals.

The drawback of orally administered testosterone is that it is poorly absorbed once in the digestive tract.

Subdermal administration. While this delivery method is more common for men, some women have testosterone pellets implanted beneath the skin. These contain 75 mg of testosterone USP and provide sustained release of the hormone. One pellet can be used for three to six months.

Natural testosterone

Natural testosterone is produced by compounding pharmacies (see the appendix), which are able to formulate a wide range of dosages. These can be prepared as a cream or a gel, the two most popular forms, or as sublingual tablets or oral capsules.

Creams. According to Madison Pharmacy Associates, a women's health-prescription compounding pharmacy, 0.2 mg/g and 0.5 mg/g testosterone creams are commonly used. One-quarter teaspoon provides 1 g of cream and 0.5 mg of testosterone. A typical dose is $^1/_8$ to $^1/_4$ tsp., used daily in the morning. The cream is applied to various sites, which are rotated, including the inner thigh, the back of the hand, the abdomen, and the arm. An advantage of testosterone cream is that, once absorbed through the skin, it immediately enters the general circulation and travels directly to target cells. Only later does the testosterone pass through the liver, which then begins to metabolize, or break down, the hormone.

Gels. The gel is normally applied to vaginal tissue, from which the testosterone is absorbed into the bloodstream.

Sublingual tablets. Sublingual tablets are well absorbed. Women usually begin with doses of 2 to 5 mg, but even a dose of only 0.5 mg may be sufficient. A reduced dose may be appropriate for a woman who is also taking estrogen, because estrogen activates testosterone receptor sites and strengthens its hormonal effect.

Oral capsules. Capsules can be prepared with no preservatives, which some people prefer. However, capsules do have a disadvantage in that, once absorbed, the testosterone must first pass through the liver before entering the general circulation. Because the liver metabolizes the hormone, a smaller quantity of less active testosterone reaches target cells.

Side effects

The downside of women supplementing with testosterone is that, when taken in high amounts, masculinization can occur. A woman's voice may deepen, she may develop more facial hair, and there may be clitoral enlargement. Acne may develop, and existing skin problems can worsen. A woman may also experience changes in her menstrual cycle, and if a woman who is pregnant takes testosterone, a female fetus can develop male sexual characteristics. However, these effects are not likely to happen when testosterone is administered in smaller dosages.

There is a possibility that testosterone may increase a woman's risk of heart disease, and if taken with estrogen, testosterone may neutralize some of the benefits of estrogen therapy. Testosterone lowers HDL cholesterol, a risk factor for cardiac problems. There is some evidence that testosterone given by injection, rather than given orally, is able to maintain more healthful levels of HDL.

It is important for anyone taking testosterone to be monitored closely by a physician so that any adverse effects can be recognized and dealt with promptly.

HERBAL SUPPORT OF TESTOSTERONE PRODUCTION AND SEXUAL FUNCTION: GINSENG

Among the herbs, ginseng has been shown to improve testosterone levels and sperm count. In fact, this herb has an almost legendary reputation for treating nearly every ailment known to man. In the 1950s, scientists began to test these claims and found that when high quantities of standardized extracts were administered, ginseng could be a very beneficial tonic and therapy. One of its primary functions is as an adaptogen, a substance that helps to maintain normal biological functions such as stamina and immunity.

The most widely used and studied type of ginseng is panax ginseng, which is either of Chinese, American, or Korean origin. When processed in its mature form, after at least six or eight years of growth, panax ginseng should contain thirteen or more hormonelike compounds called ginsenosides. Clinical studies have shown that panax ginseng minimizes the harmful effects of stress on the body, protects against damage caused by radiation, and improves liver function.

Besides these actions, ginseng also has an effect on reproductive function. Traditionally, panax ginseng was taken to enhance virility and fertility. Human studies assessing this function have yielded mixed results, but animal studies, such as one published in 1976 in the *American Journal of Chinese Medicine*, have demonstrated ginseng's ability to increase sexual and mating activity. One study, appearing in 1982 in the *Archives of Andrology*, found that a 5 percent preparation of ginseng resulted in a significant increase in blood testosterone levels. In another animal study, Siberian ginseng resulted in an increase in sperm count. Based on its traditional use and these modern studies, ginseng appears to be a suitable treatment to improve sexual function.

Suggested dosage

Ginseng and extracts of ginseng vary greatly in type and quality. The most valued are wild roots that are old and well formed, which have a high proportion of active substances. The lowest grade comes from the smaller roots of cultivated plants. Most of the ginseng products on the American market are of the lowest quality. They may contain various parts of the plant as well as additives. For this reason, it is important to use a standardized preparation that has guaranteed amounts of certain of the active ingredients. The dosage is then based on the potency of the ginseng preparation being administered. A common dosage for high-quality panax ginseng root is 4 to 6 g per day. A typical dose for Siberian ginseng extract is 100 mg three times a day. As with many therapies, it is best to start with a small dosage and increase gradually. One regimen recommends taking ginseng on a repeating schedule, with two to three weeks of ginseng followed by two weeks with no treatment.

Side effects

The documented side effects of ginseng include nervousness, hypertension, morning diarrhea, skin problems, insomnia, and euphoria. It is important that a person taking ginseng monitor themselves for these symptoms. However, given the wide range of quality of ginseng on the market, it is difficult to know which specific side effects, if any, a particular preparation may be causing.

NUTRIENTS THAT SUPPORT TESTOSTERONE PRODUCTION, NORMAL SPERM COUNT, AND HEALTHY REPRODUCTIVE FUNCTION

Many vitamins, minerals, and other nutrients support male reproductive health, including zinc, vitamin C and the other antioxidants, vitamin E, vitamin B$_{12}$, carnitine, and arginine. A diet that includes plenty of unrefined and unprocessed foods will provide more appropriate amounts of these nutrients than one consisting of many highly processed foods, but supplements may also be necessary to replenish deficiencies.

Zinc

Zinc may be the most important trace mineral for the many aspects of male sexual function because of its roles in sperm formation and motility (the power to move spontaneously) and testosterone production. In a study published in 1981 in the *Archives of Andrology*, twenty-two male patients with infertility were given zinc sulfate supplements twice a day between meals for forty to fifty days. Analyses of their blood and semen showed that treatment resulted in an increase in testosterone and sperm count. Furthermore, nine of the wives of these patients become pregnant, six within three months and three within two months of a second trial. The typical American diet does not provide sufficient daily zinc, and the soil in which we grow our produce is also often deficient. The RDA for zinc is 15 mg for men and 12 mg for women.

Vitamin C and other antioxidants

Testosterone production and sperm formation are closely associated with nutrition and antioxidant intake. Sperm are especially vulnerable to damage by free radicals through a process known as oxidation; however, vitamin C and the other antioxidant nutrients, such as vitamin E and beta-carotene, have been found to prevent free radicals from harming sperm cells. It is thought that many cases of low sperm count are caused by free-radical damage. Researchers at the University of California, Berkeley, in a study published in 1991 in the *Proceedings of the National Academy of Sciences, USA*, observed that intake of both 60 mg and 250 mg of vitamin C reduced oxidative damage to the DNA contained in the sperm nucleus. Such damage could increase the risk of genetic defects, particularly for men who smoke; however, vitamin C can be somewhat helpful in reducing sperm damage due to smoking.

Vitamin B$_{12}$

In order for cells to replicate, vitamin B$_{12}$ is required. When B$_{12}$ is deficient, a decline in sperm count and motility can occur. Even when B$_{12}$ is not deficient, supplementing with this vitamin can be effective for men with sperm counts that are less than 20 million per milliliter or who have a motility rate of under 50 percent.

Carnitine

Carnitine is an amino acid compound that plays a role in sperm development, function, and motility. Carnitine must be present for the mitochondria, the energy-producing components of cells, to break down fatty acids for fuel. These fatty acids are the primary fuel source of sperm. To help restore fertility, carnitine, in the form of L-carnitine, is recommended in dosages from 300 to 1000 mg a day.

Arginine

Normal sperm production requires the presence of the amino acid arginine. Studies have shown that having an arginine-free diet, even for a few days, can impair spermatogenesis. An Israeli study done at an infertility clinic gives evidence of the benefits of arginine supplementation. The results of this study, published in the *Journal of Urology*, reported that among the 178 male patients, 42 experienced a 100 percent increase in sperm count, resulting in 15 pregnancies soon after treatment with arginine began. In another 69 patients, there was an increase in sperm number and motility, resulting in 13 pregnancies among this group's partners.

ESTROGEN

Recently, estrogen replacement therapy (ERT) has become a popular topic of conversation and a favorite subject in the media because millions of Baby Boom women are now reaching midlife. Thirty-five million women in the United States are currently menopausal.

While physicians almost universally recommend ERT, many menopausal women are hesitant to begin taking hormones and question their benefits and safety. A 1994 Gallup poll indicated that only 30 percent of postmenopausal women in the United States use estrogen replacement therapy, dropping to as low as 8 percent in certain states. A 1997 article in *Family Practice News* stated that 25 percent of first prescriptions for estrogen are never filled, and 45 percent of women who begin taking the estrogen supplement Premarin are no longer taking the drug nine months later.

Women have a variety of reasons for not using estrogen or being non-compliant once they receive a prescription. Some women are simply not good candidates for estrogen therapy to begin with. Physicians may refuse to prescribe ERT at all or only in small doses for women with preexisting health problems such as uterine or breast cancer, heavy bleeding from uterine fibroid tumors, severe migraine headaches, or blood-clotting problems. For some women, ERT fails to control the symptoms of menopause or results in side effects that include menstrual-like bleeding, fluid retention, weight gain, breast tenderness, and depression. In addition, many women worry about developing breast cancer, particularly if they have a strong family history of this disease. Many women prefer to pursue non-drug treatment options such as nutritional therapies and acupuncture for philosophical reasons.

CONVENTIONAL ESTROGEN THERAPY

The types of estrogen therapies most readily available in the United States are composed of two potent forms of estrogen, estradiol and estrone. Estradiol is the main type of estrogen manufactured by the ovaries, and estrone, a weaker form of estrogen, is the primary type produced after menopause, by the ovaries and adrenals. In the short term, these estrogens treat and prevent a wide variety of menopausal symptoms due to hormone deficiency. They also have long-term benefits, lowering the risk of heart disease and osteoporosis. Estradiol and estrone also stimulate growth. Consequently, taking these estrogens also increases the risks of cancers of the breast and uterus.

Routes of administration and dosages

Estrogen is available as oral tablets, transdermal patches, or vaginal creams. Other routes of administration are under investigation, including injected (percutaneous) estrogen gel and vaginal rings.

Tablets. The most commonly prescribed estrogen is a tablet brand called Premarin, a conjugated equine estrogen derived from the urine of pregnant mares. Much of the medical research on estrogen is based on this product, which has been available since 1941, so the benefits and side effects of Premarin are very well understood. Premarin is available in a wide variety of doses, which allows for considerable flexibility in determining the optimal treatment dosage for each patient. There are also generic conjugated estrogen and synthetic and semisynthetic estrogen compounds available, including such products as Ogen (Abbot), which contains estrone, and Estrace (Meade-Johnson), which contains estradiol.

One drawback of oral administration of estrogen is that after ingestion, a large amount of the hormone is concentrated in the digestive tract, where intestinal bacteria transform the estrogen chemically. This phenomenon can change the type as well as the potency of the estrogen that is reabsorbed back into the body. When this estrogen reaches the liver, it is again metabolized and converted to other forms before it finally enters the general circulation. How efficiently this process occurs depends on the health of the liver. Women with a history of liver or gallbladder disease or hypertension and blood-clotting problems (which are affected by various actions in the liver) may do well to avoid oral estrogen.

The most commonly prescribed dosage of estrogen is 0.625 mg. However, some women need higher amounts, such as 0.9 or 1.25 mg, to attain relief from menopausal symptoms. The dosage can be cut to 0.3 mg to avoid side effects, but this dose may not be enough to avoid bone loss. Only trial and error will tell a woman which dose works best for her. Taking estrogen alone has been associated with an increased risk of developing cancer of the uterus. Woman who have an intact uterus should always take a formulation that includes progestin for at least ten to thirteen days of each month for cancer protection.

Transdermal patches. Transdermal estrogen, marketed under the brand name Estraderm (IBA Pharmaceuticals), was created to avoid the problems inherent in oral estrogen's first passing through the liver. In this innovative form of delivery, estrogen is absorbed into the general circulation through a medicated patch applied to the skin. This method avoids an initial pass through the digestive tract and liver. Women with liver and gallbladder disease are more likely to tolerate this form of estrogen. Another benefit of the patch is that it dispenses estrogen continuously throughout the day, rather than in one large burst like the tablet, and so more closely resembles the body's own estrogen production.

In the past, there has not been as much flexibility of dosage range with the patch as with the estrogen pill. Initially, the transdermal patch was only available in two dosages. However, newer products have been introduced to offer more dosage options. For instance, Vivelle, manufactured by Cibo Pharmaceuticals, is currently available in four dosages. As with oral estrogen, the patch is used in conjunction with progesterone if the women still has an intact uterus. The patch appears to be as effective as the estrogen pill in reducing menopausal symptoms and seems to be as protective against heart disease and osteoporosis.

Vaginal creams. Estrogen cream is primarily applied to the vagina and urethral area to prevent atrophy and breakdown of the tissues caused by lack of natural estrogen. Because of the vaginal atrophy that exists when women first begin treatment, estrogen tends to be absorbed rapidly. This can cause the blood levels of estrogen to rise significantly. As a result, side effects from using the vaginal cream, such as breast tenderness or mild fluid retention, usually occur early in the course of treatment. However, once the estrogen thickens the vaginal walls and causes the cellular pattern of the mucous membranes to change to a more youthful and healthier condition, estrogen absorption into the bloodstream slows down. Not only will estrogen thicken the vaginal wall, making it less traumatized by sexual intercourse or foreplay, but it also reduces the incidence of bladder infections. ERT may still not restore vaginal lubrication to adequate levels in some women. Thus, the use of a lubricant cream or gel during sexual activity may still be needed.

Another benefit of the vaginal cream is that it does not make an initial pass through the liver, aggravating liver and gallbladder disease. However, women with preexisting breast cancer or whose cancers are positive for estrogen receptors may not be candidates for estrogen vaginal creams.

The commonly prescribed Premarin cream comes with a calibrated applicator that allows for the use of 2 to 4 g per day. One-half to one full applicator of Premarin cream will deliver 1.25 to 2.5 mg of estrogen to the vaginal tissues. However, many women find that they function quite well at smaller doses, often with as little as one-eighth of an applicator.

Initially, a woman may want to use estrogen cream daily, at least for the first week or two. It is important that the most sore or abraded areas come directly in contact with the cream, either through placement of the applicator or by applying the cream to sore and tender areas with the fingers. After healing has begun and sexual activity is more comfortable, many women reduce usage to two or three times per week. If estrogen is taken to prevent osteoporosis or cardiovascular disease, estrogen vaginal cream is inadequate to meet these goals.

Candidates for ERT

ERT is appropriate for women with menopausal symptoms due to estrogen deficiency when these symptoms are so severe that they disrupt normal life. These women may also be unable or unwilling to make lifestyle and dietary changes that can lessen their symptoms. Other candidates for ERT include women who have had surgical removal of the ovaries and women whose ovarian hormone production is prematurely reduced or terminated through removal of the uterus or due to other causes.

Estrogen should be used cautiously. ERT may be contraindicated for women with certain preexisting medical conditions, as discussed in the following subsections.

Cancer. ERT is not advised for women with previously diagnosed or suspected cancer of the uterus or endometrium. Although estrogen itself does not cause cancer, it can cause hyperplasia (the buildup of cells of the uterine lining). In some women, hyperplasia can progress to cancer if estrogen is used without progesterone.

There has also been concern over the degree to which hormone replacement therapy increases the risk of breast cancer. A recent study, published in 1997 in the *Lancet*, provides definitive evidence that HRT increases the risk of breast cancer in postmenopausal women. British epidemiologists analyzed data from 151 studies involving more than 161,000 women. They found that for every 1000 women, aged fifty to seventy, who did not take HRT, 45 developed breast cancer. Expressing the risk another way, after taking estrogen replacement therapy for five years, there were 47 cases of breast cancer per 1000 women; after ten years, 51 cases per 1000, and after fifteen years, 57 cases per 1000. Expressed as a percentage, women using estrogen for five years or longer have a 35 percent higher risk of breast cancer than women not taking hormones.

Women with previously diagnosed or suspected breast cancer are not normally given estrogen. The concern is that estrogen replacement could help promote a recurrence of the disease, and physicians are wary of exposing patients to this risk.

Liver and gallbladder disease. Women with active liver disease, such as hepatitis, or with a history of alcohol abuse should avoid oral ERT because with these conditions, the liver is unable to perform its normal function of breaking down estrogen for safe elimination. However, these women can receive estrogen via an estrogen patch, because the hormone administered this way bypasses the liver and directly enters the general circulation. Women at risk for gallbladder disease, such as women with a Native American ethnic background, are not candidates for ERT. Replacement therapy increases the risk of developing gallstones two and a half times.

Heart disease. Estrogen is not recommended for women at risk for heart disease. The hormone can increase blood pressure and the tendency for blood to form clots (thrombophlebitis). Women who are very overweight need to take special care, as they have a greater risk of developing clots.

Diabetes. High doses of estrogen can disturb glucose levels, which should be monitored carefully. However, diabetic women are usually able to use ERT without any significant effect on carbohydrate metabolism.

Uterine fibroid tumors. Fibroid tumors occur when there is excessive growth in the muscular tissue of the uterus. These growths are usually seen in women during their menstrual years, and because these growths are stimulated by estrogen, women transitioning into menopause may experience an increase in fibroid growth. Fibroids usually shrink after menopause as estrogen levels decline, but a woman taking estrogen therapy may not experience this shrinking process.

Endometriosis. Endometriosis occurs when the uterine lining implants itself into organs and tissues of the pelvic cavity such as the ovaries, bladder, and ligaments. Normally, endometriosis tends to decline with menopause as estrogen stimulation recedes. Rarely, however, ERT may restimulate the endometrial implants, so women with this condition should be cautious in using ERT.

Side effects of ERT

Women using ERT may suffer side effects such as fluid retention, tender breasts, and weight gain, all three of which may be related. The other most common side effects include bleeding on stopping ERT as prescribed on a cyclical basis by many physicians, irregular bleeding, bloating, headaches, nausea, anxiety, heavy vaginal discharge, and estrogen allergy. Although estrogen is generally well tolerated, some women may find that they experience one or more of these side effects. When this occurs, the dosage and route of administration can be altered to minimize these uncomfortable symptoms.

Estriol: Complementary Estrogen Therapy

For those women who cannot use estrogen because of previous health conditions or are who prone to side effects with conventional therapy, a third and much less potent form of estrogen, estriol, offers another treatment option. Although estriol has been commonly prescribed in Canada and Europe for many years, in the United States its use is limited to physicians practicing complementary medicine and those practicing conventional medicine who have expanded their treatment options in response to patients' requests. Estriol must be ordered by a physician from a compounding pharmacy. Unlike pregnenolone and DHEA, the two sex hormones used in alternative medicine, estriol is not available over the counter.

Estriol is produced in the laboratory from natural ingredients such as soy and wild yam. It is commonly prescribed in pill form to reduce menopausal symptoms such as hot flashes, vaginal dryness, and mood swings. These benefits were demonstrated in a study published in 1978 in the *Journal of the American Medical Association*. The researchers selected fifty-two symptomatic postmenopausal women and administered estriol in various dosages. Twenty women were given 2 mg a day; sixteen women, 4 mg a day; eight women, 6 mg a day; and eight women, 8 mg a day. The estriol was given orally for six months. On average, the women in every group experienced a decrease in symptoms after one month of treatment, with greater improvement the higher the dosage. Furthermore, in three of the four groups, symptoms that were described as severe were now ranked as very mild. Estriol was found to be particularly useful for women with symptoms of vaginal atrophy. Physicians also prescribe it for the relief of hot flashes and mood swings. Estriol is normally prescribed in doses of 2 to 4 mg per day. It is recommended that a woman combine estriol therapy with natural progesterone, 50 to 100 mg of oral micronized progesterone once a day, for at least two weeks of every menstrual cycle. Estriol is not recommended for the prevention of osteoporosis. In order for estriol to benefit bone health, a daily dosage as high as 12 mg is necessary. However, such elevated amounts often cause nausea. No beneficial effect of estriol on cardiovascular health has been shown.

Side effects

Of the three estrogens, estriol is the weakest, and more importantly, it is probably the safest type of natural estrogen. Based on various animal and human studies, it appears that estriol is less likely to promote tissue growth and helps prevent breast and endometrial cancers. Several human studies indicate that it may be the ratio of estriol to estradiol and estrone that is protective. Women with higher amounts of estriol in relation to the other hormones were less likely to develop cancer, perhaps because estriol attaches to estrogen receptors that might otherwise bind to forms of estrogen that more readily promote cell proliferation.

DIETARY SUBSTANCES WITH ESTROGENLIKE ACTIVITY

It is possible to obtain an estrogenlike effect by eating foods such as soybeans and flaxseeds, supplementing with nutrients like vitamin E, bioflavonoids, and boron, and taking certain herbs, all of which exhibit a degree of estrogenic activity. Consuming these substances regularly in sufficient amounts can improve hormone status.

Soy-based foods

Weak estrogenic activity is found in a variety of plant foods, including grains, vegetables, legumes, nuts, and seeds. However, for therapeutic purposes, only soybeans contain sufficient active compounds to approximate the effects of estrogen produced by the body. The phytoestrogens in soybeans are two substances called genistein and daidzein, which belong to the class of chemicals called isoflavones. Soy isoflavones were first discovered during the 1930s, but their potency was not assayed until the 1950s. At that time, genistein was found to be 50,000 times weaker than estrogen. Asian women eat much more soy products, and thereby phytoestrogens, in their traditional diet (which provides between 50 and 150 mg of isoflavones per day) than American women, whose isoflavone intake is virtually zero. This was confirmed in a study published in 1992 in the *Lancet*, which found that Japanese women who regularly eat a range of soy products had 100 to 1000 times more isoflavone breakdown products in their urine than Western women, who do not commonly eat soy foods. Menopausal women in Japan are rarely troubled by symptoms such as hot flashes. Similar studies, recently conducted in the United States, that monitored soy intake and menopausal symptoms, confirmed these findings. Eating soy-based foods resulted in a reduction in the severity of hot flashes and also promoted growth of vaginal cells, counteracting the tendency of this tissue to thin after menopause.

American women can enjoy benefits similar to those seen in Asian women by increasing their intake of soy foods. Between 40 and 60 mg of soy isoflavones per day are necessary to confer protection against menopausal symptoms. Luckily, there is a wide variety of soy-based foods and supplement products currently available for women wishing to include this food in their diet.

▲▲ Susan has had many patients use soy-based foods successfully as an estrogen substitute. To receive optimal therapeutic benefits, be sure to read labels to make sure that your total soy intake is at least 30 to 50 g of soy protein per day. For example, one glass of soy milk contains between 2 and 10 g of protein, soy burgers typically contain 8 g, and soy cheeses 4 g per slice. Soy sauce, however, is of very little benefit as a phytoestrogen. For women who do not like soy foods, soy-based protein powders and capsules now contain premeasured amounts of isoflavones.

Eating soy-based foods also has several other long-term health benefits. Unlike prescription estrogen, soy does not appear to have a carcinogenic effect on uterine cells or breast tissue. In fact, it appears to be cancer-protective for several reasons. Not only does soy reduce the production of estrogen within the body, but it also directly inhibits the growth of breast cancer cells. A review article appearing in 1991 in the *Journal of the American Dietetics Association* confirmed that two compounds in soy, protease inhibitors and phytic acid, both have anticarcinogenic activity. The writers noted that soybean intake is associated with reduced rates of prostate, colon, and breast cancer. Women in Japan who regularly eat large quantities of soy foods have an incidence of breast cancer four to six times lower than that of women who do not include soy in their diet.

Other studies currently in progress suggest that soy can have a beneficial effect on both blood fats and bone metabolism. While estrogen is often prescribed to prevent heart disease and osteoporosis, soy offers a food-based approach to the same health issues.

Vitamin E

Supplementing with vitamin E offers a natural way to reduce the symptoms of menopause—such as hot flashes, night sweats, insomnia, headaches, nervousness, and irritability—with little risk of side effects. The original research on vitamin E's usefulness as an estrogen substitute was done between the 1930s and the early 1950s. Some of this research was done on breast and uterine cancer patients who were in menopause and were known to be poor candidates for estrogen replacement therapy, since it was understood that estrogen could stimulate the growth of any remaining tumor cells. Vitamin E was found to be both effective and safe in alleviating menopausal symptoms in these patients. Between 67 and 95 percent of the women followed in various studies had relief of such common menopausal symptoms as hot flashes, fatigue, mood swings, and muscle aches and pains. Vitamin E was less successful for the treatment of vaginal atrophy, being helpful in only 50 percent of the cases.

There is also interesting early research on vitamin E being used to reestablish healthy menstrual cycles in young women. Living under the stress of war is often associated with widespread disruption of menstrual cycles. This was true of women living in an internment camp in Manila during World War II. Doctors who treated these women observed that menstruation had stopped abruptly after the first bombing of Manila, before a nutritional deficiency would have been experienced. These physicians conducted a small study, published in 1944 in the *Journal of the American Medical Association*, in which ten women with amenorrhea (a lack of menstruation) were given twenty drops of wheat germ oil as a source of vitamin E. The doses were taken orally, three times a day, for a period of ten days, preceding the onset of each woman's expected menstrual flow. Of the ten women, eight began to menstruate or had uterine bleeding.

SUGGESTED DOSAGE: Although vitamin E is present in such foods as whole grains, eggs, and nuts, only supplemental amounts of vitamin E provide the quantity needed to produce health benefits comparable to hormone replacement. Vitamin E is available as an oil-based capsule providing 400 or 1000 IU of the vitamin. Most research studies use the d-alpha-tocopherol form of the vitamin. A dry form of vitamin E is also available for individuals who can not tolerate oil-based products.

Susan generally recommends that women with menopause-related symptoms take between 400 and 2000 IU of vitamin E daily. She advises starting with a lower dose and increasing this by 400 IU every two weeks until the desired effect is achieved.

Note: Oil-based capsules can also be used topically to treat irritation caused by the thinning of the vaginal walls that can occur at menopause. The capsule is opened and the vitamin oil applied directly to vaginal tissues. Susan recommends that women test the vitamin first to make sure that there is no skin reaction. A tiny amount of vitamin E can be applied over a few days before using larger doses topically.

Side effects. Vitamin E is considered extremely safe and is commonly used by millions of individuals. However, women with certain medical problems, such as hypertension, insulin-dependent diabetes, and menstrual-bleeding problems, should begin taking vitamin E at lower dosages, starting with 100 IU per day and slowly increasing the dosage. A woman with any of these health conditions should ask a knowledgeable health care professional about the advisability of supplementing with vitamin E.

Bioflavonoids

A subclass of flavonoids called flavones are commonly called bioflavonoids. Flavones are found in the peel and pulp of citrus fruits as well as in buckwheat. While bioflavonoids can be useful in helping relieve and prevent premenopausal symptoms, they can be equally useful for menopausal women. This is because bioflavonoids are weakly estrogenic and can be used as a safe, nontoxic substitute for estrogen. The potency of bioflavonoids is so low that they have no side effects for most women, yet they can relieve hot flashes as well as vaginal dryness. A study of ninety-four women at Loyola University Medical School showed the effectiveness of a bioflavonoids–vitamin C combination in controlling hot flashes for most of the women tested. In addition, bioflavonoids were suggested in this particular study as an estrogen substitute for cancer patients who cannot use traditional replacement therapy because their tumors are estrogen-sensitive.

SUGGESTED DOSAGE: 750 to 2000 mg per day. Bioflavonoids are considered very safe and have virtually no side effects.

Essential fatty acids

Essential fatty acids are critical for health and must be supplied daily by the diet, as the body cannot make them. The skin is full of fatty acids that, along with estrogen, provide moisture, softness, and smooth texture. When estrogen levels decline with menopause, moisture can continue to be provided to tissues of the skin, vagina, and bladder, as well as the hair, by increasing the intake of fatty acid–containing foods. Excellent sources of essential fatty acids are fish, nuts, and seeds, especially flaxseeds.

Both ground whole flaxseeds, which are 30 percent oil by content, and cold-pressed organic flaxseed oil used as a food supplement, are excellent sources of the two essential oils, linoleic acid and linolenic acid. Flaxseed oil is sold in opaque containers in the refrigerator section of most health food stores, as it is very sensitive to heat, light, and oxygen. It is also marketed as a meal and in capsule form. Flaxseed is unusual since it contains a double source of plant-based estrogen. Both the oil and the flax lignan (a substance contained within the celluloselike material that provides structure to plants) contained within the seed have been researched for their weakly estrogenic effect.

A study published in 1990 in the *British Medical Journal* described how shifting the diet toward phytoestrogen-containing foods can change certain menopause indicators. In this study, twenty-five menopausal women (average age: fifty-nine) were asked to supplement their normal diet with phytoestrogen-containing foods such as flaxseed oil. The women consumed these foods over a six-week period. Smears from the vaginal wall were taken every two weeks to see if the addition of estrogen-containing plant foods would cause a beneficial hormonal effect on the vagina. Typically, the vaginal mucosa thins out and becomes more prone to trauma and infections as the estrogen level drops with menopause. Interestingly, the vaginal mucosa responded significantly to the additional ingestion of flaxseed oil and soy flour but returned to previous levels eight weeks after these foods were discontinued and the women went back to their usual diet.

Seeds and whole grains also contain lignans, which make up part of the structure of plants. Once plant lignans are eaten, intestinal bacteria convert them to substances that are weakly estrogenic and can provide additional nutritional support to menopausal women deficient in this hormone. This was confirmed in a study appearing in 1995 in *Proceedings of the Society for Experimental Biology and Medicine*. Flaxseeds are 100 times richer in lignans than any other plant. Other sources of essential fatty acids include evening primrose oil, borage oil, and black currant oil. Unlike flaxseed oil, these other oils are not used as foods, but as nutritional supplements.

For women who are still having periods, flaxseed can act as a menstrual regulator. In a study conducted at the University of Minnesota, published in 1993 in the *Journal of Clinical Endocrinology and Metabolism*, eighteen women with normal menstrual cycles ate normally for three cycles and then added 10 g of flaxseed powder per day to their diet for an additional three cycles. During the time that the women did not eat flaxseed, there were three cycles when no ovulation occurred. But when flaxseed was included, all of the women in the study ovulated every menstrual cycle. Thus, ground flaxseed was found to improve the estrogen-to-progesterone ratio favoring the levels of progesterone within the body. Progesterone production occurs only in ovulatory menstrual cycles. Although Susan is in her fifties, she continues to have regular, ovulatory menstrual cycles. She has been using flaxseed oil and flaxseed meal for many years and feels that they are responsible, at least in part, for her continued excellent menstrual health.

SUGGESTED DOSAGE: 1 to 3 tbsp. per day of flaxseed oil or 3 to 6 tbsp. of the ground seed. Women who like the buttery taste of raw flaxseed oil can use it as a flavoring oil on salads, popcorn, steamed vegetables, baked potatoes, and toast. It blends well with most food flavors but should never be used for cooking. Add it to foods eaten at room temperature and to hot foods after they are heated. Discard any leftover food, as the oil will quickly go rancid. The whole seeds must be ground in a food processor or blender to break up the hard exterior shell of the seed and allow both the lignans and the oil contained within the seeds to be absorbed by the body. Never eat the whole seed. The resultant flaxseed powder or meal can be added to shakes or combined with nondairy milk or juice and stirred to create an instant cereal (see page 315).

Boron

Boron is a trace mineral found in such foods as apples, grapes, almonds, legumes, honey, and dark green leafy vegetables like kale and beet greens. There is some evidence that boron has estrogenic activity, according to a study conducted by the U.S. Department of Agriculture. When women on estrogen therapy supplemented their normally low-boron diet with 3 mg of boron, their blood levels of estrogen, specifically ß-estradiol, were significantly elevated. It appears that boron enhances and mimics some effects of estrogen. There is also anecdotal evidence that boron may reduce hot flashes. A diet plentiful in certain fruits, vegetables, and nuts can supply 1 to 3 mg of boron a day, and if combined with a 3 mg supplement, total intake will still be well below the recommended limit of 10 mg a day. Unfortunately, the foods most commonly consumed—meat, dairy products, and refined flour—are not good sources of boron, so many Americans are deficient in this forgotten mineral.

Herbs

Many herbs are estrogenlike in their activity, including common culinary herbs such as fennel and anise, as well as licorice. Other herbs, such as black cohosh and unicorn root, have been used medicinally as part of healing traditions for thousands of years. While their estrogenic activity is a small fraction of the activity of the estrogen a woman produces (at least 400 times less active), their benefit is that these herbs cause no unwanted side effects.

Black cohosh. One of the most effective of the estrogenic herbs is black cohosh. Native to America, black cohosh was well known and accepted in Native American herbal medicine and was widely prescribed in colonial times as a treatment for menstrual cramps and menopausal symptoms. Today, black cohosh is available as a standardized extract of 20 mg of black cohosh per dosage. This should contain 1 to 2.5 mg of the active component, which are triterpenes, calculated as 27-deoxyacteine per tablet. Chemically, black cohosh is similar to estriol, the weakest form of estrogen made within the body. Black cohosh has been used by millions of women in Australia and Europe and is available in the United States in health food stores and some pharmacies.

The effectiveness and safety of black cohosh are well documented. Clinical studies have shown that black cohosh reduces PMS symptoms such as mood swings, anxiety, tension, and depression. It also relieves the symptoms of pain and discomfort due to menstrual cramps. Other studies have focused on the symptoms of menopause and have found that black cohosh relieved hot flashes, night sweats, heart palpitations, headaches, and vaginal dryness and atrophy. It is also effective in relieving other symptoms such as depression, anxiety, sleep disturbances, and a decline in libido. Black cohosh is considered a safe and effective therapy.

SUGGESTED DOSAGE: The dosage for the standardized extract is 40 mg twice a day for menopause and once or twice a day for PMS.

Licorice root. Licorice root has been used medicinally for several thousand years in both Eastern and Western cultures. Prescribed for problems including respiratory infections, peptic ulcers, abdominal pain, and malaria, licorice is especially useful in treating PMS, which can be caused by a dominance of estrogen in relation to progesterone levels. A review article published in 1997 in the *American Journal of Natural Medicine* indicated that licorice root can lower estrogen while at the same time raising progesterone. Licorice promotes an increase in progesterone by inhibiting the enzyme necessary for its breakdown. The potency of licorice root is 400 times weaker than estradiol, the most potent form of estrogen created within the body.

Licorice is also useful in counteracting the common PMS symptoms of bloating and breast tenderness caused by water retention. Licorice blocks aldosterone, the adrenal hormone that limits the excretion of sodium, and as sodium attracts fluids, aldosterone can cause fluid retention (edema).

SUGGESTED DOSAGE: To treat PMS symptoms, a woman should take licorice beginning on the fourteenth day of her cycle until menstruation begins. Licorice can be taken as a fluid extract in a 1 milliliter dosage, one to three times per day. One ml is equal to one full dropperful of the herb in a 1 oz. bottle. It can also be taken in powdered form in a 400 or 500 mg capsule. The dosage is one to two capsules one to three times per day. Licorice root is not recommended for individuals with a history of kidney failure or hypertension, or who are currently taking medications made from digitalis.

Chaste tree berry (Vitex agnus castus). The chaste tree that yields these berries is native to the Mediterranean. As the name suggests, chaste tree berries were used in traditional botanical medicine to dampen libido. The berries have a unique effect on hormone function. The hypothalamus and pituitary glands in the brain help regulate hormone production, and chaste tree berry has a profound effect on these two glands. It increases the production of luteinizing hormone (LH). LH is the pituitary hormone that triggers ovulation at midcycle, thereby promoting the production of progesterone during the second half of the menstrual cycle. Chaste tree berry also inhibits the release of follicle-stimulating hormone (FSH). FSH is needed to stimulate estrogen production during the first half of the menstrual cycle. The end result is to promote the estrogen-to-progesterone ratio in favor of progesterone. Consequently, chaste tree berry can help normalize the secretion of hormones and bring estrogen and progesterone levels into a healthful balance. This makes it a useful treatment for conditions related to estrogen excess, such as PMS and perimenopause.

SUGGESTED DOSAGE: The dosage is 20 mg of the standardized extract, taken twice a day, in the early morning and evening. It is manufactured as a 10:1 extract. If taken as a liquid, a typical dose is 1 ml once or twice a day. One milliliter is equal to one full dropperful of the herb in a 1 oz. bottle. It may take a while for the benefits of chaste tree berry to manifest, typically about three months or so.

Dandelion root. To maintain a balance of estrogen and progesterone and prevent symptoms of PMS or perimenopause, it is important to support the liver in its function of breaking down and excreting hormones. The liver must produce sufficient bile, which then passes through the gallbladder and into the intestine. In traditional Chinese medicine, when this action of the liver is sluggish, the liver is said to be congested. Herbalists treat PMS with certain herbs to stimulate bile production and thereby bring hormones back into balance. Dandelion root, as well as fennel seed and milk thistle, are commonly used liver herbs.

SUGGESTED DOSAGE: Dandelion is available in 500 mg capsules. Take one to three capsules three times per day.

Dong quai. The Chinese herb dong quai has been used for thousands of years as a female health tonic and to prevent or treat symptoms of PMS and menopause. Traditionally, dong quai has been used to treat abnormal menstruation and menopausal hot flashes. Many naturopathic physicians and herbalists today regularly prescribe this herb for their female patients. However, in a recent twelve-week study involving seventy-one postmenopausal women, presented in 1997 at the annual meeting of the Pacific Coast Fertility Society, there was virtually no evidence of dong quai's purported estrogenic activity. There was no apparent thickening of tissue in the uterus or vagina and no significant reduction in hot flashes. As the Chinese herbalists normally prescribe dong quai in combination with other herbs, it may be that its action depends on several herbs working together.

SUGGESTED DOSAGE: If taken as a liquid, a typical dose is 1 ml once or twice a day. One milliliter is equal to one full dropperful of the herb in a 1 oz. bottle. Dong quai can also be taken in powdered form in a 500 mg capsule. The dosage is two capsules two to three times per day.

PROGESTERONE

Before the 1980s, all progesterone therapy had to be administered by injection in the doctor's office. The development of oral progesterones made this hormone more readily available. Initially, progesterone was combined with estrogen in birth control pills for younger women. Then progesterone's important role in preventing endometrial cancer in postmenopausal women on ERT was discovered in the 1970s. It rapidly became part of the standard hormonal regimen for postmenopausal women who still had their uterus intact. The traditional form of treatment does not, however, use the same natural form of progesterone produced by the ovaries. Instead, a synthetic form called a progestin is used. It is important to be aware that progestins and natural progesterone do not have the same chemical structure and do not behave the same biologically. They also differ in their benefits and side effects.

SYNTHETIC PROGESTINS

Progestins are helpful during the transition into menopause. Perimenopausal women may produce too much estrogen without ovulating, which can cause heavy periods lasting as long as ten to twelve days. Taking progestins alone can help prevent erratic heavy periods. Progestins also help prevent the heavy buildup of endometrial lining by making sure that the lining is completely shed each month. By promoting a regular menstrual period each month, the use of progesterone can also help reduce the number of endometrial biopsies a woman's physician needs to perform.

Routes of administration and dosages

Oral tablets of synthetic progesterone are the most widely prescribed form of progesterone. To regulate the menstrual cycle, only small doses of progestins, usually 5 to 10 mg, are needed. Some women require slightly higher or lower doses. Progestins are used ten to thirteen days per month. The most commonly used brand of progestins is Provera (Upjohn). Norlutate (Parke-Davis) is also frequently prescribed, but it may cause side effects similar to those of androgens, such as oily skin and acne. A third progestin currently on the market is Amen (Carnick).

Side effects

Some women taking progestins experience side effects that include fatigue, headaches, depression and mood changes, bloating, breast tenderness and enlargement, and increased appetite. If any of these occur, dosages should be decreased to as low as 1.25 mg per day.

Progestins can also cause more serious problems, such as an increased risk of heart disease. Researchers associated with the Oregon Health Sciences University conducted a study, published in 1997 in the *Journal of* the *American College of Cardiology*, in which monkeys were made vulnerable to coronary spasms. The researchers then treated the monkeys with estrogen, and this tendency was completely reversed. Then six monkeys were given combined treatment of estrogen plus progesterone, and six others estrogen plus progestins. The progestin treatment resulted in coronary-artery spasms in all the monkeys, while those receiving natural progesterone had no spasms.

Progestins also appear to lower the desirable HDL cholesterol associated with a lower risk of heart disease, though the results of some studies do conflict with this. In the PEPI trials (Postmenopausal Estrogen/Progestin Interventions), published in 1995 in the *Journal of the American Medical Association*, women taking estrogen and progestins had lower HDL levels, while women on estrogen and natural progesterone maintained higher levels of HDL.

There is also evidence that progestins increase the risk of birth defects if taken during the first four months of pregnancy, and may have a harmful effect on various systems of the body if taken over a long period.

NATURAL PROGESTERONE

Natural progesterone is produced from dioscorea, the active component of the Mexican wild yam, as are pregnenolone and DHEA. While synthesized in the laboratory, it has the same chemical structure and range of activity as the progesterone made by our body. Natural progesterone appears to confer an equal amount of protection against uterine cancer and functions as a diuretic and an antianxiety treatment; it can also stimulate libido. Natural progesterone also helps prevent fibrocystic breast disease and breast cancer, regulates thyroid hormone activity, stabilizes blood sugar levels, assists in normal blood clotting, is essential for the production of cortisone in the adrenal cortex, and helps convert fat to energy.

Beyond all these benefits, natural progesterone also plays an important role in the prevention and reversal of osteoporosis. In a study conducted by John Lee, published in 1991 in *Medical Hypotheses*, 100 postmenopausal women were treated with natural progesterone for a minimum of three years. Without treatment, these women would have had an expected bone loss of 4.5 percent. However, the bone density of the women was found to increase—10 percent in the first year on average, followed by a yearly increase of 3 to 5 percent thereafter.

Routes of administration and dosages

Natural progesterone can be taken in oral micronized form, as a rectal or vaginal suppository, as a skin cream, or as sublingual drops.

Oral micronized progesterone. Natural progesterone cannot be taken orally because it is destroyed during digestion and never reaches the bloodstream. However, a micronized form of progesterone is now available that is protected from destruction by stomach acid and enzymes and can be absorbed and used by the body. Susan began to prescribe natural progesterone almost two decades ago for her PMS patients, who found it helpful in controlling their anxiety and mood swings. Menopausal women are also beginning to use this form of progesterone more frequently because it causes fewer side effects than the synthetic progestins. In menopausal women, dosages of 100 to 200 mg daily can be effective, although the dose can vary in either direction. A woman needs these high doses, as 85 to 90 percent of the amount consumed will be metabolized by the liver soon after it has been ingested. Like the synthetic progestins, oral micronized progesterone is used ten to thirteen days per month.

Suppositories. Progesterone can also be taken as a rectal or vaginal suppository. Vaginal suppositories allow for excellent local intake of progesterone into the uterus and may be helpful for perimenopausal women with heavy and irregular bleeding.

Skin cream. A range of progesterone creams, available without prescription, contain from less than 2 mg to more than 400 mg of the hormone per jar. Pro-Gest cream, which contains more than 400 mg in a container, is one of the more well-known brands. The cream is applied to the skin and absorbed into the general circulation. This is in contrast to oral progesterone, which is first metabolized by the liver and converted into three different compounds. Using the cream, more progesterone reaches body tissues.

A typical dosage of natural progesterone is 20 mg a day. A 2 oz. jar should last for over one month. In perimenopausal women, the cream can be applied from day twelve to day twenty-six of the menstrual cycle. Menopausal women not taking estrogen may use progesterone for two to three weeks each month. If a woman is self-medicating herself with progesterone cream in an effort to block the cancer-promoting effect of estrogen on the uterus, she needs to make sure she is taking enough progesterone for it to be protective. Blood or saliva testing of progesterone levels will help to determine if the level of supplemental progesterone is in the therapeutic range.

The cream is used twice daily in $^1/_4$- to $^1/_2$-teaspoon amounts, generally on rising in the morning and before going to bed at night. The cream can be applied to any area of the skin. Many women rub it into their chest, abdomen, arms, or back. If the cream is absorbed rapidly (under two minutes), it means that the body needs a higher dose, and a slightly higher amount may be used. Few physicians have any experience using Pro-Gest cream to date, and it is more likely to be used by physicians knowledgeable about alternative therapies.

Note: Many progesterone products that contain wild yam extract contain only the precursor compound, diosgenin, and no progesterone. Also, progesterone delivered as a cream must suspend the hormone in a proper medium or it will not be effective. A cream containing mineral oil will not allow the progesterone to be absorbed. Some products have not stabilized the progesterone, and as a result, the hormone deteriorates over time.

Sublingual drops. Progesterone is available in a vitamin E oil. This is held under the tongue for at least a minute so that it is absorbed, rather than swallowed. The result is a quick rise in hormone levels followed by a drop three to four hours later. It is necessary to take the drops three to four times a day to maintain stable blood levels.

Side effects

When natural progesterone is taken in normally prescribed amounts, 20 to 40 mg, there are no known side effects. However, very high doses can cause drowsiness because of progesterone's sedative effect on the brain, and huge doses of the hormone can be an anesthetic or cause a person to feel drunk. During the beginning stages of supplementing with progesterone, a woman may have symptoms of estrogen dominance, such as hot flashes. This happens because progesterone can increase the sensitivity of estrogen receptor sites; however, this sensitivity will disappear after a few weeks.

Progesterone replacement in men

Throughout life, men normally have levels of progesterone equivalent to those of women after menopause. However, if a man has depressed DHEA production, supplementing with natural progesterone cream may be beneficial. There is little research on the use of progesterone therapy in men, but it is known that supplemental progesterone can increase levels of DHEA and enhance libido. However, progesterone replacement therapy is not recommended for men with prostate cancer.

NUTRIENTS THAT SUPPORT SPECIFIC BENEFITS OF HORMONE REPLACEMENT THERAPY

The benefits that hormone replacement therapy confers can be additionally supported by a wide variety of nutrients. Vitamins, minerals, and even fiber—consumed in the food we eat or taken as supplements—can support the long-term health benefits of hormone replacement therapy. They can reduce the incidence of and prevent the onset of many common problems seen after midlife, such as heart disease, bone loss, and diminished cognitive abilities. Following are some of the health conditions that specific nutrients will help to prevent.

HEART DISEASE

Antioxidants, B vitamins, and fiber all help to keep the heart healthy and prevent heart disease.

Antioxidants

Various studies have shown that higher intakes of antioxidants—such as vitamin C, beta-carotene, and vitamin E—are associated with a lower risk of developing heart disease. Antioxidants counteract free radicals, which are errant electrons that damage arteries. They also prevent LDL cholesterol (the more harmful form of cholesterol) from being oxidized. These vitamins reduce other risk factors as well.

A study conducted in Boston and mentioned in an article published in 1996 in the *Medical Tribune* showed that consuming 2000 mg of vitamin C a day improved blood flow in persons with coronary-artery disease. And two large studies documented the protective effects of vitamin E. One was the Nurses' Health Study, reported in an article appearing in 1993 in *Nutrition Reviews* and involving more than 87,000 female nurses, aged thirty-four to fifty-nine. Over an eight-year follow-up period, 552 cases of major coronary-heart disease occurred, with the majority nonfatal. The researchers found that the risk of heart disease was inversely related to an individual's total vitamin E intake. A similar study involving 40,000 males, published in 1993 in the *New England Journal of Medicine*, found similar results. And in a third study, the Cambridge Heart Antioxidant Study, conducted in England and published in 1996 in the *Lancet*, vitamin E supplements resulted in a 47 percent reduction in the risk of cardiovascular death and nonfatal heart attack.

Even in the smaller doses supplied by food alone, antioxidants are protective of heart disease. In a Finnish study published in 1994 in the *American Journal of Epidemiology*, men and women who had relatively high amounts of vitamin E in their diets had a lower incidence of fatal coronary-heart disease. The same was true for women with a high dietary intake of vitamin C and beta-carotene.

Nitric oxide

Nitric oxide is a gaseous molecule produced in the body from the amino acid arginine. As a potent vasodilator, nitric oxide enhances the flow of blood through the arteries and veins to all the tissues and cells of the body. It not only improves the health and functional capability of the heart, but also helps to support the health of the respiratory, neuroendocrine, immune, reproductive, and other systems because of its beneficial effect on circulation.

Impaired circulation due to diminished nitric oxide production can also greatly hamper one's level of performance in many important areas of life. This can lead to diminished physical and mental energy and immune-system function, erectile dysfunction (in men), diminished sexual responsiveness (in women), poor or slow recovery from exertion and injury, and impaired wound healing. Nitric oxide production enhances sports performance in activities where good muscular development and healthy circulation provide a competitive edge, such as bodybuilding, football, swimming, and cycling. Furthermore, levels of nitric oxide tend to decrease with age.

Not only does optimal production of nitric oxide increase performance capability, but its beneficial effect on peripheral circulation also contribute to the "look of success" that many peak performers have during their prime. High nitric oxide producers typically have healthy skin and hair and well-developed muscles. In contrast, elderly individuals (and even younger individuals with diminished nitric oxide production) often have thinner hair and paler, thinner skin.

Nitric oxide production can be increased through nutritional supplementation. By improving vasodilation and oxygenation, nitric oxide can greatly improve both health and performance capability. Although research studies have shown that intravenous administration of the amino acid arginine can increase nitric oxide production in humans, attempts to increase nitric oxide production through oral administration of arginine have met with limited success. However, a nutraceutical research and development company has been able to orally administer small amounts of arginine combined with other nutrients, which allows the body to increase its production of nitric oxide. This unique technology offers an effective oral supplement to support the body's production of nitric oxide.

B vitamins

Intakes of folic acid and vitamin B_6 in amounts several times higher than the RDAs for these nutrients appear to protect against heart disease. In a fourteen-year study conducted at Harvard University and published in 1998 in the *Journal of the American Medical Association*, 80,000 healthy middle-aged women were assessed for the intake of these vitamins. Those with the highest intake had a remarkable 45 percent lower incidence of heart disease, as compared with those having the lowest intake.

Fiber

Dietary fiber is valuable for maintaining a healthy heart. See chapters 3 and 4 for specific information on the different types of fiber that can be used in a dietary program.

OSTEOPOROSIS

While much attention has been given to the need for HRT to maintain strong bones after menopause, bone health also depends on having an adequate supply of a long list of nutrients. Vitamins, major minerals, and trace minerals that support bone health include calcium, magnesium, manganese, vitamin K, folic acid, boron, vitamin B_6, zinc, strontium, copper, silicon, vitamin C, and vitamin D. Some of these nutrients work in tandem with one another; for instance, calcium cannot be absorbed without the presence of sufficient magnesium. Unfortunately, the refined foods most Americans consume cause significant deficiencies of these nutrients. To insure bone health, it is important to eat unrefined, unprocessed foods and to take a supplement for bone health that contains a wide variety of essential minerals and other micronutrients that mirror the natural composition of bone.

COGNITIVE FUNCTION

Several nutrients are important for maintaining the health of the brain, thereby supporting cognitive function and benefiting mental clarity and acuity.

Ginkgo biloba

The ginkgo biloba tree originated about 250 million years ago, and a single tree can live as long as 1000 years. It is often planted in urban settings, lining fashionable streets and decorating parks, as it resists disease, insects, and pollution. Modern science is finding that this ancient plant can help prevent the brain from aging. Millions of dosages of ginkgo leaf extracts are taken each year worldwide. The extracts contain flavonols, including the primary flavonoids, quercetin, kaempferol, and isorhamnetine.

Brain cells contain the highest percentage of fragile oils of any part of the body, making the brain particularly susceptible to aging. Ginkgo biloba protects brain and nerve cells from deteriorating by stabilizing cell walls and scavenging free radicals that can destroy delicate cell structures. It also helps maintain the brain's supply of energy in the form of glucose and oxygen.

Various studies give evidence of ginkgo's ability to increase the functional capacity of the brain in illnesses such as Alzheimer's disease, especially in its early stages. The extract promotes synthesis of neurotransmitters and increases nerve transmission rate. A confirming study of the effects of ginkgo extract for dementia was published in 1997 in the *Journal of the American Medical Association*. The study was a one-year, placebo-controlled, double-blind study of 309 patients forty-five years of age or older diagnosed with mild to moderately severe dementia. A standardized extract of ginkgo biloba containing 24 percent ginkgo-flavone glycosides and 6 percent terpene lactones was used. The researchers concluded that ginkgo was safe and appeared capable of stabilizing and, in a substantial number of cases, improving the cognitive performance and social functioning of demented patients for six months to one year. Although changes were modest, they were recognized by the caregivers.

SUGGESTED DOSAGE: Ginkgo biloba extracts are standardized to contain 24 percent flavonoid glycosides and 6 percent terpene lactones. A common dosage is 40 mg, three times a day.

Phosphatidylserine

After midlife, many men and women begin to notice a slow decline in memory, mental alertness, and other cognitive functions. A substance called phosphatidylserine can be helpful in reversing this trend. This substance helps to maintain the flexibility and permeability of our cell membranes, permitting the movement of nutrients into the cell and allowing waste products to be eliminated. Phosphatidylserine levels tend to be more abundant in younger people, and levels decline with age. This can cause cell membranes to become more rigid, so that the free flow of nutrients and waste products, both into and out of the cells, becomes less efficient. High levels of phosphatidylserine are needed by the brain cells to maintain healthy cognitive function.

SUGGESTED DOSAGE Take 100 to 200 mg of phosphatidylserine per day to prevent memory loss and improve cognitive function.

Vitamin E

Vitamin E may play a role in brain function, as evidenced by a 1997 study sponsored by the National Institute on Aging and reported at the annual meeting of the American Academy of Neurology. Researchers assessed the effect of vitamin E supplementation on Alzheimer's disease. Supplementation with 2000 IU of vitamin E slowed the progression of Alzheimer's in patients in moderately severe stages of the disease.

COMPLEMENTARY THERAPIES THAT SUPPORT HORMONAL FUNCTION AT ANY AGE

In this section we discuss two intriguing and innovative methods of improving hormone status. HeartMath makes use of certain mental disciplines, and phototherapy manipulates the quality of light. Whether a person is still producing adequate hormones or their hormone production has begun to decline, these techniques offer yet another way to achieve hormonal health.

HEARTMATH TECHNIQUE

We usually think of hormone production in purely physical terms, but hormone levels are also influenced by our thoughts and emotions. This is a radical concept for Western medicine, but the notion that the mind affects the body is a premise of many natural healing techniques and traditions.

Using scientific methods, researchers at the Institute of HeartMath, in Boulder Creek, California, have done a series of experiments measuring the changes in hormones that different states of mind induce. In the chapter on stress, we gave an extensive description of the HeartMath program and its underlying principles. In essence, the HeartMath premise is that a person's state of mind triggers the heart to emit specific electrical signals, which stimulate the brain to produce certain chemicals. As the heart's electrical signals become more powerful and orderly, the hormonal system is able to function with more harmony and efficiency. This is the phenomenon known as *entrainment,* when two or more systems are locked in frequency and work at maximum efficiency.

The researchers at HeartMath have found that eliminating negative emotions and replacing them with positive feelings like appreciation and thankfulness resulted in an increase in levels of the hormone DHEA. They designed a study using twenty-eight volunteers who practiced a HeartMath technique called "cut-thru." This technique takes a person past angry and anxious thoughts to a state of peace that is heart-centered. Volunteers also listened to music specially composed to promote emotional balance. DHEA samples were taken before the volunteers began the program and after one month. The results were impressive. Among all volunteers, there was an average 100 percent increase in DHEA levels, and for some, DHEA tripled and even quadrupled. As DHEA is a precursor hormone, this means that the levels of all those hormones that arise from DHEA—specifically, testosterone, estrogen, and progesterone—also increased.

The cut-thru technique is a subtle approach to hormone treatment that may work well for those hesitant to use hormone replacement therapy who are willing to turn inward for a few minutes each day. As Susan has heard from enthusiastic fans of HeartMath, the techniques also promote better decision making, greater creativity, and heightened intuition, bonuses beyond the notable increase in hormones.

PHOTOTHERAPY

The health benefits of light have been appreciated since ancient times. More recent research has proven that natural sunlight and various types of light therapy can enhance hormone production and balance. Light that falls on the skin and strikes the retina of the eye has been found to lower hypertension, reduce depression, and treat ailments related to hormone imbalance such as premenstrual syndrome (PMS), decreased sex drive, and infertility.

How light interacts with the body

After light enters the eye, it is converted into electrical impulses through the action of millions of cells that are sensitive to light and color. The electrical impulses move along the optical nerve to the hypothalamus gland in the brain, which regulates a variety of body functions including breathing, digestion, temperature, blood pressure, mood, and sexual function. The resultant stimulatory effect that light has in the hypothalamus can affect the hypothalamus's action on the pituitary gland. The pituitary controls the secretion of many hormones, including luteinizing hormone (LH) and follicle-stimulating hormone (FSH), both involved with the menstrual cycle.

The pineal gland, located in the brain, also receives light waves through the eye, which are then transformed into nerve impulses capable of affecting hormones. The hypothalamus, through the pineal gland, also controls the body's internal clock, the circadian rhythms that pace and synchronize biological events.

Sunlight: A fundamental nutrient

Daily exposure to natural sunlight is as essential for maintaining robust health as vitamins and minerals. Sunlight consists of all wavelengths of light, those that are visible, and those we cannot see, such as the ultraviolet light associated with tanning and the infrared light associated with heating. The full range of frequencies is necessary to insure physical, mental, and emotional well-being, as the different wavelengths act on the body in specific ways. About 98 percent of the sunlight we absorb enters through the eyes, with the remaining 2 percent being absorbed through the skin.

Everyone needs around one-half to two hours of sunlight each day. However, most people, unless they have jobs that involve outdoor work, spend the majority of the day shielded from sunlight. Window glass, windshields on cars, sunglasses and tinted contacts, clothing, and suntan lotion all block sunlight. Smoggy air can also reduce our exposure. Even the coveted corner office, which can have windows on two walls, is not bright enough to be truly life-supporting. Outdoor light is about 100 times more intense than the normal lighting inside a building.

In the late 1870s, researchers found that natural light was capable of killing microorganisms such as bacteria. The health practitioners of the time began to prescribe sunlight therapy for a wide range of ailments, from tuberculosis to obesity. Much of the pioneering work on light therapy in the twentieth century was done by photobiologist John Ott. Dr. Ott did a number of interesting experiments, including research that examined the effect of various wavelengths of light on the growth cycle of plants. He also investigated the effects of ultraviolet light and radiation on humans and developed a number of full-spectrum light products. It is now known that taking in light through the eye plays a role in maintaining high energy and being able to concentrate, both important for peak performance. Having sufficient light also sustains hormone production and the health of the reproductive function in a variety of ways.

Sunlight is necessary for the timely development of secondary sexual characteristics. Boys who are blind have been observed to have delayed spermatogenesis and onset of ejaculation, and blind girls have delayed onset of menstruation. One theory of how this occurs, based on studies on hibernating animals who remain in darkness for long periods, is that the absence of light suppresses the excretion of gonadotropins (gonad-stimulating hormones) from the pituitary gland.

Most people in the workforce spend much of their time indoors working under artificial light, most of which is fluorescent. Fluorescent light is not full spectrum, as the wavelengths are not equivalent to those of sunlight. This distribution of wavelengths is particularly noticeable when you purchase clothing in a store under fluorescent lighting, only to find that the color is different in sunlight. You get the same effect of distorted wavelengths from fluorescent street lights: The colors of cars do not appear the same as they do in daylight. When you work under fluorescent light, you are in essence being undernourished lightwise because the amount of the various color wavelengths differs from that of sunlight and may even be deficient in certain parts of the light spectrum. Fluorescent lights also emit three types of harmful radiation: X-rays, radio frequencies, and extremely low frequency radiation. Working too close to or working for a long time under fluorescent lighting can reduce the activity of the immune system due to the effects of these radiations. Finally, older fluorescent lighting fixtures were underpowered, causing the lights to flicker. This flickering can cause extreme eye fatigue and affect mental and physical performance in the workplace.

Seasonal affective disorder

The short, dark days of winter also limit our access to sunlight. Some individuals are sensitive to this seasonal change. Light deprivation can cause them to feel depressed and tired as well as suffer from a reduction in mental clarity. This condition is known as seasonal affective disorder (SAD). Individuals with SAD may have difficulty getting out of bed in the morning and may tend to isolate themselves socially. They may show less interest in sex. Symptoms of PMS, such as irritability and moodiness, may also worsen. The darker winter days are also associated with decreased fertility. It is thought that these changes occur because the lack of sunlight disrupts the natural pacing of hormone production. Such changes in personality, due to hormonal alterations, can stress personal relationships and even affect job performance.

Individuals who are prone to SAD should, if possible, spend one to two hours in the sun every day during the winter months, when the sun's radiant energy is at its weakest. Indoor lighting from incandescent or halogen bulbs should also be kept bright. In addition, several therapeutic devices are available that can supplement indoor lighting. The light box emits 10,000 lux of bright indoor light. (In contrast, sunshine produces 100,000 lux.) The light spectrum used in this product provides minimal exposure to the more harmful ultraviolet and blue rays and tends to emphasize the red rays, which have a mood-elevating effect. Recommended exposure time is normally one-half hour a day. Individuals can exercise, read, or work at their desk while using the light box. Another type of light therapy called the dawn simulator is used to gradually increase the level of light that an individual with SAD is exposed to in the morning. The light exposure enables SAD sufferers to wake up more rapidly and begin their day's work with more energy. Symptom relief is rapid, usually occurring within several days.

Corporations and businesses can enhance the health and productivity of their workers by using more therapeutic wavelengths and intensities in the lighting systems in their office buildings and plants. The improvement in productivity and health of workers should more than offset the cost of converting and installing bright lighting. Businesses in northern climates might even consider having bright light boxes available for workers in the winter season, as 10 to 20 percent of the workforce may be affected by SAD.

Colored-light therapy

Different visible wavelengths of light, which we see as a particular color, have long been used to treat specific ailments. Today, many alternative health care practitioners work with light therapy, and recently such techniques are gaining more credence among physicians as well. Research studies have tested different parts of the visible light spectrum to see the effect that different types of colored light produced on individuals with SAD. It was found that green light was more effective in treating SAD than red light. Newborns with jaundice are routinely treated with full-spectrum and blue-light phototherapy.

Norman Shealy, a neurosurgeon by training and a prominent practitioner of complementary medicine, incorporates light therapy into his practice, using flashing bright light and colored light to treat depression and pain. Colored-light therapy regulates neuroendocrine and neurochemical functions. A study conducted by Shealy measured the effect of red, green, and violet light on many hormones, including DHEA and progesterone. He found that red light increased the level of fourteen out of the forty hormones and neurochemicals measured; green light, twenty out of forty; and violet light, fifteen out of forty. Red-light therapy has been used successfully to treat dysmenorrhea, PMS, frigidity, and impotence. Other research has found red light to have a stimulatory effect on the pituitary and immune systems: It is useful in improving energy and vitality in individuals suffering from chronic fatigue.

SUMMARY OF TREATMENT OPTIONS
FOR RESTORING YOUR SEX HORMONES

Pregnenolone supplementation

DHEA supplementation

Testosterone

    Conventional testosterone therapy

    Natural testosterone

    Herbal support for testosterone production and sexual function:

        Ginseng

Testosterone (cont.)
    Nutrients that support testosterone production, normal sperm
        count, and healthy reproductive function
        Zinc
        Vitamin C and other antioxidants
        Vitamin B_{12}
        Carnitine

Estrogen
    Conventional estrogen therapy
    Estriol
    Dietary substances with estrogenlike activity
        Soy foods
        Vitamin E
        Bioflavonoids
        Essential fatty acids
    Boron
        Black cohosh
        Licorice root
    Dietary substances that promote healthy hormonal balance
        Chaste tree berry (*Vitex agnus castus*)
        Dandelion root
        Dong quai

Progesterone
    Conventional progesterone therapy (progestins)
    Natural progesterone

**Nutrients that support specific benefits of hormone replacement
therapy**
    Heart disease
        Nitric-oxide enhancers
        Antioxidants
        B vitamins
        Fiber
    Osteoporosis
        Major minerals
        Trace minerals
        Vitamins C, D, K, and folic acid

Nutrients that support specific benefits of hormone replacement
therapy (cont.)
   Cognitive function
     Ginkgo biloba
     Phosphatidylserine
     Vitamin E

Complementary therapies that support healthy hormone production
   HeartMath technique
   Light therapy

PEAK-PERFORMANCE RESOURCES

CHEMISTRY OF SUCCESS PROGRAMS BY SUSAN M. LARK, MD, AND JAMES A. RICHARDS, MBA

Dr. Lark and Mr. Richards provide consulting services to organizations and individuals interested in using the principles and techniques of the Chemistry of Success to enhance performance and productivity and achieve optimal health. Their services include the following:

Trainings and seminars on the Chemistry of Success for organizations

These seminars provide organizations with essential information on how their members can support and maintain their own Chemistry of Success. This information will enable the members of your team to experience a quantum leap in their own personal performance capability and productivity, as well as achieve optimal health and well-being. These seminars can be customized to fit the needs of any size group.

Editions of the book can be customized for your organization through arrangement with the publisher (Bay Books, 800-231-4944).

Creating a Chemistry of Success environment for the office or home

Dr. Lark and Mr. Richards develop customized plans for organizations that want to enhance the peak-performance capability and productivity of their members by creating a work environment that supports the Chemistry of Success. To achieve these goals, they can assist your organization in greatly improving food services, fitness centers, and preventive health programs, as well as the quality of the air, water, and light in your physical plants and offices based on the principles of the Chemistry of Success. Their customized programs will help increase the physical and mental energy of your group members and improve their productivity, as well as assist them in achieving optimal health and well-being.

Public and private institutions, corporations, health care organizations, schools and universities, retirement and nursing care facilities, private social clubs, resort and spa facilities, and sports and athletic teams are but a few of the organizations that can benefit from creating a peak-performance environment for their members.

Similar programs can be developed to create a Chemistry of Success environment in your home.

Editions of the book can be customized for your organization through arrangement with the publisher (Bay Books, 800-231-4944).

Chemistry of Success programs for individuals

Dr. Lark and Mr. Richards also develop fully customized Chemistry of Success programs for interested individuals. These programs are designed to meet the peak-performance goals and optimal-health objectives of each client.

Individuals who can benefit from these customized programs include the following:

+ Peak performers who are currently at the height of their career and personal success and wish to continue to make incremental gains in important areas of their lives and careers

+ Individuals who have had the Chemistry of Success throughout their lives but are experiencing an age-related or health-related decline in their ability to consistently maintain their winner's edge

+ People who have never quite had the Chemistry of Success and as a result have not been able to perform to the level they desire, despite positive mental programming for success

For additional information, contact Dr. Lark and Mr. Richards:

Susan M. Lark, MD, & James A. Richards
101 First Street, Suite 499
Los Altos, CA 94022-2750
Tel: 650-559-1735
Fax: 650-941-2175
E-mail: jaroffice@netgate.net

How to receive information on new projects relating to the Chemistry of Success

Dr. Lark and Mr. Richards are constantly developing new informaiton and educational resources, programs, and products to enhance your Chemistry of Success. If you would like to be notified about these new resources, please register by sending your name, E-mail, or mailing address and phone number to Dr. Lark's and Mr. Richards' office or to the Chemistry of Success website (see Chemistry of Success Resources, following).

CHEMISTRY OF SUCCESS RESOURCES

Many of the resources and products described in this book, such as the device for creating high-pH alkaline water; ozone air, water, and spa devices; therapeutic magnets; and nutritional supplements that support the Chemistry of Success are available through

Chemistry of Success Resources
Tel: 800-941-1997 (orders only)
Tel: 650-941-2023 (for information)
E-mail: Products@ChemSuccess.com
Web: www.ChemSuccess.com

ABOUT THE AUTHORS

Susan M. Lark, MD

Susan M. Lark, MD, is one of the foremost authorities in the field of clinical nutrition and preventive medicine. A graduate of Northwestern University Medical School, she has served on the clinical faculty of Stanford University Medical School, where she continues to teach in the division of Family and Community Medicine. She is a distinguished clinician, author, innovative product developer, and lecturer. Her clinical practice has spanned twenty-four years in the field of preventive medicine and clinical nutrition.

Dr. Lark is one of the most widely referenced physicians in the world on the Internet. She has been a consultant to major corporations, including the Kellogg Company and Weider Nutrition International, one of the largest manufacturers and marketers of nutritional supplements in the United States. She is the author of a nine-book series on women's health issues and clinical nutrition, including *Premenstrual Syndrome Self Help Book, Menopause Self Help Book, Anxiety and Stress,* and *Chronic Fatigue,* among others. She has appeared on hundreds of radio and television shows. In addition, her work has been featured in most of the major magazines and newspapers in the United States, such as *Reader's Digest, McCall's, Better Homes & Gardens, Shape, Mademoiselle, Seventeen, Redbook,* the *New York Times,* the *Chicago Tribune,* and the *San Francisco Chronicle.* She presently writes a biweekly health column in the *National Enquirer.*

James A. Richards, MBA

James A. Richards, MBA, is a graduate of Yale University and received his MBA from Stanford University Graduate School of Business. He spent many years in the investment banking and brokerage field. He started his career with Lehman Brothers, one of the major investment banking and brokerage firms in the United States. He subsequently founded his own consulting business in Silicon Valley, specializing in start-up companies and the licensing of innovative products to major corporations. He is currently a founder and director of CMI Worldwide, Inc., an Internet and e-commerce company.

For the past two decades, Mr. Richards has been working with Dr. Lark on the development of this new performance model and its application to success, peak performance, and optimal health. His particular interest has been the application of this work to business success and athletic performance.

PEAK-PERFORMANCE RESOURCES BY OTHER GROUPS

Tools for Managing Stress/Accelerated Learning Technologies

Tools for Exploration
9755 Independence Avenue
Chatsworth, CA 91311
Tel: 800-456-9887
Fax: 818-407-0850
E-mail: toolsforexploration@yahoo.com
Web: www.toolsforexploration.com

The Relaxation Company
20 Lumber Road
Roslyn, NY 11576
Tel: 800-788-6670
Fax: 516-621-2750
E-mail: elliarts@aol.com
E-mail: relaxco@aol.com

Lind Institute
243 Divisadero Street
P.O. Box 14487
San Francisco, CA 94114
Tel: 800-462-3766
Fax: 415-864-1742
E-mail: lind@lind-institute.com

Superlearning, Inc.
450 Seventh Avenue, Suite 500
New York, NY 10123-0500
Tel: 212-279-8450
Fax: 212-695-9288
E-mail: superlearning@worldnet.att.net
Web: www.superlearning.com

Learning Strategies Corporation
900 East Wayzata Boulevard
Wayzata, MN 55391-1836 USA
Tel: 612-476-9200 or 800-735-8273
Fax: 612-475-2373
E-mail: Info@LearningStrategies.com
Web: www.learningstrategies.com

HeartMath LLC
14700 West Park Avenue
Boulder Creek, CA 95006-9318
Tel: 408-338-8700
Tel: 800-450-9111
Fax: 408-338-9861
E-mail: gboehmer@heartmath.ipc.net
Web: www.heartmath.com

Blender Drinks

Vita-Mix Corporation
8615 Usher Road
Cleveland, OH 44138-2199
Tel: 800-848-2649
Fax: 440-235-3726

Massage Equipment

Wellness America (The Thumper)
1010 Niagara Street
Buffalo, NY 14213-2091
Tel: 800-848-6737
Fax: 905-477-5329

Low-Acid Coffee

Coffee Bean & Tea Leaf Company
4580 Calle Alto
Camarillo, CA 93012-8578
Tel: 800-TEA-LEAF
Fax: 805-484-4874
E-mail: info@coffeebean.com
Web: www.coffeebean.com

COMPLEMENTARY MEDICAL ORGANIZATIONS FOR PHYSICIAN REFERRALS

International Oxidative Medicine Association
P.O. Box 891954
Oklahoma City, OK 73189
Tel: 405-634-1310
Fax: 405-634-7320

American College for Advancement in Medicine
23121 Verdugo Drive, Suite 204
Laguna Hills, CA 92653
Tel: 714-583-7666
Tel: 800-532-3688
Fax: 714-455-9679
E-mail: acam@acam.org
Web: www.acam.org

American Holistic Medical Association
6728 Old McLean Village Drive
McLean, VA 22101
Tel: 703-556-9245
Fax: 703-556-8729
E-mail holistmed@aol.com

American Academy of Anti-Aging Medicine
1341 West Fullerton, Suite 111
Chicago, IL 60614
Tel: 800-558-1267
Fax: 773-528-5395

International Ozone Association
31 Strawberry Hill Avenue
Stamford, CT 06902
Tel: 203-348-3542

International Bio-Oxidative Medicine Foundation
P.O. Box 13205
Oklahoma City, OK 73113-1205
Tel: 405-478-4266

LABORATORY TESTING

Saliva Tests

Aeron Biotechnology, Inc.
1933 Davis Street
San Leandro, CA 94577
Tel: 510-729-0375
Tel: 800-631-7900
Fax: 510-729-0383
E-mail: aeron@aeron.com
Web: www.aeron.com

Diagnos-Techs, Inc.
6620 South 192nd Place, Suite J-104
Kent, WA 98032
Tel: 425-251-0596
Tel: 800-878-3787
Fax: 425-251-0637
E-mail: diagnos@cnet.com
Web: www.diagnostechs.com

Nutrient Testing

SpectraCell Laboratories, Inc.
515 Post Oak Boulevard, Suite 830
Houston, TX 77027
Tel: 713-621-3101
Tel: 800-227-5227
Fax: 713-621-3231
E-mail: spec1@spectracell.com
Web: www.spectracell.com

Hair Analysis

Great Smokies Diagnostic Laboratory
63 Zillicoa Street
Ashville, NC 28801-1074
Tel: 800-522-4762
Fax: 704-252-9303
E-mail: cs@gsdl.com
Web: www.gsdl.com

pH Test Paper

Micro Essential Laboratory, Inc.
4224 Avenue H
Brooklyn, NY 11210
Tel: 718-338-3618
Fax: 718-692-4491

COMPOUNDING PHARMACIES

Women's International Pharmacy
5708 Monona Drive
Madison, WI 53716
Tel: 608-221-7800
Tel: 800-279-5708
Fax: 800-279-8011
E-mail: info@wipws.com
Web: www.wipws.com

Madison Pharmacy Associates
429 Gammon Place
P.O. Box 259690
Madison, WI 53725
Tel: 608-833-7046
Tel: 800-558-7046
Fax: 888-898-7412
E-mail: wha@womenshealth.com
Web: www.womenshealth.com

Apothecure, Inc.
13720 Midway Road
Dallas, TX 75244
Tel: 972-960-6601
Tel: 800-969-6601
Fax: 800-687-5252
E-mail: gosborn@airmail.net
Web: www.apothecure.com

COMPLEMENTARY MEDICAL INFORMATION

Magazines

Townsend Letter for Doctors & Patients
911 Tyler Street
Port Townsend, WA 98368-6541
Tel: 360-385-6021
Fax: 360-385-0699
E-mail: tldp@olympus.net
Web: www.tldp.com

Explore!
Explore Publications, Inc.
P.O. Box 1508
Mount Vernon, WA 98273
Tel: 360-424-6025
Fax: 360-424-6029
E-mail: ExplorePub@aol.com

Alternative Medicine Digest
$21^1/_2$ Main Street
Tiburon, CA 94920
Tel: 800-333-4325
Fax: 415-789-9138
E-mail: altmed@ix.netcom.net
Web: www.alternativemedicine.com

Alternative & Complementary Therapies
Mary Ann Liebert, Inc.
Two Madison Avenue
Larchmont, NY 10538
Tel: 914-834-3100
Fax: 914-834-3582
E-mail: liebert@pipeline.com

Books on Relaxation, Meditation, and Yoga

Bell, L., and E. Seyfer. *Gentle Yoga*. Berkeley, CA: Celestial Arts, 1987.

Bourne, E. J. *The Anxiety and Phobia Workbook*. Oakland, CA: New Harbinger Publications, 1990.

Davis, M. M., M. Eshelman, and E. Eshelman. *The Relaxation and Stress Reduction Workbook*. Oakland, CA: Hew Harbinger Publications, 1982.

Folan, L. *Lilias, Yoga, and Your Life*. New York: Macmillan, 1981.

Gawain, S. *Creative Visualization*. San Rafael, CA: New World Publishing, 1978.

Gawain, S. *Living in the Light*. Mill Valley, CA: Whatever Publishing, 1986.

Hanna, T. *Somatics*. Reading, MA: Addison-Wesley, 1988.

Huang, C. A. *Tai Ji*. Berkeley, CA: Celestial Arts, 1989.

Iyengar, B. K. S. *Light on Yoga*. New York: Schocken Books, 1966.

Jerome, J. *Staying Supple*. New York: Bantam Books, 1987.

Kripalu Center for Holistic Health. *The Self-Health Guide*. Lenox, MA: Kripalu Publications, 1980.

Lark, Susan M., MD. *Anxiety and Stress*. Berkeley, CA: Celestial Arts, 1993.

Lark, Susan M., MD. *Chronic Fatigue*. Berkeley, CA: Celestial Arts, 1993.

Loehr, J., and J. Migdow. *Take a Deep Breath*. New York: Villard Books, 1986.

Miller, E. *Self-Imagery*. Berkeley, CA: Celestial Arts, 1986.

Ornstein, R., and D. Sobel. *Healthy Pleasures*. Reading, MA: Addison-Wesley, 1989.

Padis, E. *Your Emotions and Your Health*. Emmaus, PA: Rodale Press, 1986.

Powell, T. *Free Yourself from Harmful Stress*. New York: DK Publishing, 1997

Solveborne, S. A., MD. *The Book About Stretching*. New York: Japan Publications, 1985.

Tobias, M., and M. Stewart. *Stretch and Relax*. Tucson, AZ: The Body Press, 1985.

Bibliography

Chapters 1 & 2

Anand, C. R., and H. M. Linskwiler. 1974. Effect of protein intake on calcium balance of young men given 500 mg calcium daily. *Journal of Nutrition* 104:695–700.

Anding, J. D., et al. 1994. Diet and health behaviors of 14- and 15-year-old adolescents during summer months. *FASEB Journal* 8(A):274.

Arruda, J. A. L., and N. A. Kurtzman. 1978. Relationship of renal sodium and water transport to hydrogen ion secretion. *Annual Review of Physiology* 40:43–66.

Bell, D. S. H., and J. Adele. 1997. Diabetic ketoacidosis. Why early detection and aggressive treatment are crucial. *Postgraduate Medicine* 101(4):193–204.

Bou-Abboud, E., and S. Nattel. 1996. Relative role of alkalosis and sodium ions in reversal of Class 1 antiarrhythmic drug-induced sodium channel blockade by sodium bicarbonate. *Circulation* 94:1954–1961.

Coronado, B. E., et al. 1995. Antibiotic induced D-lactic acidosis. *Annals of Internal Medicine* 122(11):839–842.

Costill, D. L. 1977. Sweating: Its composition and effects on body fluids. *Annals of the New York Academy of Sciences* 301:160–174.

Costill, D. L., et al. 1984. Acid-base balance during repeated bouts of exercise: Influence of HCO_3. *International Journal of Sports Medicine* 5:228–231.

Cushner, H. M., et al. 1986. Calcium citrate, a new phosphate-binding and alkalinizing agent for patients with renal failure. *Current Therapeutic Research* 40(6):998–1004.

Dale, G., et al. 1987. Fitness, unfitness, and phosphate. *British Medical Journal* 294:939.

Davey, C. L. 1960. The significance of carnosine and anserine in striated skeletal muscle. *Archives of Biochemistry and Biophysics* 89:303–308.

Dennig, H. 1937. *German Weekly Medical Journal* 63:733.

Donoghue, S. 1994. Supplements for performance: Does supercharging with supplements give your dog an edge? *Pure-Bred Dogs/American Kennel Gazette* (June):22–23.

Draper, H. H., and C. A. Scythes. 1981. Calcium, phosphorus, and osteoporosis. *Federation Proceedings* 40:2434–2438.

Ellis, F. R., et al. 1972. Incidence of osteoporosis in vegetarians and omnivores. *American Journal of Clinical Nutrition* 25:555–558.

Ettinger, B., et al. 1997. Potassium-magnesium citrate is an effective prophalaxis against recurrent calcium oxalate nephrolithiasis. *Journal of Urology* 158:2069–2073.

Farber, M. O., et al. 1984. Effect of decreased O_2 affinity of hemoglobin on work performance during exercise in healthy humans. *Journal of Laboratory and Clinical Medicine* 104(2):166–175.

Fuselier, H. A., et al. 1995. Urinary Tamm-Horsfall protein increased after potassium citrate therapy in calcium stone formers. *Urology* 45(6):942–946.

Gargan, R. A., et al. 1993. Effect of alkalinization and increased fluid intake on bacterial phagocytosis and killing in urine. *European Journal of Clinical Microbiology and Infectious Diseases* 12(7):534–539.

George, K. P., and D. P. M. MacLaren. 1988. The effect of induced alkalosis and acidosis on endurance running at an intensity corresponding to 4mM blood lactate. *Ergonomics* 31(11):1639–1645.

Gizis, F. C. 1992. Nutrition in women across the life span. *Nursing Clinics of North America* 27(4):971–982.

Hansen, K. M. 1938. Some observations with a view to possible influence of magnetism upon the human organism. *ACTA Medica Scandinavica* XCVII(III–IV): 339–364.

Harris, S. S., and B. Dawson-Hughes. 1994. Caffeine and bone loss in healthy postmenopausal women. *American Journal of Clinical Nutrition* 60:573–578.

Hegsted, M., and H. M. Linkswiler. 1981. Long-term effects on level of protein intake on calcium metabolism in young adult women. *Journal of Nutrition* 111:244–251.

Hegsted, M., et al. 1981. Urinary calcium and calcium balance in young men as affected by level of protein and phosphorus intake. *Journal of Nutrition* 111:553–562.

Hermansen, L., and J-B. Osnes. 1972. Blood and muscle pH after maximal exercise in man. *Journal of Applied Physiology* 32(3):304–308.

Hintz, H. E. 1994. Ergogenics. *Equine Practice* 16(7)(July/August):8–9.

Hong, C-Z., et al. 1982. Magnetic necklace: its therapeutic effectiveness on neck and shoulder pain. *Archives of Physical Medicine and Rehabilitation* 63:462–466.

Hong, C-Z., et al. 1986. Static magnetic field influence on rat tail nerve function. *Archives of Physical Medicine and Rehabilitation* 67:746–749.

Hong, C-Z., et al. 1987. Static magnetic field influence on human nerve function. *Archives of Physical Medicine and Rehabilitation* 68:162–164.

Hood, V. L., et al. 1988. Effect of systemic pH on pH and lactic acid generation in exhaustive forearm exercise. *American Physiological Society* F479–F485.

Horswill, C. A., et al. 1988. Influence of sodium bicarbonate on sprint performance: Relationship to dosage. *Medicine and Science in Sports and Medicine* 20(6):566–569.

Hultman, E., and H. Sjöholm. 1983. Energy metabolism and contraction force of human skeletal muscle *in situ* during electrical stimulation. *Journal of Physiology* 345:525–532.

Jacobs, I., et al. 1983. Lactate in human skeletal muscle after 10 and 30-s of supramaximal exercise. *Journal of the American Physiology Society* 365–367.

Jacobs, I., et al. 1982. Changes in muscle metabolites in females with 30-s exhaustive exercise. *Medicine and Science in Sports and Exercise* 14(6):457–460.

Johnson, J. M., and P. M. Walker. 1992. Zinc and iron utilization in young women consuming a beef-based diet. *Journal of the American Dietetics Association* 92(12):1474–1478.

Konishi, N., et al. 1993. Inhibitory effect of potassium citrate on rat renal tumors induced by n-ethyl-n-hydroxyethylnitrosamine followed by potassium dibasic phosphate. *Japanese Journal of Clinical Research* 84:128–134.

Kowalchuk, J. M., et al. 1989. The effect of citrate loading on exercise performance, acid-base balance and metabolism. *European Journal of Applied Physiology* 58:858–864.

Kraut, J. A., and J. W. Coburn. 1994. Bone, acid and osteoporosis. *New England Journal of Medicine* 330(25):1821–1822.

Kreider, R. B., et al. 1990. Effects of phosphate loading on oxygen uptake, ventilatory anaerobic threshold and in performance. *Medicine and Science in Sports and Exercise* 22:250–255.

Lake, K. D., and D. C. Brown. 1985. New drug therapy for kidney stones: A review of cellulose sodium phosphate, acetohydroxamic acid, and potassium citrate. *Drug Intelligence and Clinical Pharmacy* 19:530–539.

Lavender, G., and S. R. Bird. 1989. Effect of sodium bicarbonate ingestion upon repeated sprints. *British Journal of Sports Medicine* 23(1):41–45.

Linderman, J. K., and K. Gosselink. 1994. The effects of sodium bicarbonate ingestion on exercise performance. *Sports Medicine* 18(2):75–80.

Linkswiler, H. M., et al. 1981. Protein-induced hypercalciuria. *Federation of American Societies for Experimental Biology* 40:2429–2433.

Lutz, J. 1984. Calcium balance and acid-base status of women as affected by increased protein intake and by sodium bicarbonate ingestion. *The American Journal of Clinical Nutrition* 39:281–288.

Malnic, G., and G. Giebisch. 1972. Mechanism of renal hydrogen ion secretion. *Kidney International* 1:280–296.

Marsh, A. C., et al. 1980. Cortical bone density of adult lacto-ovo–vegetarian and omnivorous women. *Journal of the American Dietetic Association* 76:148–151.

Martini, L. A., et al. 1993. Dietary habits of calcium stone formers. *Brazilian Journal of Medical and Biological Research* 26:805–812.

Matson, L. G., and Z. Vu Tran. 1993. Effects of sodium bicarbonate ingestion on anaerobic performance. *International Journal of Sports Nutrition* 3:2–28.

McCaughton, L., and R. Cedaro. 1991. The effect of sodium bicarbonate on rowing ergometer performance in elite rowers. *Australian Journal of Science and Medicine and Sports* (September):66–69.

McCully, K. 1988. Detection of muscle injury in humans with 31-P magnetic resonance spectroscopy. *Muscle and Nerve* 11:212–216.

Merkel, J. M., et al. 1990. Vitamin and mineral supplement use by women with school-age children. *Journal of the American Dietetic Association* 90(3):426–428.

Meyer, J. H., et al. 1970. Pancreatic bicarbonate response to various acids in duodenum of the dog. *American Journal of Physiology* 219:964–970.

Miller, R. G., et al. 1988. P nuclear magnetic resonance studies of high energy phosphates and pH in human muscle fatigue. *Journal of Clinical Investigation* 81:1190–1196.

Moshal, M. G., and M. Naicker. 1978. Antacid properties of a sodium citrate preparation. *South African Medical Journal* 54:105–107

Nicklas, T. A., et al. 1993. Breakfast consumption affects adequacy of total daily intake in children. *FASEB Journal* 93(8):886–891.

Noble, B. J., et al. 1983. A category-ratio perceived exertion scale: Relationship to blood and muscle lactates and heart rate. *Medicine and Science in Sports and Exercise* 15(6):523–528.

Osnes, J-B., and L. Hermansen. 1972. Acid–base balance after maximal exercise of short duration. *Journal of Applied Physiology* 32(1):59–63.

Oster, J. R., et al. 1988. Comparison of the effects of sodium bicarbonate versus sodium citrate on renal acid excretion. *Mineral Electrolyte Metabolism* 14:97–102.

Passfall, J., et al. 1997. Effect of water and bicarbonate loading in patients with chronic renal failure. *Clinical Nephrology* 47(2):92–98.

Preminger, G. M. 1987. Pharmacologic treatment of uric acid calculi. *Urologic Clinics of North America* 14(2):335–338.

Rau, T. 1995. Using biological-regulative therapy for inflammatory-rheumatic diseases. *Explore!* 6(5):8–12.

Rau, T. 1996. Allergies, what now? *Explore!* 7(2):34–38.

Remer, T., and F. Manz. 1994. Estimation of the renal net acid excretion by adults consuming diets containing variable amounts of protein. *American Journal of Clinical Nutrition* 59:1356–1361.

Sahlin, K., et al. 1978. Acid–base balance in blood during exhaustive bicycle exercise and the following recovery period. *ACTA Physiologica Scandinavica* 104:370–372.

Schuette, S. A., et al. 1980. Studies on the mechanism of protein-induced hypercalciuria in older men and women. *Journal of Nutrition* 110:305–315.

Sebastion, A., et al. 1994. Improved mineral balance and skeletal metabolism in postmenopausal women treated with potassium bicarbonate. *New England Journal of Medicine* 330:1176–81.

Spooner, J. B. 1984. Alkalinization in the management of cystitis. *Journal of International Medical Research* 12:30–34.

Sugar, A., and G. Block. 1990. Use of vitamin and mineral supplement demographics and amounts of nutrients consumed. *American Journal of Epidemiology* 132:1091–1101.

Sutton, J. R., et al. 1981. Effect of pH on muscle glycolysis during exercise. *Clinical Science* 61:331–338.

Tannen, R. L. 1980. Control of acid excretion by the kidney. *Annual Review of Medicine* 31:35–49.

Tauchi, H., et al. 1971. Age changes in the human kidney of the different races. *Gerontologia* 17:87–97.

Tesch, P. 1980. Muscle fatigue in man with special reference to lactate accumulation during short term intense exercise. *ACTA Physiologica Scandinavica* S480:1–31.

Trock, D. H., et al. 1993. A double-blind trial of the clinical effects of pulsed electromagnetic fields in osteoarthritis. *Journal of Rheumatology* 20:456–460.

Trock, D. H., et al. 1994. The effect of pulsed electromagnetic fields in the treatment of osteoarthritis of the knee and cervical spine: Report of randomized, double-blind, placebo-controlled trials. *Journal of Rheumatology* 21:1903–1911.

Ueda, H., et al. 1978. Effect of oral administration of calcium carbonate, aluminum hydroxide gel and dihydrotachysterol on renal acidosis. *Tohoku Journal of Experimental Medicine* 124:1–11.

Vallbona, C., et al. 1997. Response of pain to static magnetic fields in postpolio patients: A double-blind pilot study. *Archives of Physical Medicine and Rehabilitation* 78:1200–1203.

Vandeursen, H., et al. 1992. Effect of alkalinization on calcium oxalate monohydrate calculi during extracorporeal shock wave lithotripsy: In-vivo experiments. *Urologia Internationalis* 48:203–205.

Warburg, O. 1956. On the origin of cancer cells. *Science* 123(3191):309–314.

Warnock, D. G., and F. C. Rector, Jr. 1979. Proton secretion by the kidney. *Annual Review of Physiology* 41:197–210.

Wilkes, D., et al. 1983. Effect of acute induced metabolic alkalosis on 800-m racing time. *Medicine and Science in Sports and Exercise* 15(4):277–280.

Williams, M. H. 1992. Ergogenic and ergolytic substances. *Medicine and Science in Sports and Nutrition* S344–S348.

Wolfe, W. S., and C. C. Campbell. 1993. Food pattern, diet quality, and related characteristics of schoolchildren in New York State. *Journal of the American Dietetics Association* 93(11):1280–1284.

CHAPTERS 3 & 4

Ambrus, J. L., et al. 1967. Absorption of exogenous and endogenous proteolytic enzymes. *Clinical Pharmacology and Therapeutics* 8(3):362–368.

Anonymous. 1970. Pancreatic extracts. *British Medical Journal* 2:161–163

Anonymous. 1977. Pancreatic enzymes. *Lancet* 2:73–75.

Austad, W. J. 1979. Pancreatitis: The use of pancreatic supplements. *Drugs* 17:480–487.

Bank, S., et al. 1977. Treatment of acute and chronic pancreatitis. *Drugs* 13:373.

Blonstein, J. L. 1960. The use of "buccal varidase" in boxing injuries. *Practitioner* 185:78–79.

Boyne, P. S., and H. Medhurst. 1967. Oral anti-inflammatory enzyme therapy in injuries in professional footballers. *Practitioner* 198(S):543–546.

Buck, J. E., and N. Phillips. 1970. Trial of chymoral in professional footballers. *British Journal of Clinical Practice* 24(9):375–377.

Caci, F., and G. M. Gluck. 1976. Double-blind study of prednisolone and papase as inhibitors of complications in oral surgery. *Journal of the American Dental Association* 93:325–327.

Cichoke, A. *Enzymes and Enzyme Therapy.* New Canaan, CT: Keats Publishing, 1994.

Clemetson, C., et al. 1980. Histamine and ascorbic acid in human blood. *Journal of Nutrition* 110:662–668.

Deodhar, S. D., et al. 1980. Preliminary studies on antirheumatic activity of curcumin (diferuloyl methane) in patients with postoperative inflammation. *International Journal of Medical Research* 71:632–634.

DiMagno, E. P., et al. 1973. Relations between pancreatic enzyme outputs and malabsorption in severe pancreatic insufficiency. *New England Journal of Medicine* 288(16):813–815.

DiMagno, E. P., et al. 1977. Fate of orally ingested enzymes in pancreatic insufficiency. *New England Journal of Medicine* 296:1318–1322.

Donath, F., et al. 1997. Dose-related bioavailability of bromelain and trypsin after repeated oral administration. *Clinical Pharmacology and Therapeutics* 61:157.

Feltin, G. 1976. Does kinen released by pineapple stem bromelain stimulate production of prostaglandin E1–like compounds. *Hawaii Medical Journal* 19:73–77.

Fiasse, R., et al. 1978. Circulating immune complexes and disease activity in Crohn's disease. *Gut* 19:611–617.

Fullgrabe, E. A. 1957. Clinical experiences with chymotrypsin. *Annals of the New York Academy of Sciences* 68:192–195.

Goldberg, D. M. 1992. Enzymes as agents for the treatment of disease. *Clinica Chimica Acta* 206:45–76.

Gordon, B. 1975. The use of topical proteolytic enzymes in the treatment of post-thrombotic leg ulcers. *British Journal of Clinical Practice* 29:143–146.

Goulart, F. S. 1997. An alternative approach to reversing asthma. *Alternative and Complementary Therapies* (June):179–182.

Graham, D. Y. 1977. Enzyme replacement therapy of exocrine pancreatic insufficiency in man. *New England Journal of Medicine* 296(23):1314–1317.

Graham, D. Y. 1979. An enteric-coated pancreatic enzyme preparation that works. *Digestive Diseases and Sciences* 24(12):906–909.

Grossman, M. I., et al. 1943. On the mechanism of the adaptation of pancreatic enzymes to dietary composition. *American Journal of Physiology* 138:676.

Hall, D. A., et al. 1982. The effect of enzyme therapy on plasma lipid levels in the elderly. *Atherosclerosis* 43:209–215.

Heinicke, R. M., et al. 1972. Effect of bromelain on human platelet aggregation. *Experientia* 28:844–845.

Hemmings, W. A., and E. W. Williams. 1978. Transport of large breakdown products of dietary protein through the gut wall. *Gut* 19:715–723.

Hodgson, H. J. F., et al. 1977. Immune complexes in ulcerative colitis and Crohn's disease. *Clinical and Experimental Immunology* 29:187–196.

Holcenberg, J. S. 1981. Enzyme therapy of cancer, future studies. *Cancer Treatment Reports* 4:61–65.

Holland, P. D., et al. 1974. The enhancing influence of proteolysis on E Rosette–forming lymphocytes (T cells) in vivo and in vitro. *British Journal of Cancer* 31:64–69.

Holt, H. T. 1969. Carica papaya as ancillary therapy for athletic injuries. *Current Therapeutic Research* 11(10):621–624.

Holtmann, G. 1989. Differential effects of acute mental stress on interdigestive secretion of gastric acid, pancreatic enzymes, and gastroduodenal motility. *Digestive Diseases and Sciences* 34(11):1701–1707.

Hunter, R. G., et al. 1957. The action of papain and bromelain on the uterus. *American Journal of Obstetrics and Gynecology* 71(4)(April):867–874.

Isaksson, G., and I. Ihse. 1983. Pain reduction by an oral pancreatic enzyme preparation in chronic pancreatitis. *Digestive Diseases and Sciences* 28:97–102.

Jacob, S. W., and R. Herschler. 1983. Introductory remarks: Dimethyl sulfoxide after twenty years. *Annals of the New York Academy of Sciences* 411:xiii–xvii.

Karani, S., et al. 1971. A double-blind clinical trial with a digestive enzyme product. *British Journal of Clinical Practice* 25(8):375–377.

Kataria, M. S., and D. Bhaskarrao. 1969. A clinical double-blind trial with a broad spectrum digestive enzyme product (Combinzym) in geriatric practice. *British Journal of Clinical Practice* 23(1):15–17.

Kelly, G. S. 1996. Bromelain: A literature review and discussion of its therapeutic applications. *Alternative Medicine Review* 1:243–247.

Kelly, G. S. 1997. Hydrochloric acid: Physiological functions and clinical implications. *Alternative Medicine Review* 2(2):116–127.

Knill-Jones R. P., et al. 1970. Comparative trial of Nutrizym in chronic pancreatic insufficiency. *British Medical Journal* 4:21–24.

Lennard-Jones, J. E. 1983. Functional gastrointestinal disorders. *New England Journal of Medicine* 308:431–435.

Lichtman, A. L. 1957. Traumatic injury in athletes. *International Recreational Medicine* 170:322–325.

Lopez, D. A. *Enzymes: The Fountain of Youth*. Germany: The Neville Press, 1994.

Luerti, M., and M. Vignali. 1978. Influences of bromelain on penetration of antibiotics in uterus, salpinx and ovary. *Drugs under Experimental and Clinical Research* 4(1):45–48.

Lund, M., and R. Royer. 1969. Carcia papaya in head and neck surgery. *Archives of Surgery* 98:180–182.

Mackie, R. D., et al. 1981. Malabsorption of starch in pancreatic insufficiency. *Gastroenterology* 80(5):1220.

Mainz, D. L., and P. D. Webster. 1977. Effect of fasting on pancreatic enzymes. *Proceedings of the Society for Experimental Biology and Medicine* 156:340–344.

Marsh, W. H., et al. 1988. Acute pancreatitis following cutaneous exposure to an organophosphate insecticide. *American Journal of Gastroenterology* 83:1158–1160.

Masson, M. 1995. Bromelain in the treatment of blunt injuries to the musculoskeletal system: A case observation study by an orthopedic surgeon in private practice. *Fortschritte Der Medizin* 113(19):303.

Messer, M., and P. E. Baume. 1976. Oral papain in gluten intolerance. *Lancet* 2(S):1022.

Meyer, J. H. 1977. The ins and outs of oral pancreatic enzymes. *New England Journal of Medicine* 296(S):1347–1348.

Miller, J. 1964. The increased proteolytic activity of human blood serum after bromelain. *Journal of Experimental Medicine and Surgery* 22(4):277–280.

Mindell, E. 1997. Sulfur sets the world of nutrition on fire. *Ah Ha!*, the quarterly newsletter of the American Holistic Medical Association 4(1):1,6.

Morita, A. H., et al. 1979. Chromatographic fractionation and characterization of the active platelet aggregation inhibitory factor from bromelain. *Archives of International Pharmacology and Therapy* 239:340–365.

Murray, M. *The 21st Century Herbal*. Bellevue: Vita-Line.

Murray, M. 1994. *Glandular Extracts*. New Canaan: Keats Publishing.

Neubauer, R. A. 1961. A plant protease for potentiation of and possible replacement of antibiotics. *Experimental Medicine & Surgery* 19:143–160.

Nordgaard, I., et al. 1996. Colonic production of butyrate in patients with previous colonic cancer during long-term treatment with dietary fiber (plantago ovata seeds). *Scandinavian Journal of Gastroenterology* 31:1011–20.

Parries, G. S., and M. Hokin-Neaverson. 1985. Inhibition of phosphatidylinositol synthases and other membrane-associated enzymes by stereoisomers of hexachlorocyclohexane. *Journal of Biological Chemistry* 260:2687–2693.

Pollack, P. J. 1962. Oral administration of enzymes from carica papaya: Report of a double-blind clinical study. *Current Therapeutic Research* 4(5):229–237.

Rahn, H-D. 1990. Efficacy of hydrolytic enzymes in surgery. Paper read at the Symposium on Enzyme Therapy in Sports Injuries, XXIV FIMS World Congress of Sport Medicine, 27 May–1 June. Amsterdam: Elsevier Science Publishers, 1134–1136.

Rathgeber, W. F. 1971. The use of proteolytic enzymes (chymoral) in sporting injuries. *South African Medical Journal* 45(S):181–183.

Rathgeber, W. F. 1973. The use of proteolytic enzymes in tenosynovitis. *Clinical Medicine* 80(S):39–41.

Regan, P. T., et al. 1977. Comparative effects of antacids, Cimetidine, and enteric coating on the therapeutic response to oral enzymes in severe pancreatic insufficiency. *New England Journal of Medicine* 297(16):854–858.

Renzinni, G., and M. Varengo. 1972. The absorption of tetracyclin in combination with bromelain by oral application. *Arzeimittel-Forschung* (Drug Research) 22:410–412.

Rimoldi, R., et al. 1978. The use of bromelain in pneumological therapy. *Drugs Under Experimental and Clinical Research* 4(1):55–66.

Ryan, R. E. 1967. A double-blind clinical evaluation of bromelains in the treatment of acute sinusitis. *Headache* 7:13–17.

Satoskar, R. R., et al. 1986. Evaluation of anti-inflammatory property of curcumin (diferuloyl methane) in patients with postoperative inflammation. *International Journal of Clinical Pharmacology, Therapy and Toxicology* 24:651–654.

Saunders, J. H. B., and K. G. Wormsley. 1975. Progress report: Pancreatic extracts in the treatment of pancreatic exocrine insufficiency. *Gut* 16:157–162.

Schafer, A., and B. Adelman. 1985. Plasmin inhibition of platelet function and of arachidonic acid metabolism. *Journal of Clinical Investigation* 75:456–461.

Seligman, B. 1962. Bromelain as an anti-inflammatory agent. *Angiology* 13:508–510.

Shaw, P. C. 1969. The use of a trypsin-chymotrypsin formulation in fractures of the hand. *British Journal of Clinical Practice* 23(1):25–26.

Soule, S. E., et al. 1966. Oral proteolytic enzyme therapy (Chymoral) in episiotomy patients. *American Journal of Obstetrics and Gynecology* 95(S):820–833.

Stauder, G., et al. 1988. The use of hydrolytic enzymes as adjuvant therapy in AIDS/ARC/LAS patients. *Biomedicine & Pharmacotherapy* 42:31–34.

Steffen, C., et al. 1985. Enzymtherapie im vergleich mit immunkomplex-bestimmungen bei chronisher polyarthritis. *Zeitschrift fur Rheumatologie* 44:51–56.

Tassman, G. C., et al. 1964. Evaluation of a plant proteolytic enzyme for the control of inflammation and pain. *Journal of the American Dental Association* 19:73–77.

Taussig, S. J. 1980. The mechanism of the physiological action of bromelain. *Medical Hypotheses* 6:99–104.

Tinozzi, S., and A. Venegoni. 1978. Effect of bromelain on serum and tissue levels of amoxycillin. *Drugs Under Experimental and Clinical Research* 4:39–44.

Vallis, C., and M. Lund. 1969. Effect of treatment with carica papaya on resolution of edema and ecchymosis following rhinoplasty. *Current Therapeutic Research* 11:356–359.

Westphal, J., et al. 1966. Phytotherapy in functional upper abdominal complaints. *Phytomedicine* 2(4):285–291.

Wigand, F., and E. Messer. 1967. Enzyme treatment of traumatic swelling in oral and maxillofacial surgery. *Clinical Medicine* 74(S): 29–31.

Yeh, T. L., and M. L. Rubin. 1977. Potency of pancreatic enzyme preparations. *New England Journal of Medicine* 297(S): 615–616.

CHAPTERS 5 & 6

Abbot, L., et al. 1994. Magnesium deficiency in alcoholism: Possible contribution to osteoporosis and cardiovascular disease in alcoholics. *Alcoholism: Clinical and Experimental Research* 18(5):1076–1082.

Akar, N., and Arcasoy, A. 1990. Alcohol and zinc deficiency: Contribution to villous atropy. *Journal of Internal Medicine* 228:412.

American Institute of Stress. 1994. Hostile cities and heart attacks. *Newsletter of the American Institute of Stress* no. 7.

Angelico, M., et al. 1994. Oral s-adenosyl-l-methionine (SAMe) administration (800 mg/d) enhances bile salt conjugation with taurine in patients with liver cirrhosis. *Scandinavian Journal of Clinical Laboratory Investigation* 54:459–464.

Ankarah, N-A., et al. 1994. Decreased cysteine and glutathione levels: Possible determinants of liver toxicity risk in Ghanian subject. *Journal of International Medical Research* 22:171–176.

Biskind, M. S. 1942. Effect of vitamin B complex deficiency on inactivation of estrone in the liver. *Endocrinology* 31:109–114.

Biskind, M. S. 1943. Nutritional deficiency in the etiology of menorrhagia, metrorrhagia, cystic mastitis and premenstrual tension; treatment with vitamin B complex. *Nutritional Deficiency in Etiology of Menstrual Disorder* 3:227–234.

Bonkovsky, H. L. 1995. Acetaminophen hepatotoxicity, fasting, and ethanol. *Journal of the American Medical Association* 276(4):301.

Britton, R. S., and B. R. Bacon. 1994. Role of free radicals and liver diseases in hepatic fibrosis. *Hepato-Gastroenterology* 41:343–348.

Buchman, A. L., et al. 1992. Lecithin increases plasma free choline and decreases hepatic steatosis in long-term total parenteral nutrition patients. *Gastroenterology* 102:1363–1370.

Buzzelli, G., et al. 1993. A pilot study on the liver protective effect of silybinphos-phatidylcholine complex (IDB1016) in chronic active hepatitis. *International Journal of Clinical Pharmacology, Therapy and Toxicology* 31(9):456–460.

Calloway, N. O., and R. S. Merrill. 1965. The aging adult liver. *Journal of the American Geriatric Society* 13:594–598.

Chen, Marianne F., et al. 1990. Effect of ascorbic acid on plasma alcohol clearance. *Journal of the American College of Nutrition* 9(3):185–189.

Corbett, R., et al. The effects of chronic ethanol administration on rat liver and erythrocyte lipid composition: Modulatory role of evening primrose oil. *Alcohol and Alcoholism* 26(4):459–464.

Cuomo, R., et al. 1993. S-adenosyl-l-methionine (SAMe)–dependent nicoti-namide methylation: A marker of hepatic damage. From *Fat-Storing Cells and Liver Fibrosis*, 71st Falk Symposium, Florence, Italy (1 July):348–353.

Day, C. E. 1976. Control of the interaction of cholesterol ester–rich lipoproteins with arterial receptors. *Atherosclerosis* 25:199–204.

Doll, R., et al. 1962. Clinical trial of a triterpenoid liquorice compound in gastric and duodenal ulcer. *Lancet* (20 October):793–796.

Epstein, M. T., et. al. 1977. Effect of eating liquorice on the renin-angiotensin aldosterone axis in normal subjects. *British Medical Journal* 1:488–490.

Faulstich, H., et al. 1980. Silybin inhibition of amatoxin uptake in the perfused rat liver. *Drug Research* 30(1):452–454.

Feinman, L., and C. S. Lieber. 1990. Nutrition and Liver Disease. *Hospital Medicine* (April):150–166.

Floersheim, G. L., et al. 1978. Effects of penicillin and silymarin on liver enzymes and blood clotting factors in dogs given a boiled preparation of amanita phal-loides. *Toxicology and Applied Pharmacology* 46:455–462.

Flynn, D. L., et al. 1986. Inhibition of 5-hydroxy-eicosatetraenoic acid (5-hete) formation in intact human neutrophils by naturally occurring diarylheptanoids: Inhibitory activities of curcuminoids and yakuchinones. *Prostaglandins, Leukotrienes and Medicine* 22:357–360.

Frezza, M., et al. 1984. Reversal of intrahepatic cholestasis of pregnancy in women after high dose s-adenosyl-l-methionine administration. *Hepatology* 4(2):274–278.

Fuchs, C. S., et al. 1995. Alcohol consumption and mortality among women. *New England Journal of Medicine* 332(19):1245–1250.

Gershon, S., and S. H. Shaw. 1961. Psychiatric sequelae of chronic exposure to organo-phosphorous insecticides. *Lancet* (24 June):1371–1374.

Gerson, M. 1941. Feeding the German Army. *New York State Journal of Medicine* (15 July):1471–1476.

Goldin, B. R., and S. L. Gorbach. 1976. The relationship between diet and rat fecal bacterial enzymes implicated in colon cancer. *Journal of the National Cancer Institute* 57:371–375.

Goldin, B. R., and S. L. Gorbach. 1984. The effect of milk and lactobacillus feeding on human intestinal bacterial enzyme activity. *American Journal of Clinical Nutrition* 39:756–761.

Gyorgy, P., and H. Goldblatt. 1942. Observations on the conditions of dietary hepatic injury (necrosis, cirrhosis) in rats. *Journal of Experimental Medicine* 75:355.

Halliday, et al. 1986. Alcohol abuse in women seeking gynecologic care. *Obstetrics and Gynecology* 68(3):322–326.

Hauser, R. A., et al. 1994. Manganese intoxication and chronic liver failure. *Annals of Neurology* 36(6):871–875.

Horrobin, D. F. 1980. A biochemical basis for alcoholism and alcohol-induced damage including the fetal alcohol syndrome and cirrhosis: Interference with essential fatty acid and prostaglandin metabolism. *Medical Hypotheses* 6:929–942.

Jenkins, P. J., et al. 1982. Use of polyunsaturated phosphatidyl choline in HBSAG-negative chronic active hepatitis: Results of prospective double-blind controlled trial. *Liver* 2:77–81.

Jensen, G. B., and B. Pakkenberg. 1993. Do alcoholics drink their neurons away? *Lancet* 342:1201–1204.

Jianjun, L., et al. 1991. Polyunsaturated lecithin prevents acetaldehyde-mediated hepatic collagen accumulation by stimulating collagenase activity in cultured lipocytes. *Hepatology* 15(3): 373–381.

Kidd, P. M. 1996. Phosphatidylcholine: A superior protectant against liver damage. *Alternative Medicine Review* 1(4):258–273.

Kojima, M., et al. 1973. A chlorella polysaccharide as a factor stimulating RES activity. *Journal of the Reticuloendothelial Society* 14:192–208.

Langdon, D. 1996. Acetaminophen hepatotoxicity. *Journal of Family Practice* 43(1):13.

Levin, H., and R. Rodnitzky. 1976. Behavioral effects of organo-phosphate pesticides in man. *Clinical Toxicology* 9(3):391–405.

Lieber, C. S., et. al. 1990. Attenuation of alcohol-induced hepatic fibrosis by polyunsaturated lecithin. *Hepatology* 12(6):1390–1398.

Lieber, C. S., 1994. Alcohol and the liver: 1994 update. *Gastroenterology* 106:152–159.

Lieber, C. S., et al. 1994. Phosphatidylcholine protects against fibrosis and cirrhosis in the baboon. *Gastroenterology* 106:152–159.

Lokken, P., et al. 1995. Effect of homeopathy on pain and other events after acute trauma: Placebo-controlled trial with bilateral oral surgery. *British Medical Journal* 310:1439–1442.

MacDonald, G. A., and M. R. Lucey. 1994. Editorial: Diet and liver disease: A glimpse into the future. *Journal of Clinical Gastroenterology* 18(4):274–276.

Magliulo, P. G., et al. 1973. Studies on the regenerative capacity of the liver in rats subjected to partial hepatectomy and treated with silymarin. *Drug Research* 23(1a):161–167.

Marques-Vidal, P., et al. 1995. Cardiovascular risk factors in alcohol consumption in France and Northern Ireland. *Atherosclerosis* 115:225–232.

Mato, J. M., et al. S-adenosylmethionine and the liver. *The Liver: Biology and Pathobiology*, 3rd edition. 27:461–470.

Molina, J. A., et al. 1994. Alcoholic cognitive deterioration and nutritional deficiencies. *ACTA Neurologica Scandinavica* 89:384–90.

Montini, Von M., et al. 1975. Kontrollierte anwendung von cynarin in der behandlung hyperlipamischer syndrome. *Arzeimittel-Forschung (Drug Research)* 25(8):1311–1314.

Munoz, S. 1991. Nutritional therapies in liver disease. *Seminars in Liver Disease* 11(4):278–291.

Negishi, T., et al. 1989. Inhibitory effect of chlorophyll on the genotoxicity of 3-amino-1-methyl-5h-pyrido (4,3-b) indole (trp-p-2). *Carcinogenosis* 10(1):145–149.

Offenkrantz, W. G. 1949. Water-soluble chlorophyll in the treatment of peptic ulcers of long duration. *Review of Gastroenterology* :359–367.

Ong, T., et al. 1986. Chlorophyllin: A potent antimutagen against environmental and dietary complex mixtures. *Mutation Research* 173:111–115.

Pahor, M., et al. 1996. Alcohol consumption and risk of deep venous thrombosis and pulmonary embolism in older persons. *Journal of the American Geriatric Society* 44(9):1030–1037.

Panizzi, L., and M. L. Scarpati. 1954. Constitution of cynarine, the active principle of the artichoke. *Nature* 174:1062.

Paz, R., et al. 1996. The effect of the ingestion of ethanol on obstruction of the left ventricular outflow tract in hypertrophic cardiomyopathy. *New England Journal of Medicine* 335(13):938–941.

Porikos, K. P., and T. B. van Itallie. 1983. Diet-induced changes in serum transaminase and triglyceride levels in healthy adult men. *American Journal of Medicine* 75:624.

Ramadasan Kuttan, P., et al. 1985. Potential anticancer activity of turmeric (curcuma longa). *Cancer Letters* 29:197–202.

Rao, D. Subba, et al. 1970. Effect of curcumin on serum and liver cholesterol levels in the rat. *Journal of Nutrition* 100:1307–1316.

Rea, W., et al. 1978. Food and chemical susceptibility after environmental chemical overexposure: Case history. *Annals of Allergy* 41:101–110.

Ross, M. H. 1977. Dietary behavior and longevity. *Nutrition Reviews* 35(10):257–265.

Sano, T., and Y. Tanaka. 1987. Effect of dried, powdered chlorella vulgaris on experimental atherosclerosis and alimentary hypercholesterolemia in cholesterol-fed rabbits. *Artery* 14(2):76–84.

Schenker, S., and A. M. Hoyumpa. 1994. Polyunsaturated lecithin and alcoholic liver disease: A magic bullet? *Alcoholism: Clinical and Experimental Research* 18(5):1286–1288.

Sjolund, K., et al. 1990. Zinc deficiency and enteropathy in alcoholics. *Journal of Internal Medicine* 228:412–413.

Srimal, R. C., and B. N. Dhawan. 1973. Pharmacology of diferuloyl methane (curcumin), a non-steroidal anti-inflammatory agent. *Journal of Pharmacology* 25:447–452.

Srivastava, R., et al. 1985. Anti-thrombotic effect of curcumin. *Thrombosis Research* 40:413–417.

Strubelt, O., et al. 1980. The influence of silybin on the hepatotoxic and hypoglycemic effects of praseodymium and other lanthanides. *Drug Research* 30(II):1690–1694.

Tamura, Y., et al. 1979. Effects of glycyrrhetinic acid and its derivatives on D4-5a- and 5b-reductase in rat liver. *Drug Research* 29(I)(4):647–649.

Taniguchi, S., et al. 1995. Acquired zinc deficiency associated with alcoholic liver cirrhosis. *International Journal of Dermatology* 34(9):651–652.

Thuluvath, P., and D. Triger. 1992. Selenium and chronic liver disease. *Journal of Hepatology* 14:176.

Urbano, B. A., et al. 1995. The greater risk of alcoholic cardiomyopathy and myopathy in women compared with men. *Journal of the American Medical Association* 274(2):149–154.

Van Gossum, A., and J. Neve. 1995. Low selenium status in alcoholic cirrhosis is correlated with aminopyrine breath test. *Biological Trace Element Research* 47:201–207.

Van Gossum, A. 1996. Deficiency in antioxidant factors in patients with alcohol-related chronic pancreatitis. *Digestive Diseases and Sciences* 41(6):1225–1231.

Vogel, G., et al. 1979. On the nephrotoxicity of a-amanitin and the antagonistic effects of silymarin in rats. *Agents and Actions* 9(2):221–226.

Wang, et al. 1994. Ethanol, immune responses, and murine AIDS: The role of vitamin E as an immunostimulant and antioxidant. *Alcohol* 11(2):75–84.

Windle, M., et al. 1995. Physical and sexual abuse and associated mental disorders among alcoholic inpatients. *American Journal of Psychiatry* 152(9):1322–1328.

Wiznitzer, T., et al. 1976. Acute necrotizing pancreatitis in the guinea pig: Effect of chlorophyll-a on survival times. *Digestive Diseases* 21(6):459–464.

Zaterka, S., and M. I. Grossman. 1966. The effect of gastrin and histamine on secretion of bile. *Gastroenterology*. 50(4):500–505.

CHAPTERS 7 & 8

Arnan, M. 1985. Effect of ozone/oxygen gas mixture directly injected into the mammary carcinoma of female C3H/HEJ mice. *Journal of Holistic Medicine* 7(1):31–37.

Baggs, A. C. 1993. Are worry-free transfusions just a whiff of ozone away? *Canadian Medical Association Journal* 148(7):1155–1160.

Balkanyi, A. 1989. The interaction between ozone therapy and oxygen radicals and their importance in practice. Ninth World Ozone Conference.

Balla, G. A., et al. 1964. Use of intra-arterial hydrogen peroxide to promote wound healing. *American Journal of Surgery* 108:621–629.

Baltin, H. 1989. The clinical efficacy of ozone therapy in endanglitis obliterans. Ninth World Ozone Conference.

Baltin, H. 1993. Immune monitoring of Buerger patients under ozone treatment. Eleventh World Ozone Conference.

Barber, E., et al. 1993. Functional renal and structural study of organs in rats treated with ozone by rectal insufflation. Eleventh World Ozone Conference.

Beck, E. G., and F. Tilkes. 1991. The influence of rectally applied ozone-oxygen mixtures on selected biochemical components in humans. Tenth World Ozone Conference.

Beck, E. G., et al. 1989. Infection control by ozonizing-aspects of medical hygiene. Ninth World Ozone Conference.

Beck, R. 1996. A few unique plus traditional uses for silver colloid. *Explore!* 7(2):54–56.

Brauner, A. W. 1991. Ozone applications in periodontology. Tenth World Ozone Conference.

Brauner, A. W. 1993. In vitro and clinical examination of the effect of ozone/oxygen gas mixture on impression material on the oral microflora. Eleventh World Ozone Conference.

Broadwater, W. T., et al. 1973. Sensitivity of three selected bacterial species to ozone. *Applied Microbiology* 26(3): 391–393.

Buckley, R. D., et al. 1975. Ozone and human blood. *Archives of Environmental Health* 30:40–43.

Burleson, G. R., et al. 1975. Inactivation of viruses and bacteria by ozone, with and without sonication. *Applied Microbiology* 29(3):340–344.

Canoso, R. T., et al. 1974. Hydrogen peroxide and platelet function. *Blood* 43(5):645–656.

Carpendale, M. T. F., and J. K. Freeberg. 1991. Ozone inactivates HIV at noncytotoxic concentrations. *Antiviral Research* 16:281–292.

Carpendale, M. T. F., et al. 1993. Does ozone alleviate AIDS diarrhea? *Journal of Clinical Gastroenterology* 17(2):142–145.

Carpendale, M. T. F., and J. Griffiss. 1993. Is there a role for medical ozone in the treatment of HIV and associated infections? Eleventh World Ozone Conference.

Chahverdiani, B., and A. Thadj-Bakhche. 1976. Ozone treatment in root canal therapy. *Acta Medica Iranica* 19(3):192–200.

Church, L. 1980. Ionozone therapy for skin lesions in elderly patients. *Physiotherapy* 66(2):50–51.

Croen, K. D. 1993. Evidence for antiviral effect of nitric oxide: Inhibition of herpes simplex virus type 1 replication. *Journal of Clinical Investigation* 91:2446–2452.

Cronheim, G. 1947. Organic ozonides as chemotherapeutic agents. II. Antiseptic properties. *Journal of the American Pharmaceutical Association, Scientific Edition* 36:278–281.

Daskalakes, D. 1972. A clinical study of ozone-oxygen therapy in periodontal diseases. *Odontiatriki* 3(May–June):222–224.

Delafons, J-C. 1989. Ozonotherapy used in sexual transmitted diseases. Ninth World Ozone Conference.

Dockrell, H. M., and J. H. L. Playfair. 1983. Killing of blood-stage murine malaria parasites by hydrogen peroxide. *Infection and Immunity* 39(1):456–459.

Dolphin, S., and M. Walker. 1973. Healing accelerated by ionozone therapy. *Physiotherapy* 65(3):153–156.

Dorstewitz, H. 1989. Application forms for ozone/oxygen mixtures in viral diseases such as hepatitis and herpes. Ninth World Ozone Conference.

Dyas, A., and B. J. Boughton. 1983. Ozone killing action against bacterial and fungal species; microbiological testing of a domestic ozone generator. *Journal of Clinical Pathology* 36:1102–1104.

Eberhardt, H. G. 1993. The efficacy of ozone therapy as an antibiotic. Eleventh World Ozone Conference.

Ekblom, B., et al. 1972. Response to exercise after blood loss and reinfusion. *Journal of Applied Physiology* 3(2)(August):175–180.

Expert Scientific Working Group. 1985. Summary of a report on assessment of the iron nutritional status of the United States population. *American Journal of Clinical Nutrition* 42(December):1318–1330.

Faglia, E., et al. 1996. Adjunctive systemic hyperbaric oxygen therapy in treatment of severe prevalently ischemic diabetic foot ulcer. *Diabetes Care* 19(12)(19 December):1338–1343.

Fahmy, Z. 1989. Ozone therapy in rheumatic diseases. Ninth World Ozone Conference.

Fahmy, Z. 1991. Influence of ozone therapy in rheumatoid arthritis. Tenth World Ozone Conference.

Farber, M. O., et al. 1984. Effect of decreased O_2 affinity of hemoglobin on work performance during exercise in healthy humans. *Journal of Laboratory and Clinical Medicine* 104(2):166–175.

Farr, C. H. 1987. The therapeutic use of IV H_2O_2. *Townsend Letter for Doctors* :177.

Feigl, E. O. 1998. Neural control of coronary blood flow. *Journal of Vascular Research* 35:85–92.

Fetner, R. H., and R. S. Ingols. 1959. Bactericidal activity of ozone and chlorine against Escherichia coli at 1° C. *Advances in Chemistry Series* 21:370–374.

Gavrilushkin, A. P., and S. P. Peretyagin. 1993. Investigation of chaos and myocardium fractals as criteria of ozone-stimulating effect on physical load. Eleventh World Ozone Conference.

Gell, A., et al. 1991. Evaluation of ozone therapy in humans and in animals infected with Giardia lambi. Tenth World Ozone Conference.

Glady, G. 1993. Diverse pathology treated in medical ozone clinic. Eleventh World Ozone Conference.

Gloor, M., and B-A. Lipphardt. 1975. Untersuchungen zur ozontherapie der akne vulgaris. *Zeitschrift für Hautkrankheiten* 51(3):97–101.

Goldstein, B. D., and O. J. Balchum. 1967. Effect of ozone on lipid peroxidation in the red blood cell. *Proceedings of the Society for Experimental Biology and Medicine* 126:356–358.

Goodhart, D. M., and T. J. Anderson. 1998. Role of nitric oxide in coronary arterial vasomotion and the influence of coronary atherosclerosis and its risks. *American Journal of Cardiology* 82:1034–1039.

Gorbunov, S. N., et al. 1993. The use of ozone in the treatment of children who suffered due to different catastrophes. Eleventh World Ozone Conference.

Greenberg, J. 1993. An autovaccine for human use produced with the aid of ozone gas, an 8 year retrospective study, clinical statistics, case presentation and methodology. Eleventh World Ozone Conference.

Grundner, H-G. 1976. Tierexperimentelle untersuchungen über die anwendung von ozon auf unbestrahlte und bestrahlte tumoren. *Strahlentherapie* 151(5):480–486.

Gumulka, J., and L. L. Smith. 1983. Ozonization of cholesterol. *Journal of the American Chemical Society* 105:1972–1979.

Haimovici, A., et al. 1970. Ozone in endodontic therapy. *Stomatologia* 17(4):303–307.

Hassett, C., et al. 1985. Murine lung carcinogenesis following exposure to ambient ozone concentrations. *Journal of the National Cancer Institute* 75(4):771–777.

Hernandez, F., et al. 1993. Effect of endovenous ozone therapy on lipid pattern and antioxidative response of ischemia cardiopath. Eleventh World Ozone Conference.

Hernuss, P., et al. 1973. Effect of ozone in radiotherapy for malignant tumors in the animal experiment. *ROFO* (supplement):196.

Hernuss, P., et al. 1974. Strahlensensibilisierender effekt von ozon im tierversuch. *Strahlentherapie* 147(1):91–96.

Hernuss, P., et al. 1974. Ozon-sauerstoff-injektionsbehandlung in der gynäkologischen strahlen therapie. *Strahlentherapie* 148 (3):242–245.

Hernuss, P., et al. 1975. Ozone and gynecologic radiotherapy. *Strahlentherapie* 150(5):493–499.

Jungersten, L., et al. 1997. Both physical fitness and acute exercise regulate nitric oxide formation in healthy humans. *Journal of Applied Physiology* 82:760–764.

Kandic, D. 1968. Use of ozone in conservative dentistry. *Stomatoloski Glasnik Srbije* 15(3):159–165.

Katzenelson, E., et al. 1979. Measurement of the inactivation kinetics of poliovirus by ozone in a fast-flow mixer. *Applied and Environmental Microbiology* 37(4):715–718.

Kendall, A. I., and A. W. Walker. 1936. The effects of ozone upon certain bacteria and their respective phages. *Journal of Infectious Diseases* :204–214.

Kessel, J. F., et al. 1943. Comparison of chlorine and ozone as virucidal agents of poliomyelitis virus. *Proceedings of the Society of Experimental Biology and Medicine* 53:71–73.

Kessel, J. F., et al. 1944. The cysticidal effects of chlorine and ozone on cysts of endamoeba histolytica, together with a comparative study of several encystment media. *American Journal of Tropical Medicine* 24:177–183.

Kief, H. 1993. The treatment of malignant diseases with AHIT. Eleventh World Ozone Conference.

Kief, H. 1993. The treatment of neurodermatitis with the auto-homologous immune therapy. Eleventh World Ozone Conference.

Klug, W., and H. Knoch. 1991. Oxygen partial pressure in the blood of the arteria carotis, ear artery and vena cava superior after rectal ozone-oxygen insufflation—animal experiment examination. Tenth World Ozone Conference.

Koller-Strametz, J., et al. 1998. Role of nitric oxide in exercise-induced vasodilation in man. *Life Sciences* 62:1035–1042.

Konrad, H. 1991. Ozone therapy for viral diseases. Tenth World Ozone Conference.

Kontorschikova, C. N. 1993. The role of lipid peroxidation in ozone correction of hypoxic impairments. Eleventh World Ozone Conference.

Kreider, R. B., et al. 1990. Effects of phosphate loading on oxygen uptake, ventilatory anaerobic threshold, and run performance. *Medicine and Science in Sports and Exercise* 22(2):250–256.

Krivatkin, S. L. 1993. The experience of ozone therapy in dermatovenereological dispensary, preliminary data. Eleventh World Ozone Conference.

Lindberg, S., et al. 1997. Low levels of nasal nitric acid (NO) correlate to impaired mucociliary function in upper airways. *Acta Otolaryngol.* 117:728–734.

Lindenschmidt, R. C., et al. 1986. Inhibition of mouse lung tumor development by hyperoxia. *Cancer Research* 46:1994–2000.

Maddali, S., et al. 1998. Postexercise increase in nitric acid in football players with muscle cramps. *American Journal of Sports Medicine* 26:820–824.

Mallams, J. T., et al. 1962. The use of hydrogen peroxide as a source of oxygen in a regional intra-arterial infusion system. *Southern Medical Journal* (March):230–232.

Martin, R., et al. 1977. Blood chemistry and lipid profiles of elite distance runners. *Annals of the New York Academy of Sciences* 301:346–360.

Maxwell, A. J., et al. 1998. Limb blood flow during exercise is dependent on nitric acid. *Circulation* 98:369–374.

Menendez, D. E., et al. 1993. Ozone therapy in ischemic cerebro-vascular disease. Eleventh World Ozone Conference.

Müller, T. E., et al. 1979. Ozone–oxygen therapy for gynecologic carcinomas. *Fortschritte der Medizin* 97(10):451–454.

Musarella, P. 1989. Interests of ozone therapy in cosmetic surgery. Ninth World Ozone Conference.

Nathan, C. F., and Z. A. Cohn. 1981. Antitumor effects of hydrogen peroxide in vivo. *Journal of Experimental Medicine* 154:1539–1553.

Nieper, H. 1979. The non-toxic long-term therapy of cancer: Necessity, state-of-the-art trends. *Journal of the International Academy of Preventive Medicine* (June):41–70.

Noa, M. 1991. Morphological observations in rats treated with ozone by intramuscular applications. Tenth World Ozone Conference.

Oliver, T. H., and D. V. Murphy. 1920. Influenza pneumonia: the intravenous injection of hydrogen peroxide. *Lancet* (21 February):432–433.

Paulesu, L., et al. 1991. Studies on the biological effect of ozone: 2. Induction of tumor necrosis factor (TNF-∂) on human leucocytes. *Lymphokine and Cytokine Research* 10(5):409–412.

Peretyagin, S. P. 1993. Extra corporeal perfusion of blood with ozone–oxygen mixtures in the treatment of hypoxic states. Eleventh World Ozone Conference.

Plowman, S., and P. McSwegin. 1981. The effects of iron supplementation on female cross-country runners. *Journal of Sports Medicine* 21:407–416.

Prieto, E., et al. 1993. Evaluation of ozone genotoxicity by cytogenetics techniques. Eleventh World Ozone Conference.

Rahmy, Z. 1993. Immunological effect of ozone (O_3/O_2) in rheumatic diseases. Eleventh World Ozone Conference.

Rodriguez, S. M., et al. 1993. Ozone therapy for senile dementia. Eleventh World Ozone Conference.

Roy, D., et al. 1981. Mechanism of enteroviral inactivation by ozone. *Applied and Environmental Microbiology* 41:718–723.

Roy, D., et al. 1982. Comparative inactivation in six enteroviruses by ozone. *American Water Works Association Journal* 74(12):660–664.

Samoszuk, M. K., et al. 1989. In-vitro sensitivity of Hodgkin's disease to hydrogen peroxide toxicity. *Cancer* 63:2111–2114.

Sanders, S. P. 1999. Asthma, viruses, and nitric oxide. *Proceedings of the Society of Experimental Biology and Medicine* 220:123–132.

Sandhaus, S. 1965. Ozone therapy in odontostomatology, especially in treatments of infected root canals. *Revue Belge de Medicine Dentaire* 20(6):633–646.

Sandhaus, S. 1968. Hydrozotomy: A therapeutic method using Fj5ne. *Schweizerische Monatsschrift fuer Zahnheilkunde* 78(6):620–623.

Sandhaus, S. 1969. The use of ozone in dentistry. *Zahnaerztliche Praxis* 20(23):265–266.

Sandhaus, S. 1969. Ozone therapy in oral surgery and clinical dentistry. *Zahnaerztliche Praxis* 20(24):277–280.

Sanseverino, E. R. 1988. Intensive medical and physical treatment of osteoporosis with the aid of oxygen-ozone therapy. *Europa Medicophysica* 24:199–206.

Sanseverino, E. R. 1989. Knee-joint disorders treated by oxygen-ozone therapy. *Europa Medicophysica* 25(3):163–170.

Sanseverino, E. R., et al. 1990. Effects of oxygen–ozone therapy on age-related degenerative retinal maculopathy. *Panminerva Medica* 32(2):77–84.

Sanseverino, E. R. 1991. Cerebral and cardiac control before, during and after ozone treatment (in the form of major autohemotherapy) in normal humans. Tenth World Ozone Conference.

Santiesteban, R. E., et al. 1993. Ozone therapy in the optic nerve dysfunction. Eleventh World Ozone Conference.

Saura, M., et al. 1999. An antiviral mechanism of nitric oxide: Inhibition of a viral protease. *Immunity* 10:21–28.

Scrollavezza, P., et al. 1993. The ozonized autohemotransfusion in halothane—anesthetized horses. Eleventh World Ozone Conference.

Seeger, P. G. 1967. The anthocyans of Beta vulgaris var. rubra (red beets), Vaccinium myrtillis (whortleberries), Vinum rubrum (red wine) and their significance as cell respiratory activators for cancer prophylaxis and cancer therapy. *Arzneimittel-Forschung* 21(2):68–78.

Setty, B. N. Y., et al. 1984. Effects of hydrogen peroxide on vascular arachidonic acid metabolism. *Prostaglandins, Leukotrienes and Medicine* 14:205–213.

Shine, J. W. 1997. Microcytic anemia. *American Family Physician* 55(7):2455–2462.

Shusterman, D. 1998. Air pollution and the upper airway: Recognizing irritant-related symptoms. *Hospital Medicine* (February):9–20.

Snell, P. G., et al. 1986. Does 100% oxygen aid recovery from exhaustive exercise? *Medicine and Science in Sports and Exercise* 18(2S):59.

Spreckhart, V. 1989. Hydrogen peroxide in malignancy with and without radiation therapy. Ed. C. Farr. *Proceedings of the First International Conference on Bio-Oxidative Medicine* :35–38.

Sunnen, G. V. 1989. Ozone in medicine: Overview and future direction. Ninth World Ozone Conference.

Sweet, F., et al. 1980. Ozone selectively inhibits growth of human cancer cells. *Science* 209:931–933.

Takahashi, Y., and T. Miura. 1987. A selective enhancement of xenobiotic metabolizing systems of rat lungs by prolonged exposure to ozone. *Environmental Research* 42:425–434.

Teske, H. J., et al. 1973. The effect of ozone on the growth of tumours and the effect of irradiation. *Strahlentherapie* 145(2):155–160.

Teske, H. J., et al. 1972. Studies on the effect of ozone on tumor growth and radiation effect. *ROFO* (supplement):12–14.

Teske. H. J., et al. 1973. Tierexperimentelle untersuchungen über die ozonwirkung auf tumorwachstum und bestrahlungseffekt. *Strahlentherapie* 145(2):155–160.

Thwaites, M. 1977. Ozone healing. *Medical Journal of Australia* 1(12):757–758.

Thwaites, M., and S. Dean. 1985. Chronic leg ulcers. Ozone and other factors affecting healing. *Australian Family Physician* 14(4):292–298.

Tietz, C. 1983. Ozontherapie als adjuvans in der onkologie. *OzoNachrichten* 2:4.

Tousoulis, D. 1997. Basal and flow-mediated nitric oxide production by atheromatous coronary arteries. *Journal of the American College of Cardiology* 29:1256–1262.

Urschel, H. C. 1967. Cardiovascular effects of hydrogen peroxide: Current status. *Diseases of the Chest* 51(2):180–192.

Urschel, H. C., et al. 1965. Cardiac resuscitation with hydrogen peroxide. *Circulation* 31–32:II–210.

Vallancien, B., and J. M. Winkler. 1989. Immunomodulating effect of great masses of ozone among patients presenting an acquired dysimmunity of viral origin. Ninth World Ozone Conference.

Warburg, O. 1956. On the origin of cancer cells. *Science* 123(3191):309–314.

Warshaw, L. J. 1953. Bactericidal and fungicidal effects of ozone on deliberately contaminated 3-D viewers. *American Journal of Public Health* 43:1558–1562.

Wells, I. C., et al. 1952. Ozonization of some antibiotic substances produced by Pseudomonas aeruginosa. *Journal of Biological Chemistry* 196:321–330.

Wells, K. H., et al. 1991. Inactivation of human immunodeficiency virus type I by ozone in vitro. *Blood* 78(7):1882–1890.

Wenzel, D. G., and D. L. Morgan. 1983. Interactions of ozone and antineoplastic drugs on rat lung fibroblasts and Walker rat carcinoma cells. *Research Communications in Chemical Pathology and Pharmacology* 40(2):279–287.

Werkmeister, H. 1991. The efficacy of O_2/O_3 low-pressure application in badly healing wounds. Tenth World Ozone Conference.

Wong, R., et al. 1991. Ozone therapy on arthrosis. Tenth World Ozone Conference.

Yoon, S. S., et al. 1998. Deaths from unintentional carbon monoxide poisoning and potential for prevention with carbon monoxide detectors. *Journal of the American Medical Association* 279(9):685–687.

Zanker, K. S. 1990. In vitro synergistic activity of 5-Fluorouracil with low dose ozone against chemoresistant tumor cell line and fresh human cells. *International Journal of Experimental and Clinical Chemotherapy* (Ninth World Ozone Conference) :36.

Zhulina, N. I., et al. 1993. Ozone therapy efficiency in the treatment of patients with atherosclerosis of coronary and cerebral vessels. Eleventh World Ozone Conference.

CHAPTERS 9 & 10

Abbey, L. C. 1982. Agoraphobia. *Journal of Orthomolecular Psychiatry* 11:243–259.

Abraham, G. E., and M. M. Lubran. 1981. Serum and red cell magnesium levels in patients with premenstrual tension. *American Journal of Clinical Nutrition* 34:2364–2366.

Aganoff, J. A., and G. J. Boyle. 1994. Aerobic exercise, mood states and menstrual cycle systems. *Journal of Psychosomatic Research* 38(3):183–192.

Alberti, K. G., and M. Nattrass. 1977. Lactic acidosis. *Lancet* 2:25–29.

Allen, K., and J. Blascovich. 1994. Effects of music on cardiovascular reactivity among surgeons. *Journal of the American Medical Association* 272(1):882–884.

Bahrke, M. S., and W. P. Morgan. 1994. Evaluation of the ergogenic properties of ginseng. *Sports Medicine* 18(4):229–248.

Benjamin, J., et al. 1995. Inositol treatment in psychiatry. *Psychopharmacology Bulletin* 31:167–175.

Benkelfat, C., et al. 1994. Mood-lowering effect of tryptophan depletion: Enhanced susceptibility in young men at genetic risk for major affective disorders. *Archives of General Psychiatry* 51:687–697.

Benton, D., and R. Cook. 1990. Selenium supplementation improves mood in a double-blind trial. *Psychopharmacology* 102:549–550.

Boivin, D. B., et al. 1997. Complex interaction of the sleep–wake cycle and circadian phase modulates mood in healthy subjects. *Archives of General Psychiatry* 54:145–152.

Bosma, H., et al. 1997. Low job control and risk of coronary heart disease in Whitehall II (prospective cohort) study. *British Medical Journal* 314:558–65.

Boulenger, J. P., et al. 1984. Increased sensitivity to caffeine in patients with panic disorders: Preliminary evidence. *Archives of General Psychiatry* 41:1067–1071.

Brook, A. 1991. Bowel distress and emotional conflict. *Journal of the Royal Society of Medicine* 84:39–42.

Brown, D. R. 1995. Valerian: Clinical overview. *Townsend Letter for Doctors* (May):150–151.

Brown, D. R., et al. 1995. Chronic psychological effects of exercise in exercise plus cognitive strategies. *Medical Science in Sports and Exercise* 27(5):765–775.

Budd, M. L. 1994. Hypoglycemia and personality. *Complementary Therapies in Medicine* 2:142–146.

Buist, R. A. 1985. Anxiety neurosis: The lactate connection. *International Clinical Nutrition Review* 5:1–4.

Buxman, K. 1991. Make room for laughter: A well-developed "humor" room can have a tremendous boost to patients' recovery—not to mention staff morale and hospital reputation. *American Journal of Nursing* (December):46–51.

Capasso, A., et al. 1996. Pharmacological effects of aqueous extracts from Valeriana adscendens. *Phytotherapy Research* 10:309–312.

Carlson, R. J. 1986. Longitudinal observations of two cases of organic anxiety syndrome. *Psychosomatics* 27(7):529–531.

Carroll, L. 1995. Exercise helped quell symptoms of menopause. *Medical Tribune* 20:20.

Chambers, M. J. 1991. Exercise: A prescription for a good night's sleep. *The Physician and Sports Medicine* 19(8):107–114.

Cheraskin, E., et al. 1976. Daily vitamin-C consumption and fatigability. *Journal of the American Geriatric Society* 24(3):136–137.

Christensen, L., and R. Burrows. 1990. Dietary treatment of depression. *Behavior Therap.* 21:183–193.

Clarkson, P. M., and E. M. Haymes. 1994. Trace mineral requirements for athletes. *International Journal of Sports Nutrition* 4:104–119.

Cleare, A. J. 1994. Effects of alterations in plasma tryptophan levels on aggressive feelings. *Archives of General Psychiatry* 51:1004–1005.

Crammer, J. L. 1977. Calcium metabolism and mental disorder. *Psychological Medicine* 7(4):557–560.

Crawford. 1993. Emotional health, cancer, and heart disease. *New Zealand Medical Journal* 106(951):87.

Croughs and T. W. A. de Bruin. 1996. Melatonin and jet lag. *Netherlands Journal of Medicine.* 49:164–166.

Davison, R. C. R., and S. Grant. 1993. Is walking a sufficient exercise for health? *Sports Medicine* 16(6):369–373.

Delgado, P., et al. 1994. Serotonin and the neurobiology of depression: Effects of tryptophan depletion in drug-free depressed patients. *Archives of General Psychiatry* 51:865–874.

Devinsky, O., et al. 1992. Aggressive behavior following exposure to cholinesterase inhibitors. *Journal of Neuropsychiatry* 4:189–194.

Dou, D., et al. 1996. Ginsenoside-1: A novel minor saponin from the leaves of panax ginseng. *Planta Medica* 62:179–181.

Driver, H. S., and S. R. Taylor. 1996. Sleep disturbances and exercise. *Sports Medicine* 21(1):1–6.

Duke, J. A. 1995. Commentary—novel psychotherapeutic drugs: A role for ethnobotany. *Psychopharmacology Bulletin* 31(1):177–182.

Edwards, C. R. W. 1991. Lessons from licorice. *New England Journal of Medicine* 325(17):1242–1243.

Elin, R. J. 1987. Assessment of magnesium status. *Clinical Chemistry* 33(11):1965–1970.

Eliot, R. S. 1994. Emotions and coronary heart disease. *Heart Disease and Stroke* (November/December):361–364.

Ellis, F. R. 1973. A pilot study of vitamin B_{12} in the treatment of tiredness. *British Journal of Nutrition* 30:277–283.

Equine Veterinary Data. 1992. Ergogenic nutrients, nonnutrients, and drugs. 13(16):271.

Etnier, J., and D. M. Landers. 1995. Brain function and exercise: Current perspectives. *Sports Medicine* 19(2):81–85.

Evans, P. D., and N. Edgerton. 1991. Life-events and mood as predictor of the common cold. *British Journal of Medical Psychology* 64:35–44.

Everson, S. A., et al. 1997. Interaction of workplace demands and cardiovascular reactivity in progession of carotid atherosclerosis: Population-based study. *British Medical Journal* 314:553–557.

Eysenck, H. J. 1992. Psychosocial factors, cancer, and ischaemic heart disease. *British Medical Journal* 305:457–459.

Family Practice News. 1992. Research is showing healthful effects of laughter. (15 May):52.

Family Practice News. 1995. Is melatonin a dream drug for insomnia? (September):17.

Farnsworth, N. R., et al. 1985. Siberian ginseng (Eleutherococcus senticosus): Current status as an adaptogen. *Economic and Medicinal Plant Research* 1:156–215.

Field, R. 1992. Melatonin may relieve sleep-cycle disorders. *Medical Tribune* (8 April):2.

Flach, J., and L. Seachrist. 1994. Mind–body meld may boost immunity. *Journal of the National Cancer Institute* 86(4):256–257.

Formica, P. E. 1962. The housewife syndrome: Treatment with potassium and magnesium salts of aspartic acid. *Current Therapeutic Research* 4:98–106.

Forwood, M. R. 1991. Endorphins and exercise: A review. *Australian Journal of Science and Medicine and Sports* (September):63–65.

Foulks, E. 1992. Psychologic sequelae of chronic toxic waste exposure. *Southern Medical Journal* 85(2):122–126.

Freund, G. 1980. Benzodiazepine receptor loss in brains of mice after chronic alcohol consumption. *Life Science* 27(11):987–992.

Gardner, G. W., et al. 1977. Physical work capacity and metabolic stress in subjects with iron deficiency anemia. *American Journal of Clinical Nutrition* 30(6):910–917.

Germaine, L. M., and R. R. Freedman. 1984. Behavioral treatment of menopausal hot flashes: Evaluation by objective methods. *Journal of Consulting and Clinical Psychology* 52(6):1072–1079.

Ginsburg, I. H., et al. 1993. Role of emotional factors in adults with atopic dermatitis. *International Journal of Dermatology* 32(9):656–660.

Goei, G. S., et al. 1982. Dietary patterns of patients with premenstrual tension. *Journal of Applied Nutrition* 34(1):4–11.

Greden, J. F. 1974. Anxiety or caffeinism: A diagnostic dilemma. *American Journal of Psychiatry* 131(October):1089–1092.

Gullette, E. C. D., et al. 1997. Effects of mental stress on myocardial ischemia during daily life. *Journal of the American Medical Association.* 277(20):1521–1526.

Guthrie, E., et al. 1991. A controlled trial of psychological treatment of irritable bowel syndrome. *Gastroenterology* 100:450–457.

Hedges, H. H. 1992. The elimination diet as a diagnostic tool. *American Family Physician* 46(5):77S–85S.

Heine, W., et al. 1995. The significance of tryptophan in human nutrition. *Amino Acids* 9:191–205.

Hicks, J. 1964. Treatment of fatigue in general practice: A double-blind study. *Clinical Medicine* (January):85.

Hoes, M. J., et al. 1981. Hyperventilation syndrome, treatment with l-tryptophan and pyridoxine: Predictive value of xanthurenic acid excretion. *Journal of Orthomolecular Psychiatry* 10(1):7–15.

Horrobin, D. F. 1983. The role of essential fatty acids and prostaglandins in the premenstrual syndrome. *Journal of Reproductive Medicine* 28(7):465–468.

Houssain, M. 1970. Neurological and psychiatric manifestations in idiopathic hypoparathyroidism: Response to treatment. *Journal of Neurology, Neurosurgery and Psychiatry* 33:153–156.

Jain, S. C., et al. 1993. A study of response patterns of non–insulin dependent diabetes to yoga therapy. *Diabetes Research and Clinical Practice* 19:69–74.

Jancin, B. 1994. IBS patients' family has more mental illness. *Family Practice News* (15 May):2, 5.

Jemmott, J. B., et al. 1983. Academic stress, power motivation and decrease in salivary secretory immunoglobulin-A secretion rate. *Lancet* 1:1400.

Jenkins, C. D. 1994. The mind and the body. *World Health* 47(2):6–7.

Judge, T. G., and N. R. Cowan. 1971. Dietary potassium intake and grip strength in older people. *Gerontologia Clinica* 13:221–226.

King, D. S. 1981. Can allergic exposure provoke psychological symptoms? A double-blind test. *Biological Psychiatry* 16(1):3–19.

Krotkiewski, M., et al. 1982. Zinc and muscle strength and endurance. *ACTA Physiologica Scandinavica* 116(3):309–311.

Kruse, C. A. 1961. Treatment of fatigue with aspartic acid salts. *Northwest Medicine* 60(6):597–603.

Kvetnansky, R., et al. 1997. Chronic blockade of nitric oxide synthesis elevates plasma levels of catecholamines and their metabolites at rest and during stress in rats. *Neurochemistry Research* 22:995–1001.

Lacaille-Dubois, M. A., and H. Wagner. 1996. A review of the biological and pharmacological activities of saponins. *Phytomedicine* 2:363–386.

Lam, R. W. 1994. Morning light therapy for winter depression: Predictors of response. *ACTA Psychiatrica Scandinavica* 89:97–101.

Lane, J. D., et al. 1990. Caffeine effects on cardiovascular and neuroendocrine responses to acute psychosocial stress and the relationship to the level of habitual caffeine consumption. *Psychosomatic Medicine* 52:320–336.

Lawlor, B. A. 1988. Hypocalcemia, hypoparathyroidism, and organic anxiety syndrome. *Journal of Clinical Psychiatry* 49(8):317–318.

Lawrence Review of Natural Products. 1996. Eleutherococcus. (May):1–3.

Leathwood, P. D., et al. 1982. Aqueous extract of valerian root (Valeriana officinalis l.) improves sleep quality in man. *Pharmacology, Biochemistry and Behavior* 17:65–71.

Leathwood, P. D., and F. Chauffard. 1985. Aqueous extract of valerian reduces latency to fall asleep in man. *Planta Medica* 54:144–148.

Lee, M. A., et al. 1988. Anxiogenic effects of caffeine on panic and depressed patients. *American Journal of Psychiatry* 145(5):632–635.

Lloyd, H. M., et al. 1994. Mood and cognitive performing effects of isocaloric lunches differing in fat and carbohydrate content. *Physiology and Behavior* 56(1):51–57.

London, R. S. 1987. Efficacy of alpha-tocopherol in the treatment of the premenstrual syndrome. *Journal of Reproductive Medicine* 32(6):400–404.

Lopez-Figueroa, M. O., et al. 1998. Nitric oxide in the stress axis. *Histology, Histopathology* 13:1243–1252.

Lynch, J., et al. 1997. Workplace demands, economic reward, and progression of carotid atherosclerosis. *Circulation* 96(1):302–307.

Malcolm, B., et al. 1992. Anxiogenic effects of caffeine in patients with anxiety disorders. *Archives of General Psychiatry* 49:867–869.

Malyshev, I. Y., and E. B. Manukhina. 1998. Stress, adaptation, and nitric oxide. *Biochemistry* 63:840–853.

Mann, D. 1997. Hopelessness, defensiveness linked to acute MI risk. *Medical Tribune* (18 September):14.

Maurer, K. 1996. Emotional kids at risk for fatal asthma attack. *Family Practice News* (1 May):37.

Mazzetti, M., et al. 1994. Psoriasis, stress, and psychiatry: Psychodynamic characteristics of stressors. *ACTA Dermatologica Venereol* 186(supplement):62–64.

McAdam, P. 1993. Job stress linked to rise in colorectal cancer rate. *Epidemiology* 4(5):407–413.

McClelland, D. C., et al. 1985. The effect of an academic examination on salivary norepinephrine and immunoglobulin levels. *Journal on Human Stress* 11:52–59.

McCraty, M., et al. 1995. IHM research update. *Institute of HeartMath* 2(1):1–4.

McCraty, M., et al. 1995. The effects of emotions on short-term power spectrum analysis of heart rate variability. *American Journal of Cardiology* 76(14):1089–1093.

McCraty, M., et al. 1996. The effects of different music on moods, tension and mental clarity. *Institute of HeartMath* :1–9.

McCraty, M., et al. 1996. Music enhances the effect of positive emotional states on salivary IgA. *Stress Medicine* 12:1–9.

McGrady, A., et al. 1991. Sustained effects of biofeedback-assisted relaxation therapy in essential hypertension. *Biofeedback and Self-Regulation* 16(4):399–410.

McKee, M. G. 1993. Stress reduction, pain and relaxation therapies. *Patient Care* (15 December):75–80.

Medical Tribune. 1992. Counseling eases stress and anxiety of cancer. (9 April):10.

Medical Tribune. 1996. Reducing stress eases arthritic pain, depression. (25 January):50.

Middleton, B. A., et al. 1996. Melatonin and fragmented sleep patterns. *Lancet* 348:551.

Moeller, F. G., et al. 1996. Tryptophan depletion and aggressive responding in healthy males. *Psychopharmacology* 126:97–103.

Mohler, H., et al. 1979. Nicotinamide is a brain constituent with benzodiazepine-like actions. *Nature* 278:563–565.

Murray, M. T. 1988. Panax ginseng: Adaptogenic and anti-stress aspects. *Phyto-Pharmica Review* 1(3):1–4.

Murray, M. T. 1989. Siberian ginseng. *Phyto-Pharmica Review.* 2(1):1–4.

Murray, M. T. 1990. Valerian: Nature's cure for insomnia. *Phyto-Pharmica Review* 3(3):1–4.

Murray, M. T. 1996. Melatonin: Miracle or hype? *American Journal of Natural Medicine* 3(1):5–7.

Newell, G. R. 1991. Stress and cancer: The interactions of mind and body. *Primary Care in Cancer* (May):29–30.

Nillson, P. M., et al. 1995. Adverse effects of psychosocial stress on gonadal function and insulin levels in middle-aged mules. *Journal of Internal Medicine* 237:479–86.

Nomura, J., et al. 1994. Thyroid function and mood: Implications for treatment of mood disorders. *CNS Drugs* 1(5):356–369.

Northrup, C. 1996. Do you care or overcare? Learn the health-enhancing difference! *Health Wisdom for Women* 3(4):5,7–8.

Nutrition Week. 1994. Diet and mood. 9(34):8.

Penland, J., and J. Hunt. 1993. Diet related to menstrual symptoms, nutritional status and menstrual-related symptomatology. *FASEB Journal* 7:A379.

Rainey, J. M., Jr. et al. 1984. Specificity of lactate infusion as a model of anxiety. *Psychopharmacology Bulletin* 20(1):45–49.

Rein, G., and M. McCraty. 1994. Long-term effects of compassion and anger on salivary IgA. *Psychosomatic Medicine* 54:171.

Rein, G., et al. 1995. The physiological and psychological effects of compassion and anger. *Journal of Advancement in Medicine* 8(2):87–105.

Reiter, R. J., et al. 1993. Antioxidant capacity of melatonin: A novel action not requiring a receptor. *Neuroendocrinology Letter* 15(1 & 2):103–116.

Replogle, W. H., and F. J. Eicke. 1989. Megavitamin therapy in the reduction of anxiety and depression among alcoholics. *Journal of Orthomolecular Medicine* 4(4):221–24.

Richardson, J. H. 1981. The effect of B_6 on muscle fatigue. *Journal of Sports Medicine and Physical Fitness* 21(2):119–121.

Roelofs, S. M. 1985. Hypreventilation, anxiety, craving for alcohol: A subacute alcohol withdrawal syndrome. *Alcohol* 2(3):501–05.

Rogers, P. J., et al. 1992. Nutritional influences on mood and cognitive performance: The menstrual cycle, caffeine and dieting. *Proceedings of the Nutrition Society* 51:343–351.

Rosen, H., et al. 1962. Effects of the potassium and magnesium salts of aspartic acid on metabolic exhaustion. *Journal of Pharmaceutical Science* 51:592.

Rozman, D., et al. 1996. A new intervention program which significantly reduces psychological symptomatology in HIV-seropositive individuals. *Complementary Therapies in Medicine* 4(4):1–8.

Rudin, D. O. 1981. The major psychoses and neuroses as omega-3 essential fatty acid deficiency syndrome: Substrate pellagra. *Biological Psychiatry* 16(9):837–850.

Sack, R. L., et al. 1990. Morning vs. evening light treatment for winter depression: Evidence that the therapeutic effects of light are mediated by circadian phase shifts. *Archives of General Psychiatry* 47:343–351.

Satterlee, D. G., et al. 1989. Vitamin C amelioration of the adrenal stress response in broiler chickens being prepared for slaughter. *Complementary Biochemistry & Physiology* 94A(4):569–574.

Schlesinger, M., and Y. Yodfat. 1991. The impact of stressful life events on natural killer cells. *Stress Medicine* 7:53–60.

Seelig, M. S., et al. 1975. Latent tetany and anxiety, marginal magnesium deficit, and normocalcemia. *Diseases of the Nervous System* 36:461–465.

Shaffer, M. 1993. Melatonin could help elderly sleep better. *Medical Tribune* (22 July):15.

Sher, L. 1996. Exercise, well-being, and endogenous molecules of mood. *Lancet* 348:477.

Sherwood, R. A., et al. 1986. Magnesium and the premenstrual syndrome. *Annals of Clinical Biochemistry* 23:667–670.

Short, R. V. 1993. Melatonin: Hormone of darkness. *British Medical Journal* 307:952–953.

Steinberg et al. 1997. Exercise, mood, and creativity. *British Journal of Sports Medicine* 31:240–245.

Steptoe, A., and N. Butler. 1996. Sports participation and emotional well-being in adolescents. *Lancet* 347:1789–1792.

Surwit, R. S., and M. S. Schneider. 1993. Role of stress in the etiology and treatment of diabetes mellitus. *Psychosomatic Medicine* 55:380–393.

Sutherland, J. E. 1991. The link between stress and illness: Do our coping methods influence our health? *Postgraduate Medicine* 89(1):159–164.

Takahashi, S., et al. 1975. Effect of L-5-hydroxytryptophan on brain monoamine metabolism and evaluation of its clinical effect in depressed patients. *Journal of Psychiatric Research* 12:177–187.

Tamkins, T. 1996. Reducing stress eases arthritis pain, depression. *Medical Tribune* 25:5.

Thomson, B. 1997. Change of heart. *Natural Health* (September/October):96–101, 155–159.

Tiller, W. A., et al. 1996. Cardiac coherence: A new noninvasive measure of autonomic nervous system order. *Alternative Therapies* 2(1):52–53.

Uhde, T. W., et al. 1984. Caffeine and behavior: Relation to psychopathology and underlying mechanisms. Caffeine: Relationship to human anxiety, plasma mhpg and cortisol. *Psychopharmacology Bulletin* 20(3):426–430.

Van der Beek, E. J. 1985. Vitamins and endurance training: Food for running or faddish claims? *Sports Medicine* 2(3):175–197.

Westphal, J., et al. 1996. Phytotherapy in functional upper abdominal complaints. *Phytomedicine* 2(4):285–291.

Weyerer, S., and B. Kupfer. 1994. Physical exercise and psychological health. *Sports Medicine* 17(2):108–116.

Whiteman, M. C., et al. 1997. Submissiveness and protection from coronary heart disease in the general population. Edinburgh Artery Study. *Lancet* 350(9077):541–545.

Wick, H., et al. 1977. Thiamine dependency in a patient with congenital lacticacidaemia. *Agents Actions* 7(3):405–410.

Williams, R. D., et al. 1943. Induced thiamine (vitamin B_1) deficiency in man: Relation of depletion of thiamine to development of biochemical defect and of polyneuropathy. *Archives of Internal Medicine* 71:38–53.

Wurtman, R. J., and I. Zhdanova. 1995. Improvement of sleep quality by melatonin. *Lancet* 346:1491.

Yeung, R. R. 1996. The acute effects of exercise on mood state. *Journal of Psychosomatic Research* 40(2):123–141.

Yun, T-K., and S-Y. Choi. 1995. Preventive effect of ginseng intake against various human cancers: A case-control study on 1,987 pairs. *Cancer Epidemiology, Biomarkers and Prevention* 4:401–408.

Zhang, D., et al. 1996. Ginseng extract scavenges hydroxyl radical and protects unsaturated fatty acids from decomposition caused by iron-mediated lipid peroxidation. *Free Radical Biology in Medicine* 20(1):145–150.

CHAPTERS 11 & 12

Adlercreutz, H., and E. Hamalainen. 1992. Dietary phyto-oestrogens and the menopause in Japan. *Lancet* 339:1233.

Akwa, Y., et al. 1991. Neurosteroids: Biosynthesis, metabolism and function of pregnenolone and dehydroepiandrosterone in the brain. *Journal of Steroid Biochemistry and Molecular Biology* 40(1–3):71–81.

Bachmann, G. A. 1985. Correlates of sexual desire in post-menopausal women. *Maturitas* 7:211–216.

Bäckström, T., and H. Carstensen. 1974. Estrogen and progesterone in plasma in relation to premenstrual tension. *Journal of Steroid Biochemistry* 5:257–260.

Baker, E. R., et al. 1995. Efficacy of progesterone vaginal suppositories in alleviation of nervous symptoms of patients with premenstrual syndrome. *Journal of Assisted Reproduction and Genetics* 12(3):205–209.

Barrett-Connor, E., et al. 1986. A prospective study of dehydroepiandrosterone sulfate, mortality, and cardiovascular disease. *New England Journal of Medicine* 315(24):1519–1524.

Baulieu, E-E. 1996. Dehydroepiandrosterone (DHEA): A fountain of youth? *Journal of Clinical Endocrinology and Metabolism* 81(9):3147–3151.

Beral, V., et al. 1997. Breast cancer and hormone replacement therapy: Collaborative reanalysis of data from 51 epidemiological studies of 52,705 women with breast cancer and 108,411 women without breast cancer. *Lancet* 350:1047–1059.

Berkman, L. F., et al. 1993. High, usual, and impaired functioning in community-dwelling older men and women: Findings from the MacArthur Foundation Research Network on Successful Aging. *Journal of Clinical Epidemiology* 46(10):1129–1140.

Bhasin, S., et al. 1996. The effects of supraphysiologic doses of testosterone on muscle size and strength in normal men. *New England Journal of Medicine* 335(1):1–7.

Bhatavdekar, J. M., et al. 1994. Levels of circulating peptide and steroid hormones in men with lung cancer. *Neoplasma* 41(2):101–103.

Birkenhager-Gillesse, E. G., et al. 1994. Dehydroepiandrosterone sulfate (DHEAS) in the oldest old, ages 85 and over. *Annals of the New York Academy of Sciences* 719:543–552.

Bowen, A. 1996. Older women may benefit from estrogen–androgen therapy. *American Family Physician* 53:939.

Buffington, C. K., et al. 1993. Case report: Amelioration of insulin resistance in diabetes with dehydroepiandrosterone. *American Journal of the Medical Sciences* 306(5):320–324.

Burris, A. S., et al. 1992. A long-term, prospective study of the physiologic and behavioral effects of hormone replacement in untreated hypogonadal men. *Journal of Andrology* 13(4):297–304.

Byers, T. 1993. Vitamin E supplements and coronary heart disease. *Nutrition Reviews* 51(11):333–336.

Cacciari, E., et al. 1990. Effects of sport (football) on growth: Auxological, anthropometric and hormonal aspects. *Journal of Applied Physiology* 61:149–158.

Carlsen, E., et al. 1992. Evidence for decreasing quality of semen during past 50 years. *British Medical Journal* 305:609–613.

Check, J. H., and H. G. Adelson. 1987. The efficacy of progesterone in achieving successful pregnancy: II. In women with pure luteal phase defects. *International Journal of Fertility* 32(2):139–141.

Chung, C. J. 1995. Estrogen replacement therapy may reduce panic symptoms. *Journal of Clinical Psychiatry* 56(11):533.

Croen, K. D. 1993. Evidence for antiviral effect of nitric oxide: Inhibition of herpes simplex virus type 1 replication. *Journal of Clinical Investigation* 91:2446–2452.

Davidson, J. M., et al. 1979. Effects of androgen on sexual behavior in hypogonadal men. *Journal of Clinical Endocrinology and Metabolism* 48(6):955–958.

Davidson, J. M., et al. 1983. Hormonal changes and sexual function in aging men. *Journal of Clinical Endocrinology and Metabolism* 57(1):71–77.

Davis, S. R., and H. G. Burger. 1996. Androgens and the postmenopausal woman. *Journal of Clinical Endocrinology and Metabolism*. 81(8): 2759–2763.

Dennerstein, et al. 1985. Progesterone and the premenstrual syndrome: a double-blind crossover trial. *British Medical Journal* 290:1617.

Editorial. 1995. Male reproductive health and environmental estrogens. *Lancet* 345:933–935.

Fahim, M. S., et al. 1982. Effect of panax ginseng on testosterone level and prostate in male rats. *Archives of Andrology* 8:261–263.

Feigl, E. O. 1998. Neural control of coronary blood flow. *Journal of Vascular Research* 35:85–92.

Ferrini, R. L., and E. Barrett-Connor. 1996. Caffeine intake and endogenous sex steroid levels in postmenopausal women: The Rancho Bernardo Study. *American Journal of Epidemiology* 144(7):642–644.

Field, B., et al. 1990. Reproductive effects of environmental agents. *Seminars in Reproductive Endocrinology* 8(1):44–54.

Flood, J. F., et al. 1992. Memory-enhancing effects in male mice of pregnenolone and steroids metabolically derived from it. *Proceedings of the National Academy of Sciences, USA* 89:1567–1571.

Flood, J. F., et al. 1995. Pregnenolone sulfate enhances post-training memory processes when injected in very low doses into limbic system structures: The amygdala is by far the most sensitive. *Proceedings of the National Academy of Sciences, USA* 92:10806–10810.

Foecking, M. K., et al. 1980. Progressive patterns in breast diseases. *Medical Hypotheses* 6:659–664.

Fraga, C. G., et al. 1991. Ascorbic acid protects against endogenous oxidative DNA damage in human sperm. *Proceedings of the National Academy of Sciences, USA* 88:11003–11006.

George, M. S. 1994. CSF neuroactive steroids in affective disorders: Pregnenolone, progesterone, and DBI. *Biological Psychiatry* 35:775–780.

Goodhart, D. M., and T. J. Anderson. 1998. Role of nitric oxide in coronary arterial vasomotion and the influence of coronary atherosclerosis and its risks. *American Journal of Cardiology* 82:1034–1039.

Gordon, G. B., et al. 1988. Reduction of atherosclerosis by administration of dehydroepiandrosterone. *Journal of Clinical Investigation* 82:712–720.

Gouchie, C., and D. Kimura. 1991. The relationship between testosterone levels and cognitive ability patterns. *Psychoneuroendocrinology* 16(4):323–334.

Gozan, H. A., et al. 1952. The use of vitamin E in treatment of the menopause. *New York State Journal of Medicine* (15 May):1289–1291.

Grodstein, F. 1996. Postmenopausal estrogen and progestin use and the risk of cardiovascular disease. *New England Journal of Medicine* 335(7):453–461.

Guazzo, E. P., et al. 1996. DHEA and DHEA-S in the CSF fluid of men: Relation to blood levels and the effects of age. *Journal of Clinical Endocrinology and Metabolism* 81:3951–3960.

Guth, L., et al. 1994. Key role for pregnenolone in combination therapy that promotes recovery after spinal cord injury. *Neurobiology* 91:12308–12312.

Haffner, S. M., et al. 1994. Decreased testosterone and dehydroepiandrosterone sulfate concentrations are associated with increased insulin and glucose concentrations in nondiabetic men. *Metabolism* 43(5):599–603.

Hakkinen, K., and A. Pakarinen. 1994. Serum hormones and strength development during strength training in middle-aged and elderly males and females. *ACTA Physiologica Scandinavica* 150:211–219.

Hall, G. M., et al. 1993. Depressed levels of dehydroepiandrosterone sulphate in postmenopausal women with rheumatoid arthritis but no relation with axial bone density. *Annals of the Rheumatic Diseases* 52:211–214.

Hermsmeyer, K. 1997. Reactivity-based coronary vasospasm independent of atherosclerosis in rhesus monkeys. *Journal of the American College of Cardiology* 29(1 March):671–680.

Henderson, E., et al. 1950. Pregnenolone. *Endocrine Review* 10: 455–474.

Herbert, J., et al. 1995. The age of dehydroepiandrosterone. *Lancet* 345:1193–1194.

Isaacson, R. L., et al. 1995. The effects of pregnenolone sulfate and ethylestrenol on retention of a passive avoidance task. *Brain Research* 689:79–84.

Jackson, J., et al. 1992. Testosterone deficiency as a risk factor for hip fractures in men: A case-controlled study. *American Journal of Medical Sciences* 304(1):4–8.

Jungersten, L., et al. 1997. Both physical fitness and acute exercise regulate nitric oxide formation in healthy humans. *Journal of Applied Physiology* 82:760–764.

Kaiser, F. E., and J. E. Morley. 1994. Gonadotropins, testosterone, and the aging male. *Neurobiology of Aging* 15(4):559–563.

Kasra, M., and M. D. Grynpas. 1995. The effects of androgens on the mechanical properties of primate bone. *Bone* 17(3):265–270.

Kavinoky, N. R. 1950. Vitamin E and the control of climacteric symptoms. *Annals of Western Medicine and Surgery* 4(1):27–32.

Kim, C., et al. 1976. Influence of ginseng on mating behavior of male rats. *American Journal of Chinese Medicine* 4(2):163–168.

Knekt, P., et al. 1994. Antioxidant vitamin intake and coronary mortality in longitundinal population study. *American Journal of Epidemiology* 139(2):1180–1189.

Knight, D. C., and J. A. Eden. 1995. Phytoestrogens: A short review. *Maturitas* 22:167–175.

Knight, D. C., and J. A. Eden. 1996. A review of the clinical effects of phytoestrogens. *Obstetrics and Gynecology* 87(5) part 2:897–904.

Koller-Strametz, J., et al. 1998. Role of nitric oxide in exercise-induced vasodilation in man. *Life Sciences* 62:1035–1042.

Kulikauskas, B. S., et al. 1985. Cigarette smoking and its possible effects on sperm. *Fertility and Sterility* 44(4):526–528.

Kurzman, I. D., et al. 1990. Reduction in body weight and cholesterol in spontaneously obese dogs by dehydroepiandrosterone. *International Journal of Obesity* 14:95–104.

Lee, J. R. 1990. Osteoporosis reversal: The role of progesterone. *International Clinical Nutrition Review* 10(3):384–389.

Lee, J. R. 1991. Is natural progesterone the missing link in osteoporosis prevention and treatment? *Medical Hypotheses* 35:316–318.

Lindberg, S., et al. 1997. Low levels of nasal nitric acid (NO) correlate to impaired mucociliary function in upper airways. *Acta Otolaryngol.* 117:728–734.

Littman, A. B., et al. 1993. Physiologic benefits of a stress reduction program for healthy middle-aged army officers. *Journal of Psychosomatic Research* 37(4):345–354.

Lu, L. J., et al. 1996. Effects of soya consumption for one month on steroid hormones in premenopausal women: Implications for breast cancer risk reduction. *Cancer Epidemiology and Biomarkers of Prevention* 5:63–70.

MacEwen, E. G., and I. D. Kurzman. 1991. Obesity in the dog: Role of the adrenal steroid dehydroepiandrosterone (DHEA). *American Institute of Nutrition* :S51–S55.

Maddali, S., et al. 1998. Postexercise increase in nitric acid in football players with muscle cramps. *American Journal of Sports Medicine* 26:820–824.

Maxwell, A. J., et al. 1998. Limb blood flow during exercise is dependent on nitric acid. *Circulation* 98:369–374.

McClure, R. D., et al. 1991. Hypogonadal impotence treated by transdermal testosterone. *Urology* 37(3):224–228.

McGavack et al. 1951. The use of Δ5-pregnenolone in various clinical disorders. *Journal of Clinical Endocrinology* 11(6):559–577.

Meikle, A. W., et al. 1990. Effects of a fat-containing meal on sex hormones in men. *Metabolism* 39:943–6.

Melchior, C. L., and R. F. Ritzmann. 1994. Dehydroepiandrosterone is an anxiolytic in mice on the plus maze. *Pharmacology, Biochemistry and Behavior* 47(3):437–441.

Meriggiola, M. C., et al. 1995. Testosterone enanthate at a dose of 200 mg/week decreases HDL-cholesterol levels in healthy men. *International Journal of Andrology* 18:237–242.

Messina, M., and V. Messina. 1991. Increasing use of soyfoods and their potential role in cancer prevention. *Journal of the American Dietetic Association* 91(7):836–840.

Moilanen, J., et al. 1993. Vitamin E levels in seminal plasma can be elevated by oral administration of vitamin E in infertile men. *International Journal of Andrology* 16:165–66.

Morales, A. J., et al. 1994. Effects of replacement dose of dehydroepiandrosterone in men and women of advancing age. *Journal of Clinical Endocrinology and Metabolism* 78(6):1360–1367.

Morely et al. 1993. Effects of testosterone replacement in old hypogonadal males: A preliminary study. *Journal of the American Geriatrics Society* 41:149–152.

Morfin, R., and G. Courchay. 1994. Pregnenolone and dehydroepiandrosterone as precursors of native 7-hydroxylated metabolites which increase the immune response in mice. *Journal of Steroid Biochemistry and Molecular Biology* 50(1/2):91–100.

Moyer, D. L., et al. 1993. Prevention of endometrial hyperplasia by progesterone during long-term estradiol replacement: Influence of bleeding pattern and secretory changes. *Fertility and Sterility* 59(5):992–997.

Mulder, J. W., et al. 1992. Dehydroepiandrosterone as predictor for progression to AIDS in asymptomatic human immunodeficiency virus–infected men. *Journal of Infectious Diseases* 165:413–418.

Nestler, J. E., et al. 1988. Dehydroepiandrosterone reduces serum low-density lipoprotein levels and body fat but does not alter insulin sensitivity in normal men. *Journal of Clinical Endocrinology and Metabolism* 66(1):57–61.

Nestler, J. E., et al. 1992. Dehydroepiandrosterone: The "missing link" between hyperinsulinemia and atherosclerosis? *FASEB Journal* 6:3073–3075.

Nestler, J. E., et al. 1994. Effects of a reduction in circulating insulin by metformin on serum dehydroepiandrosterone sulfate in nondiabetic men. *Journal of Clinical Endocrinology and Metabolism* 78(3):549–554.

Netter, A., et al. 1981. Effect of zinc administration on plasma testosterone, dihydrotestosterone, and sperm count. *Archives of Andrology* 7:69–73.

Nielsen, F. H., et al. 1992. Boron enhances and mimics some effects of estrogen therapy in postmenopausal women. *Journal of Trace Elements and Experimental Medicine* 5:237–246.

Nillson, P. M., and K. Solstad. 1995. Adverse effects of psychosocial stress on gonadal function and insulin levels in middle-aged males. *Journal of Internal Medicine* 237:479–86.

O'Carroll, R., et al. 1985. Androgens, behavior and nocturnal erection in hypogonadal men: The effects of varying the replacement dose. *Clinical Endocrinology* 23:527–538.

Opstad, P. K. 1994. Circadian rhythm of hormones is extinguished during prolonged physical stress, sleep and energy deficiency in young men. *European Journal of Endocrinology* 131:56–66.

Petitti, D. B., et al. 1998. Ischemic stroke and use of estrogen and estrogen/progestogen as hormone replacement therapy. *Stroke* 29:23–28.

Phillips, G. B., et al. 1994. The association of hypotestosteronemia with coronary artery disease in men. *Arteriosclerosis and Thrombosis* 14:7001–7006.

Phillips, S. M., and B. B. Sherwin. 1992. Effects of estrogen on memory function in surgically menopausal women. *Psychoneuroendocrinology* 17:485–495.

Phipps, W. R., et al. 1993. Effect of flax seed ingestion on the menstrual cycle. *Journal of Clinical Endocrinology and Metabolism* 77(5):1215–1219.

Pincus, G. P., and H. Hoaglund. 1944. Effects of administration of pregnenolone on fatiguing psychomotor performance. *Journal of Aviation Medicine* 15:98.

Pincus, G. P., and H. Hoaglund. 1945. Effects on industrial production of the administration of $\Delta 5$ pregnenolone to factory workers. *Psychosomatic Medicine* 7:342.

Prior, J. C. 1990. Progesterone as a bone-trophic hormone. *Endocrine Reviews* 11(2):386–398.

Reichert, R. 1996. Yam and DHEA. *Quarterly Review of Natural Medicine* :257–258.

Rimm, E., et al. 1993. Vitamin E consumption and the risk of coronary heart disease in men. *New England Journal of Medicine* 328:1450–1456.

Roberts, E. 1995. Pregnenolone: From Selye to Alzheimer and a model of the pregnenolone sulfate binding site on the GABA receptor. *Biochemical Pharmacology* 49(1):1–16.

Rudmen, D., et al. 1994. Relations of endogenous anabolic hormones and physical activity to bone mineral density and lean body mass in elderly men. *Clinical Endocrinology* 40:653–661.

Sanders, S. P. 1999. Asthma, viruses, and nitric oxide. *Proceedings of the Society of Experimental Biology and Medicine* 220:123–132.

Saura, M., et al. 1999. An antiviral mechanism of nitric oxide: Inhibition of a viral protease. *Immunity* 10:21–28.

Schachter, A., et al. 1973. Treatment of oligospermia with the amino acid arginine. *Journal of Urology* 110:311–313.

Shafagoj, Y., et al. 1992. Dehydroepiandrosterone prevents dexamethasone-induced hypertension in rats. *American Physiological Society* E210–E213.

Sharpe, R. M., and N. E. Skakkebaek. 1993. Are oestrogens involved in falling sperm counts and disorders of the male reproductive tract? *Lancet* 341:1392–1395.

Sherwin, B. B. 1985. Differential symptom response to parenteral estrogen and/or androgen administration in the surgical menopause. *American Journal of Obstetrics and Gynecology* 151(2):153–160.

Sherwin, B. B. 1990. Estrogenic effect on memory in women. *Annals of the New York Academy of Medicine* 593:213–231.

Sherwin, B. B., and G. M. Morrie. 1984. Effects of parenteral administration of estrogen and androgen on plasma hormone levels and hot flushes in the surgical menopause. *American Journal of Obstetrics and Gynecology* 148:552.

Sherwin, B. B., et al. 1985. Androgen enhances sexual motivation in females: A prospective, crossover study of sex steroid administration in surgical menopause. *Psychosomatic Medicine* 47:339–351.

Sma, R. M. The lowering of lipoprotein(a) induced by estrogen plus progesterone replacement therapy in postmenopausal women. *Archives of Internal Medicine* 153:1462–1468.

Snow, J. M. 1996. Gingko biloba L. (Ginkgoaceae). *Protocol Journal of Botanical Medicine* 2(1):9–15.

Spector, T. D., et al. 1997. Is hormone replacement therapy protective for hand and knee osteoarthritis in women? The Chingford Study. *Annals of the Rheumatic Diseases* 56:432–434.

Stahl, F., et al. 1992. Dehydroepiandrosterone (DHEA) levels in patients with prostatic cancer, heart diseases and under surgery stress. *Experimental and Clinical Endocrinology* 99:68–70.

Steeno, O. P., and A. Pangkahila. 1984. Occupational influences on male fertility and sexuality. *Andrologia* 16(1):5–22

Steiger, R., et al. 1993. Neurosteroid pregnenolone induces sleep-EEG changes in man compatible with inverse agonistic GABA a-receptor modulation. *Research* 615:267–274.

Studd, John. 1992. Gender and depression. *Lancet* 340:794.

Tenover, J. S. 1992. Effects of testosterone supplementation in the aging male. *Journal of Clinical Endocrinology and Metabolism* 75(4):1092–1098.

Tenover, J. S. 1994. Androgen administration to aging men. *Endocrinology and Metabolism Clinics of North America* 23(4):877–892.

Tousoulis, D. 1997. Basal and flow-mediated nitric oxide production by atheromatous coronary arteries. *Journal of the American College of Cardiology* 29:1256–1262.

Tierra, M. 1997. Healing the liver, healing the body. *International Journal of Alternative and Complementary Medicine* (February):23–25.

Tsitouras, P. D., and T. Bulat. 1995. The aging male reproductive system. *Endocrinology and Metabolism Clinics of North America* 24(2):297–315.

Urban, R. J., et al. 1995. Testosterone administration to elderly men increases skeletal muscle strength and protein synthesis. *Journal of the American Physiological Society* :E820–E826.

Vassilios, A. T., et al. 1978. Estriol in the management of the menopause. *Journal of the American Medical Association* 239(16):1638–1641.

Watts, N. B., et al. 1995. Comparison of oral estrogens and estrogens plus androgen on bone mineral density, menopausal symptoms, and lipid–lipoprotein profiles in surgical menopause. *Obstetrics and Gynecology* 85(4):529–537.

Whitacre, F. E., and B. Barrera. 1944. War amenorrhea. *Journal of the American Medical Association* 124(7):399–403.

Wilbur, P. 1996. The phyto-estrogen debate (part 1). *European Journal of Herbal Medicine* 2(2):20–26.

Wilbur, P. 1996. The phyto-estrogen debate (part 2). *European Journal of Herbal Medicine* 2(3):19–26.

Wilcox, G., et al. 1990. Oestrogenic effects of plant foods in postmenopausal women. *British Medical Journal* 301:905–906.

Williams, D. P., et al. 1993. Relationship of body fat percentage and fat distribution with dehydroepiandrosterone sulfate in premenopausal women. *Journal of Clinical Endocrinology and Metabolism* 77(1):80–85.

Wisniewski, T. L., et al. 1993. The relationship of serum DHEA-S and cortisol levels to measures of immune function in human immunodeficiency virus–related illness. *American Journal of the Medical Sciences* 305(2):79–83.

Wolkowitz, O. M., et al. 1997. Dehydroepiandrosterone (DHEA) treatments of depression. *Biological Psychiatry* 41:311–318.

Writing Group for the PEPI Trial. 1995. Effects of estrogen or estrogen/progestin regimens on heart disease risk factors in postmenopausal women. *Journal of the American Medical Association* 273(3):199–208

Wu, F. S., et al. Pregnenolone sulfate: A positive allosteric modulator at the N-methyl-d-aspartate receptor. *Molecular Pharmacology* 40:333–336.

Young, R. L. 1993. Androgens in postmenopausal therapy? *Menopause Management* :21–24.

INDEX

A

Acetic acid, 50
Acetyl CoA, 442
Acetylsalicylic acid. *See* Aspirin
Acid/alkaline balance
  aging and, 37, 43, 53
  benefits of, 28
  body's regulation of, 37–43
  diet and, 44–50
  getting along with people and, 28, 67
  laboratory tests for, 96–97
  lifestyle and, 50–52
  mental clarity and acuity and, 28, 65–67
  optimism and vision and, 28, 68
  physical vitality and stamina and, 28, 55–65
  recovery from illness and, 28, 68–77
  resistance to illness and, 28, 68–77
  and responding to stress, 447–448
  self-test for, 32–33
  treatment options for restoring, 164
Acidity. *See also* Acid/alkaline balance; Overacidity
  within the human body, 35–37
  measuring, 34–35
  neutralizing, 35
  theories concerning, 34
Acidosis
  metabolic, 52
  respiratory, 52, 69
Acini, 173
ACTH, 456
Adaptation energy, 6
Adrenal glands, 441, 449–450, 455
  activated by sunlight, 533
  testing function of, 479
Adrenal medulla, 441–442
Adrenaline. *See* Epinephrine
Adrenocorticotrophin. *See* ACTH
Affirmations, 471
Age discrimination, 12–13
Age-related macular degeneration. *See* AMD
Aging
  acid/alkaline balance and, 37, 43, 53
  of autonomic nervous system, 455–456
  detoxification and, 269
  DHEA production and, 558–559

digestive-enzyme production and, 185–187
  estrogen levels and, 597–598
  high-alkaline producers and, 54–55
  kidneys and, 53
  oxygen intake and, 53
  oxygenation and, 343–344
  pancreas and, 53
  progesterone and, 618
  sports and, 57
Agoraphobia, 437, 455, 499
Agriculture, development of, 133–134
AIDS, 356, 381–382
Air pollution, 344–346
Airplane travel
  acidifying effect of frequent, 51
  reducing jet lag, 502, 503
Alcohol
  ability to tolerate, 287–288
  anxiety and, 451
  calories from, 270
  cancer and, 299
  detoxification of, 266, 279–280
  estrogen levels and, 298, 599
  high rate of consumption of, 182
  liver function and, 269–270
  pancreatic disease and, 184–185
  PMS and, 285
  -related heart disease, 297–298
  sexual problems and, 298
  substitutes for, 292
  as toxin, 262
  vitamin deficiencies and, 270
  women and, 288–290
Aldosterone, 442
Alfalfa, 120
Algae, wild blue-green, 322, 323–324
Alkaline power diet
  making food substitutions, 115–120
  meal planning, 120–124
  rotating foods, 124–126
  selecting proper foods for, 101, 108–115
Alkalinity. *See also* Acid/alkaline balance; High-alkaline producers
  within the human body, 35–37
  measuring, 34–35
  neutralizing, 35
  theories concerning, 34

NOTES

NOTES

NOTES